Radiologic Pathology

Third Edition

VOLUME 1
Chest, Gastrointestinal, and Genitourinary Radiologic Pathology Correlations

2004
2005

Editors

Kelly K. Koeller, CAPT, MC, USN
Chairman and Registrar
Chief, Neuroradiology

Angela D. Levy, LTC, MC, USA
Associate Chairperson
Chief, Gastrointestinal Radiology

Paula J. Woodward, MD
Chief, Genitourinary Radiology

Geoffrey A. Agrons, MD
Chief, Pediatric Radiology

Jeffrey R. Galvin, MD
Chief, Chest Radiology

Mark D. Murphey, MD
Six Week Course Director
Chief, Musculoskeletal Radiology

Associate Editor
Jean-Claude Kurdziel, MD

Illustrators
Aletta A. Frazier, MD
Dianne D. Engelby, MAMS, RDMS
Heike Blum, MFA
James A. Cooper, MD

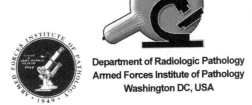

Department of Radiologic Pathology
Armed Forces Institute of Pathology
Washington DC, USA

American Registry of Pathology
Armed Forces Institute of Pathology
Washington, DC
20306-6000

Great care has been taken to guarantee the accuracy of the information contained in this
volume. However, neither the American Registry of Pathology, Armed Forces Institute of
Pathology, nor the editors and contributors can be held responsible for errors or for any
consequences arising from the use of the information contained herein.

The opinions and assertions contained herein are the private views of the authors and are
not to be construed as official nor as representing the views of the Departments of the Army,
Air Force, Navy, or Defense.

9 8 7 6 5 4 3 2 1

Library of Congress Cataloging-in-publication Data [in process]

ISBN 1-881041-91-3

Preface

This third edition of Radiologic Pathology features a new editor and several improvements to the prior editions. Geoffrey A. Agrons, M.D. is our new section chief of Pediatric Radiology and assumes all editorial duties for that section. Heartfelt thanks are extended to Gael J. Lonergan, M.D. for her dedication and diligence in preparing the Pediatric Radiology section in the first two editions. Accurate pictorial depiction of important concepts is an essential part of this syllabus and we are pleased to feature the work of Aletta A. Frazier, M.D., Dianne Engelby, MAMS, RDMS, Heike Blum, MFA, and James A. Cooper, M.D. in this edition. Based upon recommendations provided by residents attending the course, captions have now been added for nearly all illustrations to improve clarity and understanding. The paper quality has also improved with brighter more vibrant pages that provide greater visibility of the images and text. Many new lectures have been added and existing material has been substantially revised and updated. Work has begun on instituting a complete index in next year's edition. The editors and course faculty continue to strive for a concise effective review of major topics in radiology by emphasizing the concept of radiologic-pathologic correlation to improve one's understanding of the imaging appearance of disease.

Preface to the Second Edition

Following the resounding success of the first edition of Radiologic Pathology, we are pleased to present this second edition for radiologists at all levels of experience. It is our hope that this edition will fulfill even more expectations of the user and provide better understanding of the imaging appearance of disease through the use of gross pathology and histopathology. In this edition, there has been a major expansion of the number of illustrations for virtually all the presentations. Nearly every outline is now generously supplemented with the same key figures, images, and diagrams shown in the lectures. Numerous new lectures have also been added to the curriculum and significant updates and modifications have been made to existing lectures. It is the editors' intent to keep all of the material presented in the syllabus as current as possible.

Preface to the First Edition

Since 1947, the Department of Radiologic Pathology at the Armed Forces Institute of Pathology (AFIP) has utilized the concept of radiologic pathologic correlation to understand the patterns of disease seen on imaging studies. Beginning with early informal sessions at the viewbox with radiology residents, an Army radiologist, Colonel William Thompson, solicited an exchange of information between his radiological colleagues and pathologists by reviewing radiographic studies, gross pathologic specimens, and histologic findings of each case. Over time, the number of these cases with radiologic-pathologic correlation steadily increased and analysis of this material revealed certain imaging patterns that empowered the radiologist to refine the differential diagnosis or even favor a particular diagnosis based on the imaging findings alone. In the early 1970s, Colonel Thompson's successor and Navy radiologist, Captain Elias Theros, dramatically expanded the scope of this educational program based on radiologic pathologic correlation into a more formal course presented over consecutive multiple weeks. Other faculty members were added to the Department of Radiologic Pathology while guest lecturers generously provided their unique perspective to supplement the "core" material.

Today, instruction provided in the six-week AFIP course has fulfilled the training requirements in radiologic pathologic correlation for over 25,000 diagnostic radiology residents from around the world and attendance is at an all-time high. Despite the success of this educational program, one recurring comment frequently heard from residents attending a course would be: "Your lectures are great…but can't we see the same images from a lecture in the syllabus?" To that end, the Department of Radiologic Pathology is pleased to present the first edition of the syllabus in a true book format. The publication of this volume represents the culmination of two years' effort on the part of the entire course faculty to produce a major revision of the previous syllabus and is a great testament to the dedication and perseverance of these speakers. All text slides from the lectures highlight the major teaching points in each lecture and are now generously supplemented with key images and line drawings that are significantly upgraded from prior versions of the syllabus. Future editions will be updated and published for each new academic year.

It is our sincere hope that users of this material, regardless of your level of experience, will find that this new syllabus enhances your comprehension of imaging patterns and understanding of why a disease appears as it does on an imaging study. To all of us that have ever had the honor of presenting this material to tens of thousands of diagnostic radiology residents, the means to this knowledge lies in radiologic pathologic correlation.

Acknowledgements

We are indeed fortunate to have the talents and efforts of so many dedicated personnel to make this project a reality. Alethia West and Adahlia Glover collect and manage the case material, carefully compiled by the thousands of residents who attend our courses. Ingrid Jenkins not only assists the case managers but also supports the digitization process, headed by Jessica Holquin. Our department's archives are diligently maintained by Sharon Holquin. Anika Torruella, our editorial assistant, superbly accomplishes the coordination of the text submitted by faculty members. Coordination of the participation of more than 1,200 residents who attend the six-week course is capably provided by Carl Williams with assistance from Monte Grace. Donald Hatley, Ben Yohannes, and Kathy Rahimly manage myriad other administrative tasks so that distractions to the faculty are kept to a minimum. Much gratitude is extended to our associate editor, Jean-Claude Kurdziel, M.D.

Finally, we are continually grateful for the outstanding contributions of case material from residency programs worldwide for 57 years to the Department of Radiologic Pathology. Through the efforts of program directors and residents alike, our educational program continues to thrive and, hopefully, increases the comprehension of the imaging appearance of disease. Thank you all for your continued interest and support.

Faculty – VOLUME 1

Chest Radiology

Gerald F. Abbott, MD
Director of Chest Radiology
Rhode Island Hospital
and
Assistant Professor of Radiology
Brown University School of Medicine
Providence, RI

Aletta A. Frazier, MD
Physician and Medical Illustrator
and
Assistant Professor, Department of Radiology
University of Maryland
Baltimore, MD

Jeffrey R. Galvin, MD
1997-1998 Distinguished Scientist
Chief, Pulmonary and Mediastinal Radiology
Department of Radiologic Pathology
Armed Forces Institute of Pathology
Washington, DC
and
Professor of Radiology and Pulmonary Medicine
University of Maryland
Baltimore, MD

Leonard M. Glassman, MD
Clinical Professor
Department of Radiology
George Washington University Medical Center
Washington, DC

Melissa L. Rosado de Christenson, MD, FACR
Clinical Professor of Radiology
The Ohio State University
Columbus, OH
and
Adjunct Professor of Radiology
Uniformed Services University of the Health Sciences
Bethesda, MD

Rosita M. Shah, MD
Assistant Professor of Radiology
Thomas Jefferson University Hospital
Philadelphia, PA

Gastrointestinal Radiology

Robert M. Abbott, MD
Assistant Professor of Radiology
University of Maryland School of Medicine
Baltimore, MD

Bruce P. Brown, MD
Associate Professor of Radiology
University of Iowa
Iowa City, IA

Marc S. Levine, MD
Professor of Radiology
University Hospital of Pennsylvania
University of Pennsylvania
Philadelphia, PA
and
Former Distinguished Scientist
Department of Radiologic Pathology
Armed Forces Institute of Pathology
Washington, DC

Angela D. Levy, LTC, MC, USA
Asssociate Chairperson and
Gastrointestinal Radiology Section Chief
Department of Radiologic Pathology
Armed Forces Institute of Pathology
Washington, DC
and
Associate Professor of Radiology and Nuclear Medicine
Uniformed Services University of the Health Sciences
Bethesda, MD

Francis J. Scholz, MD
Radiologist, Lahey Clinic Medical Center
Burlington, MA
and
Clinical Professor of Radiology
Tufts Univeriisty School of Medicine
Boston, MA
Sponsored by an Educational Grant from E-Z-EM, Inc.

Robert K. Zeman, MD
Chairman and Professor of Radiology
George Washington University
Washington, DC

Genitourinary Radiology

Peter L.Choyke, MD, FACR
Chief Molecular Imaging Program
National Cancer Institute
Bethesda, MD
and
Professor of Radiology and Nuclear Medicine
Uniformed University of the Health Sciences
Bethesda, MD

David S. Hartman, MD
Professor of Radiology
Chief of Education Division
Department of Radiology
Pennsylvania State Geisinger Health System
M. S. Hershey Medical Center
Hershey, PA

Brent J. Wagner, MD
Staff Radiologist
West Reading Radiology Associates
West Reading, PA

Paula J. Woodward, MD
Chief, Genitourinary Radiology
Department of Radiologic Pathology
Armed Forces Institute of Pathology
Washington, DC

Jade J. Wong-You-Cheong, MD
Assistant Professor of Diagnostic Radiology
Director, Section of Ultrasound
University of Maryland School of Medicine
Baltimore, MD

Table of Contents – VOLUME 1

Chest Radiology

Jeffrey R. Galvin, MD
An Approach to Diffuse Lung Disease, Sarcoidosis 3
The Idiopathic Interstitial Pneumonias 13
Airways Disease: The Movement from Anatomic to Physiologic Assessment 22
Inhalational Lung Disease (Asbestosis and Silicosis) 40
Pulmonary Lymphoid Disorders 50
Angiitis and Granulomatosis 59
The Pulmonary Complications of Bone Marrow Transplantation 71
The Diagnosis of Pulmonary Embolism 79
Tuberculosis 90
Fungal Disease in the Thorax:Opportunistic and Primary Pathogens .98
Bronchogenic Carcinoma: Radiologic–Pathologic Correlation 110
Chest Seminar 1 120
Chest Seminar 2 125

Aletha A. Frazier, MD
Pulmonary Hypertension 130
Pulmonary Metastasis 138

Melissa L. Rosado de Christenson, MD, FACR
Differential Diagnosis of Mediastinal Masses 146
Radiologic Pathology: Unknown Case Seminar: Where is the lesion? 162
Radiologic Pathology: Unknown Case Seminar: Differential Diagnosis of Mediastinal Masses 166

Rosita M. Shah, MD
Pneumonia: Usual and Unusual Organisms 169

Gerald F. Abbott, MD
Uncommon Malignant Tumors of the Lung 181
Benign Tumors of the Lung and Tumor-like Lesions 186
Pleural Disease I 192
Pleural Disease II and Chest Wall 199

Leonard M. Glassman, MD (Mammography)
Classic Breast Lesions 205
Breast Pathology – What the Radiologist Needs to Know 213
Ductal Carcinoma in Situ (DCIS) 221

Gastrointestinal Radiology

Angela D. Levy, LTC, MC, USA
Gastrointestinal Radiology 229
Hepatic Neoplasms 231
Imaging of Diffuse Liver Disease 244
Hepatic Infections 253
Benign Biliary Disease 261
Gallbladder and Biliary Neoplasms 276
Pancreatic Neoplasms 283
Gastric Malignancies 285
Abdominal Non Hodgkin Lymphoma 306
Small Intestinal Neoplasms 313
Colorectal Carcinoma 322
Imaging of Anorectal Disease 330
Appendicitis and Beyond 338
Mesenteric Masses and Cysts 347
Seminar 1: Abdominal Gas 357
Seminar 2: Diffuse Diseases of the Stomach 362
Seminar 3: Polyposis Syndromes 367
Seminar 4: Pancreatic Duct 374
Seminar 5: Hepatic Imaging 378
Seminar 6: Complications of Meckel Diverticulum 382

Robert K. Zeman, MD
Cholelithiasis and Cholecystitis 388

Marc S. Levine, MD
Inflammatory Diseases of the Esophagus 395
Tumors of the Esophagus 401
Radiology of Peptic Ulcer Disease 406

Bruce Brown, MD
Pancreatitis: Imaging Has Made a Difference 411
Gastrointestinal Bleeding In The Age of the Endoscope. What Does a Radiologist Have To Contribute? . .420

Francis J. Scholz, MD
Small Bowel Obstruction 427
Mesenteric Ischemia 439
Malabsorption 453

Robert M. Abbott, MD
The Spleen 465
Inflammatory Bowel Disease 479

Genitourinary Radiology

Paula J. Woodward, MD
Genitourinary Radiology 493
Imaging of Uterine Disorders 495
Renal Neoplasms, Approach to Renal Masses 505
Urinary Tract Trauma 517
Retroperitoneum 524
Radiologic Evaluation of the Scrotum 531
First Trimester Ultrasound 540
Fetal CNS Malformations 548
Fetal Anomalies 553

Peter L. Choyke, MD
Cystic Diseases of the Kidney 559
Imaging of Prostate Cancer 566

Brent J. Wagner, MD
Imaging of Ovarian Masses 571
Adrenal Imaging in Adults: Radiologic-Pathologic Correlation 579
Imaging of the Urinary Bladder and Urethra 583

Jade Wong You Cheong, MD
Non-Neoplastic Disorders Of The Ovary And Adnexae 587
Imaging of Solid Organ Transplants 595

David S. Hartman, MD
The Neglected Nephrogram 603
Problem Renal Masses 606

Paula J. Woodward, MD
Seminar: MSAFP 612
Seminar: Renal Calcifications 614

Chest Radiology

An Approach to Diffuse Lung Disease, Sarcoidosis

Jeffrey R. Galvin, MD
Chief, Pulmonary and Mediastinal Radiology
Armed Forces Institute of Pathology
and
Clinical Professor Department of Radiology
University of Maryland

Describing Diffuse Lung Disease
- The Alveolar vs. Interstitial Problem
- Alveolar or Interstitial ?

An Approach to Diffuse Lung Disease
- Radiograph
  - Lung volumes
  - Opacity
  - Distribution
  - Ancillary findings
- Computed tomography
  - Opacity
  - Distribution

Lung Volumes
- Reduced *[Figure 1-1-1]*
  - Pathology distal to the airway
  - Fibrosis
  - IPF, asbestosis, sarcoidosis, chronic hypersensitivity pneumonitis
- Increased *[Figure 1-1-2]*
  - Pathology of the airway
  - Emphysema, asthma, bronchitis, constrictive bronchiolitis, LAM

Distribution: Upper vs Lower

Plain Film and CT Opacities
- Nodules
- Reticulation and Lines
- Ground glass
- Consolidation
- Cystic airspaces

Figure 1-1-1

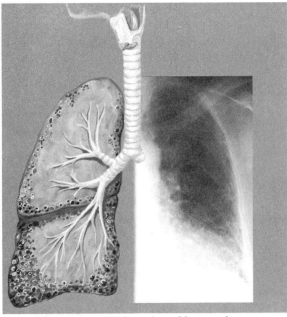

Fibrosis results in reduced lung volumes

Figure 1-1-2

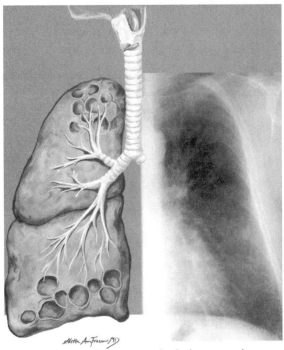

Airways disease results in increased lung volumes

Plain Film and CT Opacities

- Nodules
  - ➢ Sarcoid, silicosis, coal-workers
  - ➢ Random pattern
    - ✧ Hematogenous
    - – Miliary TB, metastasis
  - ➢ Centrilobular
    - ✧ Airway spread
    - – Acute hypersensitivity, infectious bronchiolitis, endobronchial spread of TB
- Reticulation and Lines
  - ➢ Fibrosis
    - ✧ IPF-lower, subpleural
    - ✧ Asbestosis-lower, subpleural
    - ✧ Sarcoidosis-peribronchovascular
    - ✧ Chronic hypersensitivity pneumonitis-mid and upper lung zone
- Ground glass
  - ➢ Non-specific
    - ✧ Airspace, interstitial, combined
    - – DIP, NSIP, AIP, DAD (32%)
    - ✧ Infection (32%)
    - ✧ Drug toxicity (11%)
    - ✧ Hemorrhage (3%)
    - ✧ Ground glass with reticulation
    - – Fibrosis
- Consolidation
  - ➢ Organizing Pneumonia (BOOP)
  - ➢ Chronic eosinophilic pneumonia
  - ➢ Lymphoma
  - ➢ Bronchoalveolar cell carcinoma
  - ➢ Infection
  - ➢ Hemorrhage
- Cystic airspaces
  - ➢ Mimics reticulation on plain radiographs
  - ➢ Fibrosis and honeycombing
    - ✧ IPF-Lower, subpleural
    - ✧ LAM-Diffuse
    - ✧ LCH-Upper

The Secondary Lobule [Figure 1-1-3]

- Irregular polygon
- 2-3 cms
- 3-5 bronchioles
- Lymphatics [Figure 1-1-4]
  - ➢ Bronchovascular bundles
  - ➢ Interlobular septa

Figure 1-1-3

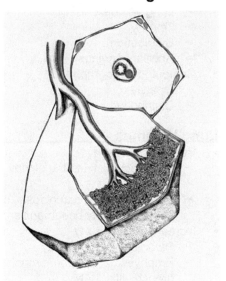

The secondary lobule

Figure 1-1-4

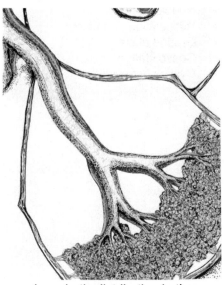

Lymphatic distribution in the secondary lobule

Abnormal Patterns
- Bronchovascular *[Figure 1-1-5 and 1-1-9]*
  - ➤ Bronchus
    - ◇ Asthma, CF, bronchitis and bronchiectasis
  - ➤ Lymphatics
    - ◇ CA, lymphoma, sarcoidosis or edema
- Centrilobular *[Figure 1-1-6]*
  - ➤ Airway related
- Panlobular *[Figure 1-1-7]*
  - ➤ Nonspecific
- Septal *[Figure 1-1-8 and 1-1-9]*
  - ➤ Lymphatic

Sarcoidosis
- Multisystem granulomatous disorder
- Unknown etiology
- Young and middle aged adults
- Bilateral hilar lymphadenopathy, pulmonary infiltration, eye and skin lesions
- Clinical and radiologic findings supported by evidence of noncaseating epithelioid granulomas
- Exclusion of granulomas of unknown cause and local sarcoid reactions

ATS Statement on Sarcoidosis 1999

Sarcoidosis: Epidemiology
- Worldwide
  - ➤ both sexes, all races, all ages
- Predilection for adults
  - ➤ under 40 years
  - ➤ peak 20-29 years
- U.S. prevalence
  - ➤ 10 per 100,000 exams
- Highest disease
  - ➤ African-American women

Sarcoidosis: Clinical Features
- Asymptomatic
  - ➤ 15-50%
- Constitutional symptoms
  - ➤ 33%
- Dyspnea, cough, chest pain
  - ➤ 33-50%
- Palpable lymph nodes
  - ➤ 33-75%
- Ocular involvement
  - ➤ 11-83%
- Cutaneous involvement
  - ➤ 20-30% Erythema nodosum, Lupus pernio

Figure 1-1-5

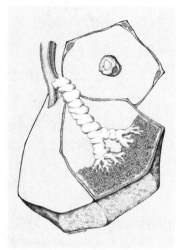

Bronchovascular pattern

Figure 1-1-6

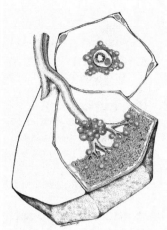

Centrilobular pattern

Figure 1-1-7

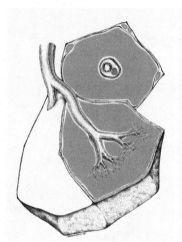

Panlobular pattern

Figure 1-1-8

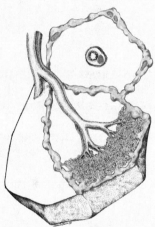

Septal pattern

Figure 1-1-9

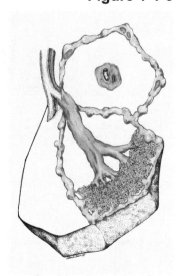

Combined septal and bronchovascular pattern

Sarcoidosis: Laboratory Abnormalities
- BAL
  - ↑ macrophages, ↓ proportions; ↑ CD4 helper cells
- Angiotensin-Converting Enzyme
  - Nonspecific Produced by granuloma/macrophage
  - ↑ 33-90%
- Hypercalcemia 10%
- Hypercalciuria 30%
  - Macrophage/granuloma extrarenal sources of 1-25 Dihydroxyvitamin D
- Anergy
- Hypergammaglobulinemia

Sarcoidosis: Respiratory System
[Figure 1-1-10]
- 100% lung involvement
- Portal of entry
  - Local lymph nodes
  - Distant organs
- Disease distribution
  - Alveolar wall
  - Secondary lobule,
  - Axial CT
  - Radiograph

Non-Caseating Granuloma and Fibrosis

Alveolar Distribution

Sarcoidosis and the Secondary Lobule *[Figure 1-1-11]*

Figure 1-1-10

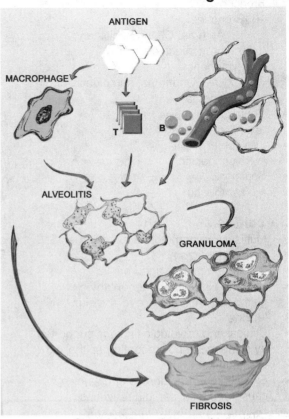

Sarcoidosis pathogenesis

Figure 1-1-11

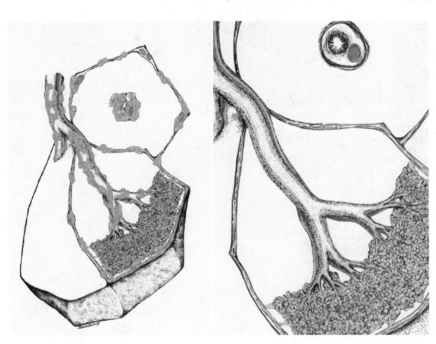

Bronchovascular distribution of granulomas in Sarcoidosis

Figure 1-1-12

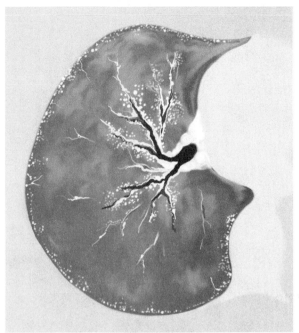

Distribution of nodules in sarcoidosis

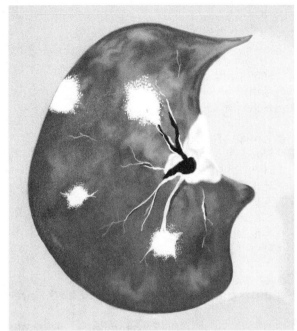

Masses in Sarcoidosis

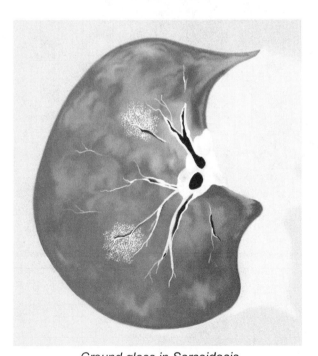

Ground glass in Sarcoidosis

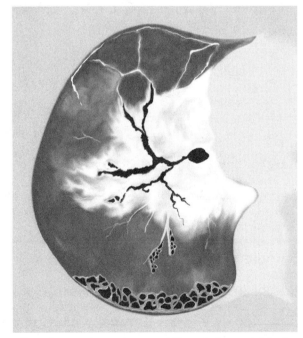

Conglomerate masses and fibrosis in sarcoidosis

Sarcoidosis: Computed Tomography *[Figure 1-1-12]*

- Nodules
- Masses
- Ground Glass
- Fibrosis
  - ➢ Conglomeration
  - ➢ Distortion
- Emphysema
- Bulla
- Honeycombing

Parenchymal Disease: Radiography
- Bilateral
- Symmetrical
- Nodules
- Reticulonodular
- Masses
- Ground Glass
- Hilar Retraction
- Bulla
- Honeycombing

Sarcoidosis: Adenopathy

Node Group	CXR	CT
Hilar	84	88
R. Paratracheal	76	100
A-P Window	72	92
Subcarinal	12	64
Ant. Med.	12	48
Post. Med.	0	16

Sarcoidosis:
Staging based on Adenopathy and Parenchyma

	Presentation	Resolution
Stage 0	8	–
➢ Normal		
Stage 1	51	65
➢ Adenopathy		
Stage 2	29	49
➢ Adenopathy & Parenchyma		
Stage 3	12	20
➢ Parenchyma		

20% develop fibrosis or Stage 4 disease

Sarcoidosis Stage I

Sarcoidosis Stage II

Sarcoidosis Stage III

Sarcoidosis Stage IV

Sarcoidosis Progression

Sarcoidosis and the Parenchyma: Computed Tomography
- Thickened Bronchovascular Bundles
- Nodules
  - ➢ Peribronchovascular
  - ➢ Pleural, subpleural and septal
- Consolidation and Large Nodules
- Ground-Glass Opacities
- Fibrosis

Thickened Bronchovascular Bundles [Figure 1-1-13]

Peribronchovascular Nodules

Figure 1-1-13

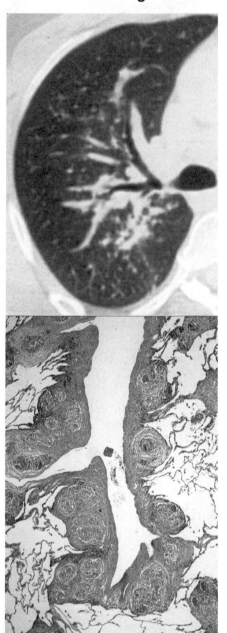

Peribronchovascular opacities in sarcoidosis

Peribronchovascular and Pleural Nodules

Septal Lines

Ground Glass Opacities

Consolidation and Large Nodules

Fibrosis

Bronchovascular Bundle Distortion *[Figure 1-1-14]*

Conglomerate Mass

Fibrosis and Emphysema

Fibrosis and Honeycombing

Sarcoidosis Resolution

Sarcoidosis: Diagnosis
- Typical clinical and radiologic manifestations
- Non-caseating granulomas
- Transbronchial Bx
- Endobronchial Bx

Sarcoidosis: Differential Diagnosis
- Infection
  - ➢ Tuberculosis, Fungal (Histoplasmosis)
- Pneumoconiosis
  - ➢ Silica, Beryllium
- Hypersensitivity Pneumonitis
- Malignancy
  - ➢ Lymphoma

Miliary Tuberculosis

Transbronchial Spread of Tuberculosis

Histoplasmosis

Silicosis

Berylliosis

Extrinsic Allergic Alveolitis

Sarcoidosis: Mortality
- Mortality range 5-10%
- Cor Pulmonale related to fibrosis
- Cardiac Arrhythmia
- Pulmonary Hemorrhage
  - ➢ Aspergilloma

Cor Pulmonale

Figure 1-1-14

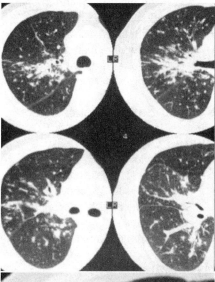

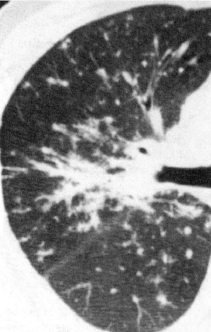

Peribronchovascular opacities and architectural distortion in sarcoidosis

Sarcoidosis: Cardiac Involvement
- Clinical involvement 5%
  - ➢ Heart block, arrhythmia, mitral regurgitation, CHF (dilated cardiomyopathy) and sudden death
- Autopsy involvement 20-30%
- Localized wall motion abnormalities
  - ➢ Anterior and apical
  - ➢ MRI, Echocardiograph, Thallium-201

Cardiac Sarcoidosis

Dilated Cardiomyopathy

Sarcoidosis: Mycetoma
- Present in 40-50% of cystic lesions
  - ➢ Bullae, cavities or bronchiectasis
- Hemorrhage
- Steroids may convert to invasive process

Mycetoma [Figure 1-1-15]

Sarcoidosis: Therapy
- Cardiac, CNS, eye involvement
- Hypercalcemia
- Corticosteroids
  - ➢ Relief of symptoms; resolution of radiologic abnormalities; improved function
- Cytotoxic agents
  - ➢ Methotrexate, Azathioprine
- Chlorambucil, cyclophosphamide, antimalarials
- Risk of recurrence

Sarcoidosis: Prognosis
- Favorable
  - ➢ Acute onset, erythema nodosum,
  - ➢ > 80% spontaneous remission
  - ➢ Löfgren syndrome
  - ➢ Low stage
- Poor
  - ➢ Chronic course, Lupus pernio
  - ➢ Older age at presentation
  - ➢ Hypercalcemia/nephrocalcinosis
  - ➢ Black race, Extrathoracic involvement

Sarcoidosis Conclusion

Figure 1-1-15

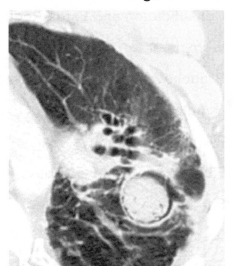

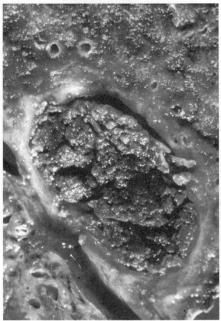

Mycetoma in a cystic space caused by sarcoidosis

Sarcoidosis Bibliography

General
1. Akira M, Hara H, Sakatani M. Interstitial lung disease in association with polymyositis- dermatomyositis: long-term follow-up CT evaluation in seven patients. Radiology 1999; 210(2):333-8.
2. Bergin CJ, Muller NL. CT of interstitial lung disease: a diagnostic approach. American Jounal of Roentgenology 1987; 148:8-15.
3. Bergin C, Roggli V, Coblentz C, Chiles C. The secondary pulmonary lobule: normal and abnormal CT appearances. American Journal of Roentgenology 1988; 15:21-25.
4. Epler GR, McLoud TC, Gaensler EA, Mikus JP, Carrington CB. Normal chest roentgenograms in chronic diffuse infiltrative lung disease. N Engl J Med 1978; 298(17):934-9.

5. Epler GR. Chest films: underused tool in interstial lung disease. Journal of Respiratory Diseases 1987; 8(6):14-24.
6. Felson B. A new look at pattern recognition of diffuse pulmonary disease. American Journal of Roentgenology 1979; 133:183-189.
7. Galvin JR, Mori M, Stanford W. High-resolution computed tomography and diffuse lung disease. Curr Probl Diagn Radiol 1992; 21(2):31-74.
8. Grenier P, Valeyre D, Cluzel P, Brauner MW, Lenoir S, Chastang C. Chronic diffuse interstitial lung disease: diagnostic value of chest radiography and high-resolution CT. Radiology 1991; 179:123-132.
9. Gruden JF, Webb WR, Naidich DP, McGuinness G. Multinodular disease: anatomic localization at thin-section CT—multireader evaluation of a simple algorithm. Radiology 1999; 210(3):711-20.
10. Gurney JW, Schroeder BA. Upper lobe lung disease: physiologic correlates. Radiology 1988; 167:359-366.
11. Heitzman ER. The lung. Second ed. St. Louis: C.V. Mosby, 1984.
12. Johkoh T, Muller NL, Cartier Y, Kavanagh PV, Hartman TE, Akira M, Ichikado K, Ando M, Nakamura H. Idiopathic interstitial pneumonias: diagnostic accuracy of thin-section CT in 129 patients. Radiology 1999; 211(2):555-60.
13. Mathieson JR, Mayo JR, Staples CA, Müller NL. Chronic diffuse infiltrative lung disease: comparison of dianostic accuracy of CT and chest radiography. Radiology 1989; 171:111-116.
14. Mayo JR, Webb WR, Gould R, Stein MG, Bass I, Gamsu G, Goldberg H. High-resolution CT of the lungs: an optimal approach. Radiology 1987; 163:507-510.
15. McLoud TC, Carrington CB, Gaensler EA. Diffuse Infiltrative lung disease: a new scheme for description. Radiology 1983; 149(2):353-363.
16. Muller NL, Miller RR. Computed tomography of chronic diffuse infiltrative lung disease. Part 2. Am Rev Respir Dis 1990; 142(6 Pt 1):1440-8.
17. Muller NL, Miller RR. Computed tomography of chronic diffuse infiltrative lung disease. Part 1. Am Rev Respir Dis 1990; 142(5):1206-15.
18. Muller NL, Coiby TV. Idiopathic interstitial pneumonias: high-resolution CT and histologic findings. Radiographics 1997; 17(4):1016-22.
19. Murata K, Itoh H, Todo G, Kanaoka M, Noma S, Itoh T, Furuta M, Asamoto H, Torizuka K. Centrilobular lesions of the lung: demonstration by high-resolution CT and pathologic correlation. Radiology 1986; 161:641-645.
20. Murata K, Khan A, Rojas KA, Herman PG. Optimization of computed tomography technique to demonstrate the fine structure of the lung. Investigative Radiology 1988; 23:170-175.
21. Murata K, Khan A, Herman P. Pulmonary parenchymal disease: evaluation with high-resolution CT. Radiology 1989; 170:629-635.
22. Müller NI, Miller RR. Computed tomography of chronic diffuse lung disease. American Review of Respiratory Disease 1990; 142:1206-1215, 1440-1448.
23. Staples CA, Müller NL, Vedal S, Abboud R, Ostrow D, Miller RR. Usual interstitial Pneumonia: correlation of CT with clinical, functional, and radiologic findings. Radiology 1987; 162:377-381.
24. Webb WR. High resolution CT of lung parenchyma. Radiologic Clinics of North America 1989; 27(6):1085-1097.
25. Weibel ER. Looking into the lung: what can it tell us? American Journal of Roentgenology 1979; 133:1021-1031.
26. Weibel ER, Bachofen H. The Fiber Scaffold of Lung Parenchyma. In: Crystal RG, West JB, eds. The Lung. New York: Raven Press, 1991; 787-794.
27. Weibel ER, Crystal RG. Structural Organization of the Pulmonary Interstitium. In: Crystal RG, West JB, eds. The Lung. New York: Raven Press, 1991; 369-380.

Sarcoidosis
1. Bergin CJ, Bell DY, Coblentz CL, Chiles C, Gamsu G, MacIntyre NR, Coleman RE, Putman CE. Sarcoidosis: correlation of pulmonary parenchymal pattern at CT with results of pulmonary function tests. Radiology 1989; 171(3):619-24.
2. Gawne-Cain ML, Hansell DM. The pattern and distribution of calcified mediastinal lymph nodes in sarcoidosis and tuberculosis: a CT study. Clin Radiol 1996; 51(4):263-7.

3. Gleeson FV, Traill ZC, Hansell DM. Evidence of expiratory CT scans of small-airway obstruction in sarcoidosis. AJR Am J Roentgenol 1996; 166(5):1052-4.

4. Hansell DM, Milne DG, Wilsher ML, Wells AU. Pulmonary sarcoidosis: morphologic associations of airflow obstruction at thin-section CT. Radiology 1998; 209(3):697-704.

5. Kuhlman JE, Fishman EK, Hamper UM, Knowles M, Siegelman SS. The computed tomographic spectrum of thoracic sarcoidosis. Radiographics 1989; 9(3):449-66.

6. Muller NL, Kullnig P, Miller RR. The CT findings of pulmonary sarcoidosis: analysis of 25 patients. AJR Am J Roentgenol 1989; 152(6):1179-82.

7. Muller NL, Mawson JB, Mathieson JR, Abboud R, Ostrow DN, Champion P. Sarcoidosis: correlation of extent of disease at CT with clinical, functional, and radiographic findings. Radiology 1989; 171(3):613-8.

8. Murdoch J, Muller NL. Pulmonary sarcoidosis: changes on follow-up CT examination. AJR Am J Roentgenol 1992; 159(3):473-7.

9. Newman LS, Rose CS, Maier LA. Sarcoidosis [published erratum appears in N Engl J Med 1997 Jul 10;337(2):139] [see comments]. N Engl J Med 1997; 336(17):1224-34.

10. Nishimura K, Itoh H, Kitaichi M, Nagai S, Izumi T. Pulmonary sarcoidosis: correlation of CT and histopathologic findings [published erratum appears in Radiology 1994 Mar;190(3):907]. Radiology 1993; 189(1):105-9.

11. Nishimura K, Itoh H, Kitaichi M, Nagai S, Izumi T. CT and pathological correlation of pulmonary sarcoidosis. Semin Ultrasound CT MR 1995; 16(5):361-70.

12. Padley SP, Padhani AR, Nicholson A, Hansell DM. Pulmonary sarcoidosis mimicking cryptogenic fibrosing alveolitis on CT. Clin Radiol 1996; 51(11):807-10.

13. Padley SP, Padhani AR, Nicholson A, Hansell DM. Pulmonary sarcoidosis mimicking cryptogenic fibrosing alveolitis on CT. Clin Radiol 1996; 51(11):807-10.

14. Rockoff SD, Rohatgi PK. Unusual manifestations of thoracic sarcoidosis. AJR Am J Roentgenol 1985; 144(3):513-28.

15. Thomas PD, Hunninghake GW. Current concepts of the pathogenesis of sarcoidosis. Am Rev Respir Dis 1987; 135(3):747-60.

16. Winterbauer RH, Belic N, Moores KD. Clinical interpretation of bilateral hilar adenopathy. Ann Intern Med 1973; 78(1):65-71.

The Idiopathic Interstitial Pneumonias

Jeffrey R. Galvin, MD
Chief Pulmonary and Mediastinal Radiology
Armed Forces Institute of Pathology
Clinical Professor Department of Radiology
University of Maryland

Figure 1-2-1

The Idiopathic Interstitial Pneumonias
Chronic Diffuse Lung Disease [Figure 1-2-1 and 1-2-2]

- Alveolar involvement
  - ➤ Surrounding airways
  - ➤ Fibrosis and/or cells
    - ✧ Alveolar wall
    - ✧ Alveolar space
- Restrictive physiology
- Decreased lung volumes
- Increased attenuation
- Subacute or chronic
  - ➤ Weeks to months

The Idiopathic Interstitial Pneumonias

- Liebow 1975
- Supporting lung structures
  - ➤ Inflammation
  - ➤ Fibrosis
- Not confined to interstitium
- Initiated within the airspace

Liebow, Prog Reps Dis 1975

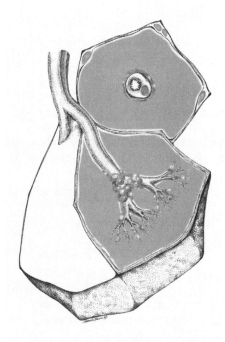

The Idiopathic Interstitial Pneumonias involve the alveolar walls and spaces

The Idiopathic Interstitial Pneumonias
Current List-ATS/ERS Consensus Classification

- Idiopathic Pulmonary Fibrosis (IPF)
  - ➤ Usual Interstitial Pneumonia (UIP)
- Respiratory Bronchiolitis-Interstitial Lung Disease (RB-ILD)
- Desquamative Interstitial Pneumonia (DIP)
- Acute Interstitial Pneumonia (AIP)
- Cryptogenic Organizing Pneumonia (COP)
- NonSpecific Interstitial Pneumonia (NSIP)

Travis et al. Am J Respir Crit Care 2002

Figure 1-2-2

Idiopathic Pulmonary Fibrosis

- Usual Interstitial Pneumonia: histologic pattern
- 5th-7th decade
  - ➤ 66% > 60 years
  - ➤ 7/100,000 women and 10/100,000 men
- Insidious onset of dyspnea
  - ➤ 6 months before diagnosis
  - ➤ Restrictive ventilatory defect
  - ➤ Rales and clubbing
- Associations:
  - ➤ Cigarette smoke
  - ➤ Dusty environments: farming, wood dust, metal dust
  - ➤ GE reflux
  - ➤ Autoantibodies common (ANA, RA)
- Median survival 2.5-3.5 years

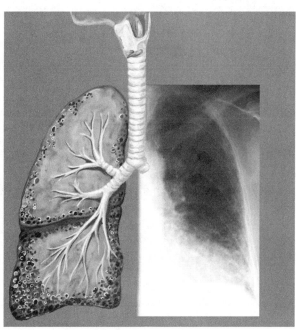

The lung volumes are low and there are areas of increased density

Usual Interstitial Pneumonia: Histology
- Geographic variation
- Temporal variation
  - Fibroblast foci
  - Mature fibrous tissue
- Extensive fibrosis
- Inflammation
  - Minimal
  - No correlation outcome
    Abnormal wound healing
- Prognosis
  - Fibroblast foci
    - Presence and extent

Katzenstein, Am J Respir Crit Care Med 1998

Selman, Ann Int Med 2001

King, Am J Respir Crit Care Med 2001

Idiopathic Pulmonary Fibrosis Imaging *[Figure 1-2-3]*
- Radiograph abnormal-95%
  - Volume loss
  - Reticulonodular opacities
  - Lower lobe
  - Honeycombing
- Computed tomography
  - Peripheral and lower lobe
  - Reticulation and ground glass
    - Progress to honeycombing
  - Ground glass in areas of
    traction bronchiectasis

Hartman, Chest 1996

IPF-Progressive Volume Loss

Idiopathic Pulmonary Fibrosis *[Figure 1-2-4]*

IPF and Emphysema

Utility of Biopsy for Diagnosis of IPF
- Prospective, multi-center study
  - 91 patients suspected of IPF
- Clinical diagnosis
  - Positive predictive value with a confident
    diagnosis-87%
- Imaging diagnosis
  - Positive predictive value with a confident
    diagnosis-96%
  - CT always abnormal in patients with proven IPF
- Histologic diagnosis
  - Agreement regarding the presence or absence
    of IPF-85%
  - Agreement in patients without IPF-48%
    - Relevance to NSIP

Hunninghake, Am J Respir Crit Care Med 2001

Figure 1-2-3

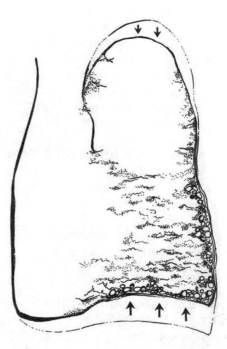

*The abnomalities are predominantly
peripheral and lower lung field.
There is progressive volume loss*

Figure 1-2-4

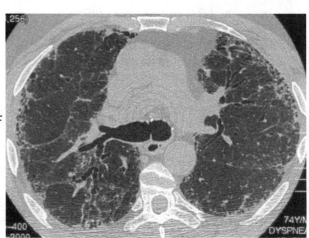

*Typical peripheral recticulation and honeycombing
and traction bronchiectasis in a patient with IPF*

Utilility of Biopsy for Diagnosis of IPF

- Uncertain diagnosis
- Discordant data
- Disease other than IPF
  - Hypersensitivity pneumonitis
  - Collagen-vascular disease
  - Infection

Hunninghake, Am J Respir Crit Care Med 2001

IPF Rad-Path Discord

Smoking Related ILD
Interstitial Lung Disease

- Respiratory bronchiolitis
  - RB
- Respiratory bronchiolits-interstitial lung disease
  - RB-ILD
- Desquamative interstitial lung disease
  - DIP

Smoking Related ILD
RB

- Clinical
  - Cigarette smoke or equivalent
  - Asymptomatic
- Pathology
  - Peribronchiolar macrophages
  - Peribronchiolar fibrosis
- Imaging
  - Centrilobular nodules
    - ⬧ Poorly defined 2-3 mm
    - ⬧ Uper lobe predominance
  - Ground glass opacity
  - Bronchial wall thickening
  - Decreased attenuation
  - Emphysema
  - Air trapping
  - Reticulation

Niewoehner, NEJM 1974 ; Remy-Jardin, Radiology 1993

Smoking Related ILD *[Figure 1-17]*
RB-ILD

- Clinical
  - Gigarette smoke or equivalent
  - Dyspnea
  - Restrictive or mixed PFT's
  - Good prognosis
- Pathology
  - Peribronchiolar macrophages
  - Peribronchiolar fibrosis
- Imaging
  - Centrilobular nodules
    - ⬧ Poorly defined 2-3 mm
    - ⬧ Uper lobe predominance
  - Ground glass opacity
  - Bronchial wall thickening
  - Decreased attenuation
  - Emphysema
  - Air trapping
  - Reticulation

Meyers, Am Rev Respir Dis 1987; Park, J Comput Assist Tomogr 2002

Smoking Related ILD
DIP

- Clinical
  - ➢ Cigarette smoke
  - ➢ 4th and 5th decade
  - ➢ Uncommon
  - ➢ 70% survival-10 years
  - ➢ Steroids
- Pathology
  - ➢ Pigmented macrophages
  - ➢ Interstitial infiltrate
    - ◇ Plasma cells and eosinophils
  - ➢ Fibrosis
- Imaging
  - ➢ Ground glass
    - ◇ Symmetrical
    - ◇ Basal predominance
  - ➢ Reticulation
  - ➢ Cysts
    - ◇ Alveolar ducts
    - ◇ Bronchioles
    - ◇ Emphysematous spaces

Carrington, NEJM 1978 ; Hartman, Radiology 1993

Figure 1-2-5

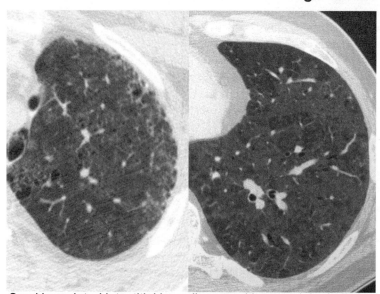

Smoking related intestitial lung disease with upper lobe indistinct nodules, reticulation and well defined emphysematous spaces combined with lowerlobe ground glass

Desquamative Interstitial Pneumonia

Dependent Density

Desquamative Interstitial Pneumonia

RB and DIP

Smoking Related ILD [Figure 1-2-5]

Acute Interstitial Pneumonia
AIP

- Hammon-Rich disease
- Rapidly progressive
- Days-weeks
- Antecedent flu-like syndrome
- Mean age 50 years
- 50% fatal at least

Vourlekis, Medicine 2000

Acute Interstitial Pneumonia
Histology

- Exudative phase
  - ➢ Hyaline membranes
  - ➢ Edema
  - ➢ Inflammation
- Collapse of alveoli
- Organizing phase
  - ➢ Type II hyperplasia
  - ➢ Loose fibrosis
- Diffuse Alveolar Damage

Katzenstein, Am J Pathol 1986 ; Ichikado, AJR 1997

Acute Interstitial Pneumonia
Radiography [Figure 1-2-6]

- Diffuse
- Airspace opacification
- Costal sparing
- Mechanical ventilation
- Resembles ARDS

Acute Interstitial Pneumonia Computed Tomography

- Exudative phase
  - Consolidation
  - Bilateral
  - Focal sparing
- Organizing phase
  - Distortion
  - Traction bronchiectasis
  - Ground glass

Johkoh, Radiology 1999;
Ichikado et al. Am J Respr Crit Care Med 2002

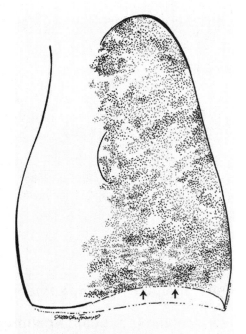

AIP involves all 5 lobes

Acute Interstitial Pneumonia

Cryptogenic Organizing Pneumonia

- Non-specific inflammatory response
- Pattern of repair
- Self-perpetuating
- Cryptogenic
- Secondary
  - Connective tissues disease, hematologic malignancy, drugs or organ transplantation
- Focal
  - Bacteria, legionella, mycoplasma, mycobacterial, or infarction

Lohr, Arch Int Med 1997

Cryptogenic Organizing Pneumonia

- Terminology problem
  - Bronchiolitis obliterans OP (BOOP), bronchiolitis obliterans (BO), bronchiolitis interstitial pneumonia (BIP)
- Subacute presentation (3 months)
- M=F
- Cough, dyspnea, weight loss, fever
- Restrictive PFT's
- Steroid responsive
- Relapse common

Epler, NEJM 1985

Cryptogenic Organizing Pneumonia Histology

- Fibroblastic plugs in alveoli
- Fibrosis in the alveolar space
- May be airway centered
  - Bronchiolitis

Cryptogenic Organizing Pneumonia [Figure 1-2-7]
Radiography
- Consolidation
  - ➢ Unlateral or bilateral
- Small Nodules
  - ➢ 10-50%
- Lung volumes
  - ➢ normal in 75%

Cryptogenic Organizing Pneumonia [Figure 1-2-8]
Computed Tomography
- Consolidation 90%
- Ground glass 75%
- Bronchial thickening and dilatation
- Small nodules along bronchvascular bundles
- Large nodules (15%)
  - ➢ Irregular margins
  - ➢ Air bronchograms
- Reverse halo

Cryptogenic Organizing Pneumonia

Nonspecific Interstitial Pneumonia
- Katzenstein
  - ➢ Described in 1994
- Does not fit definition of other IIPs
  - ➢ UIP, RB-ILD, DIP, OP, AIP
- Represents a variety of etiologies
  - ➢ Collagen vascular disease, drug reaction, inhaled antigen
  - ➢ Inadequately sampled UIP or OP
- Median age 45
- Onset gradual with wide range
  - ➢ 6 months to 3 years
- Better prognosis

Katzenstein, Am J Resp Crit Care 1994
Nicholson, Am J Respir Crit Care Med 2001

Nonspecific Interstitial Pneumonitis
Histology
- 3 categories
  - ➢ Cellular
  - ➢ Fibrosing
  - ➢ Mixed
- Prognosis=fibrosis
- OP common
- Temporally uniform

Nonspecific Interstitial Pneumonitis
Imaging
- Few reports on chest radiography
- Wide variety of CT patterns
  - ➢ Ground glass, consolidation, reticular and honeycombing
- Traction bronchiectasis=fibrosis
- CT pattern indistinguishable
  - ➢ UIP 32%
  - ➢ Hypersensitivity 20%
  - ➢ OP 14%
  - ➢ Other 12%

Hartman, Radiology 2000

Figure 1-2-7

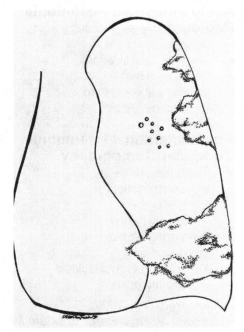

Cryptogenic organizing pneumonia is characterized by focal areas of consolidation more common in the lower lung fields

Figure 1-2-8

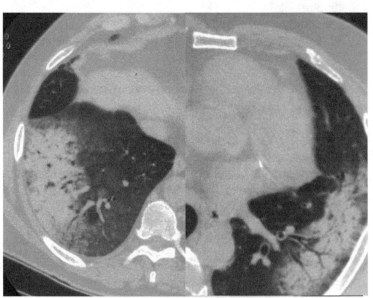

Typical findings in COP with peripheral areas of consolidation. The differential includes chronic eosinophilic pneumonia, bronchoalveolar cell carcinoma, lymphoma and infection

Nonspecific Interstitial Pneumonia

NSIP ATS Consensus Conference
- Pathologists
- Radiologists
- Pulmonalogists
- 300 cases submitted
  - ➢ 11 cases agreed to be NSIP by all pathologists
- Imaging
  - ➢ Lower lobe
  - ➢ Peribronchiolar reticulation and distortion
  - ➢ Subpleural clearing

NSIP Current View

NSIP Fibrosis with IPF Imaging
- Areas of NSIP commonly found in proven cases of UIP
- NSIP and UIP
  - ➢ Different severity of injury?
  - ➢ Different mechanism of injury?
- Prognosis in these cases is driven by the imaging

Katzenstein AA et al, Amer J of Surg Path 2002

Hypersensitivity Pneumonitis

NSIP in Cigarette Smokers

Nonspecific Interstitial Pneumonia

OP-NSIP

The Idiopathic Interstitial Pneumonias
Current List
- Idiopathic Pulmonary Fibrosis (IPF)
  - ➢ Usual Interstitial Pneumonia (UIP)
- Respiratory Bronchiolitis-Interstitial Lung Disease (RB-ILD)
- Desquamative Interstitial Pneumonia (DIP)
- Acute Interstitial Pneumonia (AIP)
- Cryptogenic Organizing Pneumonia (COP)
- NonSpecific Interstitial Pneumonia (NSIP)

Idiopathic Pulmonary Fibrosis

RB/RB-ILD

RB-ILD/DIP

Acute Interstitial Pneumonia

Acute Interstitial Pneumonia

Organizing Pneumonia

NSIP in the Literature

NSIP-IPF

NSIP-Cigarette Smokers

NSIP-Hypersensitivity Pneumonitis

NSIP-Hypersensitivity Pneumonitis

NSIP-Organizing Pneumonia

NSIP-Organizing Pneumonia

The Idiopathic Interstitial Pneumonias: Bibliography

IPF/UIP
1. Hansell DM, Wells AU. CT evaluation of fibrosing alveolitis—applications and insights. J Thorac Imaging 1996; 11(4):231-49.
2. Katzenstein AL, Myers JL. Idiopathic pulmonary fibrosis: clinical relevance of pathologic classification. Am J Respir Crit Care Med 1998; 157(4 Pt 1):1301-15.
3. Kondoh Y, Taniguchi H, Kawabata Y, Yokoi T, Suzuki K, Takagi K. Acute exacerbation in idiopathic pulmonary fibrosis. Analysis of clinical and pathologic findings in three cases. Chest 1993; 103(6):1808-12.
4. Liebow AA. Definition and classification of interstitial pneumonias in human pathology. Prog Resp Res 1975; 8:1-33.
5. Tobin RW, Pope CE, 2nd, Pellegrini CA, Emond MJ, Sillery J, Raghu G. Increased prevalence of gastroesophageal reflux in patients with idiopathic pulmonary fibrosis. Am J Respir Crit Care Med 1998; 158(6):1804-8.
6. Schurawitzki H, Stiglbauer R, Graninger W, Herold C, Pölzleitner D, Burghuber OC, Tscholakoff D. Interstitial lung disease in progressive systemic sclerosis: high-resolution CT versus radiography. Radiology 1990; 176(755-759).
7. Coxson HO, Hogg JC, Mayo JR, Behzad H, Whittall KP, Schwartz DA, Hartley PG, Galvin JR, Wilson JS, Hunninghake GW. Quantification of idiopathic pulmonary fibrosis using computed tomography and histology. Am J Respir Crit Care Med 1997; 155(5):1649-56.
8. Gay SE, Kazerooni EA, Toews GB, Lynch JP, 3rd, Gross BH, Cascade PN, Spizarny DL, Flint A, Schork MA, Whyte RI, Popovich J, Hyzy R, Martinez FJ. Idiopathic pulmonary fibrosis: predicting response to therapy and survival. Am J Respir Crit Care Med 1998; 157(4 Pt 1):1063-72.
9. Bjoraker JA, Ryu JH, Edwin MK, Myers JL, Tazelaar HD, Schroeder DR, Offord KP. Prognostic significance of histopathologic subsets in idiopathic pulmonary fibrosis. Am J Respir Crit Care Med 1998; 157(1):199-203.

DIP
1. Gaensler EA, Goff AM, Prowse CM. Desquamative interstitial pneumonia. N Engl J Med 1966; 274(3):113-28.

DAD/AIP
1. Bone RC. The ARDS lung. New insights from computed tomography [editorial; comment]. Jama 1993; 269(16):2134-5.
2. Desai SR, Wells AU, Rubens MB, Evans TW, Hansell DM. Acute respiratory distress syndrome: CT abnormalities at long-term follow-up. Radiology 1999; 210(1):29-35.
3. Greene R. Adult respiratory distress syndrome: acute alveolar damage. Radiology 1987; 163(1):57-66.
4. Ichikado K, Johkoh T, Ikezoe J, Takeuchi N, Kohno N, Arisawa J, Nakamura H, Nagareda T, Itoh H, Ando M. Acute interstitial pneumonia: high-resolution CT findings correlated with pathology. AJR Am J Roentgenol 1997; 168(2):333-8.
5. Johkoh T, Muller NL, Taniguchi H, Kondoh Y, Akira M, Ichikado K, Ando M, Honda O, Tomiyama N, Nakamura H. Acute interstitial pneumonia: thin-section CT findings in 36 patients. Radiology 1999; 211(3):859-63.
6. Katzenstein AL, Myers JL, Mazur MT. Acute interstitial pneumonia. A clinicopathologic, ultrastructural, and cell kinetic study. Am J Surg Pathol 1986; 10(4):256-67.
7. Olson J, Colby TV, Elliott CG. Hamman-Rich syndrome revisited [see comments]. Mayo Clin Proc 1990; 65(12):1538-48.
8. Primack SL, Hartman TE, Ikezoe J, Akira M, Sakatani M, Muller NL. Acute interstitial pneumonia: radiographic and CT findings in nine patients [see comments]. Radiology 1993; 188(3):817-20.

NSIP

1. Cottin V, Donsbeck AV, Revel D, Loire R, Cordier JF. Nonspecific interstitial pneumonia. Individualization of a clinicopathologic entity in a series of 12 patients. Am J Respir Crit Care Med 1998; 158(4):1286-93.
2. Katzenstein AL, Fiorelli RF. Nonspecific interstitial pneumonia/fibrosis. Histologic features and clinical significance. Am J Surg Pathol 1994; 18(2):136-47.
3. Kim TS, Lee KS, Chung MP, Han J, Park JS, Hwang JH, Kwon OJ, Rhee CH. Nonspecific interstitial pneumonia with fibrosis: high-resolution CT and pathologic findings. AJR Am J Roentgenol 1998; 171(6):1645-50.

BOOP/Organizing Pneumonia

1. Akira M, Yamamoto S, Sakatani M. Bronchiolitis obliterans organizing pneumonia manifesting as multiple large nodules or masses. AJR Am J Roentgenol 1998; 170(2):291-5.
2. Carlson BA, Swensen SJ, O'Connell EJ, Edell ES. High-resolution computed tomography for obliterative bronchiolitis. Mayo Clin Proc 1993; 68(3):307-8.
3. Chandler PW, Shin MS, Friedman SE, Myers JL, Katzenstein AL. Radiographic manifestations of bronchiolitis obliterans with organizing pneumonia vs usual interstitial pneumonia. AJR Am J Roentgenol 1986; 147(5):899-906.
4. Epler GR, Colby TV, McLoud TC, Carrington CB, Gaensler EA. Bronchiolitis obliterans organizing pneumonia. N Engl J Med 1985; 312(3):152-8.
5. Gosink BB, Friedman PJ, Liebow AA. Bronchiolitis obliterans. Roentgenologic-pathologic correlation. Am J Roentgenol Radium Ther Nucl Med 1973; 117(4):816-32.
6. Haddock JA, Hansell DM. The radiology and terminology of cryptogenic organizing pneumonia. Br J Radiol 1992; 65(776):674-80.
7. Katzenstein AL, Myers JL, Prophet WD, Corley LS, 3rd, Shin MS. Bronchiolitis obliterans and usual interstitial pneumonia. A comparative clinicopathologic study. Am J Surg Pathol 1986; 10(6):373-81.
8. Lau DM, Siegel MJ, Hildebolt CF, Cohen AH. Bronchiolitis obliterans syndrome: thin-section CT diagnosis of obstructive changes in infants and young children after lung transplantation. Radiology 1998; 208(3):783-8.
9. Lee KS, Kullnig P, Hartman TE, Muller NL. Cryptogenic organizing pneumonia: CT findings in 43 patients. AJR Am J Roentgenol 1994; 162(3):543-6.
10. Lohr RH, Boland BJ, Douglas WW, Dockrell DH, Colby TV, Swensen SJ, Wollan PC, Silverstein MD. Organizing pneumonia. Features and prognosis of cryptogenic, secondary, and focal variants. Arch Intern Med 1997; 157(12):1323-9.
11. McLoud TC, Epler GR, Colby TV, Gaensler EA, Carrington CB. Bronchiolitis obliterans. Radiology 1986; 159(1):1-8.
12. Muller NL, Guerry-Force ML, Staples CA, Wright JL, Wiggs B, Coppin C, Pare P, Hogg JC. Differential diagnosis of bronchiolitis obliterans with organizing pneumonia and usual interstitial pneumonia: clinical, functional, and radiologic findings. Radiology 1987; 162(1 Pt 1):151-6.
13. Muller NL, Staples CA, Miller RR. Bronchiolitis obliterans organizing pneumonia: CT features in 14 patients. AJR Am J Roentgenol 1990; 154(5):983-7.

Airways Disease: The Movement from Anatomic to Physiologic Assessment

Jeffrey R. Galvin, MD
Chief Pulmonary and Mediastinal Radiology
Armed Forces Institute of Pathology
Clinical Professor Department of Radiology
University of Maryland

Figure 1-3-1

Assessment of Dyspnea
A Common Clinical Problem
- 55 million adult smokers
- 15 million meet criteria for bronchitis
- 5 million with airway obstruction
- 10 million with asthma

Gordon Snyder

Differential Diagnosis of Airways Obstruction
- Common
  - ➤ Emphysema, bronchitis, bronchiectasis, asthma
- Uncommon
  - ➤ LAM, BO, panbronchiolitis, sarcoid, alpha-1 deficiency, ABPA

Diseases with Obstructive Physiology

The Changing Role of Imaging
- Diagnosis
- Functional assessment

Why Pulmonary Functions are Insensitive
- PFT's based on wide range of normal
  - ➤ 80-120% predicted
- Diseases with opposing physiologic processes
- The "silent zone" of the lungs

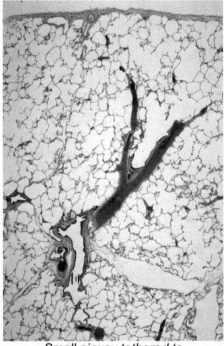

*Small airway tethered to
the pleural surface by alveolar walls*

The "Silent Zone" of the Lungs
[Figure 1-3-1 and 1-3-2]
"Small Airways"
- Peter Macklem
  - ➤ 1970's
- No cartilage
  - ➤ <2mm physiologists
  - ➤ 1mm pathologists
- Tethered
  - ➤ fiber skeleton
  - ➤ pleura

Weibel

Figure 1-3-2

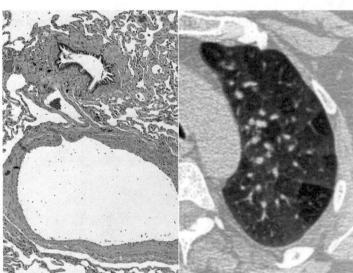

*Mosaic attenuation on an expiratory CT in patient with
constrictive bronchiolitis*

Diffuse Lung Disease
Airways [Figure 1-3-3]
- Airways involvement
- Obstructive physiology
- Increased lung volumes
- Decreased attenuation

Airways Disease
Direct Signs [Figure 1-3-4]
- Changes
  - Airway wall
  - Airway lumen
- Opacities
  - Tubular
  - Nodular
  - Branching

Airways Disease
Indirect Signs
- Mosaic density
  - Air trapping
- Subsegmental atelectasis
- Ground glass

Airways Disease
- Emphysema
- Emphysema and Fibrosis
- Alpha-1 deficiency
- Langherhans Cell Histiocytosis
- Bronchiectasis
- Asthma
- Allergic Bronchopulmonary Aspergillosis
- Sarcoidosis
- Diffuse Panbronchiolitis
- Bronchiolitis Obliterans
- Lymphangioleiomyomatosis

Emphysema
ATS Definition
- Permanent enlargement of airspaces distal to the terminal bronchiole, accompanied by destruction of the walls without obvious fibrosis

Emphysema

Emphysema
Classification
- Proximal Acinar
  - Centrilobular
  - Resp bronchiole
  - Cigarette smoke
  - Upper lobes
- Panacinar
  - Entire acinus
  - Alpha-1 deficiency
  - Lower lobes
- Distal Acinar
  - Paraseptal
  - Distal acinus
  - Subpleura
  - Pneumothorax

Figure 1-3-3

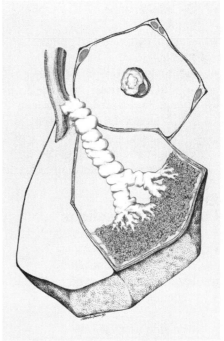

Airways involvement at the level of the secondary lobule

Figure 1-3-4

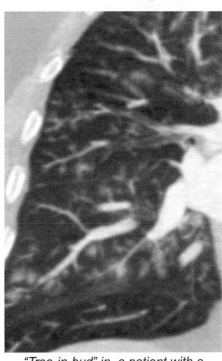

"Tree-in-bud" in a patient with a respiratory infection

Emphysema
Clinical Presentation
- Symptoms after 20-30 years of smoking
- Cough, dyspnea and sputum production
- Hemoptysis rare
  - R/O cancer
- Symptomatic air flow obstruction
  - After age 50, 20-30 years of smoking
- Cor pulmonale (late) related to hypoxemia and loss of capillary bed

Emphysema
Pulmonary Functions
- Important to identify patients at risk
- Reduction in Fev1
  - Most reproducible
- RV increases followed by TLC
- Volumes and flows
  - Insensitive to early changes
- Diffusing capacity
  - Sensitive but non-specific
- Small airways tests

Emphysema
Radiographic Feature
- Hyperinflation
  - Concave diaphragm
  - Increased A-P diameter
  - Retrosternal airspace
- Arterial deficiency pattern
- Bulla
  - Cystic airspaces > 1cm
- Radiography is insensitive
  - 41% of moderate disease
  - 66% of severe disease

Saber Trachea [Figure 1-3-5]

Emphysema and Computed Tomography [Figure 1-3-6]

The Diagnosis of Mild Emphysema Correlation of CT and Pathology Scores
- HRCT detects emphysema
  - Before there is airflow limitation on PFT's
- HRCT excludes emphysema
  - Patients with moderate to severe airflow limitation

Kuwano et al, Am Rev Respir Dis 1990

Early Emphysema

Figure 1-3-5

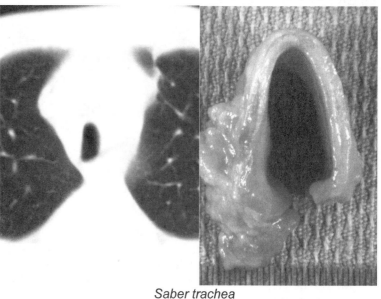

Saber trachea

Figure 1-3-6

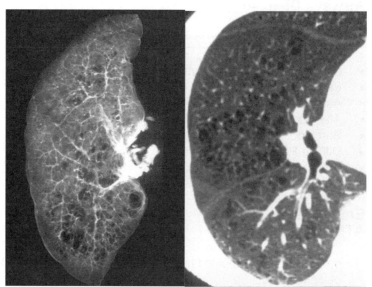

Typical low attenuation lesions of emphysema

Respiratory Bronchiolitis [Figure 1-3-7]
"Smoker's Bronchiolitis"
- Common change
  - all smokers
- Pigmented macrophages
  - In respiratory bronchioles
  - Surrounding alveoli
- Upper lobe predominance
- Usually asymptomatic
  - May cause symptoms

Relationship of RB and Emphysema
- Prospective study
- 111 subjects
  - Followed for 5 years
    - ✧ Imaged at inception TO and 5 years T1
  - Smokers, nonsmokers and quitters
- Micronodules at TO predisposes to the development of emphysema at T1
- Micronodules and emphysema at TO predicts more rapid decline in lung function

Remy-Jardin, Radiology 2001

Relationship of RB and Emphysema
Remy-Jardin, Radiology 2001

Emphysema and Fibrosis
- 42 smokers
- 13 nonsmokers
- RB 100% smokers
- Respiratory and bronchiolar fibrosis related to chronic cigarette use

Adekunle, Am Rev Resp Dis 1990

Emphysema and Fibrosis
- 14 patients
- Scanning electron microscopy
- Thick and thin walls
  - Both fibrotic

Nagai & Thurlbeck, Am Rev Resp Dis 1985

Emphysema and Fibrosis
- Normal lung volumes and
- Normal flow rates
- Reduced diffusing capacity
  - Severe
- Minimal pulmonary reserve

Emphysema and Fibrosis
- TLC   119%
- VC   126%
- RV   109%
- FEV1/FVC   88%
- D/Va   28%

Emphysema and Fibrosis [Figure 1-3-8]

Idiopathic Pulmonary Fibrosis

Figure 1-3-7

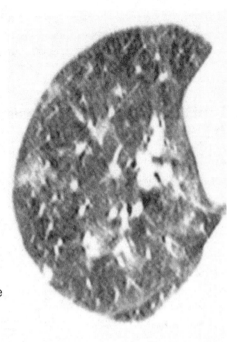

Respiratory bronchiolitis

Figure 1-3-8

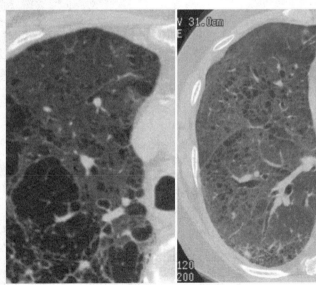

Emphysema and fibrosis

Langerhans Cell Histiocytosis
Clinical Presentation
- Almost exclusively cigarette smokers
- Slight male preponderance
- Cough and dyspnea most common
- May be asymptomatic
- Occasional bone lesion

Langerhans Cell Histiocytosis
Histology [Figures 1-3-9]
- Nodular
  - Interstitial lesions
  - Located near bronchioles
- Histiocytes, eosinophils, plasma cells and lymphocytes
- Diagnosis requires Langerhans cells
  - Large histiocytes
  - Folded nuclei
  - Eosinophilic cytoplasm
- Path DDX
  - Eos pneumonia, DIP,UIP

Langherhans Cell Histiocytosis
[Figures 1-3-10 and 1-3-11]

Langherhans Cell Histiocytosis
Radiographic Features
- Varies over time
- Upper lobe
  - Predominance
- Nodules
  - 0.5-1.0 cm in upper lobes
  - Early
- Cysts replace nodules
  - Later
- Honeycomb lung
- Pneumothorax 15%
- Adenopathy and effusion are unusual

Langerhans Cell Histiocytosis
EM and Immunohistochemistry
- Immunoperoxidase staining
  - CD1a, S-100 protein
- Cells in clusters in interstitium
- EM
  - X-bodies
  - Langerhans cell granules
  - Birbeck granules

Langerhans Cell Histiocytosis
Clinical Course
- Clinical resolution
  - Common
- Radiographic abnormalities
  - Persist
- Occasional progression
  - Fibrosis and honeycombing
- May be fatal
  - Rapid progression

Figure 1-3-9

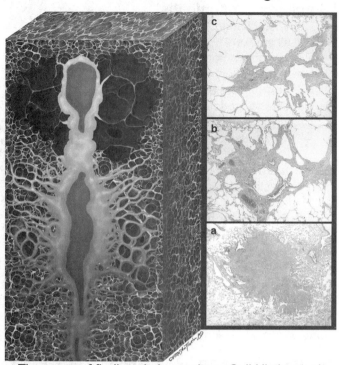

The range of findings in Langerhans Cell Histiocytosis

Figure 1-3-10

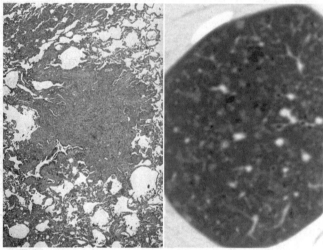

Typical nodules in LCH

Figure 1-3-11

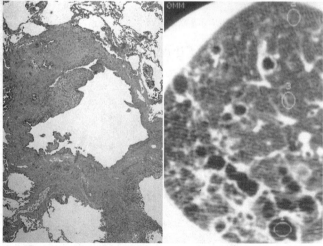

Cystic lesions in LCH

Langherhans Cell Histiocytosis

Alpha-1 Antitrypsin Deficiency
Pathophysiology
- 1-2% of emphysema in the US
- Alpha-1 antitrypsin inactivates neutrophil elastase
- Production controlled by 2 genes
- Level of antitrypsin dependent on allele
- ZZ homozygotes most severe
- Smoking accelerates the destruction

Alpha-1 Antitrypsin Deficiency
Imaging Features
- Radiograph may be normal
- Lower lobe predominance
- Panacinar emphysema
- CT
  - ➢ Upper lobe involvement
  - ➢ Bronchiectasis
  - ➢ Airway thickening common
- CT more sensitive

Alpha-1 Antitrypsin Deficiency [Figure 1-3-12]

Bronchiectasis
Pathophysiology
- Dilatation of bronchi
- Reversible form
  - ➢ Infection
  - ➢ Atelectasis
- Congenital
  - ➢ tracheobronchomalacia
- Post-inflammatory
- Postobstructive
- Fibrotic
  - ➢ IPF
  - ➢ Sarcoid

Williams-Campbell [Figure 1-3-13]

Mounier-Kuhn Syndrome

Bronchiectasis
Postinflammatory
- Primary Ciliary Dyskinesia
  - ➢ Kartagener's
- Immunodeficiency
- Postinfectious
  - ➢ TB, Measles, pertussis, viral
- Post-toxic bronchitis
  - ➢ gastric acid aspiration
- Immunologic
  - ➢ ABPA

Primary Ciliary Dyskinesia

Figure 1-3-12

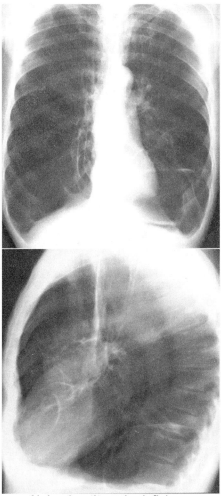

Alpha-1 antitrypsin deficiency

Figure 1-3-13

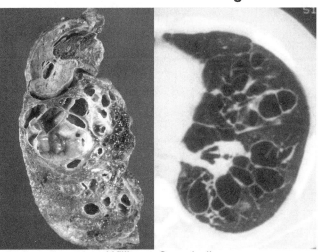

Williams-Campbell

Post Obstructive Bronchiectasis [Figure 1-3-14]

- Neoplasm
- Foreign body
- Broncholith
- Lymph node enlargement

Bronchiectasis
Clinical Presentation

- Cough
- Purulent sputum
- Hemoptysis (50%)
- Dyspnea
- Rare
  - clubbing, brain abscess, amyloidosis

Bronchiectasis
Radiographic Features

- Prominent markings
- Crowding of Vessels
- "Tram Tracks"
- Loss of volume
- Cystic spaces

Bronchiectasis
CT Features

- Bronchi in the periphery
- "Signet Rings"
- "Tram Tracks"
- Sensitivity
  - Collimation

Emphysema [Figure 1-3-15]

RB/RB-ILD [Figure 1-3-16]

Emphysema and Fibrosis [Figure 1-3-17]

Langherhans Cell Histiocytosis [Figures 1-3-18 to 1-3-20]

Figure 1-3-14

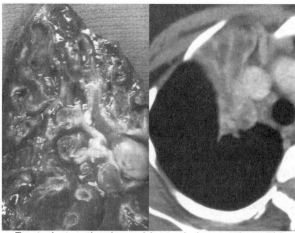

Post obstructive bronchiectasis in a patient with mucoepidermoid carcinoma

Figure 1-3-15

Figure 1-3-16

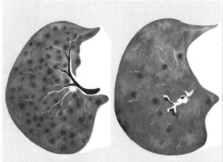
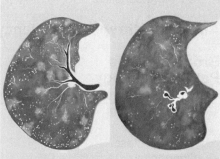

Upper lobe smoking related emphysema

RB-ILD

Figure 1-3-17

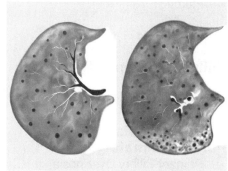

Emphysema and fibrosis

Figure 1-3-18

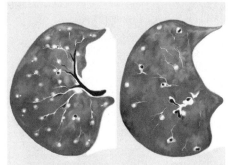

Early LCH nodules

Figure 1-3-19

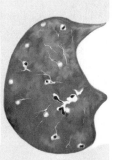

Late LCH Cysts and nodules

Figure 1-3-20

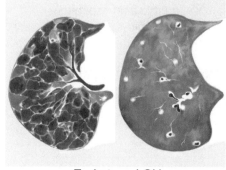

End-stage LCH

Alpha-1 Antitrypsin Deficiency [Figure 1-3-21]

Figure 1-3-21

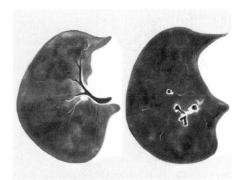

Lower lobe predominance in Alpha-1 antitrypsin

Diffuse Lung Disease
Airways
- Airways involvement
- Obstructive physiology
- Increased lung volumes
- Decreased attenuation

Asthma
ATS Definition
- Reversible airway disease
- Increased airway responsiveness
- Persistent airflow obstruction occurs in chronic asthmatic
  - Why?
- 6% in the American population
  - Rate has doubled in 20 years
  - Higher incidence in large cities

Asthma
Extrinsic
- Family history atopy
- Early onset <30 years
- Seasonal symptoms
- Increased IGE
- Positive skin tests
- Often remits

Asthma
Intrinsic
- No atopy
  - Absence of external triggers
- Older age group
- Increased blood eosinophils
- Increased sputum eosinophils
- Fixed airway obstruction
  - Progressive

Asthma
Pathology
- Airway smooth muscle
  - Hypertrophy
- Airway wall
  - Inflammation
  - Edema
- Airway plugging
  - Mucus
  - Inflammatory exudate

Asthma
Radiographic Features [Figure 1-3-22]
- Chest roentgenogram
  - Often normal
- Airway thickening
  - Chronic disease
- Rapid attenuation of vessels
  - hypoxemia
- Pneumomediastinum
  - pneumothorax
- Hyperinflation
  - Adaptive
  - Later air trapping

Figure 1-3-22

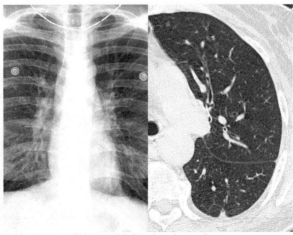

Airway thickening in asthma

Asthma-Hyperinflation [Figure 1-3-23]

Figure 1-3-23

Asthma [Figure 1-3-24]
CT Features
- More sensitive than CXR
- Reversible
  - ➢ Consolidation
  - ➢ Atelectasis
  - ➢ Mucoid impaction
  - ➢ Airway Narrowing
  - ➢ Air Trapping
- Permanent
  - ➢ Bronchial wall thickening
  - ➢ Bronchiectasis
  - ➢ Emphysema

Allergic Bronchopulmonary Aspergillosis
Primary Criteria
- Asthma
- Eosinophilia
- Immediate skin test reactivity
- Precipitating antibodies (IgG)
- Elevated serum (IgE)
- Pulmonary infiltrates
- Central bronchiectasis

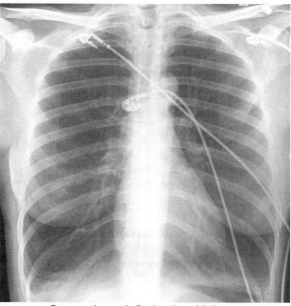

Severe hyperinflation in which you can see the slips of the diaphragm as it inverts

Figure 1-3-24

Allergic Bronchopulmonary Aspergillosis
Presentation & Pathology
- Atopic individuals
  - ➢ Most common
- Cystic fibrosis
- Airways filled
  - ➢ Fungus
  - ➢ Inspissated mucous
- Presentation with
  - ➢ cough, fever
  - ➢ Hemoptysis
  - ➢ worsening asthma
- Seen in stable asthmatics
- Good response to steroids

Allergic Bronchopulmonary Aspergillosis
Imaging [Figure 1-3-25 and 1-3-26]
- Bifurcating opacities
  - ➢ "Gloved-finger"
  - ➢ Mucous filled airways
- Central Bronchiectasis
- Fleeting infiltrates
- Pleural disease
  - ➢ Uncommon

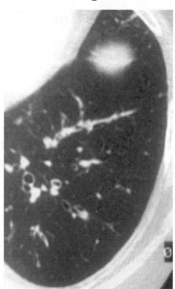

Mucoid impaction in severe asthma

Figure 1-3-25

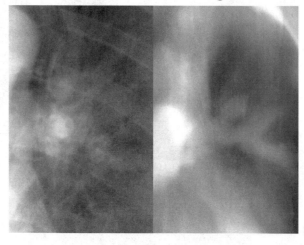

Mucoid impaction in ABPA

Sarcoidosis and the Airways
Computed Tomography

- Functional evidence of airways obstruction
  - Obstructive PFT's are common
- Endobronchial biopsies find granulomas
- Obstructive physiology correlates with
  - Decreased attenuation on expiratory scans (small airways)
  - Reticular pattern and advanced fibrotic disease (large airways)

Hansell et al, Radiology 1998

Figure 1-3-26

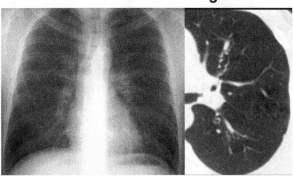

Central bronchiectasis in ABPA

Endobronchial Granulomas

Small Airway Distortion

Reticular Pattern and Fibrosis

Diffuse Panbronchiolitis

- Japan most common
  - Rarely: Korea, China, Europe and North America
  - HLA BW54
  - M-F 2:1
- Presentation
  - Dyspnea
  - Cough
- Obstructive PFT's
- Slowly progressive
  - 15 yr mean survival
- Erythromycin
  - May not be an antibacterial effect

Diffuse Panbronchiolitis
Pathology

- Discrete nodules
- Early infiltration
  - Interstitium
  - Respiratory bronchioles
  - Alveolar ducts
  - Foamy histiocyte, lymphocyte and plasma cells
- Late secondary ectasia
  - Proximal terminal bronchioles

Diffuse Panbronchiolitis
Imaging Early

- Radiography
  - Nodules 5mm
  - Hyperinflation
- Computed Tomography
  - Centrilobular nodules
  - Branching opacities
  - Mosaic attenuation

Diffuse Panbronchiolitis
Imaging Late *[Figures 1-3-27]*
- Radiography
  - Nodules
  - Cysts and bulla
  - Hyperinflation
- Computed Tomography
  - Centrilobular nodules
  - Bronchiolectasis
  - Bronchiectasis

Constrictive Bronchiolitis
Introduction
- Confusing Terminology
  - Obliterative Bronchiolitis
  - Bronchiolitis Obliterans
  - Bronchiolitis Obliterans Organizing Pneumonia
    - ◇ Different disease
    - ◇ Cryptogenic organizing pneumonia
- Small Airways
  - Fibrosis
  - Inflammation
- Response to
  - Inflammatory disorders
  - Infectious disorders

Constrictive Bronchiolitis
Clinical Presentation
- Cough, dyspnea and malaise
- History
  - prior infection
  - exposure
- Hypoxemia
- Airway obstruction

Constrictive Bronchiolitis
Classification
- Infection
  - RSV, adenovirus and mycoplasma
- Toxic Inhalation
  - Ammonia, acid and NO
- Aspiration: gastric acid
- Collagen Vascular: RA
- Organ Transplantation
- Unknown

Constrictive Bronchiolitis
Histology *[Figures 1-3-28]*
- Obstruction
  - Terminal bronchiole
  - Respiratory bronchioles
- Polyps of fibrosis
- Cellular infiltration
  - Lymphs
  - Plasma cells
  - Histiocytes

Figure 1-3-27

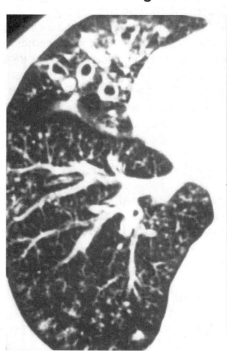

Severe airway involvement in panbronchiolitis

Figure 1-3-28

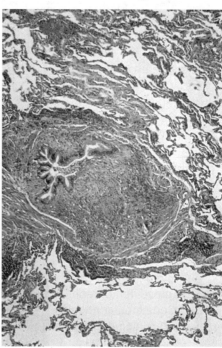

Constrictive bronchiolitis

Constrictive Bronchiolitis

Imaging *[Figures 1-3-29 and 1-3-30]*

- Hyperinflation
  - ➤ Localized
  - ➤ Diffuse
- Discrete nodules
  - ➤ Airway associated
- Mosaic pattern
- Airway thickening
- Bronchiectasis
- Air trapping

Swyer-James Syndrome

Swyer-James Syndrome-Adenovirus

Swyer-James Syndrome *[Figures 1-3-31 and 1-3-32]*

Figure 1-3-29

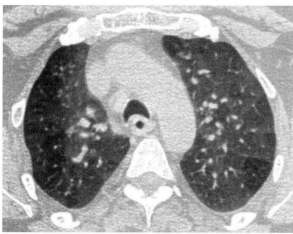

Mosaic attenuation in constrictive bronchiolitis

Figure 1-3-30

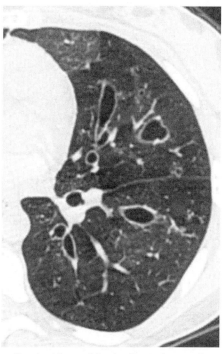

Central bronchiectasis and mosaic attenuation in constrictive bronchiolitis

Figure 1-3-31

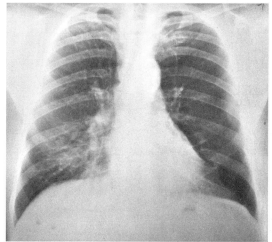

Unilateral hyperlucent lung in a patient with Swyer-James

Figure 1-3-32

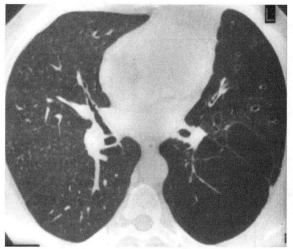

Swyer-James Syndrome

Lymphangioleiomyomatosis
Clinical Presentation
- Exclusively women
- Reproductive years
- Progressive dyspnea
- Chylous pleural effusions
- Hemoptysis
- Massive hemorrhage

Lymphangioleiomyomatosis
Function
- Obstructive defect
- FEV1 is decreased
- TLC and RV increased
- DLCO reduced
- Hypoxemia
- Hypocapnia

Lymphangioleiomyomatosis
Histology
- Smooth muscle proliferation
  - Disorderly
  - Bronchioles, alveolar septa, arteries, veins and lymphatics
- Small air filled cysts
  - Air trapping

Lymphangioleiomyomatosis
Gross Features [Figure 1-3-33 and 1-3-34]
- Cysts
  - 0.2-2cm
- Diffuse involvement
- Enlarged thoracic duct
- Enlarged lymph nodes

Lymphangioleiomyomatosis
Radiographic Features
- Reticulonodular opacities
  - Basilar
- Lung volume
  - Normal
  - Increased
- Pleural effusion
  - 60-75%
- Pneumothorax
- Honeycombing late

Lymphangioleiomyomatosis
CT Features [Figure 1-3-35]
- Thin-walled cysts
  - More sensitive than plain film
- Diffuse
- Bilateral involvement
- Adenopathy

Figure 1-3-33

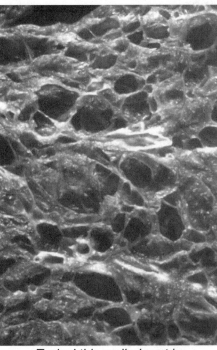

Typical thin-walled cyst in lymphangioleiomyomatosis

Figure 1-3-34

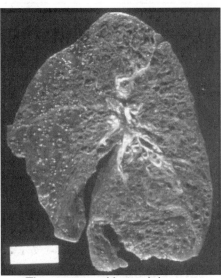

The upper and lower lobes are equally involved in LAM

Figure 1-3-35

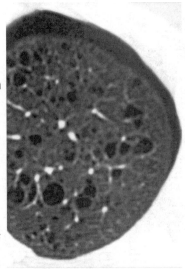

Thin-walled cysts and a pneumothorax in patient with lymphangioleiomyomatosis

Lymphangioleiomyomatosis
Therapy and Prognosis

- Slowly progressive course
  - Variable
- Progression
  - Cor pulmonale
  - Respiratory insufficiency
- 50-80% 5 year survival
  - Average survival 10 years
- Hormonal therapy
  - Oophorectomy, progesterone

Tuberous Sclerosis

Emphysema

Emphysema and Fibrosis

Langherhans Cell Histiocytosis

Alpha-1 Antitrypsin Deficiency

Asthma

ABPA *[Figure 1-3-36]*

Sarcoidosis *[Figure 1-3-37]*

Diffuse Panbronchiolitis *[Figure 1-3-38]*

Constrictive Bronchiolitis *[Figure 1-3-39]*

Swyer-James Syndrome

LAM *[Figures 1-3-40]*

Figure 1-3-36

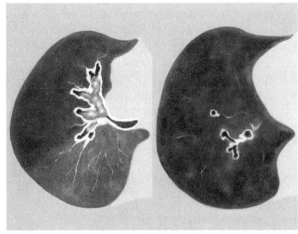

ABPA

Figure 1-3-37

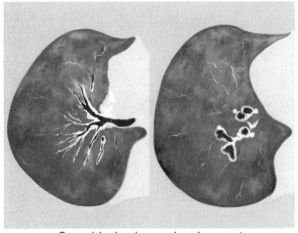

Sarcoidosis airways involvement

Figure 1-3-38

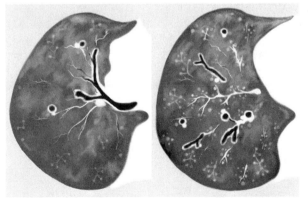

Diffuse Panbronchiolitis

Figure 1-3-39

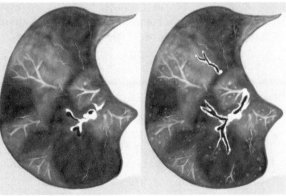

Mosaic attenuation in constrictive bronchiolitis

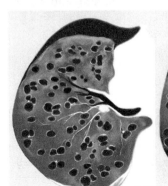

Figure 1-3-40

Typical findings in LAM

Physiologic Measurement
An Integral Part of Imaging
- Imaging provides physiologic information
  - ➤ not available from pulmonary functions
- Air content and blood flow can be quantified

Airways Disease
- Emphysema
- Emphysema and Fibrosis
- Alpha-1 deficiency
- Histiocytosis-X
- Bronchiectasis
- Asthma
- Allergic Bronchopulmonary Aspergillosis
- Sarcoidosis
- Diffuse Panbronchiolitis
- Bronchiolitis Obliterans
- Lymphangioleiomyomatosis

Diffuse Lung Disease
Airways
- Airways involvement
- Obstructive physiology
- Increased lung volumes
- Decreased attenuation

Airways Bibliography

General
1. Hartman T, Primack S, Lee K, Swensen S, Muller N. CT of bronchial and bronchiolar diseases. RadioGraphics 1994; 14:991-1003.
2. Hogg JC, Macklem PT, Thurlbeck WM. Site and nature of airway obstruction in chronic obstructive lung disease. N Engl J Med 1968; 278(25):1355-60.
3. King GG, Muller NL, Pare PD. Evaluation of airways in obstructive pulmonary disease using high- resolution computed tomography. Am J Respir Crit Care Med 1999; 159(3):992-1004.
4. Lucidarme O, Coche E, Cluzel P, Mourey-Gerosa I, Howarth N, Grenier P. Expiratory CT scans for chronic airway disease: correlation with pulmonary function test results. AJR Am J Roentgenol 1998; 170(2):301-7.
5. Macklem PT. Obstruction in small airways—a challenge to medicine. Am J Med 1972; 52(6):721-4.
6. Muller NL, Miller RR. Diseases of the bronchioles: CT and histopathologic findings. Radiology 1995; 196(1):3-12.
7. Naidich D, McCauley DI, Khouri NF, al e. Computed tomography of bronchiectasis. Journal of Computer Assisted Tomography 1982; 6:437-444.
8. Neeld DA, Goodman LR, Gurney JW, Greenberger PA, Fink JN. Computerized tomography in the evaluation of allergic bronchopulmonary aspergillosis. American Review of Respiratory Disease 1990; 142:1200-1205.
9. Snider GL. Distinguishing among asthma, chronic bronchitis, and emphysema. Chest 1985; 87(1,supplement):35S-39S.
10. Stern EJ, Swensen S, Hartman T, Frank M. Ct mosaic pattern of lung attenuation: distinguishing different causes. American Journal of Roentgenolgoy 1995; 165:813-816.
11. Teel G, Engeler C, Tahsijain J, duCret R. Imaging of small airways disease. RadioGraphics 1996; 16:27-41.
12. Weibel ER, Bachofen H. The Fiber Scaffold of Lung Parenchyma. In: Crystal RG, West JB, eds. The Lung. New York: Raven Press, 1991; 787-794.
13. Weibel ER, Crystal RG. Structural Organization of the Pulmonary Interstitium. In: Crystal RG, West JB, eds. The Lung. New York: Raven Press, 1991; 369-380.

14. Worthy SA, Muller NL, Hartman TE, Swensen SJ, Padley SP, Hansell DM. Mosaic attenuation pattern on thin-section CT scans of the lung: differentiation among infiltrative lung, airway, and vascular diseases as a cause. Radiology 1997; 205(2):465-70.

Emphysema

1. Bankier AA, De Maertelaer V, Keyzer C, Gevenois PA. Pulmonary emphysema: subjective visual grading versus objective quantification with macroscopic morphometry and thin-section CT densitometry. Radiology 1999; 211(3):851-8.
2. Coxson HO, Rogers RM, Whittall KP, D'Yachkova Y, Pare PD, Sciurba FC, Hogg JC. A quantification of the lung surface area in emphysema using computed tomography. Am J Respir Crit Care Med 1999; 159(3):851-6.
3. Gelb AF, Hogg JC, Muller NL, Schein MJ, Kuei J, Tashkin DP, Epstein JD, Kollin J, Green RH, Zamel N, Elliott WM, Hadjiaghai L. Contribution of emphysema and small airways in COPD. Chest 1996; 109(2):353-9.
4. Kinsella M, Muller NL, Staples C, Vedal S, Chan-Yeung M. Hyperinflation in asthma and emphysema. Assessment by pulmonary function testing and computed tomography. Chest 1988; 94(2):286-9.
5. Kinsella M, Müller NL, Abboud RT, Morrison NJ, DyBuncio A. Quantitation of emphysema by computed tomography using a "density mask" program and correlation with pulmonary function tests. Chest 1990; 97:315-321.
6. Klein JS, Gamsu G, Webb WR, Golden JA, Muller NL. High-resolution CT diagnosis of emphysema in symptomatic patients with normal chest radiographs and isolated low diffusing capacity. Radiology 1992; 182(3):817-21.
7. Kondoh Y, Taniguchi H, Yokoyama S, Taki F, Takagi K, Satake T. Emphysematous change in chronic asthma in relation to cigarette smoking: assessment by computed tomography. Chest 1990; 97:845-849.
8. Kuwano K, Matsuba K, Ikeda T, Murakami J, Araki A, Nishitani H, Ishida T, Yasumoto K, Shigematsu N. The diagnosis of mild emphysema. Correlation of computed tomography and pathology scores. Am Rev Respir Dis 1990; 141(1):169-78.
9. Miller RR, Müller NL, Vedal S, Morrison NJ, Staples CA. Limitations of computed tomography in the assessment of emphysema. American Review of Respiratory Disease 1989; 139:980-983.
10. Muller NL, Thurlbeck WM. Thin-section CT, emphysema, air trapping, and airway obstruction [editorial;comment]. Radiology 1996; 199(3):621-2.
11. Müller NL, Staples CA, Miller RR, Abboud RT. "Density Mask" An objective method to quantitate emphysema using computed tomography. Chest 1988; 94:782-787.
12. Nagao M, Murase K, Yasuhara Y, Ikezoe J. Quantitative analysis of pulmonary emphysema: three-dimensional fractal analysis of single-photon emission computed tomography images obtained with a carbon particle radioaerosol. AJR Am J Roentgenol 1998; 171(6):1657-63.
13. Park KJ, Bergin CJ, Clausen JL. Quantitation of emphysema with three-dimensional CT densitometry: comparison with two-dimensional analysis, visual emphysema scores, and pulmonary function test results. Radiology 1999; 211(2):541-7.
14. Remy-Jardin M, Remy J, Gosselin B, Becette V, Edme J. Lung parenchymal changes secondary to cigarette smoking: pathologic-ct correlations. Radiology 1993; 186:643-651.
15. Snider GL, Kleinerman J, Thurlbeck WM, Bengali ZH. The definition of emphysema. Report of the National Heart, Blood and Lung Institute, Division of Lung Diseases Workshop. American Review of Respiratory Diseases 1985; 132:182-185.
16. Sutinen S, Christoforidis AJ, Klugh GA, Pratt PC. Roentgenologic criteria for the recognitiion of nonsymptomatic pulmonary emphysema. American Review of Respiratory Disease 1965; 91:69-76.
17. Uppaluri R, Mitsa T, Sonka M, Hoffman EA, McLennan G. Quantification of pulmonary emphysema from lung computed tomography images. Am J Respir Crit Care Med 1997; 156(1):248-54.

Alpha-1 Antitrypsin

1. Brantly ML, Paul LD, Miller BH, Falk RT, Wu M, Crystal RG. Clinical features and history of the destructive lung disease associated with alpha-1-antitrypsin deficiency of adults with pulmonary symptoms. Am Rev Respir Dis 1988; 138(2):327-36.
2. Brantly M, Nukiwa T, Crystal RG. Molecular basis of alpha-1-antitrypsin deficiency. Am J Med 1988; 84(6A):13-31.
3. Guest PJ, Hansell DM. High resolution computed tomography (HRCT) in emphysema associated with alpha-1-antitrypsin deficiency. Clin Radiol 1992; 45(4):260-6.
4. Kueppers F, Black LF. Alpha1-antitrypsin and its deficiency. Am Rev Respir Dis 1974; 110(2):176-94.

Eosinphilic Granuloma

1. Brauner MW, Grenier P, Mouelhi MM, Mompoint D, Lenoir S. Pulmonary histiocytosis X: evaluation with high-resolution CT. Radiology 1989; 172(1):255-8.
2. Friedman PJ, Liebow AA, Sokoloff J. Eosinophilic granuloma of lung. Clinical aspects of primary histiocytosis in the adult. Medicine (Baltimore) 1981; 60(6):385-96.
3. Lacronique J, Roth C, Battesti JP, Basset F, Chretien J. Chest radiological features of pulmonary histiocytosis X: a report based on 50 adult cases. Thorax 1982; 37(2):104-9.
4. Moore AD, Godwin JD, Muller NL, Naidich DP, Hammar SP, Buschman DL, Takasugi JE, de Carvalho CR. Pulmonary histiocytosis X: comparison of radiographic and CT findings. Radiology 1989; 172(1):249-54.
5. Stern EJ, Webb WR, Golden JA, Gamsu G. Cystic lung disease associated with eosinophilic granuloma and tuberous sclerosis: air trapping at dynamic ultrafast high-resolution CT. Radiology 1992; 182(2):325-9.

Asthma

1. Backman KS, Greenberger PA, Patterson R. Airways obstruction in patients with long-term asthma consistent with 'irreversible asthma'. Chest 1997; 112(5):1234-40.
2. Brown RH, Herold CJ, Hirshman CA, Zerhouni EA, Mitzner W. In vivo measurements of airway reactivity using high-resolution computed tomography. Am Rev Respir Dis 1991; 144(1):208-12.
3. Haraguchi M, Shimura S, Shirato K. Morphometric analysis of bronchial cartilage in chronic obstructive pulmonary disease and bronchial asthma. Am J Respir Crit Care Med 1999; 159(3):1005-13.
4. Kinsella M, Muller NL, Staples C, Vedal S, Chan-Yeung M. Hyperinflation in asthma and emphysema. Assessment by pulmonary function testing and computed tomography. Chest 1988; 94(2):286-9.
5. Martin J, Powell E, Shore S, Emrich J, Engel LA. The role of respiratory muscles in the hyperinflation of bronchial asthma. Am Rev Respir Dis 1980; 121(3):441-7.
6. Paganin F, Trussard V, Seneterre E, Chanez P, Giron J, Godard P, Senac JP, Michel FB, Bousquet J. Chest radiography and high resolution computed tomography of the lungs in asthma. Am Rev Respir Dis 1992; 146(4):1084-7.

Allergic Bronchopulmonary Aspergillosis

1. Neeld DA, Goodman LR, Gurney JW, Greenberger PA, Fink JN. Computerized tomography in the evaluation of allergic bronchopulmonary aspergillosis. Am Rev Respir Dis 1990; 142(5):1200-5.

Lymphangioleiomyomatosis

1. Aberle DR, Hansell DM, Brown K, Tashkin DP. Lymphangiomyomatosis: CT, chest radiographic, and functional correlations. Radiology 1990; 176(2):381-7.
2. Chu SC, Horiba K, Usuki J, Avila NA, Chen CC, Travis WD, Ferrans VJ, Moss J. Comprehensive evaluation of 35 patients with lymphangioleiomyomatosis. Chest 1999; 115(4):1041-52.

3. Corrin B, Liebow AA, Friedman PJ. Pulmonary lymphangiomyomatosis. A review. Am J Pathol 1975; 79(2):348-82.
4. Lenoir S, Grenier P, Brauner MW, Frija J, Remy-Jardin M, Revel D, Cordier J. Pulmonary lymphangiomyomatosis and tuberous sclerosis: Comparison of radiographic and thin-section CT findings. Radiology 1990; 175:329-334.
5. Muller NL, Chiles C, Kullnig P. Pulmonary lymphangiomyomatosis: correlation of CT with radiographic and functional findings. Radiology 1990; 175(2):335-9.
6. Sullivan EJ. Lymphangioleiomyomatosis: a review. Chest 1998; 114(6):1689-703.

Inhalational Lung Disease (Asbestosis and Silicosis)

Jeffrey R. Galvin, MD
Chief Pulmonary and Mediastinal Radiology
Armed Forces Institute of Pathology
Clinical Professor Department of Radiology
University of Maryland

Figure 1-4-1

Pneumonokoniosis
- "It will then be necessary to embrace under a single title all essentially identical forms of disease
- ...the pneumonokoniosis (from Konis, dust) recommends itself"

Zenker 1866 Hematite Mining

Inorganic Dusts
- Silica
- Asbestos
- Coal
- Iron
- Beryllium

Pneumoconiosis
The accumulation of dust in the lungs and the tissue reaction to its presence
- Dust macules
- Diffuse interstitial fibrosis
- Diffuse alveolar damage
- Alveolar proteinosis
- Giant cell (GIP)
- Granulomatous inflammation

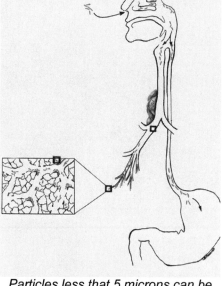

Particles less that 5 microns can be deposited beyond the conducting airways in the alveolar spaces.

Types and Sizes of Common Aerosols

Particle Deposition
Inertial impaction, sedimentation and diffusion [Figure 1-4-1]
- 10,000-20,000 liters/day
- Deposition related to particle size
- >10 microns deposit in nasopharynx and large airways (100%)
- 1-5 micron particles deposit in lung parenchyma (20%)

Figure 1-4-2

Airway Velocity
Inertial impaction, sedimentation and diffusion

Early Basal Deposition

Particle Clearance [Figure 1-4-2]
Cough, tracheobronchial and alveolar transport
- Most important
  - ➢ Deposition less critical
- Mucociliary escalator
  - ➢ Outer gel, inner liquid sol
- 90% of particles removed within 2 hrs
- Alveolar transport
  - ➢ Dissolution, engulfed by macrophages, removed to lymphatics

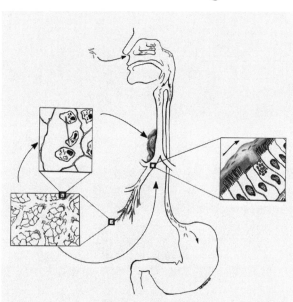

Macrophages remove small particles to regional lymph nodes.

Removal to Lymph Nodes

Physiologic Gradients-Airflow FRC [Figure 1-4-3]

Physiologic Gradients-Airflow TLC [Figure 1-4-4]

Figure 1-4-3   **Figure 1-4-4**

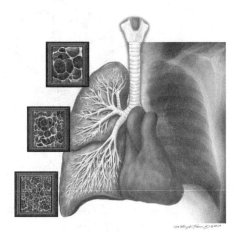

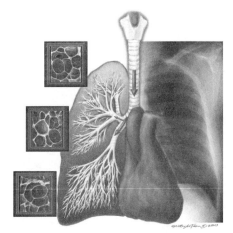

Alveoli in the bases are smaller than those in the apex.

The smaller alveoli in the bases enlarge to a greated degree than those in the apex. Therefore most airflow is directed towards the bases

Physiologic Gradients-Blood Flow [Figure 1-4-5]

Physiologic Gradients-Lymphatic Flow [Figure 1-4-6]

Figure 1-4-5   **Figure 1-4-6**

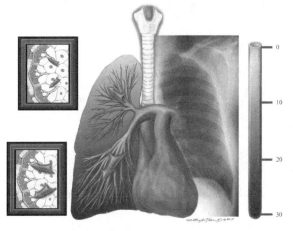

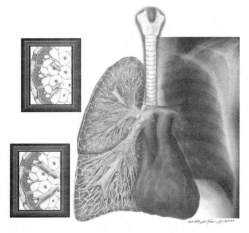

There is increased blood flow and hydrostatic pressure in the dependent vessels

The lymphatics are driven by hydrostatic pressure. Therefore lymphatic flow is best in the dependent lung.

Removal to Lymph Nodes [Figure 1-4-7]

Physiologic Gradients
Particle deposition and removal

- Lung bases
  - ➤ Increased ventilation
  - ➤ Increased perfusion
  - ➤ Increased lymphatic flow
- Basal deposition of particles
- Minimal apical clearance
- TB, histo, silica, sarcoid

Figure 1-4-7

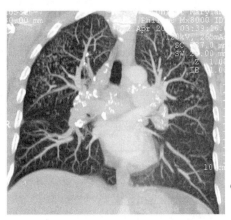

This explains the tendency for chronic diseases to be upper lobe

Edema

Tuberculosis

Silicosis
Mineralogy
- Silicon
  - ➤ Element
- Silica (SiO2)
  - ➤ Mineral
- Silicone
  - ➤ Synthetic polymer

Figure 1-4-8

Silicosis Adenopathy

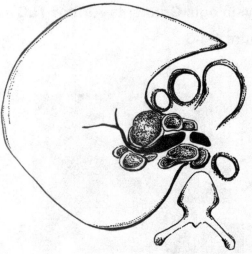

Adenopathy with peripheral calcification is a hallmark of silicosis

Figure 1-4-9

Silicosis Upper

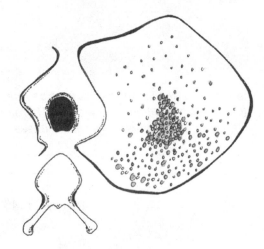

Nodules with an upper lobe predominance is typical

Figure 1-4-10

Silicoproteinosis

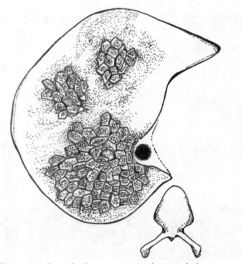

Silicoproteinosis is an acute lower lobe process

Figure 1-4-11

Tuberculosis

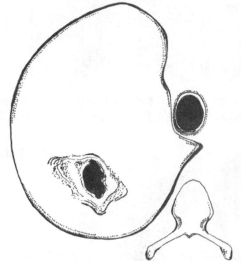

Silicosis predisoposes a patient to having active tuberculosis

Silicosis
Epidemiology
- Occupational exposure predominates
  - 3 million workers
- Mining, stonecutting, engraving and foundry work
- Males more commonly affected
- Degree of exposure underestimated
- Increased risk of neoplasia and scleroderma

Silicosis
Pathogenesis
- 5 million particles/cubic foot-lower threshold
- 100 million particles/cubic foot-100% affected
- > 5 micron particle removed in nares and upper airways
- 80% of particles removed in hours to days
- Retained particles consistently .5-.7 microns

Silicosis
Pathogenesis
- Macrophages and polys concentrate
- Macrophages generate oxygen-free radicals
- Macrophages generate fibrogenic proteins
- Immune related tissue damage
  - Rheumatoid factor, ANA and gamma globulin

Silicosis [Figures 1-4-8 to 1-4-11]
Clinical manifestations
- Diagnosis
  - Typical imaging pattern of adenopathy and nodules
  - Exposure to high concentration of silica
  - 10-20 years of exposure
- Simple silicosis
  - Asymptomatic
- Symptoms with PMF
- Intense exposure
  - Silicoproteinosis
- TB and cancer

Simple Silicosis
Pathology
- Collections of dust laden macrophages
  - Peribronchiolar
  - Interlobular septa
  - Pleural

Simple Silicosis
Pathology [Figure 1-4-12]
- Progress to mature nodules: 3 zones
  - Central dense fibrosis
  - Mid-zone concentric collagen
  - Peripheral dust laden cells

Simple Silicosis
Imaging manifestations [Figure 1-4-13]
- Adenopathy common
- Calcification 10-20%
- Calcification 5-10%
  - Eggshell pattern

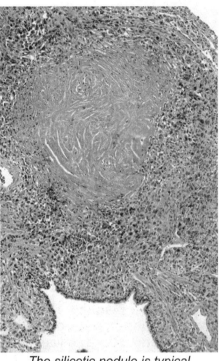

Figure 1-4-12

The silicotic nodule is typical response to inhaled silica

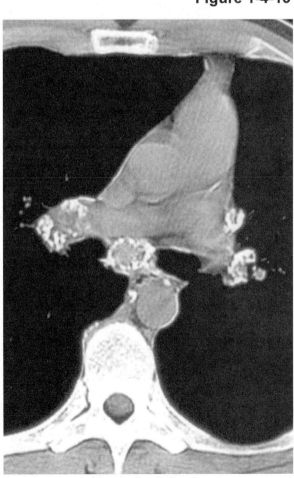

Figure 1-4-13

Eggshell calcification

Simple Silicosis
Imaging manifestations
- Well-circumscribed nodules
  - 1-10 mm
- Upper lobe and posterior
  - Lymphatic gradient
  - CT more sensitive
- Pleural lesions
  - Candle-wax or pseudoplaques

Progressive Massive Fibrosis
Pathology
- Conglomeration of nodular lesions
- Pathology definition
  - 2 cm
- Radiology definition
  - 1 cm
- Upper lung zones
  - Posterior

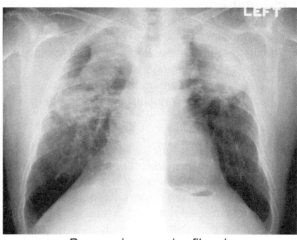

Figure 1-4-14

Progressive massive fibrosis

Progressive Massive Fibrosis
Imaging manifestations [Figure 1-4-14]
- Progression after exposure
- May fill entire upper lobe
  - Posterior
- Usually bilateral
- Carcinoma mimic
  - Solitary
  - Lower lobe
- Associated emphysema
  - Not always smoking related
  - Scar emphysema

Silicotic Alveolar Proteinosis
Pathology
- High concentration of particulate silica
- Acute onset
  - Weeks-months
- Alveoli filled with PAS+ material
- Similar to surfactant
- Type II cell hyperplasia

Silicosis and Tuberculosis [Figure 1-4-15]

Silicosis
Computed tomographic technique
- Thick sections of value in nodular diseases
  - Small nodules easier to differentiate from vessels
- Thin sections 1-2 mm collimation at 10 mm intervals or 3-5 selected images with prior thick section CT
- High spatial frequency algorithm
- Supine
- No contrast

Silica and Lung Disease
- Adenopathy
- Nodules
- PMF
- Silicoproteinosis
- Tuberculosis
- Cancer

Figure 1-4-15

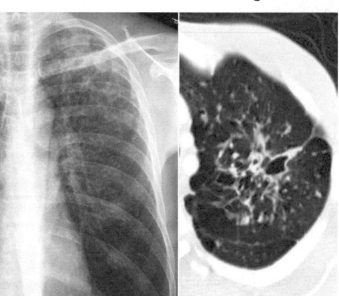

Tuberculosis in a patient with silicosis

Asbestos
Introduction
- Group of naturally occurring mineral fibers
  - Hydrated fibrous silicate
- Flexible and strong
- Corrosion, thermal and electrical resistance
- 500 tons - 3 million tons
  - 60 years
- 9 million people exposed
  - Primary (mining)
  - Secondary (industrial)
  - Nonoccupational (air)

Nonoccupational Exposure

Asbestos Bodies [Figures 1-4-16 and 1-4-17]
- Indicates exposure
- Transparent fiber core
- Iron and mucopolysaccharide coat
- Predominantly amphiboles
- Longer fibers are coated
  - < 20 microns not coated
  - Uncoated fibers are pathogenic
  - 7-5000 X's more uncoated fibers
- Fibers cannot be removed
- Lower posterior disease

Figure 1-4-16

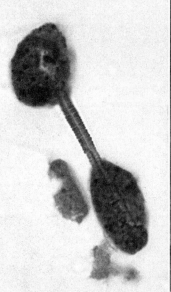

Asbestos bodies are commonly found in urban dwellers

Figure 1-4-17

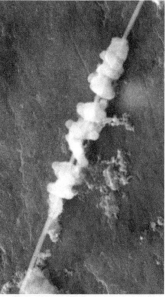

Asbestos fibers are much larger than macrophages and therefore cannot be removed to regional lymph nodes

Asbestos
Serpentine: chrysotile
- 95% of commercial use
- Curly and pliable
- Textile manufacture
- Fragments easily
- Chemically unstable
  - Dissolves easily
- Less pathogenic

Asbestos
Amphiboles: amosite, crocidolite, anthophilite, tremolite and actinolite
- 5% of commercial use
- Straight, broad fiber
- Do not fragment easily
- Long fibers (>20 microns)
  - Not cleared
- More likely coated
- Higher carcinogenic potential

Asbestos Related Chest Disease
[Figures 1-4-18 to 1-4-20]
- Pleural effusions
- Pleural plaques
- Round atelectsis
- Pleural thickening
  - Diffuse
- Mesothelioma
- Asbestosis
- Lung cancer

Figure 1-4-18

Pleural Effusion

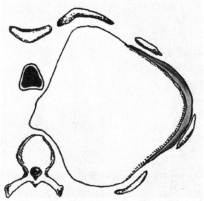

Pleural effusions are the most common early complication of asbestos exposure

Figure 1-4-19

Rounded Atelectasis

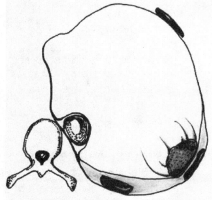

Rounded atelectasis is usually preceded by a pleural effusion

Asbestosis

Figure 1-4-20

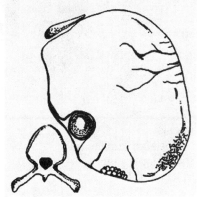

Asbestosis is a lower lobe subpleural process

Pleural Plaques
Pathology

- Common autopsy finding
  - ➢ (50-10%)
- Dense bands of collagen
  - ➢ "Basket weave"
- Asbestos bodies absent
- Uncoated fibers in dissolved lung tissue
- Dose response
  - ➢ Between parenchymal asbestos bodies and presence of plaques
- Pathogenesis uncertain

Pleural Plaques

- Postero-lateral parietal pleura
- Central Diaphragm
- Absent
  - ➢ Apices and costophrenic angles
- Almost always bilateral
- Sharply demarcated
- Millimeters to 10 cm
- May calcify extensively
- Highly suggestive of asbestos exposure

Roberts, AJCP 1971

Pleural Anatomy [Figure 1-4-21]

Pleural Plaques
Imaging

- Radiography insensitive
  - ➢ (8-40% of autopsy cases)
- Companion shadows
  - ➢ Fat and muscle
- HRCT
  - ➢ Best sensitivity and specificity

Pleural Fat

Pleural Plaques [Figure 1-4-22]

Diffuse Pleural Thickening

- Smooth pleural density
  - ➢ CXR: > 25% of the length of the chest wall
  - ➢ CT: 3 mm thick, 8 cm wide, 5 cm craniocaudal
- Posteromedial lower lobes
- Involves costophrenic angle
- Mediastinal pleural involvement
  - ➢ Rare
  - ➢ Suggests mesothelioma
- Visceral and parietal pleura
  - ➢ Adhesions
- Sequela of prior effusion?

Pleural Effusion
Definition

- History of exposure to asbestos
- Confirmation of effusion
  - ➢ Imaging of thoracentesis
- Absence of other disease related to effusion
- Absence of malignant tumor for 3 years

Epler, JAMA 1982

Figure 1-4-21

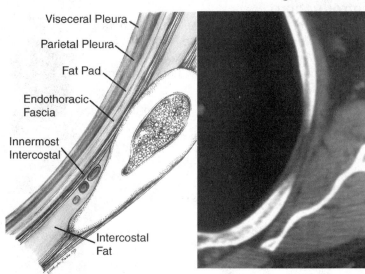

Visceral Pleura
Parietal Pleura
Fat Pad
Endothoracic Fascia
Innermost Intercostal
Intercostal Fat

The visceral pleural stripe is best seen between the ribs

Figure 1-4-22

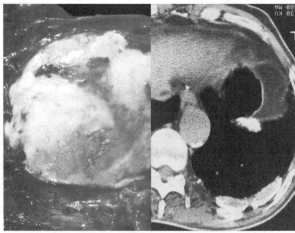

Visceral pleural plaques

Pleural Effusion
Clinical presentation
- Most common abnormality
  - First 20 yrs
- 3% prevalence
  - Asbestos exposed
- Small < 500 ml
- Serosanguinous
- Persist for weeks to 6 months
- 66% asymptomatic
- 28% recur

Pleural Effusion
Differential diagnosis
- Benign asbestos effusion
- Tuberculosis
- Mesothelioma
- Lung cancer

Round Atelectasis
- Described 1928 Loeschke
- Usually asymptomatic
- Folded lung vs inflammatory reaction
- Associated conditions
  - Asbestos exposure, CHF, infarct, TB and histoplasmosis
- Preceded by effusion

Round Atelectasis
Histology
- Irregular fibrous thickening of the visceral pleura
- Extensive pleural folding beneath the fibrosis
- Layers of invaginated pleura bound by fibrous adhesions
- Surrounding lung collapsed or fibrotic

Menzies, AJSP 1987

Round Atelectasis
Imaging criteria [Figure 1-4-23]
- Well-circumscribed
- Round or oval opacity
- "Comet tail" sign
- Pleural thickening
- Volume loss

Asbestosis
Pathologic definition
- Interstitial fibrosis
  - Associated with asbestos bodies
- Biopsy
  - Not the standard of practice

Asbestosis
- Dose-response relationship
- Probable exposure threshold
- Latency period inversely proportional to exposure level
- Latency is several decades
- Cigarette smoke may act synergistically

Figure 1-4-23

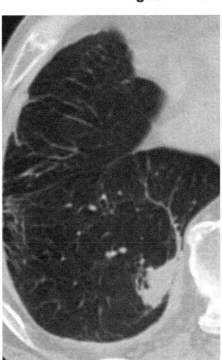

Round atelectasis

Asbestosis
ATS criteria 1986
- Reliable history of exposure
- Latency of at least 10 years
- Restrictive pulmonary functions
  - DLco and VC <80%
- Appropriate physical findings
  - Inspiratory crackles, clubbing
- Chest radiographic abnormalities
  - ILO perfusion > 1/0 (s, t or u)

Asbestosis
Histology
- Early
  - Fibrosis of respiratory bronchioles
- Progression
  - Terminal bronchioles, alveolar ducts and alveolar septa
- Minimum 2 asbestos bodies in area of fibrosis

Craighead, Arch Pathol Lab Med, 1982

Asbestosis
Chest radiography
- Lower lobe
  - Irregular opacities
  - Nonspecific
  - Associated pleural disease
- Large inter-observer variation
  - Low perfusion
- Normal in 26% of path proven cases

Asbestosis and Cigarette Smoking
Small irregular opacities
- Small opacities are related to
  - Dust exposure, cigarette smoke, age, radiographic technique and obesity
- Cigarette smoke causes
  - Interstitial fibrosis
  - Emphysema
  - Bronchiolar thickening
- Asbestos causes
  - Interstitial fibrosis
- Asbestos workers who smoke
  - Have more opacities
  - Related to dust exposure and cigarettes

Asbestosis
High-resolution CT
- Lower lobe and posterior
  - Reticulonodular opacities
  - Parenchymal bands
  - Curvilinear subpleural line
  - Interstitial short lines
  - Honeycombing
- High sensitivity
- Nonspecific
- Specificity increases with # of abnormalities
- Prone imaging is key!

Parenchymal Bands [Figure 1-4-24]

Figure 1-4-24

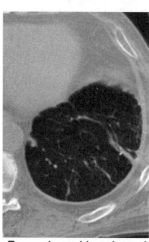

Parenchymal bands and round atelectasis in a patient with asbestosis

Reticulonodular Opacites

Curvilinear Subpleural Line

Short Lines

Honeycombing

Asbestosis vs UIP
- Asbestos exposure in the last 30 years is low
- Clinical asbestosis requires substantial exposure
- Asbestos exposed individuals can have other interstitial lung diseases
- Band like opacities merging with the pleura are rare in UIP
- Upper zone fibrosis and ground glass are rare in asbestosis

Gaensler, ARRD, 1991 – Al-Jarad, Thorax, 1992

Asbestosis
High-resolution CT
- Short lines and parenchymal bands are statistically most significant
- Strong association with diffuse pleural disease
- Multifocal
- HRCT finds asbestosis in exposed individuals with normal radiographs and PFT's
- Obstructive PFT's correlate with emphysema

Aberle, AJR, 1988 – Aberle, Radiology, 1988 – Staples, ARRD, 1989

Asbestosis
Dependent density
- Posterior blood flow
  - 5X's greater
- Posterior alveoli
  - Smaller or collapsed
  - Less steep ventilatory gradient
  - Closing volumes
    (10-40% of VC)

Asbestosis
Computed tomographic technique
- 1.5-2 mm collimation
- 10 mm interval
- High spatial frequency algorithm
- Prone
- Thick section supine: CA screen?

Asbestos Related Chest Disease

Asbestosis

Silicosis

Particle Deposition and Clearance
Cough, tracheobronchial and alveolar transport

Pulmonary Lymphoid Disorders

Jeffrey R. Galvin, MD
Chief, Pulmonary and Mediastinal Radiology
Armed Forces Institute of Pathology
and
Clinical Professor Department of Radiology
University of Maryland

The Pulmonary Lymphoid System
- Lymphatics
- Lymph nodes
- BALT
  - ➤ Bronchus Associated Lymphoid Tissue
- Lymphoid aggregates
- Lymphocytes
- Dendritic cells
- Langerhans cells

The Pulmonary Lymphoid System
[Figures 1-5-1 and 1-5-2]
- Lymphatics
  - ➤ Originate in the pleura
  - ➤ Valves
  - ➤ Drain towards hilum
  - ➤ Follow interlobular septa
  - ➤ Accompany blood vessels
- Lymph Nodes
- BALT
- Lymphoid aggregates
- Lymphocytes
- Dendritic cells
- Langerhans cells

The Pulmonary Lymphoid System
[Figures 1-5-3 and 1-5-4]
- Lymphatics
- Lymph Nodes
  - ➤ Encapsulated lymph nodes
    - ✧ Proximal bronchi
    - ✧ Bifurcations
  - ➤ Reactive lymph nodes
    - ✧ Peripheral and septal
    - ✧ Cigarettes or dust
- BALT
- Lymphoid aggregates
- Lymphocytes
- Dendritic cells
- Langerhans cells

Figure 1-5-1

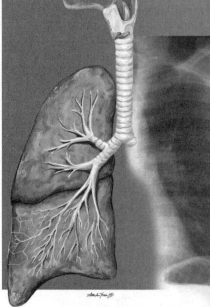

One set of lymphatics enter the lung and follow the interloblular septa in the periphery of the lung

Figure 1-5-2

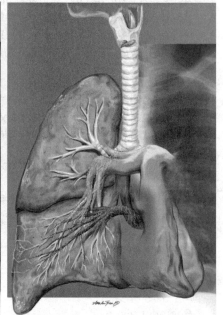

These lymphatic channels continue along the pulmonary veins to the hilum. A second set of lymphatics originates near the center of the secondary lobule and follows the pulmonary arteries

Figure 1-5-3

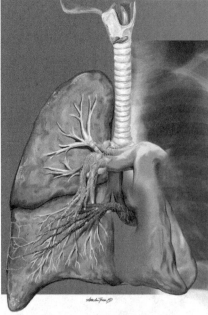

Classic encapsulated intrapulmonary lymph nodes are found at the bifurcations of the first 3-4 orders of bronchi and are demonstrated adhering to the right main pulmonary

Figure 1-5-4

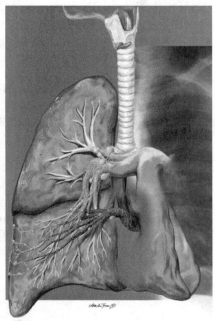

The majority of intrapulmonary lymph nodes are probably not visible radiographically. Almost all of these lymph nodes are subpleural and inferior to the carina

Reactive Lymph Nodes

The Pulmonary Lymphoid System
- Lymphatics
- Lymph nodes
- BALT
  - Bronchus Associated Lymphoid Tissue
- Lymphoid aggregates
- Lymphocytes
- Dendritic cells
- Langerhans cells

BALT – The organizing principle [Figure 1-5-5]
- Lymphoid Collections
  - Bronchial epithelium
  - Bifurcations
- Absent in the normal adult
  - Absent at birth
  - Common in young children
- Reappears with antigenic stimulation
  - Cigarette smoke
  - Connective tissue disease
  - AIDS
- Basis of pulmonary lymphoid disorders

Pulmonary Lymphoid Disorders – Derivations of BALT
- Hyperplasias of BALT
  - Follicular Hyperplasia
    - ✧ Follicular Bronchitis
  - Diffuse Hyperplasia
    - ✧ Lymphoid Interstitial Pneumonia
  - Nodular Lymphoid Hyperplasia
    - ✧ Pseudolymphoma
- Non-Hodgkin's Lymphomas
  - Low-Grade B Cell Lymphomas
  - Lymphomatoid Granulomatois
- Immune Impairment
  - PTLD, AIDS and other

Koss, Sem Diag Pathol 1995

Follicular Hyperplasias of BALT – Hyperplasia of BALT
[Figure 1-5-6]
- Follicular Bronchitis and Bronchiolitis
- Pathologic Features
  - Antigenic stimulation of BALT
  - Lymphoid aggregates
  - Peribronchial
  - Reactive follicles
  - Minimal alveolar extension
- Clinical

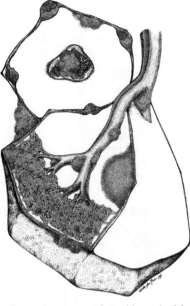

Figure 1-5-5

Bronchus associated lymphoid tissue or BALT is found along the bronchiole, interlobular septa and pleura. It is normally found only in young children.

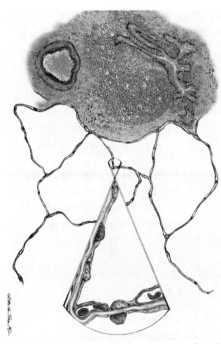

Figure 1-5-6

Follicular bronchitis is characterized by hyperplastic lymphoid follicles with reactive germinal centers distributed along bronchioles and to a lesser extent bronchi.

Follicular Hyperplasias of BALT – Hyperplasia of BALT

- Pathologic features
- Clinical
  - ➢ Young adults (44 yrs.)
  - ➢ Cough and dyspnea
    - ✧ Fever and weight loss
  - ➢ Immune deficiencies
    - ✧ AIDS
    - ✧ Congenital
  - ➢ Collagen vascular diseases
    - ✧ Sjogren's
    - ✧ Rheumatoid arthritis
  - ➢ Uncertain Etiology
    - ✧ Hypersensitivity reactions?

Figure 1-5-7

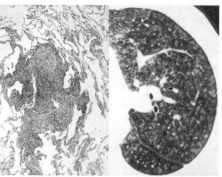

Almost all patients with follicular bronchitis have centrilobular nodes that are less than 3mm. These nodules correlate with the peribrochiolar distirbution of hyperplastic lymphoid follicles shown on the histology section to your left

Follicular Hyperplasias of BALT – Hyperplasia of BALT: Imaging

[Figure 1-5-7]

- Radiography
  - ➢ Diffuse
  - ➢ Reticulonodular
- CT
  - ➢ Nodules 3-12 mm
    - ✧ Centrilobular
    - ✧ Peribronchial
  - ➢ Ground Glass
  - ➢ Air Trapping

Figure 1-5-8

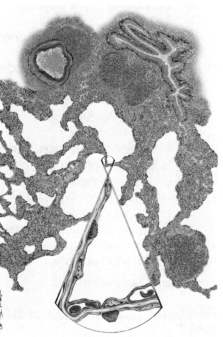

LIP is characterized by diffuse infiltration of the alveolar septa

Follicular Hyperplasia – Differential Diagnosis

- Cystic Fibrosis
- Panbronchiolitis
- Sarcoidosis
- Respiratory Bronchiolitis
- Extrinsic Allergic Alveolitis

Diffuse Hyperplasias of BALT – Hyperplasia of BALT

[Figure 1-5-8]

- Lymphocytic Interstitial Pneumonia
- Pathologic Features
  - ➢ Alveolar septal infiltration
    - ✧ Lymphocytes (T-cells)
    - ✧ Diffuse
  - ➢ Lymphoid follicles (B-cells)
    - ✧ Germinal centers
    - ✧ Peribronchial distribution
    - ✧ Spectrum with follicular hyperplasia of BALT (Follicular Bronchitis)
- Clinical

Diffuse Hyperplasias of BALT – LIP- Hyperplasia of BALT

- Pathologic features
- Clinical
  - ➢ Women>men
  - ➢ 4th-6th decade
  - ➢ Cough and dyspnea
  - ➢ Collagen vascular disease
    - ✧ Sjogrens, RA, and SLE
  - ➢ Bone marrow transplantation
  - ➢ AIDS rare in adults
    - ✧ Common in children
  - ➢ Dysproteinemia
  - ➢ Restrictive lung functions

Diffuse Hyperplasia of BALT – Hyperplasia of BALT: Imaging   Figure 1-5-9

[Figures 1-5-9 and 1-5-10]

- Radiography
  - ➤ Lower lung zone
  - ➤ Reticulonodular
- CT
  - ➤ Ground Glass
  - ➤ Nodules
    - ✧ Centrilobular
    - ✧ Poorly defined
  - ➤ Cystic air spaces
  - ➤ Thickened BVB's
  - ➤ Adenopathy

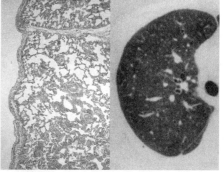

The lung windows demonstrate diffuse hazy ground glass that correlates with diffuse alveolar wall thickening. The alveolar wall thickening is primarily the result of lymphoid infiltation

LIP vs Lymphoma

	LIP	Lymphoma
Cysts	82%	2%
Consolidation	18%	66%
Large Nodules	6%	41%
Effusions	0%	25%

Nodular Lymphoid Hyperplasia – Hyperplasia of BALT   Figure 1-5-10

[Figure 1-5-11]

- Pseudolymphoma
- Pathologic Features
  - ➤ Solitary, subpleural mass
  - ➤ Lymphoid proliferation
    - ✧ Interstitial
    - ✧ Perivascular
    - ✧ B and T cells
    - ✧ Polyclonal pattern
      - – Benign
  - ➤ Reactive germinal centers
  - ➤ Difficult to separate from lymphoma
- Clinical

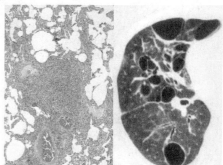

Thin walled cysts are often found deep within the lung parenchyma. Previous reports have suggested that airway narrowing or obliteration results in these cystic lesions. The histology on the left demonstrates complete obliteration of the bronchiole by lymphoid infiltration. The accompanying arteriole is identified by its typical wall.

Nodular Lymphoid Hyperplasia – Hyperplasia of BALT

- Pseudolymphoma
- Pathologic features
- Clinical
  - ➤ Rare entity
  - ➤ Most cases were lymphomas
    - ✧ Monoclonal B cell proliferation
  - ➤ Middle age
    - ✧ Asymptomatic
  - ➤ Autoimmune Diseases 15%
    - ✧ Sjorgren
    - ✧ SLE
    - ✧ Transverse myelitis
  - ➤ Surgical excision curative

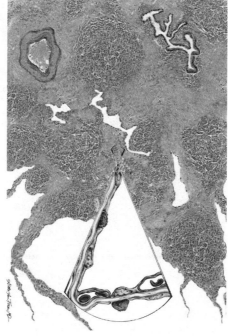

Figure 1-5-11

Nodular lymphoid hyperplasia or pseudolymphoma presents as a solitary subpleural mass of lymphoid tissue with numerous reactive germinal centers

Nodular Lymphoid Hyperplasia
Hyperplasia of BALT: Imaging

[Figures 1-5-12 and 1-5-13]
- Radiography
  - ➢ Solitary Nodule
  - ➢ Focal Consolidation
- CT
  - ➢ Air bronchograms
    - ✧ 100%
  - ➢ Indistinct margins
  - ➢ Occasionally multiple
  - ➢ Adenopathy and/or effusion suggests lymphoma

Pulmonary Lymphoid Disorders
Derivations of BALT
- Hyperplasias of BALT
- Non-Hodgkin's Lymphomas
  - ➢ Low-Grade B Cell Lymphomas
  - ➢ Lymphomatoid Granulomatosis
- Immune Impairment

Low-Grade B-Cell Lymphoma
- Pathologic Features
  - ➢ Lymphocytic infiltration
  - ➢ Small lymphocytes
    - ✧ Alveolar wall
    - ✧ Peribronchiolar
    - ✧ Perivascular
  - ➢ Immunologic evidence of malignancy
    - ✧ Monoclonality
    - ✧ B-cell markers CD20
  - ➢ Germinal Centers

Low-Grade B-Cell Lymphoma
- Clinical
  - ➢ Similar presentation to nodular lymphoid hyperplasia
  - ➢ 5th-6th decade
  - ➢ Male=Female
  - ➢ Asymptomatic 50%
  - ➢ 5 year survival 85-95%
  - ➢ Surgical resection
    - ✧ Rare recurrence

Low-Grade B-Cell Lymphoma
[Figure 1-5-14
- Imaging
  - ➢ Radiography
    - ✧ Solitary nodule/mass
      - – Multiple
    - ✧ Consolidation
    - ✧ Air Bronchogram
      - – 50%
    - ✧ Slow Growth
  - ➢ CT
    - ✧ Consolidation
    - ✧ Air Bronchograms
    - ✧ Airway narrowing or "stretching"

Figure 1-5-12

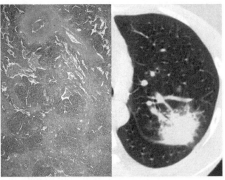

The CT demonstrates the typical sub-pleural, solitary lesion with indistinct margins. The bulk of the lesion consists of a mass of lymphoid tissue with multiple reactive germinal centers.

Figure 1-5-13

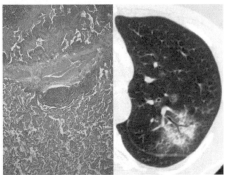

Air bronchograms are universally present and the lymphoid infiltration gradually diminishes resulting in the classical indistinct margin

Figure 1-5-14

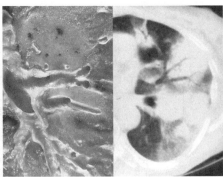

Grossly low grade B-cell lymphoma usually presents as a single white tan lesion that can be either well circumscribed or indistinct. This is well demonstrated by the gross specimen on the left from the AFIP archive. The disease can, however, be multifocal as shown on the right and has been reported as a primarily endobronchial lesion.

Primary Tracheal Lymphoma
- Extremely rare
- BALT derivative
- Extensive at diagnosis
- Potentially curable

Lymphomatoid Granulomatosis
[Figure 1-5-15]
- Pathologic Features
  - ➢ Majority of cases are B-cell lymphomas
  - ➢ Reactive small T-cells
  - ➢ Malignant B Cells
    - ✧ Majority of infiltrate
  - ➢ Epstein-Barr Virus
  - ➢ Angiocentric infiltration
  - ➢ Necrosis
    - ✧ Peribronchovascular
    - ✧ Peripheral

Lymphomatoid Granulomatosis
- Clinical
  - ➢ 7-85 years (mean 48 yrs)
  - ➢ Male:Female (2:1)
  - ➢ Malaise and weight loss
  - ➢ Lung involvement 100%
  - ➢ Cough and dyspnea
  - ➢ Skin 39-53%
    - ✧ Nodules, ulcers and rash
  - ➢ CNS 37-53%
  - ➢ Renal 32-40%
  - ➢ High mortality rate 53-90%
  - ➢ Most proceed to lymphoma

Lymphomatoid Granulomatosis
- Imaging
  - ➢ Nodules 80%
    - ✧ Multiple
    - ✧ Bilateral (80%)
  - ➢ Mid and lower lobes
  - ➢ Cavitation 20%
  - ➢ Large masses
    - ✧ Correspond to infarcts
  - ➢ Diffuse reticulonodular opacities
  - ➢ Hilar adenopathy 25%

LYG *[Figure 1-5-16]*

Pulmonary Lymphoid Disorders – Derivations of BALT
- Hyperplasias of BALT
- Non-Hodgkin's Lymphomas
- Immune Impairment
  - ➢ Posttransplantation Lymphoproliferative Disease (PTLD)
  - ➢ AIDS
  - ➢ Other forms of prolonged immune suppression

Figure 1-5-15

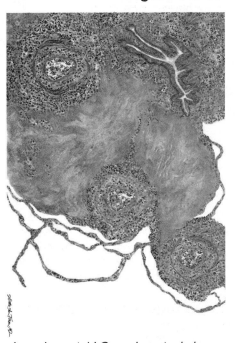

Lymphomatoid Granulomatosis is an angiocentric B-cell lymphoma which often demonstrates areas of necrosis.

Figure 1-5-16

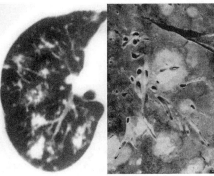

Chest CT on the left demonstrates a bronchovascular distribution of nodules that are shown to be areas of infarction on gross examination.

Lymphoma and Immune Impairment [Figure 1-5-17]

- Pathologic Features
  - B-cell non-Hodgkin's lymphoma
    - Driven by Epstein-Barr Virus infection
    - Diffuse polyclonal expansion
      - Reduced T-cell control
    - Malignant transformation

Lymphoma and Immune Impairment

- Clinical
  - Spectrum of benign to malignant
    - Infectious mono-like
    - PTLD polymorphic
    - PTLD monomorphic
  - Cyclosporin shortens induction (<1 year)
  - May respond to reduction in immunosuppression, anti-virals and surgery
  - Chemotherapy should be avoided
  - Heart-Lung up 20%

Lymphoma and Immune Impairment

- Imaging
  - Nodules
    - May cavitate
    - Halo
    - Along bronchovascular bundles
  - Lymph node
  - Ground glass
  - Septa thickening
  - Consolidation
  - Effusion

PTLD

[Figure 1-15-18]

Bone Marrow Transplant

Prolonged Chemotherapy

Pulmonary Lymphoid Disorders Derivations of BALT

- Hyperplasias of BALT
- Non-Hodgkin Lymphomas
- Immune Impairment
  - PTLD
  - AIDS
  - Other

Figure 1-5-17

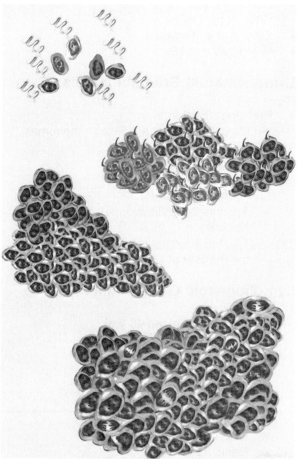

Post transplant lymphomas are driven by Epstein-Barr virus, reduced T-cell surveillance and malignant transformation. Genetic mutation may eventually result in malignant transformation of one of these clones, represented in purple.

Figure 1-5-18

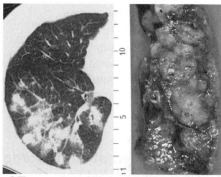

CT reveals multiple multiple indistinct nodules in a characteristic distribution along the bronchovascular bundles

Follicular Hyperplasia [Figure 1-5-19]

Diffuse Hyperplasia of BALT-LIP [Figure 1-5-20]

Nodular Lymphoid Hyperplasia [Figure 1-5-21]

Low-Grade B-Cell Lymphoma [Figure 1-5-22]

LYG [Figure 1-5-23]

Figure 1-5-19

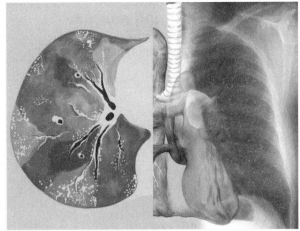

Follicular Bronchitis.

Figure 1-5-20

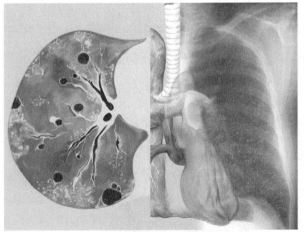

Lymphocytic Interstitial Pneumonia (LIP).

Figure 1-5-21

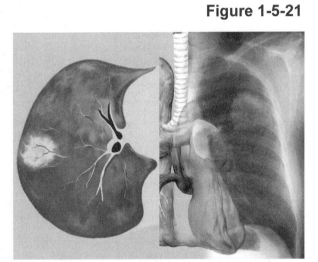

Nodular Lymphoid Hyperplasia which was formerly known as Pseudolymphoma.

Figure 1-5-22

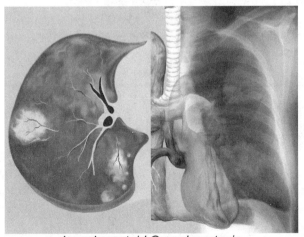

Lymphomatoid Granulomatosis

Figure 1-5-23

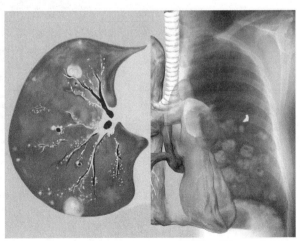

Low grade B-cell Lymphoma

Figure 1-5-24

BALT - The organizing principle
- Lymphoid collections
- Basis of pulmonary lymphoid disorders

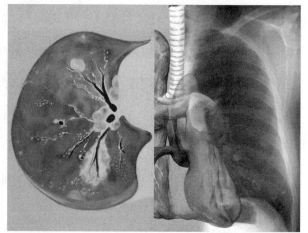

Post Transplant Lymphoproliferative Disorder

Angiitis and Granulomatosis

Jeffrey R. Galvin, MD
Chief, Pulmonary and Mediastinal Radiology
Armed Forces Institute of Pathology
and
Clinical Professor Department of Radiology
University of Maryland

Angiitis and Granulomatosis
- First characterized by Averill Liebow 1973
- Unknown etiology
- Angiitis
  - ➢ Cellular infiltration of blood vessel
- Granulomatosis
  - ➢ Necrosis of lung parenchyma not related to blood vessel occlusion

Angiitis and Granulomatosis: Current List
- Wegener's granulomatosis
- Churg-Strauss syndrome
  - ➢ Allergic granulomatosis
- Necrotizing sarcoid granulomatosis
- Bronchocentric granulomatosis
- Lymphomatoid granulomatosis

Angiitis and Granulomatosis: General Concepts
- Etiology remains unknown
- Inflammatory vs. lymphoproliferative
- Clinical and laboratory findings key to Dx
- Adequate tissue samples are important
- Must R/O infection: mycobacterial or fungal

Pathogenesis of Vasculitis

Wegener's Granulomatosis – Classic Pathology Triad
- Vasculitis described 1852
  - ➢ Von Rokitansky
- Wegener described 1936
  - ➢ Wegener's
- Focal vasculitis of
  - ➢ arteries and veins
- Necrotising granulomas
  - ➢ Upper and lower airways
- Necrotising glomerulitis
  - ➢ Focal

Wegener's Granulomatosis – Gross Pathology
[Figure 1-6-1 and 1-6-2]
- Necrotic nodules
  - ➢ With and without cavitation
- Parenchymal consolidation
- Massive hemorrhage
- Airway narrowing

Figure 1-6-1

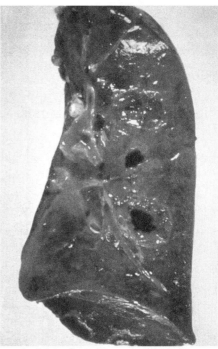

Solid and cavitary nodules often coexist in patients with Wegener's granulomatosis

Figure 1-6-2

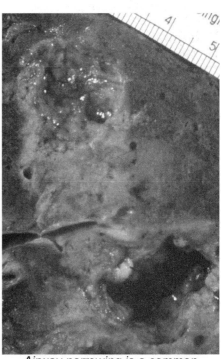

Airway narrowing is a common complication

Wegener's Granulomatosis – Demographics
- Rare
  - 3/100,000 in US
- 2nd-8th decades of life
- Average age-50 years
- Male=Female
  - Slight male predominance (4:3)
- May occur in children

Wegener's Granulomatosis – Limited
- Involvement of lungs alone
- Clinical sparing
  - Kidneys
  - Upper respiratory tract
- Biopsy positive
  - When clinically normal
- Better prognosis

Wegener's Granulomatosis – Clinical Presentation
- Classic triad
  - Sinusitis
  - Pulmonary symptoms
  - Renal insufficiency
- Variable onset and course
- Chronic URI symptoms
  - May persist for years before pulmonary disease
- Overwhelming vasculitis
  - Diffuse

Upper Airway
- Chronic nasal obstruction
  - Chronic discharge
- Destruction of cartilaginous nasal septum
- "Saddle nose deformity"
- Laryngeal involvement
  - Subglottic stricture
- Eustachian tube obstruction
- Otitis media
- Cochlear nerve vasculitis

Pulmonary
- Most commonly affected (94%)
- Multiple bilateral nodules or masses
- Cavitation common (30-50%)
- Occasionally solitary mass or nodule
  - Dx difficult
  - All patients progress
- Less common
  - Diffuse alveolar hemorrhage
- Pleural lesion and effusions are rare

Renal
- Tempo: insidious to explosive
- Segmental necrotizing glomerulonephritis
- UA: erythrocyte casts and proteinuria
- Large vessel vasculitis

Wegener's Granulomatosis: Other Organ Involvement

- Skin (50%)
  - ➢ Symmetric papulonecrotic lesion of extremities
- Eye and orbit (30%)
  - ➢ Scleritis, conjunctivitis, optic nerve and retro-orbital mass
- Nervous system (30%)
  - ➢ Mononeuritis multiplex
- Joints
  - ➢ Acute arthritis follows activity of disease (+RA latex)

Wegener's Granulomatosis: Airway Involvement
[Figure 1-6-3]

- Endobronchial abnormalities
  - ➢ 59% bronchoscopy
- Subglottic stenosis
- Tracheobronchitis
  - ➢ Ulcerating
- Tracheal or bronchial stenosis
- Often multifocal
  - ➢ Variable length of involvement
- CT key for evaluation
  - ➢ CXR often normal

Wegener's Granulomatosis: Radiography

- Earliest lesions
  - ➢ Bilateral reticulo-nodular opacities
- Multifocal nodules
  - ➢ Bilateral
  - ➢ 5mm-10cm
- Sharply marginated
- Cavitation 20-50%
- Evolution
  - ➢ Thick walls to thin walled cysts with treatment
- Airspace consolidation

Changing Presentation

Necrosis and Hemorrhage *[Figure 1-6-4]*

Figure 1-6-3

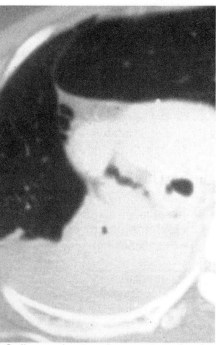

Collapse due to airway narrowing in Wegener's

Figure 1-6-4

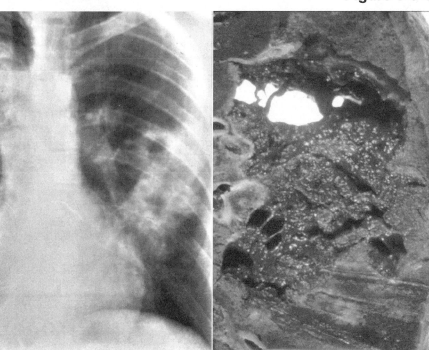

Massive necrosis and hemorrhage in Wegener's

Evolution with Treatment [Figure 1-6-5]

Wegener's Granulomatosis: Computed Tomography [Figure 1-6-6]

- Feeding vessels
  - ➢ 88%
- Cavitation
  - ➢ Nodules greater than 2cm
- Subpleural location
  - ➢ Predominant
- CT "halo sign"
- Pleural based lesions
  - ➢ Mimic infarcts
- Reveals more nodules

Diffuse Pulmonary Hemorrhage: Capillaritis
[Figure 1-6-7]

- Common
  - ➢ Microscopic polyangiitis
  - ➢ Wegener's granulomatosis
  - ➢ SLE
- Uncommon
  - ➢ Goodpastures
    - ✧ Anti-GBM
  - ➢ Collagen vascular
  - ➢ Idiopathic pulmonary hemorrhage
  - ➢ Churg Strauss syndrome
  - ➢ Behcet's syndrome
  - ➢ IgA Nephropathy

Figure 1-6-5

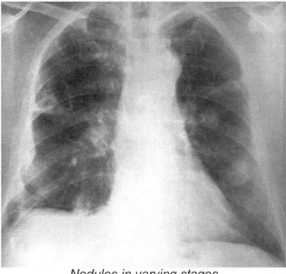

Nodules in varying stages

Figure 1-6-6

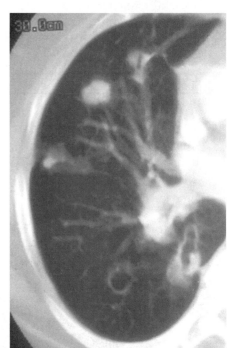

Nodules with feeding vessels are common in vasculitis

Figure 1-6-7

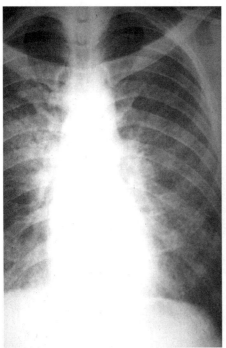

Pulmonary hemorrhage in capillaritis

Microscopic Polyangiitis

[Figure 1-6-8]
- Microscopic polyarteritis nodosa
- Most common cause of pulmonary-renal syndrome
- 5th decade
- Male > Female
- Renal, muskuloskeletal, pulmonary, GI and cutaneous

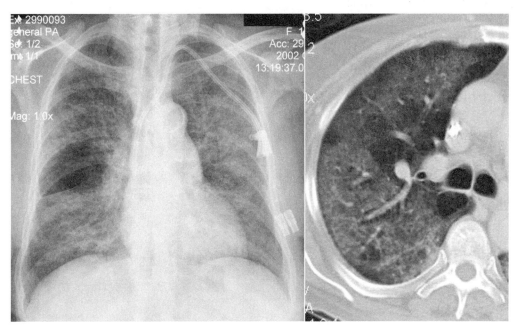

Figure 1-6-8

Microscopic polyangiitis

Wegener's Granulomatosis: Laboratory
- ANCA
  - Serum Antineutrophil Cytoplasmic Autoantibody
- c-ANCA cytoplasmic pattern
  - Proteinase 3
  - 99% specificity and 96% sensitivity in active disease
  - Positivity drops to 30% in remission
- p-ANCA perinuclear pattern
  - Reacts with myeloperoxidase
  - positive in collagen vascular diseases

Wegener's Granulomatosis: Treatment and Prognosis
- Universally fatal without treatment
- Trimethoprim/Sulfa effective in localized disease
- Steroids and cyclophosphamide
  - Remission in 93%
- 5 year survival 90-95%
- Infectious complications
  - Relapse and drug toxicity require close monitoring and follow-up imaging
- Relapse has different manifestations from presentation

Churg-Strauss Syndrome: Allergic Angiitis and Granulomatosis
- Described by Churg and Strauss
  - 1951
- True systemic vasculitis
- Associated
  - Asthma
  - Allergic rhinitis
  - Blood eosinophilia
- Hypersensitivity response to inhaled antigen?

Churg-Strauss Syndrome: Pathology
- Necrotizing vasculitis
- Eosinophilic tissue infiltration
- "Allergic granulomas"
  - ➢ Extravascular
  - ➢ Eosinophils
  - ➢ Multinucleated giant cells

Churg-Strauss Syndrome: Demographics
- 2nd-4th decades
- 28 years mean age of onset
- Male=Female
- Excellent response to steroids

Churg-Strauss Syndrome: Background
- Late onset asthma
  - ➢ 100%
- Precedes CSS by weeks to years (30)
- Severe rhinitis and sinusitis
  - ➢ 70%

Churg-Strauss Syndrome: Prodromal Stage
- Infiltration of tissues with eosinophils
- Blood eosinophilia
- Elevated IgE
- + rheumatoid factor
- Progressive asthma, sinus pain, myocardial involvement
- Loffler's like fleeting infiltrates
- Abdominal pain
  - ➢ Diarrhea and eosinophilic peritonitis
- Myalgias and neuritis

Churg-Strauss Syndrome: Vasculitic Stage
- Increasingly severe and widespread symptoms
- Lung
  - ➢ Eosinophilic consolidation, miliary to 2 cm nodules (without cavitation), and diffuse hemorrhage
- Cardiac
  - ➢ Coronary vasculitis and eosinophilic myocarditis (50% of mortality)
- GI
  - ➢ Ulcerations, perforations and peritonitis

Churg-Strauss Syndrome: Computed Tomography
- Parenchymal opacification
  - ➢ Predominantly peripheral 59%
  - ➢ Effusions
- Nodules
  - ➢ 12%
- Bronchial thickening
- Dilatation
  - ➢ 12%
- Interlobular septal thickening
  - ➢ 6%

Worthy et. Al. AJR Feb. 1998

Churg-Strauss Syndrome: Comparison with Wegener's
- CSS
  - ➢ High incidence of asthma
  - ➢ High incidence of cardiac involvement (47%)
  - ➢ Less severe renal and sinus disease
  - ➢ Associated with P-ANCA

Churg-Strauss Syndrome: Therapy and Prognosis
- Prognosis relates to early diagnosis and therapy
- High dose steroids usually effective
- Cyclophosphamide in resistant cases
- Therapy stopped after 6-12 months of remission

Necrotizing Sarcoid Granulomatosis
How is this related to sarcoidosis?
- A distinct entity?
  - ➢ Katzenstein
- Some reported cases are undiagnosed infections
- Those with extrapulmonary involvement
  - ➢ Sarcoidosis

Necrotizing Sarcoid Granulomatosis: Demographics
- 3rd to 7th decades
- Mean age 49 years
- Female:male
  - ➢ 2.2:1

Necrotizing Sarcoid Granulomatosis: Pathology
- Non-caseating granulomas
  - ➢ Similar to sarcoidosis
- Vasculitis
  - ➢ Pulmonary arteries
  - ➢ Pulmonary veins
  - ➢ Found in areas away from parenchymal granulomas
- Coagulative Necrosis
  - ➢ Widespread
  - ➢ Main distinction from sarcoidosis

Necrotizing Sarcoid Granulomatosis: Clinical Presentation
- 100% lung involvement
- Cough most common symptom
- Chest pain, fever and dyspnea
- Weight loss and fatigue
- May be asymptomatic
  - ➢ 15-40%
- Rare extrapulmonary involvement
  - ➢ 13%
- Aspergillus antigens in some patients

Koss et al, Human Pathology 1980

Necrotizing Sarcoid Granulomatosis: Imaging
[Figure 1-6-9]
- Hilar adenopathy
  - ➢ Variable
  - ➢ Up to 79%
- Nodules
  - ➢ Cavitation is common
  - ➢ Subpleural
  - ➢ Perivascular
- Parenchymal opacities
  - ➢ Same distribution

Necrotizing Sarcoid Granulomatosis: Prognosis and Therapy
- May require no therapy
- Prompt response to steroids
- No reported deaths

Figure 1-6-9

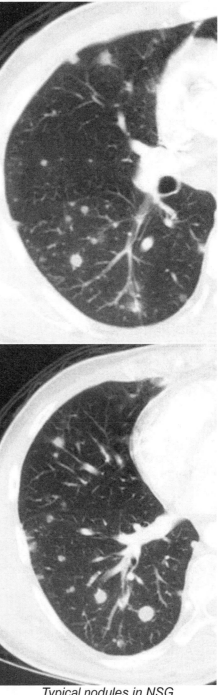

Typical nodules in NSG

Lymphomatoid Granulomatosis: Etiology and Demographics
- Majority of cases are B-cell lymphomas
- Epstein-Barr Virus
- Reactive small T-cells
  - Majority of infiltrate
- Malignant B Cells
- Age range
  - 7-85 years
- Mean age of onset
  - 48 years
- Male:Female (2:1)

Lymphomatoid Granulomatosis: Pathology
- Angiocentric infiltration
  - Mixed cell population
    - Atypical lymphocytes, plasma cells, histiocytes
- Vascular invasion
- Vascular destruction
- Necrosis
  - Peribronchovascular
  - Peripheral

Lymphomatoid Granulomatosis: Clinical Presentation
- Lung involvement
  - 100%
  - Cough and dyspnea
- Skin
  - 39-53%
  - Nodules, ulcers and rash
- CNS
  - 37-53%
- Renal
  - 32-40%
- Malaise and weight loss
  - 35%

Lymphomatoid Granulomatosis: Imaging
[Figure 1-6-10]
- Nodules
  - 80%
  - Multiple
  - Bilateral (80%)
- Mid and lower lobes
- Cavitation
  - 20%
- Large masses
  - Correspond to infarcts
- Diffuse reticulonodular opacities
- Hilar adenopathy
  - 25%

Figure 1-6-10

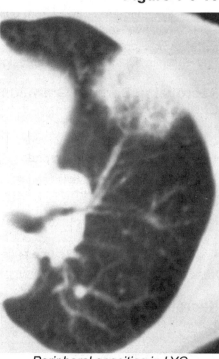

Peripheral opacities in LYG

Lymphomatoid Granulomatosis: Treatment and Prognosis
- Mortality rate
  - 53-90%
- Long term remissions reported
  - Cyclophosphamide and steroids
- All who fail therapy proceed to develop lymphoma
  - 12-47%

Bronchocentric Granulomatosis
Clinical and Demographics – Asthmatics
- Average age 22 years
- Tissue manifestation of ABPA
- Dyspnea, cough, fever, malaise and hemoptysis
- Peripheral and tissue eosinophilia
- No extrapulmonary findings

Bronchocentric Granulomatosis
Clinical and Demographics – Non-Asthmatics
- Average age 50 years
- Males=Females
- Fungal infections
  - ➤ Histo, Blastomyces, Aspergillus
- Mycobacterial infections
- Rheumatoid Arthritis
- Wegener's granulomatosis
- Idiopathic

Bronchocentric Granulomatosis: Pathology
- Nonspecific reaction
- Early invasion of mucosa
  - ➤ Histiocytes
  - ➤ Eosinophils
    - ✧ Asthmatics
  - ➤ Neutrophils
    - ✧ Non-asthmatics
- Secondary involvement of adjacent arteries
- Granulomatous destruction
  - ➤ Bronchial walls
- Bronchopneumonia
  - ➤ Distal to affected airways

Bronchocentric Granulomatosis: Imaging [Figure 1-6-11]
- Most often unilateral
  - ➤ 75%
- Multiple or solitary nodules
- Parenchymal consolidation
  - ➤ Upper lobe predominance
- Associated findings of ABPA
  - ➤ Bronchiectasis
  - ➤ Mucoid impaction

BCG and Tuberculosis

Bronchocentric Granulomatosis: Treatment and Prognosis
- Asthmatics respond to steroids
- Some cases remit without treatment
- Must rule out treatable infection and Wegener's

Angiitis and Granulomatosis: Differential
Multiple nodules and masses with cavitation
- Metastatic disease
  - ➤ squamous
- Multifocal infection
  - ➤ Fungus, TB, bacteria
- Septic abscesses
- Multiple pulmonary infarcts
- Lymphoma
- Rheumatoid nodules
- Langerhans' cell histiocytosis

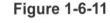

Figure 1-6-11

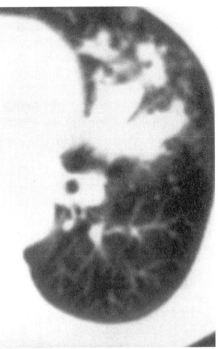

Mucoid impaction in patients with BCG

BCG?

Fungal Infection ?

Angiitis and Granulomatosis: Conclusion
- Wegener's granulomatosis
- Churg-Strauss syndrome
  - ➤ Allergic granulomatosis
- Necrotizing sarcoid granulomatosis
- Bronchocentric granulomatosis
- Lymphomatoid granulomatosis

"Until specific causes are found ....we must devise syndromes"
- Etiology
- Prognosis
- Therapy

Angiitis and Granulomatosis Bibliography
1. Thurlbeck WM, Churg AM, eds. Pathology of the lung, second edition. New York: Thieme Medical Publishers, 1995; 401-435.
2. Godman GC, Churg J. Wegener's granulomatosis: Pathology and review of the literature. A.M.A. Arch Pathol, 1954; 58(6): 533-553
3. Churg A, Brallas M, Cronin SR, Churg J. Formes frustes of Churg-Strauss syndrome. Chest 1995; 108(2):320-323.
4. Liebow AA. The J. Burns Amberson Lecture: pulmonary angiitis and granulomatosis. Am Rev Respir Dis 1973; 108:1-18.
5. Travis WD, Fleming MV. Vasculitis of the lung. Pathology: State of the Art Reviews 1996; 4(1): 23-41.
6. Travis WD. Pathology of pulmonary granulomatous vasculitis. Sarcoidosis Vasc and Diffuse Lung Dis 1996; 13:14-27.
7. Leavitt RY, Fauci AS. Pulmonary vasculitis. Am Rev Respir Dis 1986; 134:149-166.
8. Fauci AS, Haynes BF, Katz P, Wolff SM. Wegener's granulomatosis: Prospective clinical and therapeutic experience with 85 patients for 21 years. Ann Intern Med 1983; 98:76-85.
9. Kornblut AD, Fauci AS. Conversations on allergy and immunology; Cutis 1985; 35:27-34.
10. McDonald TJ, DeRemee RA. Wegener's granulomatosis. Laryngoscope 1983; 93: 220-231.
11. Cordier JF, Valeyre D, Guillevin L, Loire R, Brechot JM. Pulmonary Wegener's granulomatosis: a clinical and imaging study of 77 cases. Chest 1990; 97:906-912.
12. Daum TE, Specks U, Colby TV, et al. Tracheobronchial involvement in Wegener's granulomatosis. Am J Respir Crit Care Med 1995; 151: 522-526.
13. Aberle DR, Gamsu G, Lynch D. Thoracic manifestations of Wegener granulomatosis: diagnosis and course. Radiology 1990; 174:703-709.
14. Nölle B, Specks U, Lüdemann J, Rohrbach MS, DeRemee RA, Gross WL. Anticytoplasmic autoantibodies: Their immunodiagnostic value in Wegener granulomatosis. Ann Intern Med 1989; 111:28-40.
15. Travis WD, Carpenter HA, Lie JT. Diffuse pulmonary hemorrhage: an uncommon manifestation of Wegener's granulomatosis. Am J Surg Pathol 1987; 11(9): 702-708.
16. Staples CA. Pulmonary angiitis and granulomatosis. Radiol Clin North Am 1991; 29(5): 973-982.
17. Kornblut AD, Wolff SM, DeFries HO, Fauci AS. Symposium on granulomatous disorders of the head and neck: Wegener's granulomatosis. Otol Clin North Am 1982; 15(3):673-683.
18. Allen NB, Bressler PB. Diagnosis and treatment of the systemic and cutaneous necrotizing vasculitis syndromes. Med Clin North Am 1997; 81(1):

243-259.

19. Travis WD, Hoffman GS, Leavitt RY, Pass HI, Fauci AS. Surgical pathology of the lung in Wegener's granulomatosis: review of 87 open lung biopsies from 67 patients. Am J Surg Pathol 1991; 15(4): 315-333.

20. Katzenstein AA, Locke WK. Solitary lung lesions in Wegener's granulomatosis: Pathologic findings and clinical significance in 25 cases. Am J Surg Pathol 1995; 19(5): 545-552.

21. Feigin DS. Vasculitis in the lung. J Thorac Imag 1988; 3(1):33-48.

22. Epstein DM, Gefter WB, Miller WT, Gohel V, Bonavita JA. Spontaneous pneumothorax: an uncommon manifestation of Wegener granulomatosis. Radiol 1980; 135:327-328.

23. Fraser RS, Pare JAP, Fraser PD, eds. Synopsis of diseases of the chest, second edition. Philadelphia: WB Saunders Company, 1994; 411-419.

24. Farrelly CA. Wegener's granulomatosis: a radiological review of the pulmonary manifestations at initial presentation and during relapse. Clin Radiol 1982; 33:545-551.

25. Lee SJ, Berry GJ, Husari AW. Wegener's granulomatosis presenting as right middle lobe obstruction. Chest 1993; 103(5):1623-1624.

26. Travis WD, Colby TV, Lombard C, Carpenter HA. A clinicopathologic study of 34 cases of diffuse pulmonary hemorrhage with lung biopsy confirmation. Am J Surg Pathol 1990; 14(12):1112-1136.

27. Wadsworth DT, Siegel MJ, Day DL. Wegener's granulomatosis in children: chest radiographic manifestations. AJR 1994;163:901-904.

28. McHugh K. Wegener's granulomatosis in children. [Letter] AJR 1995; 165(3):743.

29. Maguire R, Fauci AS, Doppman JL, Wolff SM. Unusual radiographic features of Wegener's granulomatosis. AJR 1978; 141:233-238.

30. Maskell GF, Lockwood CM, Flower CDR. Computed tomography of the lung in Wegener's granulomatosis. Clin Radiol 1993; 48:377-380.

31. Papiris SA, Manoussakis MN, Drosos AA, Kontogiannis D, Constantopoulos SH, Moutsopoulos HM. Imaging of thoracic Wegener's granulomatosis: the computed tomographic appearance. Am J Med 1992; 93: 529-536.

32. Jaspan T, Davison AM, Walker WC. Spontaneous pneumothorax in Wegener's granulomatosis. Thorax 1982; 37:774-775

33. Grotz W, Mundinger A, Würtemberger G, Peter HH, Schollmeyer P. Radiographic course of pulmonary manifestations in Wegener's granulomatosis under immunosuppressive therapy. Chest 1994;105(2):509-513.

34. Weir IH, Muller NL, Chiles C, Godwin JD, Lee SH, Kullnig P. Wegener's granulomatosis: findings from computed tomography of the chest in 10 patients. Can Assoc Radiol J 1992; 43(1):31-34.

35. Kuhlman JE, Hruban RH, Fishman EK. Wegener granulomatosis: CT features of parenchymal lung disease. J Comput Assist Tomogr 1991; 15(6):948-952.

36. Erzurum SC, Underwood GA, Hamilos DL, Waldron JA. Pleural effusion in Churg-Strauss syndrome. Chest 1989; 95(6):1357-1359.

37. Primack SL, Hartman TE, Lee KS, Müller NL. Pulmonary nodules and the CT halo sign. Radiol 1994; 190:513-515.

38. Connolly S, Manson D, Eberhard A, Laxer RM, Smith C. CT appearance of pulmonary vasculitis in children. AJR 1996; 167:901-904.

39. Foo SS, Weisbrod GL, Herman SJ, Chamberlain DW. Wegener granulomatosis presenting on CT with atypical bronchovasocentric distribution. J Comput Assist Tomogr 1990; 14(6):1004-1006.

40. Stokes TC, McCann BG, Rees RT, Sims EH, Harrison BDW. Acute fulminating intrapulmonary haemorrhage in Wegener's granulomatosis. Thorax 1982; 37:315-316.

41. Dugowson CE, Aitken ML. Unusual presentation of recurrent Wegener's granulomatosis. Chest 1991; 99(3):781-784.

42. Erzurum SC, Underwood GA, Hamilos DL, Waldron JA. Pleural effusion in Churg-Strauss syndrome. Chest 1989; 95 (6):1357-1359.

43. Amundson DE. Cavitary pulmonary cryptococcosis complicating Churg-

Strauss vasculitis. Southern Med J 1992; 85(7):700-702.

44. Buschman DL, Waldron JA, King TE. Churg-Strauss pulmonary vasculitis: high-resolution computed tomography scanning and pathologic findings. Am Rev Respir Dis 1990; 142:458-461.

45. Liebow AA, Carrington CRB, Friedman PJ. Lymphomatoid granulomatosis. Hum Pathol 1972; 3(4):457-558.

46. Katzenstein AA, Carrington CB, Liebow AA. Lymphomatoid granulomatosis: a clinicopathologic study of 152 cases. Cancer 1979; 43:360-373.

47. Fauci AS, Haynes BF, Costa J, Katz P, Wolff SM. Lymphomatoid granulomatosis: prospective clinical and therapeutic experience over 10 years. N Engl J Med 1982; 306(2):68-74.

48. Bragg DG, Chor PJ, Murray KA, Kjeldsberg CR. Lymphoproliferative disorders of the lung: histopathology, clinical manifestations, and imaging features. AJR 1994; 163:273-281.

49. Fauci AS, Haynes BF, Katz P. The spectrum of vasculitis: clinical, pathologic, immunologic, and therapeutic considerations. Ann Intern Med 1978; 89(1):660-676.

50. Dee PM, Arora NS, Innes DJ. The pulmonary manifestations of lymphomatoid granulomatosis. Radiol 1982; 143: 613-618.

51. Prenovault JMN, Weisbrod GL, Herman SJ. Lymphomatoid granulomatosis: a review of 12 cases. J Can Assoc Radiol 1988; 39:263-266.

52. Koss MN. Pulmonary lymphoid disorders. Semin Diag Pathol 1995; 12(2):158-171.

53. Guinee D, Jaffe E, Kingma D, Fishback N, et al. Pulmonary lymphomatoid granulomatosis: evidence for a proliferation of Epstein-Barr virus infected B-lymphocytes with a prominent T-cell component and vasculitis. Am J Surg Pathol 1994; 18(8): 753-764.

54. Hicken P, Dobie JC, Frew E. The radiology of lymphomatoid granulomatosis in the lung. Clin Radiol 1979; 30: 661-664.

55. Scully RE, Mark EJ, McNeely WF, Ebeling SH. Case records of the Massachusetts General Hospital. New Engl J Med 1996; 335(20):1514-1521.

56. Niimi H, Hartman TE, Müller NL. Necrotizing sarcoid granulomatosis: computed tomography and pathologic findings. J Comput Assist Tomogr 1995;19(6):920-923.

57. Warren J, Pitchenik AE, Saldana MJ. Granulomatous vasculitides of the lung: a clinicopathologic approach to diagnosis and treatment. South Med J 1989; 82(4):481-491.

58. Chittock DR, Joseph MG, Paterson NAM, McFadden RG. Necrotizing sarcoid granulomatosis with pleural involvement: clinical and radiographic features. Chest 1994; 106:672-676.

59. Weisbrod GL. Pulmonary angiitis and granulomatosis: a review . J Can Assoc Radiol 1989; 40:138-134.

60. Sadoun D, Kambouchner M, Tazi A, et al. Granulomatose necrosante sarcoid-like: à propos de 4 observations. Ann Med Interne 1994; 145(4) 230-233.

61. Myers JL, Katzenstein AA. Granulomatous infection mimicking bronchocentric granulomatosis. Am J Surg Pathol 1986; 10(5):317-322.

62. Koss MN, Robinson RG, Hochholzer L. Bronchocentric granulomatosis. Hum Pathol 1981; 12(7):632-638.

63. Sulavik SB. Bronchocentric granulomatosis and allergic bronchopulmonary aspergillosis. Clin Chest Med 1988; 9(4):609-621.

64. Berendsen HH, Hofstee N, Kapsenberg PD, Siewertsz Van Reesema DR, Klein JJ. Bronchocentric granulomatosis associated with seropositive polyarthritis. Thorax 1985; 40:396-397.

65. Clee MD, Lamb D, Urbaniak SJ, Clark RA. Progressive bronchocentric granulomatosis: case report. Thorax 1982; 37:947-949.

66. Felson B, Reeder MM. Gamuts in radiology, second edition. Cincinnati: Audiovisual Radiology of Cincinnati, Inc, 1967: 561-562.

67. Albelda SM, Gefter WB, Epstein DM, Miller WT. Diffuse pulmonary hemorrhage: a review and classification. Radiology 1985; 154: 289-29

The Pulmonary Complications of Bone Marrow Transplantation

Jeffrey R. Galvin, MD
Chief, Pulmonary and Mediastinal Radiology
Armed Forces Institute of Pathology
and
Clinical Professor Department of Radiology
University of Maryland

Introduction
- First performed late 1960's
- 38,000 procedures in 1998
- Standard therapy
  - Aplastic anemia, acute and chronic leukemia and lymphoma
- Encouraging results
  - hemoglobinopathies, immunodeficiency disorders and multiple myeloma
- Not proven in breast cancer
- Younger age group

Pulmonary Complications in 40-60% – Multifactorial Cause
- Underlying disease
- Therapy for underlying disease
- Graft-vs-host disease
- Conditioning regimen
  - Chemotherapy and radiation

Early Pulmonary Complications
- Pulmonary edema
- Fungal infection
- Diffuse alveolar hemorrhage
- Bacterial infection
- Viral infection
  - CMV and herpes
- Pneumocystis carinii
- Acute graft-vs-host disease
- Idiopathic pulmonary syndrome
  - ARDS, DAD

Late Pulmonary Complications
- Chronic graft-vs-host
- Obstructive airways disease
  - Bronchiolitis obliterans
- Organizing Pneumonia
  - BOOP
- Restrictive ventilatory defect
- Late bacterial infections
  - Sinopulmonary
- Herpes varicella zoster

Pretransplant Considerations
- Residual tumor
- Occult infection

Operative Technique [Figure 1-7-1]
- Donor aspiration
  - ➢ General anesthesia
- 150-200 aspirates
- Marrow strained
- Immunocompetent T-cells
  - ➢ Depleted with monoclonal reagents
- Infusion of marrow
  - ➢ 400-800 ml

Immunologic Impact
- Profound neutropenia
- Prolonged depression
  - ➢ Cellular function
  - ➢ Humoral function
- Graft-vs-host
  - ➢ Direct effect
  - ➢ Steroids

Bone Marrow Transplant: Typical Schedule [Figure 1-7-2]

Figure 1-7-1

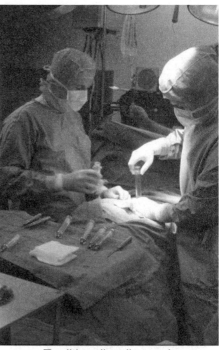

Traditionally, allogeneic transplantation used bone marrow grafts. From 1999-2002 there was a steady increase in peripheral blood stem cell grafts

Figure 1-7-2

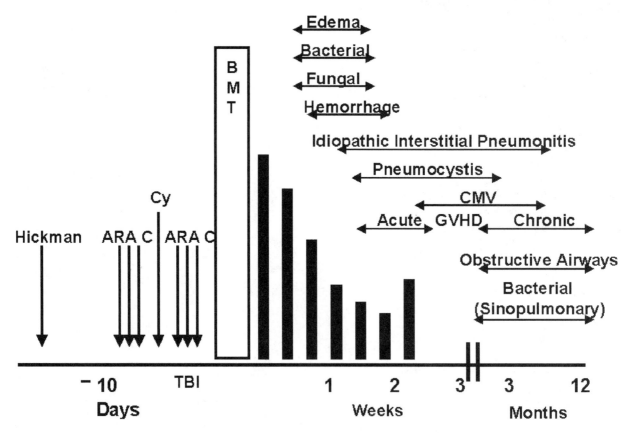

Complications are usually separated into those that occur before and after there first 100 day

Pulmonary Edema [Figure 1-7-3]

- Common complication
- 2nd-3rd week posttransplantation
- Rapid onset
  - ➢ Dyspnea and hypoxemia
- Reticulo-nodular markings
- Fluid overload
  - ➢ Blood products, antibiotics and TPN
- Cardiac
- Renal dysfunction
- Decreased albumin
- Often accompanied by fever

Fungal Infections

- Up to 45% of BMT patients
  - ➢ 85% mortality
- Aspergillus is most common
- Occurs in the first 30 days posttransplantation
- Symptoms:
  - ➢ Fever, dyspnea, cough, chest pain and hemoptysis
- Predisposition
  - ➢ Prolonged granulocytopenia
  - ➢ Broad spectrum antibiotics
- Nodules
- Early "Halo-Sign"
- Late "Air Crescent"

Fungal Infections [Figure 1-7-4; 1-7-5, 1-7-6]

Figure 1-7-4

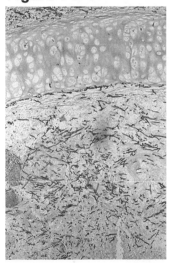

Fungi normally invade the lung via the airway

Figure 1-7-3

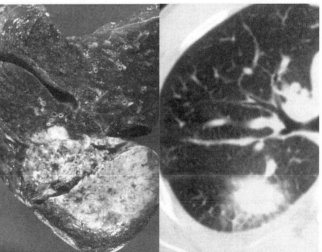

Pulmonary edema in a bone marrow transplant patient demonstrating interlobular septal thickening and enlarged pulmonary veins

Figure 1-7-5

Typical infarct with a halo of blood in an aspergillus infection

Figure 1-7-6

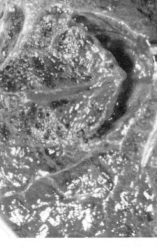
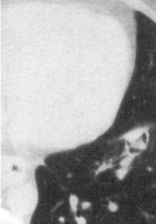
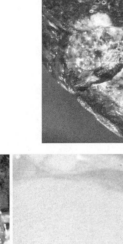

Air-crescent sign in a patient with recovering cell counts

Invasive Aspergillosis - Diagnosis

Figure 1-7-7

-
  - ➢ BAL (69%)
  - ➢ Tissue Biopsy (60%)
  - ➢ Antigen (83%)
  - ➢ Computed Tomography (92%)

Caillot, J Clin Oncol. 1997

Imaging and Survival – Invasive Aspergillosis

Caillot, J Clin Oncol. 1997

Pulmonary Hemorrhage

- 21% of BMT patients
- 12th day posttransplantation
- Neutrophil recovery
- Sudden onset:
  - ➢ Dyspnea, cough, fever and hypoxemia
- Rare hemoptysis
- Mortality 50-80%
- Radiographic abnormalities before symptoms
- Bilateral ground glass opacities
  - ➢ May be localized

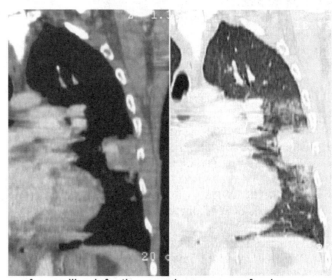

Aspergillus infection may be a cause of pulmonary hemorrhage

Pulmonary Hemorrhage   [Figure 1-7-7]

Cytomegalovirus Pneumonia

- 10-40% of BMT patients
- 6-12 weeks posttransplantation
- Mortality rate of 85%
- Reactivation of latent virus in 70%
  - ➢ Remainder infected by "CMV positive" blood products
- Anti-viral therapy improves prognosis

Pneumocystis Jiroveci Pneumonia

- <10% of BMT patients
- Effective prophylaxis
  - ➢ Trimethoprim/sulfa
- Rapid progression
- Severe dyspnea
- Bilateral perihilar
- Ground-glass opacities

Noninfectious Pulmonary Complication

- Late-onset Noninfectious Pulmonary Complications
  - ➢ LONIPC's
  - ➢ After the first 3 months
  - ➢ 10-23% of allogeneic grafts
- Idiopathic pulmonary syndrome
  - ➢ Diffuse alveolar damage (DAD)
- Bronchiolitis obliterans
- Organizing pneumonia
  - ➢ BOOP
- Associate with GVHD
  - ➢ Sicca syndrome
  - ➢ Acive donor T-cells

Sakaida, Blood Vol 102 2003

Idiopathic Pulmonary Syndrome

- Diffuse lung injury posttransplantation
- Histology
  - Interstitial mononuclear infiltrate
  - DAD
- 12% of allogenic BMT
- 40-80 days posttransplantation
- Risk factors
  - GVHD
  - Radiation
- Fever, cough and hypoxemia
- Mortality rate of 70%
- Diffuse Opacities

Idiopathic Pulmonary Syndrome

[Figure 1-7-8 to 1-7-10]

Figure 1-7-8

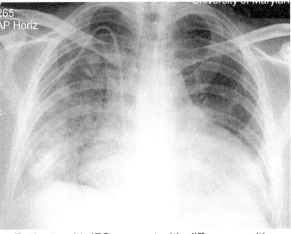

Patients with IPS present with diffuse opacities involving all 5 lobes

Figure 1-7-9

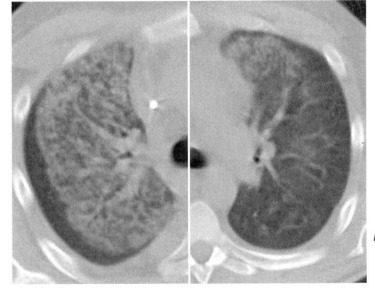

In the early phase (exudative) there is diffuse consolidation and ground glass often with peripheral clearing

Figure 1-7-10

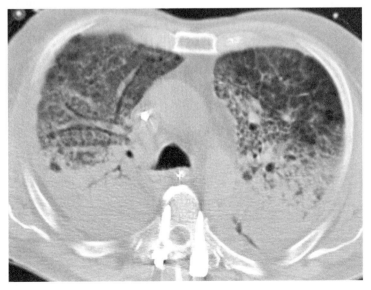

The late phase of IPS demonstrates traction bronchiectasis consistent with fibrosis

Diffuse Alveolar Damage
- Infectious agents
  - Legionella, mycoplasma, viruses
- Inhalants
  - Ammonia, chlorine, HS
- Drugs
  - Cytoxan, BCNU, Bleomycin
- Ingestants
  - Kerosene, Paraquat
- Shock/trauma
- Sepsis
- Radiation
- Idiopathic
  - Hammon-Rich or AIP

Viral Infection

Graft-vs-Host Disease (GVHD) : Donor T-lymphocytes recognize the recipient's tissue as foreign
- Acute GVHD
  - 20-100 days posttransplantation
  - 25-75% of patients
  - skin, gut and liver dysfunction
  - 10% mortality
- Chronic GVHD
  - 1> 100 days posttransplantation
  - 20-45% of patients
  - Features of autoimmune diseases
  - Sjogren's, scleroderma, biliary cirrhosis and airway obstruction

GVHD and IPS

GVHD and Infection

GVHD and IPS

Radiation Pneumonitis
- Related to dose of TBI
- Presents within 90 days
- Cough, fever, and dyspnea
- Threshold lowered by chemotherapy

Mediastinal Emphysema
- Correlates
  - Idiopathic Interstitial Pneumonia
- Increased likelihood with more radiation
- Not a serious complication by itself
- May be a harbinger of pneumothorax

Secondary Malignancies
- 0.02% incidence
- 7X's increase
  - Over the general population
- 1 year after transplantation
  - Median
- Hodgkin's 45%
- Leukemia 17%
- Solid tumors 38%

Lymphoma and Immune Impairment

- Pathologic Features
  - B-cell non-Hodgkin 's
    - Driven by Epstein-Barr virus infection
    - Diffuse polyclonal expansion
      - Reduced T-cell control
    - Malignant transformation

Bone Marrow Transplant

Bronchiolitis Obliterans

- 2-13% of BMT's
- Low immunoglobulin level
- Chronic GVHD
  - Sicca syndrome
- 100 days posttransplantation
- Gradual deterioration of PFT'S
- Airflow obstruction
  - Fixed
- Reduction in diffusing capacity
- Imaging
  - Mosaic attenuation
  - Expiratory accentuation
  - Centrilobular nodules
  - Patchy consolidation

Bronchiolitis Obliterans *[Figure 1-7-11 to 1-7-13]*

Figure 1-7-12

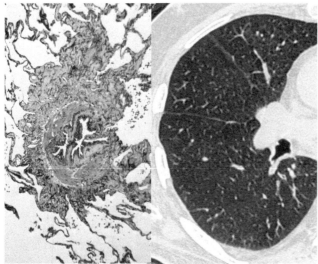

Bronchiolitis obliterans demonstrating indistinct nodules and branching opacities

Figure 1-7-11

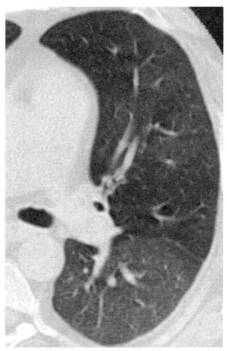

Bronchiolitis obliterans demonstrating mosaic attenuation

Figure 1-7-13

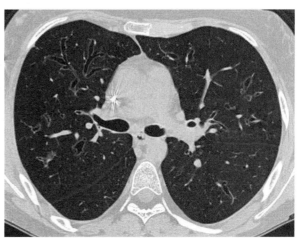

Bronchiolitis obliterans demonstrating bronchiectasis

Segmental or Lobar Consolidation
- Infection

Diffuse Opacities
- Pulmonary Edema
- Hemorrhage
- Diffuse Alveolar Damage
- Viral Pneumonia
- Pneumocystis Pneumonia

Rapid Progression Over 24 Hours
- Bacterial Pneumonia
- Pulmonary Edema
- Hemorrhage

Progression Over Days
- Aspergillus
- Pneumocystis
- Diffuse Alveolar Damage
- CMV

Diffuse Opacities

Fluid Overload

Organizing Pneumonia

BMTP: dyspnea and cough

BMTP Lymphangitic Spread

BMTP

BMTP Aspergillus

BMTP: dyspnea and cough

BMTP: Edema

Bone Marrow Transplant – Typical Schedule

The Diagnosis of Pulmonary Embolism
A Rational Approach to Familiar Tests and New Technologies

Jeffrey R. Galvin, MD
Chief, Pulmonary and Mediastinal Radiology
Armed Forces Institute of Pathology
and
Clinical Professor Department of Radiology
University of Maryland

Pulmonary Embolus
- Frequent
- Potentially fatal
- Largely undiagnosed

Baglin, J Clin Path, 1997

Pulmonary Embolus: Epidemiology
- 5 million episodes of DVT
- 300,000 embolic events
- 50,000 deaths
- 100/100,000 new cases

The "Clinical Picture" of PE
- Predisposing factors
- Pathology
- Signs and symptoms
- Radiography
- Arterial blood gases
- V/Q scanning
- Computed tomography
- Arteriography

Pulmonary Embolism is a Complication of Deep Venous Thrombosis

Sources of Pulmonary Emboli
- Majority of clots
  - ➢ Lower extremity veins
- Increasing number of clots
  - ➢ Upper extremities, cardiac chambers and catheters
- A negative venous study
  - ➢ Does not rule out PE
- < 50% of PE patients
  - ➢ Positive lower extremity study

Kelly, Ann Int Med, 1991

Embolic Events - Predisposing Causes
- Stasis
- Trauma
- Hypercoagulable states

Predisposing Causes
- 1° Thrombophlebitis   39%
- Bed rest   32%
- Recent surgery   31%
- Venous insufficiency   25%
- Recent fracture   15%
- Myocardial infarction   12%
- Malignancy   8%
- CHF   5%
- No Predisposition   6%

PE and Malignancy
- 10-15% of unexplained phlebitis
  - ➢ Gastrointestinal
  - ➢ Pulmonary
  - ➢ Genitourinary

The History and Physical are Non-Specific

Symptoms in Patients with non-fatal PE
- Chest Pain   88%
- Dyspnea   84%
- Apprehension   59%
- Cough   53%
- Hemoptysis   30%
- Sweats   27%
- Syncope   13%

Signs in Patients with non-fatal PE
- RR> 16   92%
- Rales   58%
- HR> 100   44%
- T> 37.8°C   43%
- Diaphoresis   36%
- Gallop   34%
- Phlebitis   32%
- Murmur   23%
- Cyanosis   19%

PE and Underlying Lung Disease

The History and Physical are Insensitive

We do not know the prevalence of PE.

Diagnostic Algorithm and Clinical Suspicion [Figure 1-8-1]

"Among the various causes of an incorrect diagnosis, most important are: the failure to suspect PE and, the protean nature of the disease."

Morpurgo, Chest 1995

History and Physical

The Role of Clinical Suspicion
- Less than 35% of fatal emboli were diagnosed antemortem

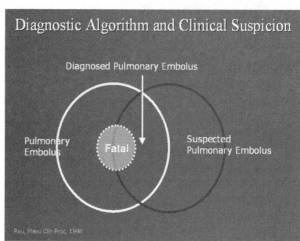

Figure 1-8-1

Diagnostic Algorithm and Clinical Suspicion

Diagnosed Pulmonary Embolus

Pulmonary Embolus

Fatal

Suspected Pulmonary Embolus

Ryu, Mayo Clin Proc, 1998

The clinical diagnosis of PE is unreliable. Many patients are symptomatic

Symptoms in Patients with Fatal PE

- Dyspnea   59%
- Syncope   27%
- Altered Mentation 20%
- Apprehension   17%
- Chest Pain   10%
- Sweatiness   9%
- Pleuritic Pain   8%
- Cough   3%
- Hemoptysis   3%
- Arrest   8%

Signs in Patients with Fatal PE

- RR> 16   66%
- HR> 100   54%
- Rales   42%
- T> 37.8°C   30%
- Edema   26%
- Hypotension   20%
- Cyanosis   12%
- Gallop   10%
- Diaphoresis   10%
- Phlebitis   7%

The Chest X-Ray is Usually Abnormal

The Chest X-Ray in Pulmonary Embolism

- 84% had abnormal radiographs

	PE(%)	NoPE(%)
Atelectasis/Infiltrate	68	48
Pleural Effusion	48	31
Pleural Opacity	35	21
Elevated Diaphragm	24	19
Decreased Vascularity	21	12
Prominent PA	17	28
Cardiomegaly	12	11
Westermark's Sign	7	2
Pulmonary Edema	4	13

Pioped

Common Radiographic Abnormalities

- Infiltrate   54%
- Pleural Effusion   51%
- Atelectasis   27%
- Diaphragm Up   17%
- 2 or More   44%
- CHF   17%
- Focal Oligemia   2%
- Normal   7%

Chest CT Findings

- Atelectasis   100%
- Consolidation   57%
- Hampton's hump   50%
- Ground glass   57%
- Pleural Effusions 87%
- Mosaic attenuation

Truong, ARRS, 1998

Radiographic and CT Findings *[Figure 1-8-2]*

Figure 1-8-2

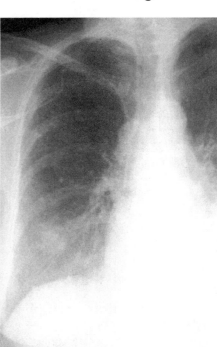

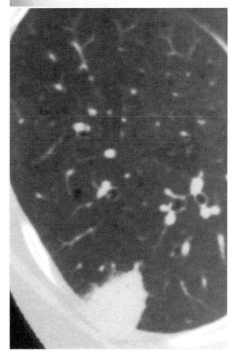

Peripheral opacities may raise suspicion for clinically unsuspected PE

Pathology *[Figure 1-8-3]*
- Edema
- Hemorrhage
- Infarction

Normal Arterial Oxygenation Does Not Exclude Pulmonary Embolism

Arterial Blood Gases
- 10-15% will have a PO2 >85mm HG
- A low arterial PO2 is non-specific
- A respiratory alkalosis is most common

The Physiology of Pulmonary Embolism
- V/Q abnormalities
  - ➢ Variable
- Complete vascular occlusion
  - ➢ Rare
- Complete shunt 2° to
  - ➢ Atelectasis
  - ➢ Hemorrhage
- Autoregulation
  - ➢ Hypoxic vasoconstriction
  - ➢ Hypocapnic bronchoconstriction

Levy, JAP, 1974
Dantzker, Circulation Res, 1974
Dantzker, Chest Vol. 91 no. 5

Physiologic Change with Heparinization
- Ventilation
  - ➢ Returns more rapidly than perfusion
- Perfusion
  - ➢ May return before ventilation

Santolicandro, Am J Res Crit Care Med, 1995

V/Q Physiology

Ventilation/Perfusion Scanning

Figure 1-8-3

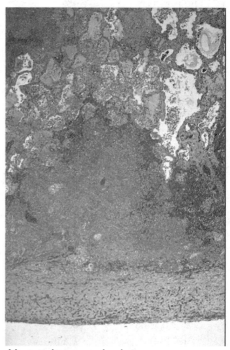

Hemorrhage and edema are common sequela of PE. Infarct is less common and is more likely to occur in patients with CHF

	Clinical Science Probability (%)				
	80-100	20-79	0-19	All Probabilities	
• High	96%	88%	56%	87%	(103/118)
• Intermediate	66%	28%	16%	30%	(104/345)
• Low	40%	16%	4%	14%	(40/296)
• Normal	0%	6%	2%	4%	(5/128)
• Total	68%	30%	9%	28%	(252/887)

Pioped Data

The Basis of "Clinical Science Probability"

	PE(%)	No PE(%)
• Dyspnea	73	72
• Pleuritic Pain	66	59
• Cough	37	36
• Leg Swelling	28	22
• Hemoptysis	13	8
• Palpitations	10	18
• Wheezing	9	11
• "Angina"	4	6

Traditional Approach [Figure 1-8-4]

Figure 1-8-4

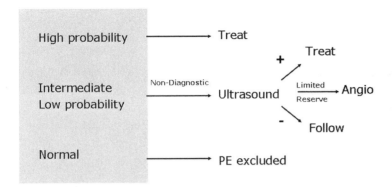

The Low-Probability Lung Scan
- "There is an 8% mortality rate in patients with a "low probability" V/Q scan and limited cardiopulmonary reserve." *Hull, Archives of Internal Medicine, 1995*
- "There is a 25%-30% disagreement between expert readers in interpreting INTERMEDIATE and LOW probability V/Q scans." *PIOPED, JAMA, 1990*
- A Potentially Lethal Reading
  - ➤ "Pulmonary embolism cannot be diagnosed on clinical grounds; it can only be suspected." *Bone, Archives of Internal Medicine, 1993*

The Goal of Imaging – Visualization of the clot

The Role of Pulmonary CT Angiography
- Initial screening
- Detection of unexpected emboli
- Detection of other pathology

The Ideal Diagnostic Test
- Accurate
- Safe
- Readily Available
- Cost Effective
- Widely Accepted

CT Angiography

Pulmonary CT Angiography – Sensitivity and Specificity
- Accurately identifies emboli
  - ➤ Main, lobar and segmental vessels
- Misses many subsegmental emboli
- Indeterminate 8-10%
- Related to collimation and scan speed

Remy-Jardin, Radiology, 1992; Goodman, AJR, 1995; Remy-Jardin, Radiology, 1996; Van Rossum, Radiology, 1996; Mayo, Radiology, 1997; Garg, Radiology, 1998; Drucker, Radiology, 1998; Kim, Radiology, 1999

Pulmonary CT Angiography – Sensitivity and Specificity
- 3mm visualizes 40% of subsegmental arteries
- 3mm visualizes 75% of segmental arteries
- 1.25mm visualizes 75% of subsegmental arteries
- 1.23mm visualizes 90% of segmental arteries

Patel, Radiology, 2003

Patient Outcome Studies – What is the significance of small emboli?

- Good outcome
  - ➢ Patients with "negative angio"
- 1.5% embolize when followed 1 year
  - ➢ 691 patients

Novelline, Radiology, 1978; Henry, Chest, 1995

Distribution of Pulmonary Emboli

- Multiple locations
  - ➢ > 55%
- Marked preference for
  - ➢ Right lung and lower lobes
- Subsegmental only
  - ➢ 6-30%

PIOPED, JAMA, 1990; Oser, Radiology, 1996; Morpurgo, Chest, 1995; Monye, Radiology, 2000

Pulmonary CT Angiography – Negative Predictive Value of a Normal CT

- No prospective, consecutive studies
- "The safety of withholding anticoagulants…is uncertain"

Rathbun, Ann Int Med, 2000

Pulmonary CT Angiography – Negative Predictive Value of a Normal CT

	n	Follow-up	NPV
Mayo	69	3m	97%
Feretti	109	3m	97%
Garg	78	6m	99%
Loomis	81	6m	100%
Goodmann	198	3m	99%
Remy-Jardin	71	3m	97%
Tillie-Leblond	185	12m	98%
Kavanagh	85	9m	99%

Pulmonary CT Angiography – Intra and Interobserver Variability

- Radiology's Achilles' Heel
- Related to clot size
- Exacerbated by poor exam
- Related to reader experience

Mayo, Radiology, 1997; Chartrand-Lefebre, AJR, 1999; Drucker, Radiology, 2000

Pulmonary CT Angiography

- Alternate diagnoses
  - ➢ 11-33%
- Unexpected emboli
  - ➢ 1-1.5%

Winston, Radiology, 1996; Gosselin, Radiology, 1998

Alternative Diagnoses [Figure 1-8-5 and 1-8-6]

Figure 1-8-5

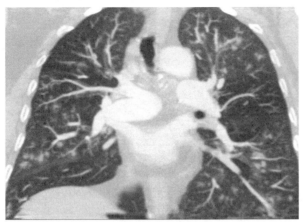

Pulmonary infection is a common alternative diagnosis is patients suspected of pulmonary embolus

Figure 1-8-6

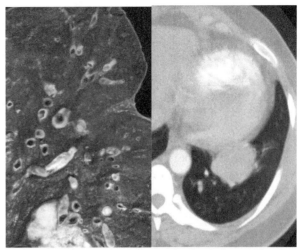

Adenocarcinoma is an important predisposition for hypercoaguability and PE

Pitfalls in Helical CT [Figure 1-8-7 and 1-8-8]
- Partial volume
  - ➢ Obliquely oriented arteries
- Suboptimal contrast enhancement
- Breathing artifacts
- Lymph nodes

Figure 1-8-7

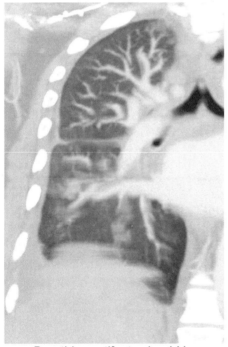

Breathing artifacts should be assessed before reading a CTA for PE

Figure 1-8-8

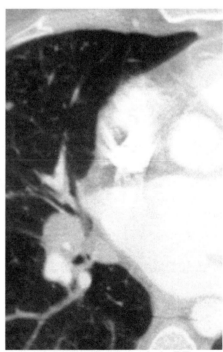

Adenopathy can mimic PE

Technical Improvements
- Multi-channel CT
- Narrower collimation: 1mm
- Subsecond scanning
- Contrast timing
  - "Smart prep"
  - Test bolus: peak + 5 sec
  - 20 seconds normal cardiac output
  - Caudal-cranial scanning
- Workstation viewing
  - Cine Mode (PACS or Workstation)
  - Adjust window and levels for each case
  - Multi-planar reconstruction
  - Breathing artifact-coronal lung windows

16 Channel CT *[Figure 1-8-9]*

Paddlewheel Reformation
Chiang et al, Radiology, 03

Figure 1-8-9

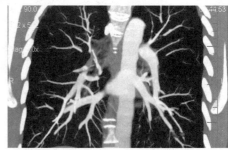

Coronal reconstruction helps separate pulmonary arteries and veins

Combined Pulmonary CTA and Venography

	Year	N	Sensitivity	Specificity
Loud	00	150	97%	100%
Duwe	00	74	89%	94%
Garg	00	70	100%	97%
Cham	00	116	100%	96%
Peterson	01	136	71%	93%

A Diagnostic Algorithm for Pulmonary Embolism

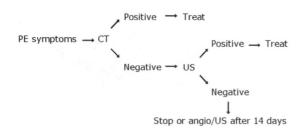

PE symptoms → CT
- Positive → Treat
- Negative → US
  - Positive → Treat
  - Negative → Stop or angio/US after 14 days

Goodman, Radiology, 1996

Pulmonary Embolus and Prognosis
The prognosis in PE patients is closely related to the presence and extent of clot in the peripheral veins

Hull, Arch Int Med, 1994

Chest Pain-Dyspnea Screening

Conclusion
- The clinical diagnosis of PE is unreliable
- The chest radiograph is usually abnormal
- V/Q readings restricted to "reliable categories"
- Small clots are a problem for all modalities
- Outcome studies are key
- CT angiography is the modality of choice

Schoepf & Costello, Radiology, 04

Pulmonary Embolus Bibliography

General

1. Robin E, D. Overdiagnosis and overtreatment of pulmonary embolism: the emperor may have no clothes. Annals of Internal Medicine 1977; 87(6):775-781.
2. Morgenthaler TI, Ryu JH. Clinical characteristics of fatal pulmonary embolism in a referral hospital. Mayo Clinic Proceedings 1995; 70(5):417-424.
3. Baglin TP, White K, Charles A. Fatal pulmonary embolism in hospitalised medical patients. J Clin Pathol 1997; 50(7):609-10.
4. Goldhaber SZ. Pulmonary embolism. N Engl J Med 1998; 339(2):93-104.
5. Huisman MV, Buller HR, ten Cate JW, van Royen EA, Vreeken J, Kersten M-J, Bakx R. Unexpected high prevalence of silent pulmonary embolism in patients with deep venous thrombosis. Chest 1989; 95(3):498-502.
6. Patriquin L, Khorasani R, Polak JF. Correlation of diagnostic imaging and subsequent autopsy findings in patients with pulmonary embolism [see comments]. AJR Am J Roentgenol 1998; 171(2):347-9.
7. Shatz DV. Statewide, population-based, time-series analysis of the frequency and outcome of pulmonary embolus in 318,554 trauma patients [letter; comment]. J Trauma 1998; 44(1):239.

Physiology

1. Dalen JE, Haffajee CI, Alpert JS, Howe JP, Ockene IS, Paraskos JA. Pulmonary embolism, pulmonary hemorrhage and pulmonary infarction. New England Journal of Medicine 1977; 296(25):1431-1435.
2. Dantzker DR, Bower JS. Clinical significance of pulmonary function tests: alterations in gas exchange following pulmonary thromboembolism. Chest 1982; 81(4):495-501.
3. Dantzker DR. Ventilation-perfusion inequality in lung disease. Chest 1987; 91:749-754.
4. Santolicandro A, Prediletto R, Fornai E, Formichi B, Begliomini E, Giannella-Neto A, Giuntini C. Mechanisms of hypoxemia and hypocapnia in pulmonary embolism. Am J Respir Crit Care Med 1995; 152(1):336-47.

Radiography

1. Moses DC, Silver TM, Bookstein JJ. The complementary roles of chest radiography, lung scanning, and selective pulmonary angiography in the diagnosis of pulmonary embolism. Circulation 1974:179-188.
2. Bynum LJ, Wilson JE. Radiographic features of pleural effusions in pulmonary embolism. American Review of Respiratory Disease 1978; 117:829-834.
3. Buckner CB, Walker CW, Purnell GL. Pulmonary embolism: chest radiographic abnormalities. Journal of Thoracic Imaging 1989; 4(4):23-27.
4. Sasahara AA, Hyers TM. The urokinase pulmonary embolus trial-A national cooperative study. Circulation 1973; 47(suppl 2):1-108.

Scintigraphy

1. Alderson PO, Rujanavech N, Secker-Walker RH, Mcknight RC. The role of 133Xe ventilation studies in the scintigraphic detection of pulmonary embolism. Radiology 1976; 120(633-640).
2. Hirsh J. Diagnosis of venous thrombosis and pulmonary embolism. American Journal of Cardiology 1990; 65:45C-49C.
3. Hull RD, Hirsh J, Carter CJ, Jay RM, Dodd PE, Ockelford PA, Coates G, Gill G, Turpie AG, Doyle DJ, Buller HR, Raskob GE. Pulmonary angiography, ventilation lung scanning, and venography for clinically suspected pulmonary embolism with abnormal perfusion lung scan. Annal of Internal Medicine 1983; 98(6):891-899.
4. Hull RD, Hirsh J, Carter CJ, Raskob GE, Gill GJ, Jay RM, Leclerc JR, David M, Coates G. Diagnostic Value of ventilation-perfusion lung scanning in patients with suspected pulmonary embolism. Chest 1985; 88(6):819-828.
5. Hull R, Raskob G, Ginsberg J. A noninvasive strategy for the treatment of patients with supected pulmonary embolism. Archives of Internal Medicine 1994; 154:289-97.

6. Hull RD, Raskob GE, Coates G, Panju AA. Clinical validity of a normal perfusion lung scan in patients with suspected pulmonary embolism. Chest 1990; 97(1):23-26.
7. Hull R, Raskob G, Pineo G, Brant R. The low-probability lung scan: a need for change in the nomenclature. Archives of Internal Medicine 1995; 155(1845-1851).
8. Schluger N, Henschke C, King T, Russo R, Binkert B, Rackson M, Hayt D. Diagnosis of pulmonary embolism at a large teaching hospital. Journal of Thoracic Imaging 1994; 9:180-184.
9. Pioped Investigators. Value of the ventialtion/perfusion scan in acute pulmonary embolism. Journal of The American Medical Association 1990; 263:2753-2759.

Angiography
1. Novelline R, Baltarowich O, Athanasoulis C, Greenfield A, McKusick K. The clinical course of patient with suspected pulmonary embolism and a negative pulmonary angiogram. Radiology 1978; 126:561-567.
2. Quinn MF, Lundell CJ, Klotz TA, Finck EJ, Pentecost M, McGehee WG, Garnic JD. Reliability of selective pulmonary arteriography in the diagnosis of pulmonary embolism. American Journal of Roentgenology 1987; 149:479-471.
3. Stein PD, Athanasoulis C, Alavi A, Greenspan RH, Hales CA, Saltzman HA, Vreim CE, Terrin ML, Weg JG. Complications and validity of pulmonary angiography in acute pulmonary embolus. Circulation 1992; 85(462-468).
4. Stein PD, Henry JW, Gottschalk A. Reassessment of pulmonary angiography for the diagnosis of pulmonary embolism: relation of interpreter agreement to the order of the involved pulmonary arterial branch. Radiology 1999; 210(3):689-91.

Computed Tomography
1. Beigelman C, Chartrand-Lefebvre C, Howarth N, Grenier P. Pitfalls in diagnosis of pulmonary embolism with helical CT angiography. AJR Am J Roentgenol 1998; 171(3):579-85.
2. Balakrishnan J, Meziane MA, Siegelman SS, Fishman EK. Pulmonary infarction: CT appearance with pathologic correlation. Journal of Computer Assisted Tomography 1989; 13(6):941-945.
3. Coche EE, Muller NL, Kim KI, Wiggs BR, Mayo JR. Acute pulmonary embolism: ancillary findings at spiral CT. Radiology 1998; 207(3):753-8.
4. Falashci F, Palla A, Formichi B, Sbragia P, Petruzzelli S, Guintini C, Bartolozzi C. CT evaluation of chronic thromboembolic pulmonary hypertension. Journal of Computer Assisted Tomography 1992; 16:897-903.
5. Garg K, Welsh CH, Feyerabend AJ, Subber SW, Russ PD, Johnston RJ, Durham JD, Lynch DA. Pulmonary embolism: diagnosis with spiral CT and ventilation-perfusion scanning—correlation with pulmonary angiographic results or clinical outcome. Radiology 1998; 208(1):201-8.
6. Gefter W, Hatabu H, Holland G, Gupta K, Henschke C, Pavelsky H. Pulmonary Thromboembolism: recent developments in diagnosis wtih CT and MR imaging. Radiology 1995; 197:561-574.
7. Geraghty JJ, Stanford W, Landas S, Galvin J. Ultrafast computed tomography in experimental pulmonary embolism. Investigative Radiology 1991; 27:60-63.
8. Goodman LR, Curtin JJ, Mewissen MW, Foley WD, Lipchik RJ, Crain MR, Sagar KB, Collier BD. Detection of pulmonary embolism in patients with unresolved clinical and scintigraphic diagnosis: helical ct versus angiography. American Journal of Roentgenology 1995; 164:1369-1374.
9. Goodman LR, Lipchik RJ. Diagnosis of acute pulmonary emoblism: time for a new approach. Radiology 1996; 199:25-27.
10. Goodman LR, Lipochik RJ, Kuzo RS. Acute pulmonary embolism: the role of computed tomographic imaging. Journal of Thoracic Imaging 1997; 12(2):83-86.
11. Goodman LR. Helical CT for initial imaging of pulmonary embolus. AJR Am J Roentgenol 1998; 171(4):1153-4.
12. Gurney JW. No fooling around: direct visualization of pulmonary embolism. Radiology 1993; 188:618-619.

13. Kim KI, Muller NL, Mayo JR. Clinically suspected pulmonary embolism: utility of spiral CT. Radiology 1999; 210(3):693-7.
14. Mayo JR, Remy-Jardin M, Muller NL, Remy J, Worsley DF, Hossein-Foucher C, Kwong JS, Brown MJ. Pulmonary embolism: prospective comparison of spiral CT with ventilation-perfusion scintigraphy. Radiology 1997; 205(2):447-52.
15. Remy-Jardin M, Remy J, Wattinne L, Giraud F. Central pulmonary thromboembolism: diagnosis with spiral volumetric ct with single-breath-hold technique-comparison with pulmonary angiography. Radiology 1992; 185:381-387.
16. Remy-Jardin M, Remy J, Deschildre F, Artaud D, Beregi JP, Hossien-Foucher C, Marchdise X, Duhamel A. Diagnosis of pulmonary embolism with spiral ct: comparison with pulmonary angiography and scintigraphy. Radiology 1996; 200:699-706.
17. Remy-Jardin M, Remy J, Artaud D, Deschildre F, Fribourg M, Beregi JP. Spiral CT of pulmonary embolism: technical considerations and interpretive pitfalls. J Thorac Imaging 1997; 12(2):103-17.
18. Ren H, Kuhlman JE, Hruban RH, Fishman EK, Wheeler PS, Hutchins GM. CT of inflation-fixed lungs: wedge-shaped density and vascular sign in the diagnosis of infarction. Journal of Computer Assisted Tomography 1990; 14(1):82-86.
19. Teigen C, Maus TP, Sheedy PF, Johnson CM, Stanson AW, Welch TJ. Pulmonary embolism: diagnosis with electon-beam ct. Radiology 1993; 188:839-845.
20. Teigen CL, Maus TP, Sheedy PF, Stanson AW, Johnson CM, Breen JF, McKusick MA. Pulmonary embolism: diagnosis with contrast-enhanced electron-beam ct and comparison with pulmonary angiography. Radiology 1995; 194:313-319.
21. Van Rossum AB, Pattynama PMT, Tjin ER, Treurniet FE, Arndt J-W, van Eck B, Kieft GJ. Pulmonary embolism: validation of spiral ct angiography in 149 patients. Radiology 1996; 201:467-470.
22. Winston C, Wechsler RJ, Salazar AM, Kurtz AB, Spirn PW. incidental pulmonary emboli detected at helical ct: effect on patient care. Radiology 1996; 201:23-27.
23. Van Erkel A, van Rossum A, Bloem J, Mali W, Pattynama P. Cost-effectiveness of the us of spiral CT angiography to determine suspected pulmonary embolism. Radiology 1995; 197(P):303-304.
24. Tardivon AA, Musset D, Maitre S, Brenot F, Dartevelle P, Simonneau G, Lobrune M. Role of ct in chronic pulmonary embolism: comparison with pulmonary angiography. Journal of Computer Assisted Tomography 1993; 17:345-351.

Magnetic Resonance

1. Hatabu H, Gaa J, Kim D, Li W, Prasad PV, Edelman R. Pulmonary perfusion and angiography: evaluation with breath-hold enhanced three-dimensional fast imaging steady-state precession mr imaging with short tr and te. AJR 1996; 167:653-655.
2. Hatabu H, Gaa J, Kim D, Li W, Prasad P, Edelman RR. Pulmonary perfusion: qualitative assessment with dynamic contrast-enhanced mri using ultra short TE and inversin recovery turbo FLASH. Magnetic Resonance in Medicine 1996; 36:503-508.
3. Gefter W, Hatabu H, Holland G, Gupta K, Henschke C, Pavelsky H. Pulmonary Thromboembolism: recent developments in diagnosis with CT and MR imaging. Radiology 1995; 197:561-574.
4. Gefter WB, Hatabu H, Dinsmore BJ, Axel L, Palevsky H, Reichik N, Schiebler ML, Kressel HY. Pulmonary vascular cine MR imaging: a noninvasive approach to dynamic imaging of the pulmonary circulation. Radiology 1990; 176(3):761-770.
5. Meaney JFM, Weg JG, Chenevert TL, Stafford-Johnson D, Hamilton BH, Prince MR. Diagnosis of pulmonary embolism with magnetic resonance angiography. The New England Journal Resonance 1997; 336:1422-1427.

Tuberculosis

Jeffrey R. Galvin, MD
Chief, Pulmonary and Mediastinal Imaging
Armed Forces Institute of Pathology
Clinical Professor, Department of Radiology
University of Maryland

Tuberculosis

- Leading cause of death from infectious disease
- 8-10 million new cases/year
- 2-3 million deaths/year
- 1/3 of world population infected
- > 90% of new cases in developing countries
- 80% 15-59 years of age
- Highest incidence
  - Southeast Asia: 247/100,000
  - Sub-Saharan Africa: 191/100,000
    - HIV co-infection: 60% of children, 70% of adults

Tuberculosis
History

- Ancient disease
- 1882: Robert Koch
  - Isolation of *M. tuberculosis*
- 1944: streptomycin
- 1952: INH

Tuberculosis Pre-Antibiotic Era

Tuberculosis
United States

- 1953: 84,304 cases
  - 19,707 deaths
- 1985: 22,201 cases
  - 1,752 deaths
- 1986-1992: 20% increase in reported cases
  - HIV
  - Immigration
  - Congregate settings
  - Deteriorating TB services
  - MDR-TB
  - Decreasing TB research

Tuberculosis
United States

- 2002: 15,075 cases
  - 5.2/100,000
  - 43% decrease from 1992
  - 4-6% of population infected
    - 15 million people
- 51% Foreign-born
  - Mexico, the Philippines, Vietnam, India and China
- U.S. -born
  - African Americans 25% of all cases
  - homeless, immunocompromised, elderly
- Urban areas, coastal states, states bordering Mexico

NMWR,March 21, 2003 Vol 52

Mycobacteria
- Tuberculosis complex
  - ➢ *M. tuberculosis, M. bovis, M. africnum, M. microti*
- *M. tuberculosis* and *M. bovis*
  - ➢ ≥ 95% of pulmonary mycobacterioses
- Slow growth
- Person-to-person transmission

M. tuberculosis
Pathologic features
- Gram positive pleomorphic rod
- Acid fast:
  - ➢ Resists decolorization with acid alcohol
- Virulence related to cell wall
  - ➢ No endotoxin or enzymes
- Caseous necrosis
- Caseating granuloma
  - ➢ Central caseous necrosis
  - ➢ Rim of histiocytes, giant cells

Caseous Necrosis *[Figure 1-9-1]*

Tuberculosis - Pathogenesis
- Inhaled bacteria *[Figures 1-9-2]*
  - ➢ Mid to lower lung zones
  - ➢ Ghon focus

Figure 1-9-2

Initial Infection

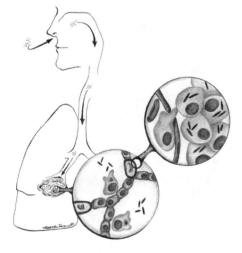

Even though we tend to think of TB as an upper lobe disease, we inhale most bacteria into the mid and lower lung zones

Physiologic Gradients-Airflow FRC

Tuberculosis
Pathogenesis
- Inhaled bacteria
  - ➢ Mid to lower lung zones
  - ➢ Ghon focus
- Regional lymph node spread *[Figures 1-9-3]*
  - ➢ Ranke complex
- Lymphatic/hematogenous dissemination
- Cell-mediated immunity
- Delayed hypersensitivity
  - ➢ Caseous necrosis
  - ➢ 2-10 weeks
- Healing

Figure 1-9-1

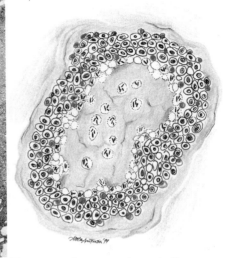

The caseating granuloma is the hallmark of TB. The actively growing bacilli reside in the macrophages in the periphery

Figure 1-9-3

Primary Tuberculosis

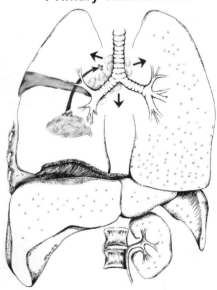

In primary tuberculosis the ineffective macrophages carry bacteria to regional lymph nodes where they proliferate and disseminate

Tuberculosis
Pathogenesis
- Latent TB infection
  - +PPD
  - No active signs of infection
- Survival of organisms *[Figures 1-9-4]*
  - Apical/posterior upper lobe
  - Superior segment lower lobe
    - ✧ Oxygen gradient
    - ✧ Lymphatic gradient
    - ✧ Bucket handle rib motion
- Active TB infection *[Figures 1-9-5]*
  - 5% within 2 years
  - 5-10% lifetime risk
  - HIV: 50% within 2 years
  - Pulmonary fibrotic lesions, underweight, silicosis, DM, renal failure, gastrectomy, jejuno-ileal bypass, transplantation, head and neck cancer, prolonged immunosuppressive therapy

Tuberculosis
Clinical features
- Primary TB
- Postprimary TB
- Disseminated TB

Primary Tuberculosis
Clinical features
- Asymptomatic 65%
  - Nonspecific symptoms when present
- Progressive primary complex
  - Fever, cough, hemoptysis, weight loss
- Pleural effusion

Primary Tuberculosis
Radiologic features
- Lymphadenopathy *[Figure 1-9-6]*
  - Children 95%, young adults 43%, elderly 10%
  - Right paratracheal, hilar
  - Peripheral enhancement, central low-attenuation
- Atelectasis, overinflation
  - Children
  - Anterior segements upper lobes
  - Medial segment middle lobe
- Consolidation
- Pleural effusion
- Consolidation
  - Unifocal 75%
  - Segmental, lobar, multifocal
  - Homogeneous, patchy, linear, nodular
- Pleural effusion
  - Adults 38%, children 11%

Figure 1-9-4

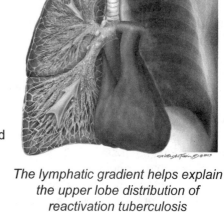

The lymphatic gradient helps explain the upper lobe distribution of reactivation tuberculosis

Figure 1-9-5

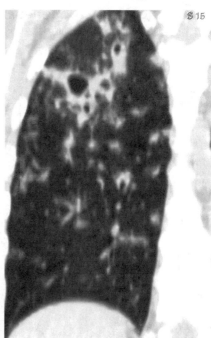

The lymphatic gradient helps explain the upper lobe distribution of reactivation tuberculosis

Figure 1-9-6

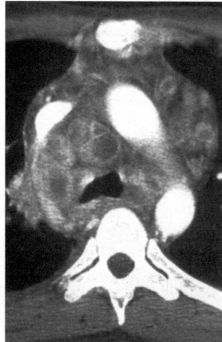

Lymphadenopathy is hallmark of primary TB and is more common in children

Primary Tuberculosis
Radiologic features
- Lymphadenopathy
- Atelectasis, overinflation *[Figure 1-9-7]*
- Consolidation
- Pleural effusion

Leung, Radiology 1999, Vol 210

Primary Tuberculosis Atelectasis

Postprimary Tuberculosis
Clinical Features
- Reactivation
  - ➢ Fever, malaise, anorexia, weight loss, anorexia, night sweats
  - ➢ Dyspnea, cough, chest pain, hemoptysis
- Active TB infection
  - ➢ 5% within 2 years
  - ➢ 5-10% lifetime risk
  - ➢ HIV: 50% within 2 years
  - ➢ Pulmonary fibrotic lesions, underweight, silicosis, DM, renal failure, gastrectomy, jejuno-ileal bypass, transplantation, head and neck cancer, prolonged immunosuppressive therapy

Postprimary Tuberculosis *[Figure 1-9-8 and 1-9-9]*
Pathogenesis
- Delayed hypersensitivity
- Liquifaction
- Cavitation
  - ➢ Airway
  - ➢ Vessel
  - ➢ Pleura

Figure 1-9-7

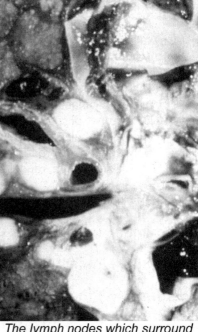

The lymph nodes which surround airways may cause narrowing that results in atelectasis

Figure 1-9-8

Postprimary TB implies reactivation of dormant bacilli. It is characterized by tissue destruction

Figure 1-9-9

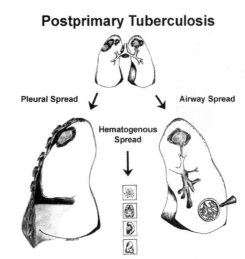

Postprimary Tuberculosis

Pleural Spread

Airway Spread

Hematogenous Spread

Cavitation and necrosis enables spread via the airway, blood stream or pleura

Postprimary Tuberculosis - Radiologic features
- Consolidation 50-70%
- Cavitation 40-45%
- Nodules
- Airways involvement

Postprimary Tuberculosis
Radiologic features
- Consolidation 50-70%
  - ➤ Heterogeneous, nodular, linear
  - ➤ Apical, posterior 85%, Superior segments 14%
- Cavitation 40-45%
  - ➤ Thin or thick walls, air-fluid levels 20%
- Nodules
  - ➤ Tuberculoma
    - ◇ SPN: variable borders, satellite lesions, upper lobes
  - ➤ Endobronchial spread *[Figure 1-9-10]*
    - ◇ Centrilobular, tree-in-bud, 100% by CT
  - ➤ Hematogenous spread
    - ◇ Miliary 1-3mm, random
- Airways involvement
  - ➤ Bronchiectasis, bronchitis, airway narrowing

Postprimary Tuberculosis-Consolidation

Postprimary Tuberculosis-Cavitation

Postprimary Tuberculosis-Tuberculoma

Postprimary Tuberculosis-Nodules *[Figures 1-9-11 and 1-9-12]*

Figure 1-9-10

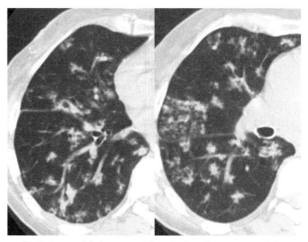

Endobronchial spread leads to airways nodules

Figure 1-9-11

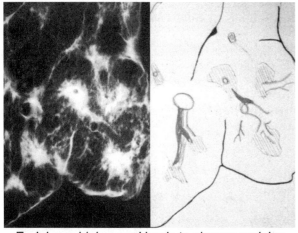

Endobronchial spread leads to airways nodules

Figure 1-9-12

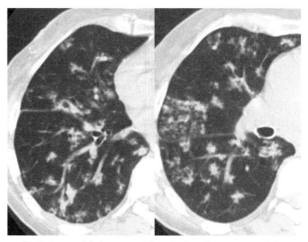

Endobronchial spread leads to airways nodules

Thoracoplasty

Oleothorax

Plumbage *[Figure 1-9-13]*

Postprimary Tuberculosis-Nodules

Postprimary Tuberculosis-Airways

Figure 1-9-13

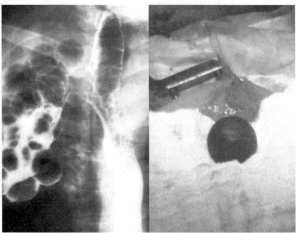

Complication associated with plumbage

Postprimary Tuberculosis
Assessment of Activity
- Cannot discern activity from a single film
- Inactive disease
  - ➢ radiographic stability
  - ➢ 6mos
- Negative cultures
- Suggestive of active disease
  - ➢ Cavitation
  - ➢ Consolidation
  - ➢ Ground glass
  - ➢ Centrilobular opacities

Lee et al, Chest, 1996

Tuberculosis
Complications
- End-stage disease
- Hemoptysis
  - ➢ Bronchial arteries in chronic cavities
  - ➢ Mycetoma
  - ➢ Rassmussen (pulmonary artery) aneurysm
- Chest wall involvement
- Pericardial involvement
- Empyema
  - ➢ BPF, empyema necessitatis

Tuberculosis
Complications
- End-stage disease

Tuberculosis
Complications
- End-stage disease
- Hemoptysis
  - ➢ Bronchial arteries in chronic cavities

Hemoptysis-Bronchial Artery

Tuberculosis
Complications
- End-stage disease
- Hemoptysis
  - ➢ Bronchial arteries in chronic cavities
  - ➢ Mycetoma

Hemoptysis-Mycetoma

Tuberculosis
Complications
- End-stage disease
- Hemoptysis
  - ➢ Bronchial arteries in chronic cavities
  - ➢ Mycetoma
  - ➢ Rassmussen (pulmonary artery) aneurysm

End-Stage Lung

Tuberculosis
Complications
- End-stage disease
- Hemoptysis
  - ➢ Bronchial arteries in chronic cavities
  - ➢ Mycetoma
  - ➢ Rassmussen (pulmonary artery) aneurysm
- Chest wall involvement

Tuberculosis-Chest Wall

Tuberculosis
Complications
- End-stage disease
- Hemoptysis
  - ➢ Bronchial arteries in chronic cavities
  - ➢ Mycetoma
  - ➢ Rassmussen (pulmonary artery) aneurysm
- Chest wall involvement
- Percardial involvement

Tuberculosis-Pericardial

Tuberculosis
Complications
- End-stage disease
- Hemoptysis
  - ➢ Bronchial arteries in chronic cavities
  - ➢ Mycetoma
  - ➢ Rassmussen (pulmonary artery) aneurysm
- Chest wall involvement
- Percardial involvement
- Empyema
  - ➢ BPF, empyema necessitatis

Tuberculosis
HIV/AIDS
- CD4>200
  - ➢ Well formed granulomas
  - ➢ Upper lobe cavities, consolidation and nodules
- CD4<200
  - ➢ Poorly formed granulomas
  - ➢ Adenopathy, consolidation and miliary disease
- CD4<60
  - ➢ No hypersensitivity reaction
  - ➢ Organisms spread from GI tract
  - ➢ Miliary Disease

Tuberculosis and AIDS

Tuberculosis and AIDS-Low CD4

Tuberculosis
Diagnosis
- Conventional methods
  - ➢ Acid-fast smear: 1 day
  - ➢ Culture: 1-2 weeks
  - ➢ Identification: 2-3 weeks
  - ➢ Drug susceptibility testing: 3-4 weeks
- Radiometric methods
- Polymerase chain reaction (PCR)
- HPLC

Summary

- Primary TB
  - ➢ Consolidation
  - ➢ Ipsilateral lymphadenopathy
  - ➢ Pleural effusion
- Postprimary TB
  - ➢ Consolidation
  - ➢ Cavitation
  - ➢ Apical/posterior upper lobe nodules
  - ➢ Tracheobronchial spread

Tuberculosis Pre-Antibiotic Era

Fungal Disease in the Thorax: Opportunistic and Primary Pathogens

Jeffrey R. Galvin, MD
Chief Pulmonary and Mediastinal Radiology
Armed Forces Institute of Pathology
Clinical Professor Department of Radiology
University of Maryland

Fungal Disease in the Thorax
Overview
- Opportunistic invaders
  - ➢ Aspergillus species
  - ➢ Candida
  - ➢ Mucormycosis
- Primary pathogens
  - ➢ Histoplasma capsulatum
  - ➢ Blastomyces dermatitidis
  - ➢ Coccidioides immitis

Opportunistic Invaders
- Immunocompromised host
  - ➢ Mucosal disruption
  - ➢ Reduced cellular and/or humoral immunity
- Ubiquitous
- Lack dimorphism
- Multiple organisms may occur

Primary Pathogens
- May infect healthy individuals
- Dimorphism
  - ➢ Saprophytes in the soil
  - ➢ Spores via germination
- Most disease mild or subclinical
- Fulminant or chronic disease may occur
- Specific geographic regions
  - ➢ Endemic

Coccidioidomycosis

Blastomycosis

Histoplasmosis

Histoplasmosis
Epidemiology and Ecology
- Endemic fungal disease
  - ➢ Ohio, Mississippi and St. Lawrence river valleys
  - ➢ Reported worldwide but relatively rare outside of the United States
  - ➢ Infection rate up to 95% in endemic areas
  - ➢ Point sources associated with aerosolization
    - ✧ Earth moving, bird husbandry and spelunking
- Dimorphic fungus
- Clinical

Histoplasmosis
Epidemiology and Ecology
- Endemic fungal disease
- Dimorphic fungus
  - Mycelial form in high nitrogen soil
    - Guano from birds and bats
  - Yeast within the infected host
- Clinical

Histoplasmosis [Figure 1-10-1]

Histoplasmosis
Pathology [Figure 1-10-2]
- Early sequence of infection
  - Mycelia produce micronidia
  - Micronidia reach alveolar spaces
    - 2-5 microns

Figure 1-10-1

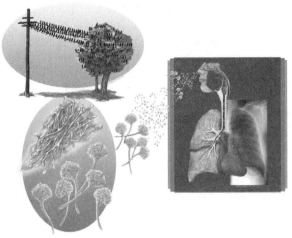

The mycelial form of Histoplasmosis is found in soil that has been enriched with bird droppings. The fungus then releases conidia or spores

Figure 1-10-2

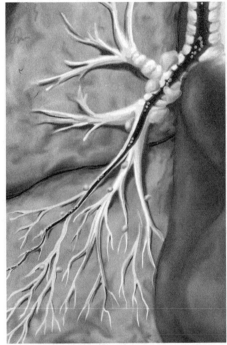

The fungal spores are able to reach the alveolar level, bypassing the upper airway defenses because of their small size which is less than 5 microns

Figure 1-10-3

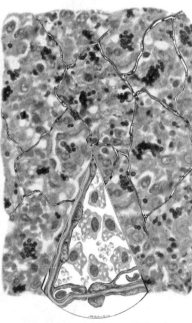

From three to 5 days following inhalation the spores germinate and release yeast forms. The yeast within the alveoli are rapidly phagacytosed by macrophages

Figure 1-10-4

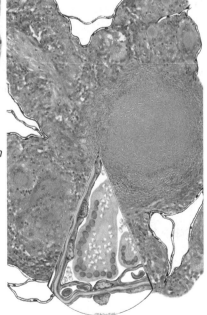

Lymphocyte-mediated cellular immunity develops at 10-14 days controlling the infection through a necrotizing granulomatous response

Histoplasmosis]
Pathology [Figure 1-10-3 and 1-10-4]
- Early sequence of infection
  - Lymphocytes and macrophages replace polys
  - Micronidia transform to conidia or spores
  - Spores transform into budding yeast
  - Macrophages phagocytose and kill yeast
- Late sequence of infection
  - Lymphocyte-mediated cellular immunity
  - Granulomatous inflammation
  - Necrosis
  - Fibrosis

Histoplasmosis
Pathology

- Distinction from tuberculosis
  - ➢ Histoplasmosis relatively benign
  - ➢ Immunity to histoplasmosis short lived
    - ✧ 20% lose immunity each year
    - ✧ Continuous reinfection
      - – Primary and postprimary not appropriate

Histoplasmosis
Clinical

- Asymptomatic
  - ➢ 95-99% of infection in endemic areas
  - ➢ Parenchymal opacities in 10-25%
  - ➢ Small inoculum or prior infection (cellular immunity) and moderate inoculum
- Symptomatic
  - ➢ Acute
    - ✧ Moderate vs large inoculum
  - ➢ Chronic
  - ➢ Disseminated
- Late complications
  - ➢ Histoplasmoma
  - ➢ Broncholithiasis
  - ➢ Mediastinal granuloma
  - ➢ Medistinal fibrosis

Histoplasmosis
Acute Clinical

- Signs and symptoms
  - ➢ "Flulike": fever, chills, cough
  - ➢ Retrosternal pain
    - ✧ Mediastinal lymph node involvement
  - ➢ Erythema nodosum in women
  - ➢ Arthralgia
- Shorter incubation with prior exposure

Histoplasmosis
Acute Radiology

- Poorly defined areas of consolidation
  - ✧ Single or multiple
- Hilar lymph node enlargement
- Numerous discrete nodular shadows in heavy exposure
  - ✧ 3-4 mm
  - ✧ Symptoms precede radiographic change
  - ✧ Nodules change to punctate calcifications

Acute Histoplasmosis [Figure 1-10-5]

Acute Histoplasmosis – large inoculum

Acute Histoplasmosis [Figure 1-10-6]

Figure 1-10-5

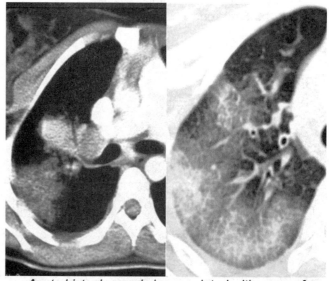

Acute histoplasmosis is associated with areas of consolidation and ipsilateral hilar and mediastinal enlargement

Figure 1-10-6

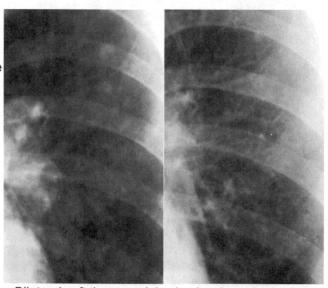

Bilateral soft tissue nodules imply a large innoculum. The nodules disappear over months leaving behind small calcific densities

Histoplasmosis
Chronic Pulmonary Histoplasmosis

- Emphysema and bullous disease a common predisposition
- Upper lobe predominance
- Two possible mechanisms
  - ➤ Hypersensitivity reaction in preexisting emphysematous space
    - ✧ Few organisms
    - ✧ Colonization or minimal invasion
    - ✧ Thick walled bulla filled with fluid may clear spontaneously
    - ✧ Progressive loss of volume
  - ➤ Similar to TB
    - ✧ Fibrosis, cavitation and granulomatous inflammation

Chronic Histoplasmosis [Figure 1-10-7]

Histoplasmosis
Disseminated
- Clinical
  - ➤ Rare entity (1/100,000-1/500,000)
  - ➤ Most patients immunocompromised
    - ✧ 30% infants < 2 years
    - ✧ 20% immunocompromised
    - ✧ 50% apparently normal (transient compromise)
  - ➤ Reduced macrophage function
    - ✧ Parasitization of macrophages
    - ✧ Intracellular survival and multiplication
  - ➤ Radiology
    - ✧ Miliary nodules (1-3 mm)
    - ✧ 50% of disease associated with AIDS purely extrathoracic
      - – Normal radiograph
      - – Positive blood or bone marrow biopsy

Disseminated Histoplasmosis [Figure 1-10-8]

Histoplasmosis
Late Complications
- Histoplasmoma
- Broncholithiasis
- Mediastinal granuloma
- Mediastinal fibrosis

Histoplasmosis
Histoplasmoma
- Solitary nodule (.5-3 cm)
  - ➤ Sharply defined
  - ➤ Smaller satellite lesions
  - ➤ Central or diffuse calcification
    - ✧ Diagnostic of benign lesion if less that 3 cm
  - ➤ May increase in size
    - ✧ Similar reaction to fibrosing mediastinitis
- Hilar calcification common on ipsilateral side
- Fungal nodules account for 30% of all solitary nodules
- 87% are less than 2.5 cm in diameter

Figure 1-10-7

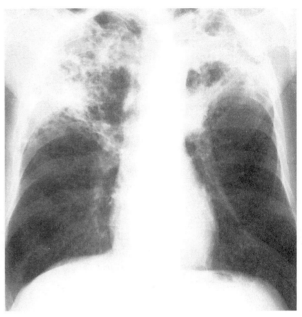

Chronic histoplasmosis resembles post-primary TB but usually represents a hypersensitivity reaction in patients with emphysema

Figure 1-10-8

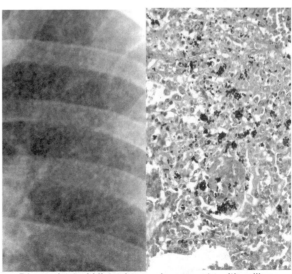

Disseminated Histoplasmosis presents with miliary nodules and macrophages filled with organisms

Histoplasmoma [Figure 1-10-9]

Figure 1-10-9

Broncholith

Histoplasmosis
Mediastinal granuloma

- Pathology
  - ➤ Direct infection of hilar and mediastinal lymph nodes
- Clinical
  - ➤ Often asypmtomatic with discovery of a mediastinal mass on chest radiograph
  - ➤ SVC or esophageal obstruction less common
- Radiology
  - ➤ Middle mediastinal mass
    - ✧ Subcarinal or paratracheal
  - ➤ Enhancing capsule with low attenuation center
  - ➤ Mass may be low signal on T2 weighted MR because of fibrous tissue or calcification

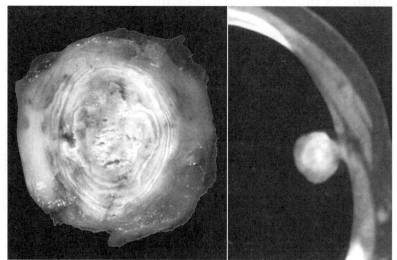

Histoplasmomas are the residua of a prior area of pneumonitis. They typically demonstrate concentric rings of calcification but may remain uncalcified especially in older individuals

Figure 1-10-10

Mediastinal Granuloma [Figure 1-10-10]

Histoplasmosis
Fibrosing Mediastinitis

- Pathology
  - ➤ Proliferation of acellular collagen and fibrous tissue within the mediastinum
  - ➤ Most cases in the United States are an immunological response to H. capsulatum
    - ✧ Focal form: paratracheal and subcarinal
    - ✧ Calcification
  - ➤ Idiopathic form
    - ✧ Diffuse, infiltrating
    - ✧ Noncalcified
    - ✧ Multiple mediastinal compartments
- Clinical
  - ➤ Signs and symptoms of obstruction to mediastinal structures
    - ✧ Superior vena cava, pulmonary veins or arteries, central airway or esophagus

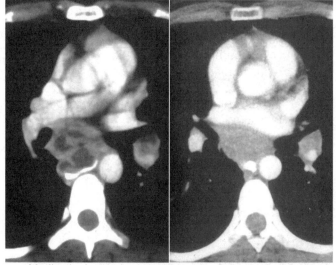

Mediastinal granuloma is the result of direct infection of mediastinal lymph nodes. Acutely the lymph nodes demonstrate low attenuation with an enhancing capsule

Fibrosing Mediastinitis

Blastomycosis

Blastomycosis
Epidemiology and Ecology

- Ecological niche
  - ➤ Difficult to establish
  - ➤ Saprophyte in an unidentified resevoir within reach of man and dogs
  - ➤ Survives only in wet soil with a high PH and high organic content
  - ➤ Soil probably contaminated rather than the natural resevoir
  - ➤ Point sources in dead and decaying material near rivers, streams and swamps
- Dimorphic fungus
- Clinical

Blastomycosis
Epidemiology and Ecology

- Ecological niche
- Dimorphic fungus
  - Mycelium in natural habitat
  - Releases spores (conidia) into the air
  - Budding yeast
    - (8-15 microns) in vivo
    - Broad based
- Clinical

Blastomycosis
Epidemiology and Ecology

- Ecological niche difficult to establish
- Dimorphic fungus
- Clinical
  - Less common than Histoplasmosis
  - High risk of symptomatic disease although most cases are probably asymptomatic
  - Males more commonly affected (3:1-15:1)
  - Exposure in heavily wooded areas
  - Variable course
    - Symptoms of acute pneumonia
      - Abrupt onset, fever, chills, cough and pleuritic pain
      - Occasional rapid progression
        - Hematogenous dissemination: skin, bone and genitourinary tract
        - ARDS
    - Chronic disease similar to tuberculosis

Blastomycosis
Pathology

- Initial inflammatory response is neutrophilic
  - Small collections of cells to hundreds of milliliters of pus
- Rapidly followed by chronic inflammatory response
  - Lymphocyte, histiocytes and plasma cells
  - Langhans' giant cells
  - Granulomas
- Both responses may coexist
  - Organisms more common in supperative area
- Progression
  - Coalescence of patchy consolidation
  - Airway perforation
  - Cavitation
- Ulcerative bronchitis is common

Blastomycosis
Pathology

- Initial response is neutrophilic
- Chronic inflammatory response
- Both responses may coexist
- Progression
  - Coalescence of patchy consolidation
  - Airway perforation
  - Cavitation
- Ulcerative bronchitis is common

Blastomycosis
Radiologic Manifestations
- Consolidation most common
  - Upper lobe 2:1
  - Rounded, ill-defined
  - Masslike opacities
    - Central or paramediastinal
    - Carinoma mimic
    - Solitary nodules
  - Air bronchograms (88% CT)
  - Cavitation
- Nodules
  - Intermediate size
  - Remote from consolidation
  - Satellite lesions
- Miliary disease
  - Hematogenous dissemination

Asymptomatic Mass

Consolidation

Solitary Pulmonary Nodule

Similar to Postprimary TB

Disseminated Disease

Mass and Dissemination

Blastomycosis
Treatment
- Pulmonary disease may be self-limited even if extensive
- Extrapulmonary disease requires treatment
- Amphotericin B IV or oral Keotconazole

Coccidioidomycosis
Epidemiology and Ecology
- Ecological niche
- Dimorphic fungus
- Clinical
  - Acute Disease
    - 100,000 new cases each year, essentially all in the southwest
    - No racial, sex or age predilection in acute disease
    - Most inhabitants of the endemic area infected in the first year of exposure
    - Incubation period 10-16 days
    - 60% are asymptomatic
    - Symptoms when present include
      - Fever, pleuritic chest pain, cough
      - Valley Fever: allergic form with erythema nodosum or multiforme
    - Severity of disease related to immune status and race
      - Filipinos, African Americans and Hispanics more likely to suffer dissemination

Coccidioidomycosis
Epidemiology and Ecology
- Ecological niche
- Dimorphic fungus
- Clinical
  - Chronic Disease (5%)
    - Symptoms persist without dissemination
    - May be mildly immunocompromised
  - Dissemination
    - Rare occurrence
      - Immunocompromise
      - Non-Caucasian (Filipino, African American and Hispanic)
      - Early dissemination more common and carries a poor prognosis
      - Mortality rate or 50% even with early treatment

Coccidioidomycosis
Pathology
- Lung the usual portal of entry
- Neutrophilic response early
  - Especially in response to ruptured spherules
  - Spherules ingested by macrophages

Coccidioidomycosis
Pathology
- Lung the usual portal of entry
- Neutrophilic response early
  - Especially in response to ruptured spherules
  - Spherules ingested by macrophages
- Granulomatous and giant cell reaction follows
- Necrosis may occur

Coccidioidomycosis
Radiologic Manifestations
- Acute Disease
  - Consolidation most common (75%)
    - Usually unilateral, hilar or basal
    - Segmental or lobar
  - Multifocal nodular or patchy opacities
  - Peribronchiolar thickening
  - Hilar or mediastinal adenopathy (20%)
    - Mediastinal adenopathy may herald dissemination
  - Pleural effusion 20%
    - Small, unilateral
- Coccidioidoma

Acute Disease

Coccidioidoma

Coccidioidomycosis
Radiologic Manifestations
- Acute Disease
- Coccidioidoma
  - Area of prior consolidation
  - Round and well circumscribed
  - 1.5cm average (up to 6cm)
  - Usually single
  - Marked enhancement with contrast CT
  - Caseating chronic granulomatous inflammation

Coccidioidomycosis
Radiologic Manifestations
- Chronic Disease
  - ➤ Cavitation
    - ✧ Occur in areas of consolidation
    - ✧ May be thin or thick walled
    - ✧ Pneumothorax or empyema may result
  - ➤ Chronic progressive pneumonia

Chronic Coccidioidomycosis

Coccidioidomycosis
Radiologic Manifestations
- Chronic Disease
  - ➤ Cavitation
  - ➤ Chronic progressive pneumonia
    - ✧ Indolent course similar to TB
    - ✧ Biapical fibronodular lesions
    - ✧ Hilar and mediastinal adenopathy
    - ✧ Hilar retraction
    - ✧ Persistently positive sputum
    - ✧ High complement fixing antibody titer
    - ✧ Non-Caucasian

Coccidioidomycosis
Radiologic Manifestations
- Disseminated Disease
  - ➤ Miliary or reticular nodular pattern
    - ✧ Less well circumscribed that TB
  - ➤ Lymphadenopathy is common
  - ➤ Pericardial effusion
  - ➤ Skin, bone, meninges or upper genitourinary tract

Dissemination – Miliary Nodules

Histoplasmosis

Acute Histoplasmosis: Figure 1-10-11
Symptomatic patients with acute histoplasmosis may present with solitary or multifocal areas of consolidation and associated adenopathy

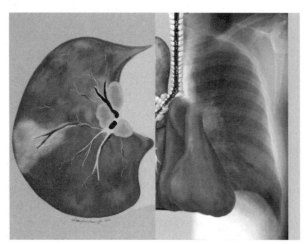

Histoplasmosis – Solitary Nodule : Figures 1-10-12 and 1-10-13

As the infection heals the inflammatory area rounds up and is surrounded by a fibrous capsule. Over a prolonged period calcification may develop in the nodule and regional lymph nodes

The nodule may enlarge by adding fibrous tissue to the periphery

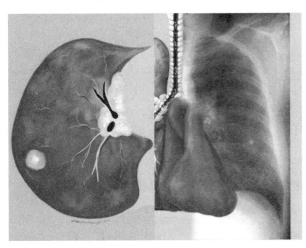

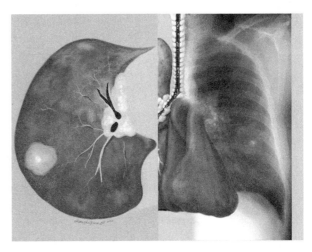

Histoplasmosis – large inoculum: Figure 1-10-14

If the patient inhales a large number of spores then numerous patches of consolidation may round up into well circumscribed nodules

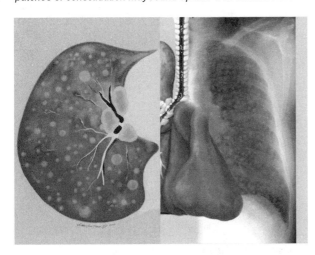

Histoplasmosis: Figure 1-10-15

As they heal the patient will be left with numerous calcifications

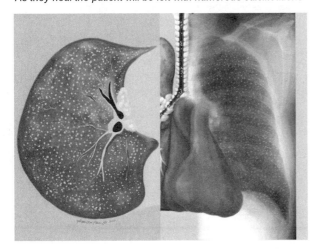

Disseminated Histoplasmosis: Figure 1-10-16

Patients with reduced immune function may present with
hematogenous spread of disease and miliary nodules

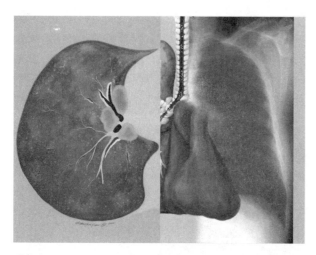

Chronic Histoplasmosis: Figure 1-10-17

Patients with underlying emphysema may develop chronic histoplasmosis which in most cases
represents a hypersensitivity reaction to a small number of organisms

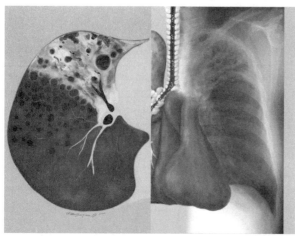

Fibrosing Mediastinitis: Figure 1-10-18

Fibrosing mediastinitis represents an exuberant fibrous reaction within the mediastinum which may
result in damage to mediastinal structures. Most focal cases of fibrosing mediastintis in the United
States are due to H. capsulatum

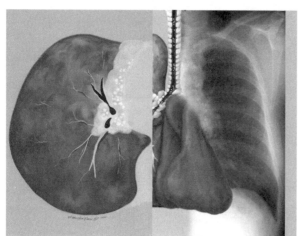

Blastomycosis

Coccidioidomycosis

Fungal Disease in the Thorax
Overview
- Opportunistic invaders
  - Aspergillus species
  - Candida
  - Mucormycosis
- Primary pathogens
  - Histoplasma capsulatum
  - Blastomyces dermatitidis
  - Coccidioides immitis
  - Paracoccidioides brasiliensis

Bronchogenic Carcinoma Radiologic–Pathologic Correlation

Jeffrey R. Galvin, MD
Chief, Pulmonary and Mediastinal Radiology
Armed Forces Institute of Pathology
and
Clinical Professor Department of Radiology
University of Maryland

A 20th Century Disaster

Histological Classification of Tumors
- World Health Organization
- Lung tumor editions
  - 1967
  - 1981
  - 1999
- Improve communication
- Consistent treatment
- Basis for comparative studies
- Prognosis

What's New in the 1999 WHO?
- Subclasses of adenomas
- Preinvasive lesions
- Adenocarcinoma
- Definition of BAC
- Neuroendocrine tumors
- Biphasic and pleomorphic tumors

Incidence of Lung Cancer

Histological Typing of Lung Tumors
- Based on light microscopic criteria
- Classified by the best differentiated region
- Graded by the most poorly differentiated region
- Histologic heterogeneity is the "rule"

Histological Typing of Lung Tumors
- Prognosis: Small cell vs. non-small cell
- Stage determines prognosis in non small cell
- >95% of 1° lung tumors
  - Adeno
  - Squamous
  - Large cell
  - Small cell
  - Combination of above

Lung Cancer Demographics
- Most common cancer in males world-wide
- Leading cause of cancer mortality in women and men (United States)
- Mortality rates in women began increasing in 1935 and surpassed breast ca in 1987

Age-Adjusted Cancer Death Rates – Males vs Females

Age-Adjusted Cancer Incidence – Females

Lung Cancer Etiology – Cigarette smoking
- 85-90% of lung cancer deaths
- 25% of lung cancer in non-smokers attributed to passive smoke
- Risk related to:
  - Number of cigarettes smoked
  - Depth of inhalation
  - Age at which smoking began

Clinical Presentation
- Central tumors
  - Cough
  - Wheezing
  - Hemoptysis
  - Pneumonia
- Extrapulmonary invasion
  - Pain
  - Pancoast Syndrome
  - SVC Syndrome
- Metastases
- Paraneoplastic Syndromes
- Asymptomatic 10%

Paraneoplastic Syndromes
- Cachexia, malaise and fever
- Ectopic hormone production
  - ACTH
  - ADH
  - Hypercalcemia
- Clubbing and HPO
- Thrombotic endocarditis
  - Non-bacterial
- Migratory thrombophlebitis

Lung Cancer and Clotting

Squamous Cell Carcinoma
- Terminology
  - Squamous
    - ✧ Flattened cells
  - Epidermoid
    - ✧ Mimics differentiation of the epidermis
- Rapid local growth
- Distant metastases later
- Strong association
  - Cigarette smoking

Squamous Cell Carcinoma
- Pancoast Syndrome
- Hyperparathyroidism
  - Parathyroid-like substance
- Most common to present as radiographically occult

Preinvasive Lesions – Squamous Dysplasia
- Similar to cervical Ca
- Squamous metaplasia
- Progression
  - ➤ Dysplastic epithelium
- Carcinoma in situ
  - ➤ Full thickness dysplasia
- Precursor
  - ➤ Invasive squamous cell Ca

Squamous Cell Carcinoma – Microscopic features
- Individual cell keratinization
  - ➤ Eosinophilia
- Keratin pearls
  - ➤ Well differentiated tumors
- Intercellular bridges

Squamous Cell Carcinoma – Gross Features [Figure 1-11-1]
- Central lesion
  - ➤ Polypoid, endobronchial, exophytic growth
- Central necrosis common
- Bronchial wall invasion
  - ➤ Common
  - ➤ Positive cytology
- Proximal growth
  - ➤ Along bronchial mucosa

Squamous Cell Carcinoma – Radiologic Features
- Hilar or perihilar mass
- Bronchial wall thickening
  - ➤ Often focal
- Consolidation
  - ➤ Must clear completely
- Atelectasis
- Peripheral nodule or mass
  - ➤ 30%
- Cavitation

Atelectasis [Figures 1-11-2 and 1-11-3]

Figure 1-11-1

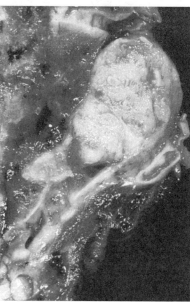

The majority of squamous cell cancers are central lesions

Figure 1-11-2

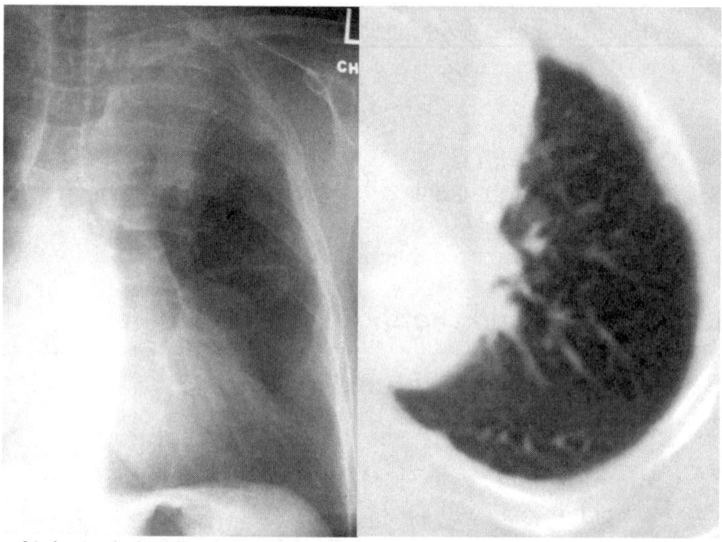

Atelectasis in an adult smoker is lung cancer until proven otherwise

Figure 1-11-3

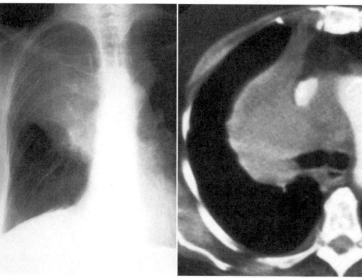

Golden's S sign

Cavitation [Figure 1-11-4]

Pancoast Tumor – Superior Sulcus Tumor
- Characteristic pain
  - 8th cervical
  - 2nd thoracic trunk
- Horner's Syndrome
- Destruction of bone
- Hand muscle atrophy

Pancoast, JAMA, 1992

Small Cell Lung Cancer
- Rapid growth
- Considered metastatic at presentation
- Poorest survival
- Strongest association with cigarette smoking

Small Cell Lung Cancer
- Small cell carcinoma
  - Pure histology
- Variant
  - Combined
- Elimination
  - Oat cell
  - Intermediate type

WHO, 1999

Small Cell Lung Cancer: Microscopic Features
- Small, uniform cells
- Scant cytoplasm
- Necrosis is common
  - Often extensive
- 10 mitosis per 10 HPF
  - Average 60-70
- Neuroendocrine morphology
- Neuroendocrine markers
  - 75%
- Light microscopy diagnosis

Small Cell Lung Cancer – Gross Features [Figure 1-11-5]
- Large
- Central mass (90%)
- Bronchial compression
- No endobronchial lesion
- Proximal growth
  - Along submucosa
- Extensive necrosis
- Hemorrhage

Figure 1-11-4

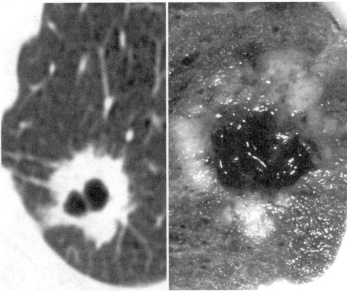

Cavitation is most common in squamous cell cancer

Figure 1-11-5

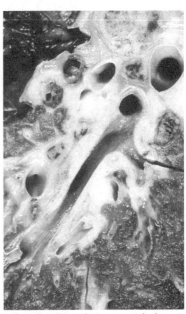

Small cell tends to spread along the peribronchovascular lymphatics

Small Cell Lung Cancer – Radiologic Features [Figure 1-11-6]

- Hilar or perihilar mass
- Mediastinal adenopathy
- Primary tumor
  - Rarely evident
- Cavitation
  - Extremely rare

Small Cell Lung Cancer

- Cushing Syndrome
- SIADH
- Eaton Lambert
- Most common cause
  - SVC Syndrome

Small Cell Lung Cancer – Therapy

- Response to chemotherapy and radiotherapy
- Untreated: median survival 2-4 months
- Treated: median survival 9-18 months
- Limited stage – 15-25% survive 2 years

Figure 1-11-6

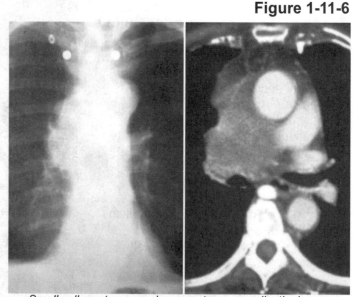

Small cell most commonly presents as a mediastinal mass

Large Cell Carcinoma

- Rapid growth
- Location
  - Segmental
  - Subsegmental
- Early metastases
- Poor prognosis
- Strong association with cigarette smoking

Large Cell Carcinoma – Microscopic Features

- Large cells
- Prominent nucleoli
- Poorly differentiated
- Diagnosis of exclusion
- Neuroendocrine features

Large Cell Carcinoma – Gross Features

- Large and bulky
  - Greater that 3 cm
- Soft
- Large areas of necrosis

Figure 1-11-7

Large Cell Carcinoma – Radiologic Features

- Usually peripheral
- 70% of tumors
  - > 4 cm at presentation

Large Cell Carcinoma [Figure 1-11-7]

Adenocarcinoma – Etiology

- Cigarette smoke causatively linked to lung cancer
  - 1950
  - Squamous cell 18X's Adeno
  - Squamous cell: central

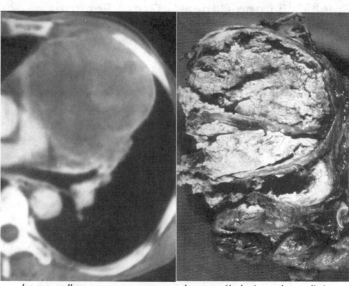

Large cell cancers are commonly necrotic but rarely cavitate

Adenocarcinoma – Etiology [Figure 1-11-8]

- Cigarette smoke causatively linked to lung cancer
- Adenocarcinoma most common
  - ➢ Peripheral
- Filtered low-yield cigarettes
  - ➢ Smaller particles
  - ➢ Reduced nicotine
  - ➢ Greater depth of puffs
  - ➢ Increased number of puffs
  - ➢ N-nitrosamines
- Other factors - 10%
  - ➢ Passive smoke
  - ➢ Particulates
  - ➢ Cooking practices

Adenocarcinoma – Microscopic Features

- Glands
- Papillary structures
- Mucin
  - ➢ Intracellular
  - ➢ Extracellular
- Prominent nucleoli
- Moderate cytoplasm
- Desmoplastic reaction
- "Scar carcinoma"
  - ➢ Rare!

Adenocarcinoma – Radiologic Features

- Peripheral (75%)
- Solitary mass or nodule
- Upper lobes 3:2
- Right lung 3:2
- Lobulated
- Borders
  - ➢ Ill-defined
  - ➢ Well-defined
- Spiculated
- Obstructive pneumonitis (25%)

Spiculation and Retraction [Figure 1-11-9]

Scar Carcinoma [Figure 1-11-10]

Figure 1-11-8

Adenocarinoma, the most common lung cancer is predominantly a peripheral lesion

Figure 1-11-9

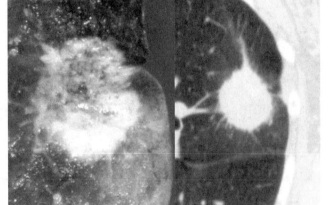

Adenocarinomas are commonly spiculated peripheral nodules

Figure 1-11-10

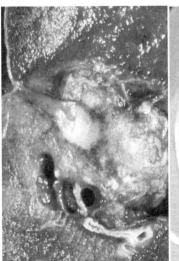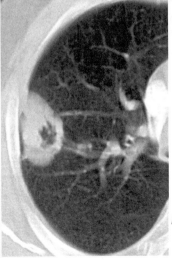

In scar carcinomas the scar is usually a reaction to the malignancy

Necrosis

Air Bronchogram *[Figure 1-11-11]*

Slow Growth

Atypical Adenomatous Hyperplasia – Preinvasive lesion
- Atypical cuboidal epithelium
  - ➢ Lining alveoli
  - ➢ Lining bronchioles
- Found in lung cancer resection specimens
- Probable precursor
  - ➢ BAC
  - ➢ Invasive adenocarcinoma
- Patchy ground glass
- 5mm or less

Kitamura, AJCP, 1999

AAH

Bronchioloalveolar Carcinoma – Microscopic Features
- Lepidic growth pattern
- No evidence
  - ➢ Stromal invasion
  - ➢ Vascular invasion
  - ➢ Pleural invasion
- Diagnosis cannot be made on a small biopsy
- Requires thorough sampling of resected specimen

WHO, 1999

Bronchioloalveolar Carcinoma – Mucinous Type
- Alveolar spaces distended with mucin
- Aerogenous spread is common
- Multifocal consolidation

Bronchioloalveolar Carcinoma – Non-mucinous Type
- Alveoli lined with
  - ➢ Clara cells
  - ➢ Type II cells
- Central alveolar fibrosis
  - ➢ Common
- Close association
  - ➢ AAH

Bronchioloalveolar Carcinoma – Gross Features
[Figure 1-11-12]
- Consolidation
  - ➢ Focal
  - ➢ Multifocal
- Architecture
  - ➢ Preserved

Figure 1-11-11

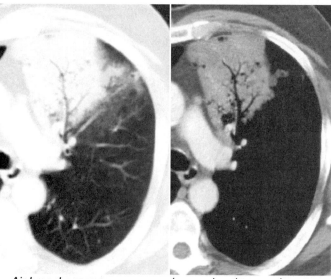

Air bronchograms are commonly seen in adenocarcinomas

Figure 1-11-12

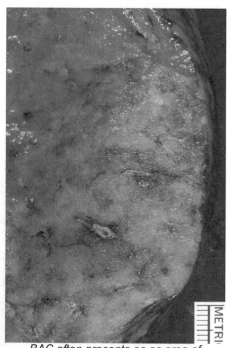

BAC often presents as as area of consolidation

Bronchioloalveolar Carcinoma – Radiologic Features
- Solitary nodule
  - ➢ Excellent prognosis
  - ➢ Resection
- Consolidation
  - ➢ May be multifocal
- Ground glass
- Multiple nodules
- May cavitate?

Noguchi, Cancer 1995

Bronchioloalveolar Carcinoma

BAC Recurrence

BAC vs Adenocarcinoma

BAC - Adenocarcinoma – CT, Histology and Doubling Time
- Type A
- Ground glass
- Localized BAC
- Doubling time
  - ➢ Mean: 880 days
  - ➢ Range: 662-1486 days

Aoki et al, AJR, 2000

BAC - Adenocarcinoma – CT, Histology and Doubling Time
- Type B
- Ground glass
- Focal increased attenuation
- Localized BAC
- Doubling time
  - ➢ Mean: 880 days
  - ➢ Range: 662-1486 days

Aoki et al, AJR, 2000

BAC - Adenocarcinoma – CT, Histology and Doubling Time
- Type C
- Solid attenuation
- Focal ground glass
- Spiculation
- Pleural tag
- Localized BAC
  - ➢ Active fibroblastic proliferation
- Doubling time
  - ➢ Range: 42-1346 days

Aoki et al, AJR, 2000

Aoki et al, AJR, 2000

BAC - Adenocarcinoma – CT, Histology and Doubling Time
- Type D
- Solid attenuation only
- Spiculation
- Pleural tag
- Poorly differentiated adenocarcinoma
- Doubling time
  - ➢ Mean: 252 days
  - ➢ Range: 124-402 days

Aoki et al, AJR, 2000

AdenoCa Appearance and Prognosis

Adenocarcinoma

BAC

AAH [Figure 1-11-13]

BAC [Figure 1-11-14]

Adenocarcinoma - BAC Prognosis [Figure 1-11-15]

Figure 1-11-13

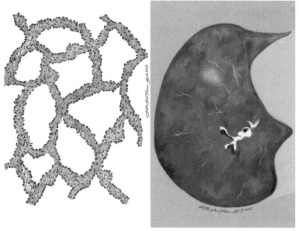

The precursor lesion to BAC is AAH

Figure 1-11-14

BAC demonstrates lepidic growth and presents as an area of ground glass and/or consolidation

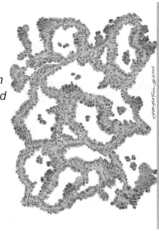
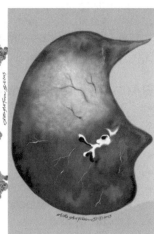

Figure 1-11-15

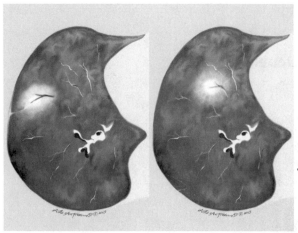

Survival decreases with increasing amount of consolidation and less ground glass opacity

Bronchogenic Carcinoma Bibliography

1. Travis W, Colby T, Shimasato Y, Brambilla E. Histological Typing of Lung and Pleural Tumors., International Classification of Tumors. Third ed. Berlin: Springer Verlag, 1999.
2. Colby T, Koss M, Travis W. Tumors of the Lower Respiratory Tract, Atlas of Tumor Pathology. Third ed. Washington, DC: Armed Forces Institute of Pathology, 1999.
3. Patel AM, Peters SG. Clinical manifestations of lung cancer. Mayo Clin Proc 1993; 68(3):273-7.
4. Davila DG, Williams DE. The etiology of lung cancer. Mayo Clin Proc 1993; 68(2):170-82.
5. Travis WD, Lubin J, Ries L, Devesa S. United States lung carcinoma incidence trends: declining for most histologic types among males, increasing among females. Cancer 1996; 77(12):2464-70.
6. Travis WD, Travis LB, Devesa SS. Lung cancer [published erratum appears in Cancer 1995 Jun 15;75(12):2979]. Cancer 1995; 75(1 Suppl):191-202.
7. Pisani RJ. Bronchogenic carcinoma: immunologic aspects. Mayo Clin Proc 1993; 68(4):386-92.
8. Whitesell PL, Drage CW. Occupational lung cancer. Mayo Clin Proc 1993; 68(2):183-8.
9. Patel AM, Davila DG, Peters SG. Paraneoplastic syndromes associated with lung cancer [see comments]. Mayo Clin Proc 1993; 68(3):278-87.
10. Morabia A, Wynder EL. Cigarette smoking and lung cancer cell types. Cancer 1991; 68(9):2074-8.
11. Ko YC, Lee CH, Chen MJ, Huang CC, Chang WY, Lin HJ, Wang HZ, Chang PY. Risk factors for primary lung cancer among non-smoking women in Taiwan. Int J Epidemiol 1997; 26(1):24-31.
12. Kitamura H, Kameda Y, Ito T, Hayashi H. Atypical adenomatous hyperplasia of the lung. Implications for the pathogenesis of peripheral lung adenocarcinoma [see comments]. Am J Clin Pathol 1999; 111(5):610-22.
13. Karsell PR, McDougall JC. Diagnostic tests for lung cancer. Mayo Clin Proc 1993; 68(3):288-96.
14. Dalager NA, Pickle LW, Mason TJ, Correa P, Fontham E, Stemhagen A, Buffler PA, Ziegler RG, Fraumeni JF, Jr. The relation of passive smoking to lung cancer. Cancer Res 1986; 46(9):4808-11.
15. Charloux A, Hedelin G, Dietemann A, Ifoundza T, Roeslin N, Pauli G, Quoix E. Prognostic value of histology in patients with non-small cell lung cancer. Lung Cancer 1997; 17(1):123-34.
16. Charloux A, Quoix E, Wolkove N, Small D, Pauli G, Kreisman H. The increasing incidence of lung adenocarcinoma: reality or artefact? A review of the epidemiology of lung adenocarcinoma. Int J Epidemiol 1997; 26(1):14-23.
17. Muller NL, Miller RR. Neuroendocrine carcinomas of the lung. Semin Roentgenol 1990; 25(1):96-104.
18. Travis WD, Rush W, Flieder DB, Falk R, Fleming MV, Gal AA, Koss MN. Survival analysis of 200 pulmonary neuroendocrine tumors with clarification of criteria for atypical carcinoid and its separation from typical carcinoid. Am J Surg Pathol 1998; 22(8):934-44.
19. Hardy J, Smith I, Cherryman G, Vincent M, Judson I, Perren T, Williams M. The value of computed tomographic (CT) scan surveillance in the detection and management of brain metastases in patients with small cell lung cancer. Br J Cancer 1990; 62(4):684-6.
20. Sone S, Takashima S, Li F, Yang Z, Honda T, Maruyama Y, Hasegawa M, Yamanda T, Kubo K, Hanamura K, Asakura K. Mass screening for lung cancer with mobile spiral computed tomography scanner [see comments]. Lancet 1998; 351(9111):1242-5.

Chest Seminar 1

Jeffrey R. Galvin, MD
Chief Pulmonary and Mediastinal Radiology
Armed Forces Institute of Pathology
Clinical Professor Department of Radiology
University of Maryland

Case1: This 57 year old male with a long history of smoking cigarettes.
He now complains of and a chronic cough

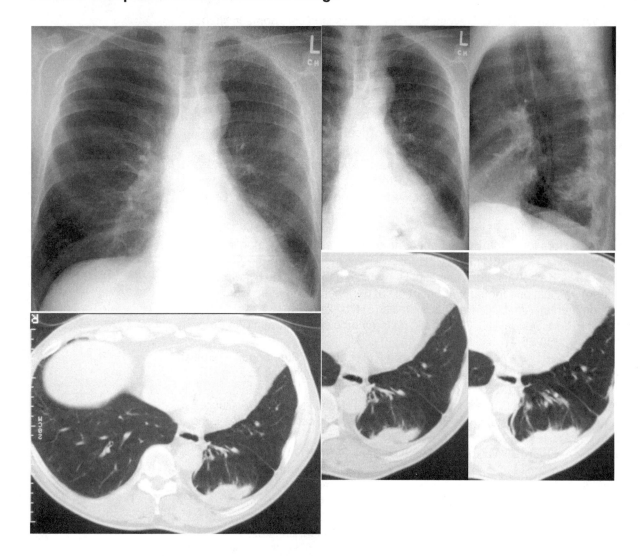

Case 2: This 20 year old Caucasian female presented 7 years prior to the current admission with sudden onset of shortness of breath. The original chest radiograph revealed a pneumothorax.

The patient now presents with increasing shortness of breath.

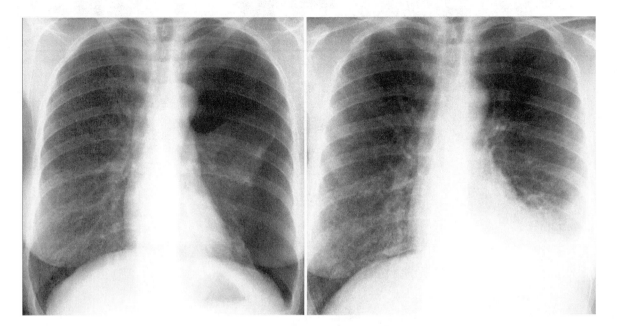

Case 3: This 58 year old Caucasion female presented with a one month history of hemoptysis

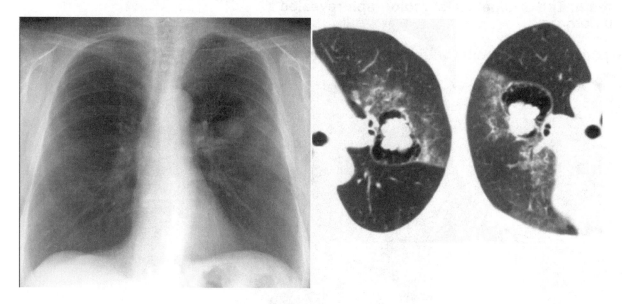

**Case 4: This 38 year old African American female presented
with a history of chronic asthma and increasing cough and
shortness of breath**

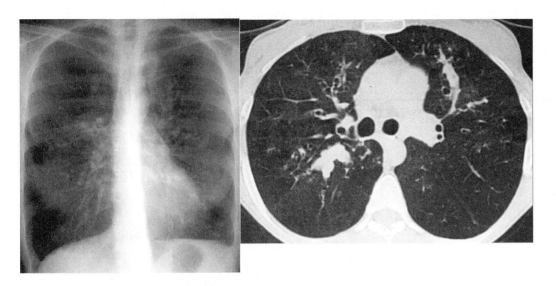

Case 5: This 72 year old Caucasian female presented with cough and occasional fever. She was treated intermittently with antibiotics for 6 months. Open biopsy was obtained because of progressive symptoms.

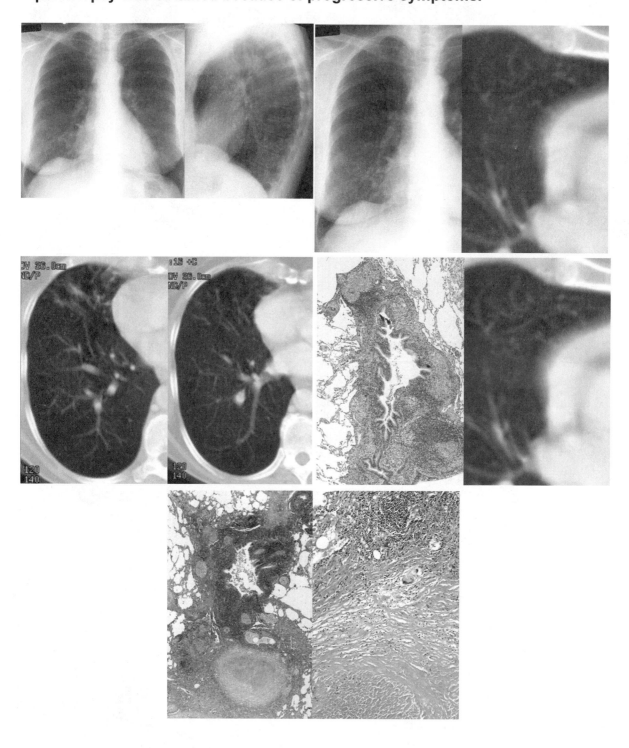

Chest Seminar 2

Jeffrey R. Galvin, MD
Teri J. Franks, MD
Department of Radiologic Pathology
and
Department of Pulmonary and Mediastinal Pathology
Armed Forces Institute of Pathology

Case 1: 15 year old female was admitted to the ER with an overdose of Nefazodone and other unknown pills. Activated charcoal was administered after which she developed vomiting and gagging. Respiratory distress required intubation. Bronchial lavage was performed and immunosuppressants were started. The patient developed progressive dyspnea and obstructive pulmonary functions over the next 6 months.

Bilateral lung transplantation was done 19 months later.

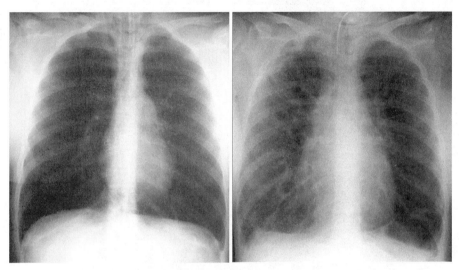

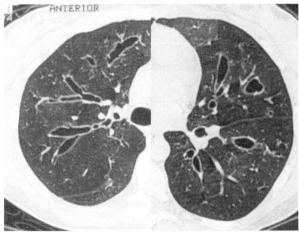

Case 2: 59 year old Caucasian female with history of breast cancer 12 years prior to admission and local recurrence treated with radiation 7 years later. She presented with a right lung mass.

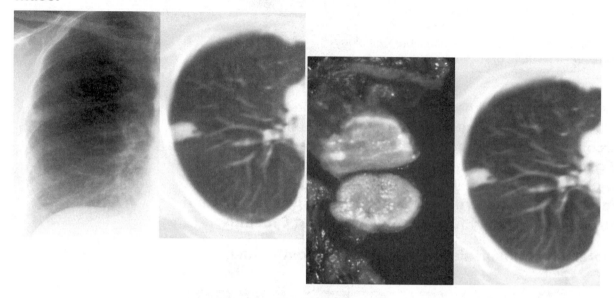

Case 3: 46 year old Caucasian male with long standing year history of shortness of breath. He presents with a 3 months of worsening dyspnea.

He demonstrated a mild leukocytosis and an increase in serum LDH.

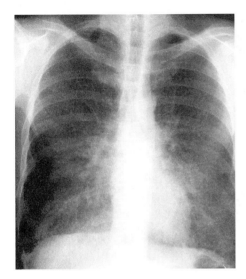
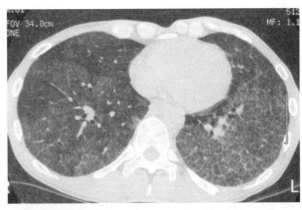
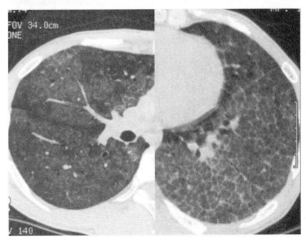

Case 4: 57 year old Caucasian male with a new history of cough and a new abnormality on chest radiograph.

A chest CT was done based on the abnormalities found on the chest radiograph.

A bronchoscopy was performed.

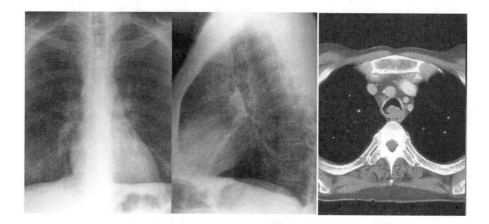

Case 5: 61 year old female worked as a hospital storage room manager.

She presented to the ER complaining of fatigue, increasing shortness of breath, chest pain, and cough productive of blood tinged sputum.

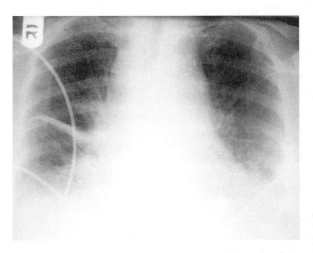
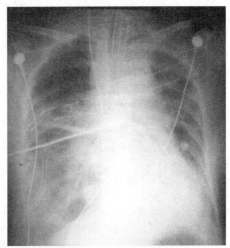

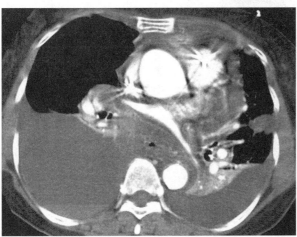

Pulmonary Hypertension

Aletta Ann Frazier, M.D.
Jeffrey R. Galvin, MD

Department of Radiologic Pathology
Armed Forces Institute of Pathology
Washington, DC
Department of Diagnostic Radiology
University Hospital
University of Maryland Medical System
Baltimore, MD

Learning Objectives
- To review the classic imaging findings of pulmonary hypertension, and to recognize how they may distinguish precapillary (arterial) from postcapillary (venous) disease
- To define the underlying vascular histopathology and secondary cardiac changes of pulmonary hypertension
- To highlight the clinical characteristics of both idiopathic and secondary conditions within the spectrum of pulmonary hypertension

Normal Pulmonary Circulation
- Low pressure system with high degree of capacitance (recruitment and distension)
- Less than one tenth the resistance to flow in comparison to systemic circulation (low vasomotor tone)
- Right ventricle expends minimal energy to perfuse the pulmonary vascular bed

Precapillary Pulmonary Circulation [Figure 1-14-1]

Figure 1-14-1

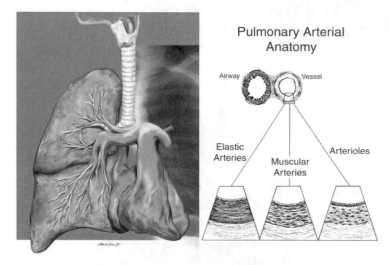

Precapillary (arterial) pulmonary circulation and vascular anatomy. Arterial vessels accompany the dichotomously branching airways of the lung

Postcapillary Pulmonary Circulation [Figure 1-14-2]

Figure 1-14-2

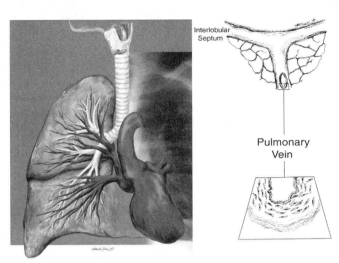

Postcapillary (venous) circulation drains the capillary beds of the alveoli. Venules and veins course back to the left atrium within interlobular septa

Precapillary (Arterial) Pulmonary Hypertension

- Insidious, subtle clinical onset
- Signs and symptoms of right heart pressure overload due to elevated pulmonary arterial pressure (cor pulmonale) are only expressed in advanced disease
- Imaging findings alone may reflect underlying anatomic change in the earlier - and potentially reversible - stages of pulmonary hypertension

Pulmonary Hypertension: Hemodynamic Criteria

National Institutes of Health Registry

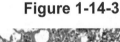

Figure 1-14-3

- Mean pulmonary artery pressure (mPAP) obtained at right heart cardiac catheterization:
  - ➢ > 25mm HG at rest (normal 10)
  - ➢ > 30mm HG with exercise (normal 15)

Pulmonary Hypertension: Cor Pulmonale

- World Health Organization: ..."alteration in the structure and function of the right ventricle resulting from diseases affecting the structure and/or function of the lungs"
- Signs of right heart pressure overload due to elevated pulmonary vascular resistance characterize the clinical presentation of pulmonary hypertension

Histologic Changes:
Precapillary Pulmonary Hypertension [Figure 1-14-3]

- Medial Hypertrophy
- Intimal Proliferation
- Arteritis
- Thrombosis ("in situ" or embolic)
- "Plexiform Lesions"
  - ➢ Primary Pulmonary Hypertension
  - ➢ Eisenmenger Physiology

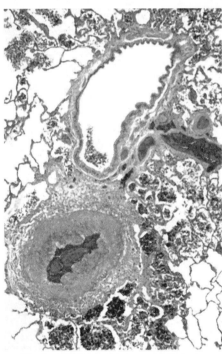

Photomicrograph demonstrates a muscular artery (adjacent to an airway) narrowed by medial hypertrophy and obstructed by intravascular thrombosis

Precapillary Hypertension: Imaging Features

- Dilatation of central pulmonary arteries
- Cor pulmonale
- Pruned vascularity
- Mosaic perfusion
- Atherosclerosis of central pulmonary arteries

Central Pulmonary Artery Dilatation [Figure 1-14-4]

Measurement of PA Dilatation [Figure 1-14-5]

Normal Heart vs Cor Pulmonale

Cor Pulmonale [Figure 1-14-6]

Vascular "Pruning" [Figure 1-14-7]

Mosaic Perfusion [Figure 1-14-8]

Figure 1-14-5

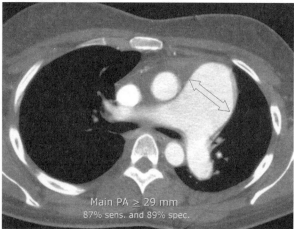

CT criteria for an enlarged main PA: transverse diameter exceeds 29 mm

Figure 1-14-7

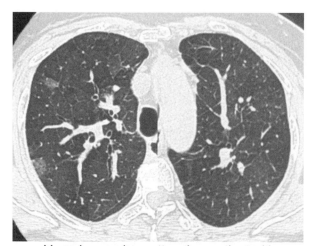

Vascular pruning pattern in a patient with pulmonary hypertension due to chronic thromboembolic disease

Figure 1-14-4

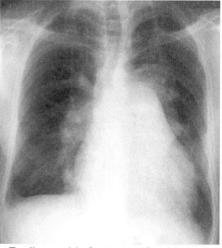

Radiographic features of pulmonary hypertension: enlarged main pulmonary artery, dilated central hilar vessels, and peripheral oligemia

Figure 1-14-6

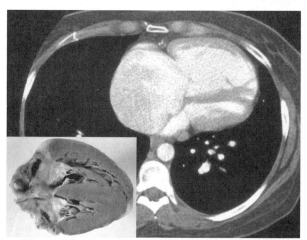

CT manifestations of cor pulmonale: dilated RA and RV, thickened anterior RV wall, and flattened interventricular septum

Figure 1-14-8

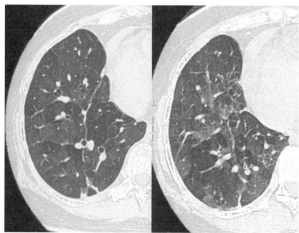

Mosaic perfusion pattern reflects geographic variations in parenchymal blood flow

Atherosclerosis of the Pulmonary Artery

Pulmonary Hypertension: Precapillary Etiologies
- Idiopathic
  - "Primary Pulmonary Hypertension"
- Secondary
  - Congenital heart disease (Eisenmenger)
  - Chronic thromboembolic disease
  - Embolization of tumor cells, parasites, talc
  - Mediastinal fibrosis
  - Collagen vascular disease
  - Chronic hypoxia (COPD, lung fibrosis, obesity-hypoventilation syndrome)

Primary Pulmonary Hypertension
- Rare disorder with no direct cause yet identified
- Mean age 45 (range 15-66 years), F>M (3:1)
- 6% of cases are "familial"
  - Autosomal dominant with incomplete penetrance
- Associated conditions
  - HIV infection
  - Appetite suppressants (dexfenfluramine, aminorex)
  - Cocaine
  - Portal hypertension
- Fatal outcome 2-3 years after diagnosis without transplantation

Atrial Septal Defect [Figure 1-14-9]

Eisenmenger Physiology of Congenital Heart Disease

Figure 1-14-9

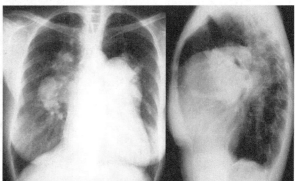

Precapillary hypertension in a patient with longstanding uncorrected atrial septal defect and Eisenmenger physiology
[Courtesy of Melissa Rosado de Christenson, MD]

- Acquired right-to-left intracardiac shunt following sustained, progressive elevation in pulmonary vascular resistance
- Ventricular septal defect (most commom)
- Atrial septal defect
- Patent ductus arteriosus
- Endocardial cushion defect

Chronic Thromboembolic Disease

Chronic Thromboembolic Disease
- Follows less than 1% of cases acute PE
- Five-year survival rate <35% without surgery
- V/Q scan typically high probability
- Up to 24% of patients have a lupus anticoagulant
- Associated inherited conditions (approx 5%)
  - Protein C deficiency
  - Protein S deficiency
  - Antithrombin III deficiency
  - Sickle Cell Disease

"Recanalized" Thrombus in Pulmonary Arterioles

"Organizing" Central Thrombus

Surgical Thromboendarterectomy

Other Thromboembolic Materials

Tumor Embolism
- Tumor cells and thrombus lodge in arterioles
- Tumor may spread to interstitium and lymphatics

Tumor Embolism
- Common malignancies: stomach, breast, prostate, liver, ovary, lymphoma, atrial myxoma
- Heralds rapid clinical deterioration
- Imaging
  - CXR: often normal
  - CT: "beading" of peripheral pulmonary arteries, mosaic perfusion, wedge-shape opacities (infaction)

Intravenous Talcosis
- Chronic IV injection of crushed tablets (Methadone, amphetamines)
- Thromboembolism induced by pharmaceutical binding agent: magnesium silicate
- Exuberant granulomas form in lung which coalesce the birefringent particles

Intravenous Talcosis: Imaging
- EARLY
  - Diffuse micronodular opacities
- LATE
  - Fibrosis
  - High density perihilar masses
  - Emphysema

Intravenous Talcosis

Mediastinal Fibrosis

Mediastinal Fibrosis
- Idiopathic or due to prior granulomatous infection
- Exuberant fibrous tissue replaces fat, encases central structures
- May constrict pulmonary arteries and/or veins

Mediastinal Fibrosis: Imaging
- Mediastinal contours abnormal
- Calcium
- Soft tissue replaces mediastinal fat
- Constriction of pulmonary arteries and/or veins, airways, esophagus

Collagen Vascular Disease

Scleroderma

Collagen Vascular Disease
- Scleroderma is the most common CVD to produce PAH
- Typical patient is female, age 35-45 years
  - 1/3 of all patients develop PAH, typically with CREST syndrome
  - Only 40% survival at 2 years

Collagen Vascular Disease
- Scleroderma
- Systemic Lupus Erythematosus
- Rheumatoid Arthritis
- Polymyositis-Dermatomyositis
- Mixed Connective Tissue Disease
- Progressive Systemic Sclerosis
- Disease mechanism for PAH probably multifactorial
  - Vasculopathy
  - Recurrent thromboembolism
  - Fibrotic lung disease

COPD - Emphysema
- 50% of COPD patients >50 y.o will develop PAH
- Significant relationship between arterial oxygen tension (ABG) and progression of PAH
- Disease mechanism multifactorial
  - Chronic alveolar hypoxia
  - Muscular arteries: smooth muscle cell hypertrophy & proliferation
  - Hyperviscosity state (polycythemia)
  - Lung destruction (loss of recruitable vessels)

Postcapillary Pulmonary Circulation: Anatomic Overview

Pulmonary Venous Hypertension
- Clinical onset may be acute or chronic
- Elevated pulmonary capillary wedge pressure (but there are exceptions)
- PAH may develop with sustained PVH

Histologic Changes - Postcapillary Pulmonary Hypertension
- Venous dilatation
- Intimal thickening
- Expanded interlobular septa
- Capillary congestion

Postcapillary Pulmonary Hypertension: Imaging Features
- Prominent interlobular septa
- Subpleural edema
- Pleural effusion

Pulmonary Hypertension: Postcapillary Etiologies
- Idiopathic
  - Pulmonary Veno-occlusive Disease" (variant; "Capillary Hemangiomatosis")
- Secondary
  - Left ventricular failure
  - Mitral stenosis
  - Mediastinal fibrosis
  - Left atrial mass/thrombus
  - Pulmonary venous constriction or invasion by neoplasm

Pulmonary Veno-occlusive Disease
[Figure 1-14-10]

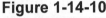

Figure 1-14-10

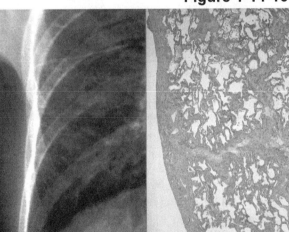

(left) Coned radiograph of a patient with postcapillary pulmonary hypertension due to PVOD demonstrates Kerley B (septal) lines and subpleural edema.

(right) Photomicrograph at the lung periphery illustrates edema expanding the interlobular septum perpendicular to the pleural surface

Pulmonary Hypertension: Postcapillary Etiologies
- Rare, idiopathic
- One third pediatric
- 2:1 M:F (Adults)
- 2/3 die within 2 years without transplantation
- Clinical
  - ➢ Evidence of both CHF and PAH
  - ➢ Normal pulmonary capillary wedge pressure
- Associations
  - ➢ Prior viral illness
  - ➢ Chemotherapy
  - ➢ HIV infection

Histologic Hallmark of PVOD
- Thrombosis, recanalization of intrapulmonary venules
- Obliterative fibrous tissue is loose, paucicellular
- Distribution of occlusive changes widespread

Pulmonary Veno-occlusive Disease
- A MISSED DIAGNOSIS may lead to life-threatening pulmonary edema if patient given vasodilators for presumptive PAH
- PRETHERAPEUTIC HRCT
  - ➢ Septal lines
  - ➢ Pleural effusion (+/-)
  - ➢ Left atrium normal or small

Left Ventricular Failure

Mitral Stenosis [Figure 1-14-11]

Mediastinal Fibrosis [Figure 1-14-12]

Left Atrial Mass

Precapillary Pulmonary Hypertension
- Enlarged central pulmonary arteries
- Cor pulmonale
- Pruned peripheral vascularity
- Mosaic perfusion
- PA atherosclerosis

Precapillary Pulmonary Hypertension: Summary
- Conditions directly involving the pulmonary arteries
- Elevated mPAP leads to vascular dilatation & cor pulmonale
- Idiopathic
  - ➢ "Primary Pulmonary Hypertension"
- Secondary
  - ➢ Congenital heart disease (Eisenmenger)
  - ➢ Chronic thromboembolic disease
  - ➢ Embolism of talc, tumor cells, parasites
  - ➢ Mediastinal fibrosis
  - ➢ Collagen vascular disease
  - ➢ Chronic hypoxic states

Figure 1-4-11

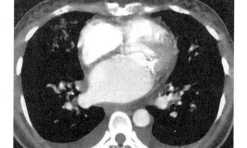

Postcapillary hypertension in a patient with mitral stenosis demonstrates bilateral pleural effusions and left atrial enlargement

Figure 1-4-12

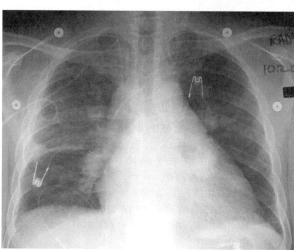

Postcapillary hypertension due to mediastinal fibrosis: constriction of right pulmonary venous drainage produces septal lines, subpleural edema and a small right pleural effusion

Postcapillary Pulmonary Hypertension
- Prominent interlobular septa
- Subpleural edema
- Pleural effusion

Postcapillary Pulmonary Hypertension: Summary
- Conditions involving pulmonary veins or the left heart
- Sustained disease produces precapillary changes
- Idiopathic
  - "Pulmonary Veno-occlusive Disease" (variant: "Capillary Hemangiomatosis")
- Secondary
  - Left ventricular failure
  - Mitral stenosis
  - Mediastinal fibrosis
  - Left atrial mass or thrombus
  - Venous constriction or invasion by neoplasm

LIST OF REFERENCES

1. Frazier AA, Galvin J, Franks T, Rosado-de-Christenson M. Pulmonary hypertension: hypertension and infarction. RadioGraphics 2000; 20:491-524.

2. Burke A, Virmani R. Mini-symposium: pulmonary pathology-evaluation of pulmonary hypertension in biopsies of the lung. Curr Diagn Pathol 1996; 3:14-26.

3. Worthy SA, Muller NL, Hartman TE, Swensen SJ, Padley SPG, Hansell DM. Mosaic attenuation pattern on thin-section CT scans of the lung: differentiation among infiltrative lung, airway, and vascular diseases as a cause. Radiology 1997; 205:465-470.

4. Primack SL, Muller NL, Mayo JR, Remy-Jardin M, Remy J. Pulmonary parenchymal abnormalities of vascular origin: high-resolution CT findings. RadioGraphics 1994; 14:739-746.

5. Bergin CJ, Sirlin CB, Hauschildt JP, et al. Chronic thromboembolism: diagnosis with helical CT and MR imaging with angiographic and surgical correlation. Radiology 1997; 204:695-702.

6. Shephard JA, Moore EH, Templeton PA, McLoud TC. Pulmonary intravascular tumor emboli: dilated and beaded peripheral arteries at CT. Radiology 1993; 187:797-801.

7. Dufour B, Maitre S, Humbert M, Capron F, Simonneau G, Musset D. High-resolution CT of the chest in four patients with pulmonary capillary hemangiomatosis or pulmonary venoocclusive disease. Am J Roentgenol 1998; 171:1321-1324.

8. Espinosa RE, Edwards WD, Rosenow EC, Schaff HV. Idiopathic pulmonary hilar fibrosis: an unusual cause of pulmonary hypertension. Mayo Clin Proc 1993; 68:778-782.

Pulmonary Metastases

Aletta Ann Frazier, M.D.
Special Acknowledgements: Melissa L. Rosado de Christenson, M.D., Jeffrey R.Galvin, M.D., Robert D. Pugatch, M.D.

Departement of Radiologic Pathology
Armed Forces Institute of Pathology
Washington, DC
Department of Diagnostic Radiology
University Hospital
University of Maryland Medical System
Baltimore, MD

Learning Objectives
- To review the pathogenesis of metastatic spread of extrathoracic malignancy to the lung parenchyma
- To illustrate the spectrum of radiological manifestations and corresponding histopathology of pulmonary metastatic disease
- To enumerate the malignant cell types which may produce characteristic patterns of pulmonary metastases
- To identify radiologic findings which may assist in distinguishing pulmonary metastases from other diseases in the chest

Metastatic Disease to the Lung
- Most common lung neoplasm
- Overall incidence: 20-50% of all patients dying from malignancy
- Lung is the ONLY site of metastatic disease in 15-25% of patients with lung metastases
- Routes of entry
  - ➢ Pulmonary or bronchial arteries
  - ➢ Lymphaties
  - ➢ Airways

What is most likely primary source of pulmonary metastases? •
- Breast
- Colon
- Pancreas
- Stomach
- Skin
- Kidney
- Ovary
- Prostate
- Uterus

Which malignancies have the greatest tendency to produce pulmonary metastases?
- Choriocarcinoma
- Osteosarcoma
- Testicular tumors
- Melanoma
- Ewing's sarcoma
- Thyroid carcinoma

Figure 1-15-1

"Generalizing Sites"

- Certain tumors cells may seed the lung directly, others pass through another filtration organ before entering pulmonary circulation
- Tumors with venous drainage directly to lung:
  - ➤ Melanoma
  - ➤ Osteosarcoma/ chondrosarcoma
  - ➤ Thyroid
  - ➤ Kidney, Testis, Adrenal
  - ➤ Head & neck
- Tumors with venous drainage via liver (portal vein)
  - ➤ Colon
  - ➤ Pancraes
  - ➤ Stomach
- Tumor with venous drainage via bone (Batson plexus)
  - ➤ Prostate
- Tumors with dual venous drainage
  - ➤ Kidney
  - ➤ Rectum

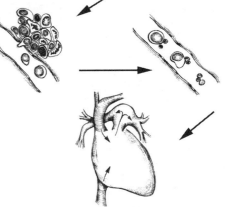

Pathogenesis of Hematogenous Metastases

[Figure 1-15-1]

- Primary tumor cells penetrate capillaries, venules, lymphatics
- Cells enter the systemic venous circulation
- Venous return to right heart - transports cells into the pulmonary arterial circulation

Hematogenous metastases arise from tumor cells which penetrate vessels and lymphatics at the primary site, and are transported via venous circulation to the right heart

Pathogenesis of Hematogenous Metastases

[Figure 1-15-2]

- Cells arrest in distal arteries and arterioles
- Factors may promote adherence and extravation
- Expansile growth in intersitium and alveolar air spaces
- Vascular supply
  - ➤ Pulmonary arteries
  - ➤ Bronchial circulation
  - ➤ Transpleural collaterals

Figure 1-15-2

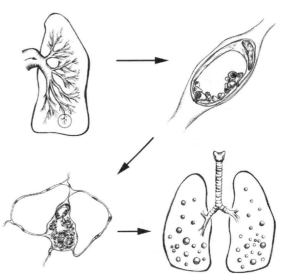

Parenchymal Nodules:
Histology - Microscopic

- well-defined focus of tumor cells
- Homogeneous cell population
- Alveolar septa typically compressed, obliterared
- Adjacent to small peripheral arteries and arterioles - may contain emboli

Parenchymal Nodules:
Histology - Gross

- Multiple well-circumscribed, rounded or coalescent multilobulated lesions
- Mixed areas of viability and necrosis
- Unusual: hemorrhagic
- Wide range of sizes
- eripheral
- Basilar >> Apical

Bloodborne tumor cells arrest in distal arterioles of the pulmonary circulation, extravasate into the interstitium, and establish nodules by focal expansile growth

Parenchymal Nodules:
Imaging Features, Chest Radiography

- Multiple
- Spherical
- Range of opacities:
  - ➢ Cannonball
  - ➢ Micronodular
  - ➢ Coalescent and/or multilobulated
- Sharply marginated or ill-defined
- Peripheral (80-90%)
- Lower lobe

Parenchymal Nodules:
Imaging Features, Chest CT

- Sensitive for nodules > 3mm, but not specific
  - ➢ Granulomatous diseases
  - ➢ Intrapulmonary lymph nodes
  - ➢ Opportunistic infection
  - ➢ Drug reaction

Parenchymal Nodular Metastases: [Figure 1-15-3]
HRCT-Pathologic Correlation: Nodules <1cm

- Peribronchovascular (12%)
- Perilobular (20-28%)
- Intermediate (60-68%)
- "Larger" nodules 3-9mm:
  - ➢ Directly-centered feeding vessel (18%)
  - ➢ Eccentric feeding vessel, pushed to one edge of nodule (58%)

Parenchymal Nodules: [Figure 1-15-4]
Imaging Features, Chest CT

- Spherical (larger nodules - lobulated or irregular margins)
- Multiple (variation in size)
- Peripheral
- Lower lung zones
- Angiocentric ("feeding vessel sign")
- "Random" pattern
- Ground glass halo (if hemorrhagic)
  - ➢ Angiosarcoma
  - ➢ Choriocarcinoma
  - ➢ Post therapy

"Cannonball" Metastases [Figure 1-15-5 and 1-15-6]

- Coloretal carcinoma
- Renal cell carcinoma
- Sarcomas
- Melanoma

Figure 1-15-6

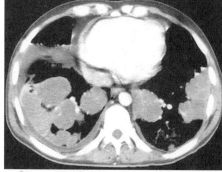

*Cannonball metastases in a young
adult male with testicular cancer*

Figure 1-15-3

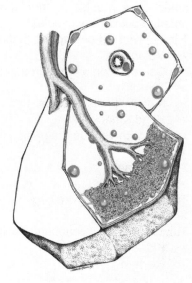

*Secondary pulmonary lobule:
hematogenous metastases may be
angiocentric but are chiefly random in
distribution with respect to this unit of
pulmonary architecture*

Figure 1-15-4

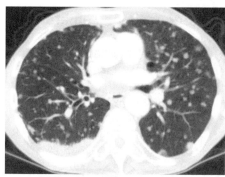

*CT image of hematogenous
metastases (colon carcinoma).*

Figure 1-15-5

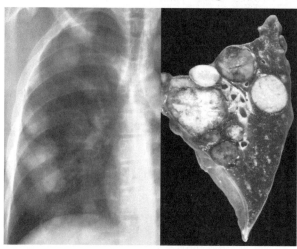

*Cannonball metastases in
a young adult male with sarcoma*

Micronodular Metastases [Figure 1-15-7]
- Widespread opacities
- Malignancies
  - ➢ Thyroid CA (papillary)
  - ➢ Choriocarcinoma
- Opacities may persist post-treatment
- DDX
  - ➢ Miliary tuberculosis
  - ➢ Viral pneumonia
  - ➢ Sarcoidosis

Atypical Pulmonary Metastases
- Parenchymal nodules which are:
  - ➢ Cavitary
  - ➢ Calcified
  - ➢ Solitary
- Lymphangitic carcinomatosis
- Tumor thromboembolism
- Endobronchial tumor

Cavitation in Metastases
- Specific malignancies
  - ➢ Squamous cell neoplasms (head and neck)
  - ➢ Genitourinary tract neoplasms (women)
  - ➢ Sarcomas
  - ➢ Adenocarcinomas (colon, breast)
- Post radiation or chemotherapy
- Incidence
  - ➢ 4% in metastases (vs. 9-16% primary lung CA)

Cavitation in Metastases [Figure 1-15-8]
- Wall thickness
  - ➢ Not reliable indicator malignancy vs. benignity
  - ➢ Thin walls - typical of sarcomas
- Spontaneous pneumothorax
  - ➢ Necrosis & excavation of subpleural metastasis
  - ➢ Characteristic of osteosarcoma (5%) and other aggressive sarcomatous tumors

Calcification in Metastases
- Specific malignancies
  - ➢ Osteosarcoma
  - ➢ Chondrosarcoma
  - ➢ Synovial sarcoma
  - ➢ Papillary/mucinous adenocarcinomas (ovary, thyroid)
- Post-chemotherapy (esp. testicular CA)
- Post-radiation
- Variable content
  - ➢ Bone in osteoid matrix
  - ➢ Dystrophic calcification
  - ➢ Psammoma body formation

Figure 1-15-7

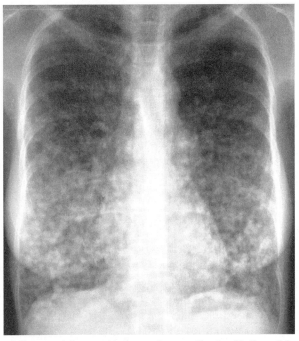

Micronodular metastases in a patient with thyroid cancer

Figure 1-15-8

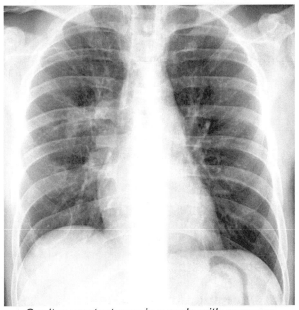

Cavitary metastases in a male with sarcoma

Figure 1-15-9

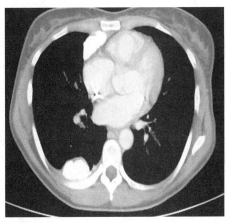

Large calcified metastases in a patient with ovarian cancer

Calcification in Metastases: Specimen Radiograph

Solitary Metastasis
- Account for 1-5% of all metastatic lesions
- 3-9% of all SPNs are solitary metastases
- "In patients with known primary malignancies and single parenchymal nodules, the overall incidence of second primary lung carcinoma is greater than that of solitary metastases

Coppage et al: J Thorac Imaging 1987; 2(4):24-37

Solitary Metastasis vs. Lung Primary
- "The likelihood of a primary lung cancer versus a metastasis depends on the histologic characteristics of the extrapulmonary neoplasm and the patient's smoking history

Quint et al: Radiology 2000; 217: 257-61

Solitary Metastasis vs. Lung Primary
- A SPN is more likely to be bronchogenic CA than a solitary met if the patient has carcinoma of:
  - Head and neck
  - Bladder
  - Esophagus
  - Breast
  - Cervix
  - Bile Ducts
  - Ovary
  - Prostate
  - Stomach

Solitary Metastasis vs. Lung Primary
- The incidence is fairly equal in patients with carcinoma of:
  - Kidney
  - Colon
  - Adrenal gland
  - Uterus
  - Salivary or parotid gland
  - Thyroid gland
- SPN is more likely solitary metastasis in:
  - Melanoma
  - Sarcoma
  - Testicular carcinoma

Solitary Metastasis

Lymphangitic Carcinomatosis
- Reported incidence varies: 6-55%
- Secondary to adenocarcinomas in 80%:
  - Lung
  - Breast
  - Stomach
  - Pancreas
  - Prostate
  - Colon
- Symptoms of dyspnea, cough
- PFT's: reduced lung compliance & diffusing capacity
- Dismal prognosis: fatal within a year

Lymphangitic Carcinomatosis [Figure 1-15-10]

- Blood-borne tumor cells extravasate into peribronchovascular interstitium, spread along lymphatic channels
- Tumor cells may also enter "retrograde" through lymphatics via involved mediastinal lymph nodes
- Lymphatics further expand with edema secondary to obstruction
- Clusters or cords of tumor in lymphatics of the interlobular septa and peribronchovascular interstitium
- Edema and desmoplastic reaction accentuate interstitial thickening
- Pleural involvement: 2/3
- Nodal involvement: 1/3

Lymphangitic Carcinomatosis: Imaging Features - Chest radiograph

- Normal chest radiograph
- Septal lines
- Reticulonodular opacities
- Subpleural edema
- Bilateral or unilateral
- If unilateral, usually right-sided (primary lung CA most likely)
- Pleural effusion (60%)
- Hilar lymphadenopathy (<25%)

Lymphangitic Carcinomatosis Imaging Features: Chest CT [Figure 1-15-11]

- Smooth or nodular thickening of
  - Bronchovascular bundles
  - Interlobular septa
  - Lobar fissures
- Focal or unilateral distribution (50%)
- "Polygonal arcades" (50%)
- Pleural effusion
- Hilar lymphadenopathy (up to 50%)
- DDX
  - Pulmonary edema
  - Lymphoma
  - Sarcoidosis
  - Drug toxicity

Tumor Embolism

- Tumor cells lodge in smaller pulmonary arteries and arterioles
- Accompanied by thrombosis
- Pulmonary hypertension and infarction may result with widespread obstruction
- +/- Parenchymal or lymphatic tumor involvement

Tumor Embolism [Figure 1-15-12]

- Malignancies
  - stomach, breast, prostate, liver, ovary, lymphoma, atrial myxoma
- Imaging
  - CXR often normal
  - CT
    "beading" of pulmonary arteries
    mosaic perfusion
    wedge-shaped peripheral opacities

Figure 1-15-10

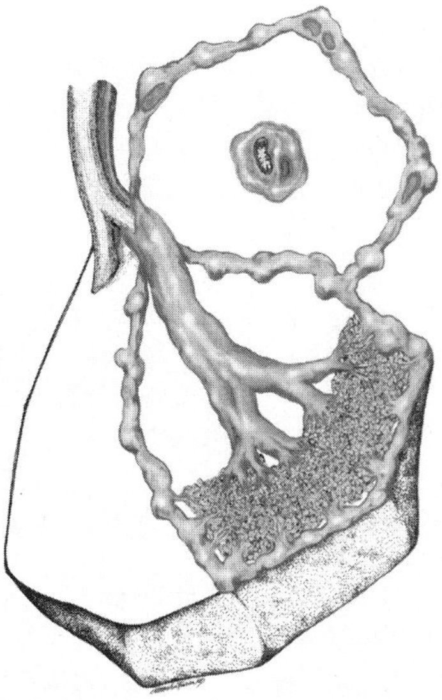

Secondary pulmonary lobule: lymphangitic carcinomatosis may produce both smooth and nodular expansion of bronchovascular bundle sheaths and interlobular septa

Figure 1-15-11

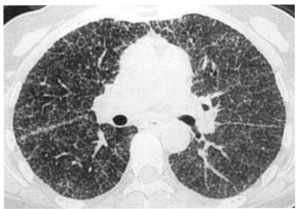

Lymphangitic carcinomatosis: widespread septal lines, delicate reticulonodular opacities, and nodular thickening of the interlobar fissures

Figure 1-15-12

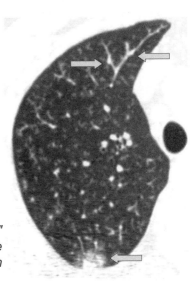

Tumor thromboembolism may produce "beading" along peripheral bronchovascular bundle as well as pulmonary infarction

Endobronchial Metastases
- May arise from aerial seeding or from tumor transported via pulmonary or bronchial arteries
- Unusual (incidence < 5% if contiguous airway invasion excluded): bronchial mucosa resistant to tumor implantation
- Typical primary sources
  - Breast
  - Pancreas
  - Colon, Rectum
  - Kidney
  - Melanoma
- Symptoms (cough, hemoptysis, wheezing) DON'T usually precede diagnosis of primary malignancy

Endobronchial Metastases: Imaging Features
[Figure 1-15-13]
- Post-obstructive atelectasis and/or consolidation
- Intraluminal soft tissue mass
- Serpiginous or nodular opacities (mucoid impaction)
- Hilar mass (if contiguous tumor invasion of hilum)
- DDX: bronchogenic carcinoma

Pleural Metastases
- Develop via lymphangitic or vascular invasion
- Typical primary malignancies
  - Lung
  - Stomach
  - Breast (50% of patients)
  - Ovary
  - Lymphoma
- 60% with pleural mets have pleural effusion
  - If exudate: hemorrhagic (consistent with pleural implants)
  - If serous: lymphatic obstruction of nodes (+/- pleural implants)

Pleural Metastases
- Scattered nodules on pleural surface
- Visceral & parietal pleura typically both involved
- DDX: asbestos exposure; splenosis; mesothelioma

Metastatic Disease to the Lung
- Entry points
  - Pulmonary arteries
  - Bronchial circulation
  - Lymphatic channels
  - Airways

- Pathogenesis
  - Invasion - venules, lymphatics
  - Transport
  - Arrest
  - Adherence
  - Extravasation
  - Proliferation - homogeneous cell population

Patterns of Metastatic Disease to the Lung
- Parenchymal nodules
  - Common: well-circumscribed, angiocentric, basilar>apical
  - Atypical: cavitary, calcified, solitary
- Lymphangitic carcinomatosis

Figure 1-15-13

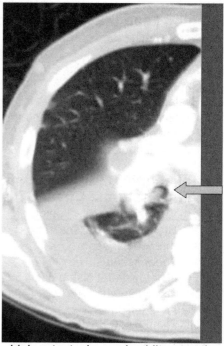

Endobronchial metastasis nearly obliterates the airway lumen in a patient with renal cancer

- ➢ Septal lines, thickened fissures
- ➢ Pleural effusion
- ➢ Lymphadenopathy
- Tumor thromboembolism
  - ➢ Beading of peripheral arteries
  - ➢ Mosaic perfusion
  - ➢ Pleural-based opacity (infarction)

Patterns of Metastatic Disease to the Lung
- Endobronchial nodule
  - ➢ Rounded defect in airway, or cut-off of airway lumen
  - ➢ Post-obstructive atelectasis, pneumonia, mucoid impaction
- Pleural-based metastases
  - ➢ Nodules located on pleural surface
  - ➢ Variation: rind-like pattern which mimics mesothelioma
  - ➢ Pleural effusion common

REFERENCES

1. Milne EC, Zerhouni EA. Blood supply of pulmonary metastases. J Thorac Imag 1987; 2(4):15-23.

2. Coppage L, Shaw C, Curtis A. Metastatic disease to the chest in patients with extrathoracic malignancy. J Thorac Imag 1987; 2(4):24-37.

3. Seo JB, Im J, Goo JM, Chung MJ, Kim M. Atypical pulmonary metastases: spectrum of radiologic findings. RadioGraphics 2001; 21:403-417.

4. Hirakata K, Nakata H, Haratake J. Appearance of pulmonary metastases on high-resolution CT scans: comparison with histopathologic findings on autopsy specimens. Am J Roentgenol 1993; 161:37-43.

5. Murata K, Takahashi M, Mori M, Kawaguchi N et al. Pulmonary metastatic nodules: CT-pathologic correlation. Radiology 1992; 182:331-335.

6. Davis S. CT evaluation for pulmonary metastases in patients with extrathoracic malignancy. Radiology 1991; 180:1-12.

7. Libshitz HI, North LB. Pulmonary metastases. Radiol Clin North Am 1982; 20:437-451.

8. Quint L, Park C, Iannettoni M. Solitary pulmonary nodules in patients with extrapulmonary neoplasms. Radiology 2000; 217:257-261.

9. Poste G, Fidler I. The pathogenesis of cancer metastasis. Nature 1980; 283:139-145.

10. Marglin S, Mortimer J, Castellino R. Radiologic investigation of thoracic metastases from unknown primary sites. J Thorac Imag 1987; 2(4):38-43.

Differential Diagnosis of Mediastinal Masses

Melissa L. Rosado de Christenson, MD, FACR

Clinical Professor of Radiology
The Ohio Sate University
Columbus, OH

Adjunct Professor of Radiology
Uniformed Services University
Bethesda, MD

The majority of mediastinal masses encountered in clinical practice relate to mediastinal metastases from primary lung cancer, lymphoma and other extrathoracic primary malignant neoplasms as well as vascular lesions and variants. Primary mediastinal tumors are rare. Most primary mediastinal neoplasms are thymomas (20%) and neurogenic tumors (20%) occurring in the anterior and posterior mediastinal compartments respectively. Congenital mediastinal cysts (20%) are also frequent among primary mediastinal masses and affect the middle mediastinum. Mediastinal goiter, lymphoma, mature teratoma and granulomatous lymphadenopathy represent approximately 30% of primary mediastinal lesions. Miscellaneous conditions related to endocrine disorders, the esophagus, infections and systemic disorders also affect the mediastinum. Radiographic localization of a mass in one of three mediastinal compartments allows the formulation of a focused differential diagnosis, which is refined based on cross-sectional imaging features. The radiologist plays an important role in diagnosis by identifying pathognomonic lesions and by helping clinicians decide whether a specific lesion should be biopsied or excised.

Learning Objectives:
- To describe the mediastinal compartments and common mediastinal masses
- To define clinical and cross-sectional imaging features that allow a focused differential diagnosis
- To differentiate neoplastic from non-neoplastic conditions
- To describe lesions best diagnosed by mediastinal biopsy and those that should be surgically excised
- To describe lesions with pathognomonic radiologic features

The Mediastinum [Figure 1-16-1]
- Space between the pleural surfaces and lungs
- Bound by sternum (anteriorly) and vertebrae (posteriorly)
- From thoracic inlet to diaphragm
- Thymus, lymph nodes, heart, great vessels,trachea, esophagus, nerves, other soft tissues
- Arbitrary division into compartments - no anatomic boundaries

Outline
- The mediastinal compartments
- Thymic neoplasms / enlargement
- Lymphadenopathies
- Cysts
- Neurogenic neoplasms
- Endocrine lesions
- Vascular lesions
- Esophageal lesions
- Miscellaneous conditions

Figure 1-16-1

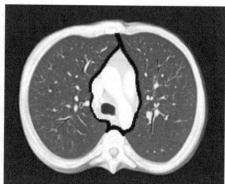

The mediastinum - space between pleural surfaces and lungs

The Mediastinal Compartments [Figures 1-16-2 to 1-16-4]

- Anatomic - Superior, anterior, middle, posterior (excludes paravertebral areas)
- Surgical - Superior, anterior, middle, posterior (includes paravertebral areas)
- Radiographic (Felson) - Anterior, middle, posterior
- Radiographic (Fraser, Müller, Colman, Paré - Anterior, middle-posterior, paravertebral

Figure 1-16-2

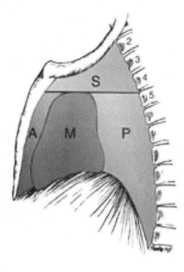

Anatomic mediastinal compartments

Figure 1-16-3

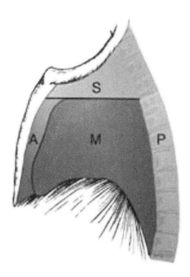

Surgical mediastinal compartments

Figure 1-16-4

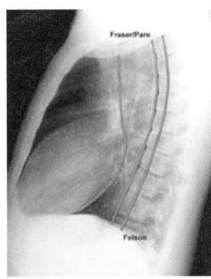

Radiographic mediastinal compartments Felson / Fraser, Müller, Colman, Paré

Mediastinal Masses – Mayo Clinic (N=1064)

- Neurogenic tumor   20%
- Thymoma   19%
- Cysts   18%
- Lymphoma   30%
  Teratoma
  Granuloma
  Mediastinal goiter

Wychulis et al. J. Thorac Cardiovasc Surg 1971

Mediastinal Masses

- Patients are often asymptomatic
- 83% of asymptomatic masses are benign
- 57% of symptomatic masses are malignant
- Approximately 1/3 are malignant
- Approximately 1/10 are vascular

The Thymus [Figure 1-16-5]

- Origin: 3rd and 4th pharyngeal pouches
- Prevascular, bilobed, encapsulated
- Thymic lobules; cortex and medulla

Thymic Masses

- Thymoma
- Thymic malignancy
  - Carcinoid
  - Carcinoma
- Thymolipoma
- Thymic enlargement / Hyperplasia
- Germ cell neoplasms

Figure 1-16-5

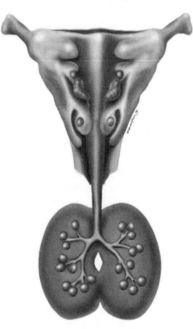

Embryology of the thymus

Thymoma

- Epithelial neoplasm, most common primary thymic neoplasm
- Slow growth, "benign" behavior
- M=F; 70% in the 5th and 6th decades
- Most patients asymptomatic
- 25-30% with symptoms of compression/invasion
- Associated parathymic syndromes:
  - ➢ Myasthenia gravis
  - ➢ Pure red cell aplasia
  - ➢ Hypogammaglobulinemia

Thymoma and Myasthenia Gravis

- Myasthenia gravis (MG) – autoimmune neurological disorder
- 85% of patients with MG have follicular thymic hyperplasia
- 15% of patients with MG have a thymoma
- Of all patients with thymoma, 30-50% have MG

Thymoma: Pathologic Features *[Figures 1-16-6 and 1-16-7]*

- Lymphocytes and epithelial cells in varying proportions
- WHO 1999 classification (morphology and lymphocyte-to-epithelial cell ratios)
  Types A, AB, B1, B2, B3
- Tumor lobules compartmentalized by fibrous septa / tumor capsule
- Spherical mass, variable size
- Encapsulated vs Invasive
- Invasive thymoma - microscopic documentation of capsular invasion
- Spherical mass, variable size, lobular contours, typically encapsulated
- Hemorrhage, necrosis, cystic change
- Local invasion, tumor implants, metastases

Thymoma: Imaging Features *[Figure 1-16-8]*

- Anterior mediastinal mass
- Well-marginated, lobular, unilateral
  Spherical shape, variable size
- Irregular or ill-defined contours suggest invasion
- Normal radiographs in 25% (occult)

Thymoma: Imaging Features

- CT
  - ➢ Well-defined, prevascular, spherical, lobular
  - ➢ Homogeneous or heterogeneous
    Calcification (peripheral or central), necrosis, cystic change (mural nodules)
  - ➢ No lymphadenopathy
  - ➢ Exclusion of local invasion to fat, cardiovascular structures, lung
    Pleural implants, diffuse pleural thickening
- MR *[Figures 1-16-9 and 1-16-10]*
  - ➢ T1 – intermediate signal
  - ➢ T2 – increased signal
  - ➢ Enhancement
  - ➢ Heterogeneous, fibrous septa, cystic areas

Figure 1-16-6

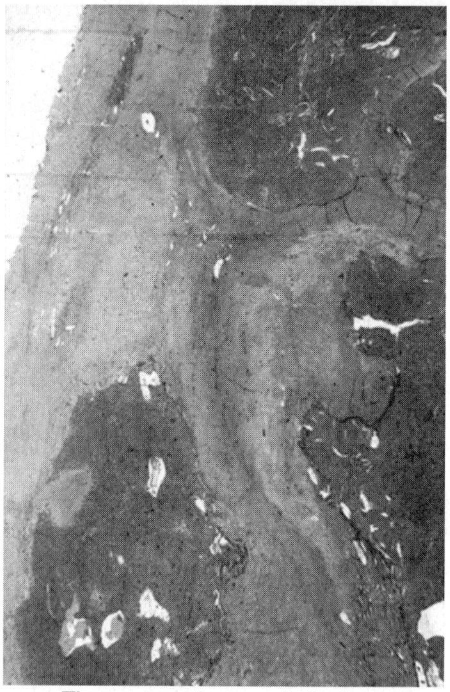

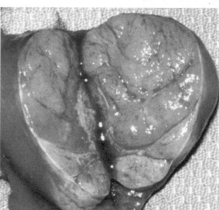

Thymoma; microscopic features

Figure 1-16-7

Thymoma; gross features

Figure 1-16-8

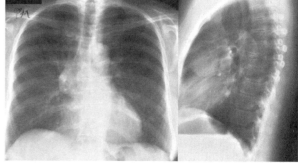

Thymoma; lobular right anterior mediastinal mass

Figure 1-16-9

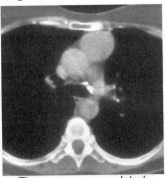

Figure 1-16-10

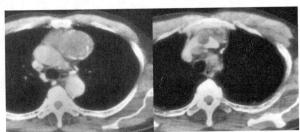

Thymoma; invasive - mediastinal and vascular invasion

*Thymoma; encapsulated -
Homogeneous spherical
left anterior mediastinal
mass*

Thymoma: Staging (Masaoka) /Survival (10-year)
I   Encapsulated / no microscopic capsular invasion (86-100%)
II   Microscopic invasion into surrounding fat / mediastinal pleura, microscopic capsular invasion (55-100%)
III   Macroscopic invasion into adjacent organs (pericardium, great vessels, lung) (47-60%)
IVa Pleural / pericardial dissemination (0-11%)
IVb Lymphogenous or hematogenous dissemination

Thymoma: Therapy / Prognosis
- Encapsulated; complete excision
  - ➢ Best prognosis
  - ➢ Occasional local recurrence, distant metastases
- Post-operative radiation in invasive thymoma to decrease local recurrence
- Chemotherapy for progression after surgery and unresectable lesions

Thymic Malignancy: Carcinoid / Carcinoma
- Rare malignant epithelial neoplasms
- Symptomatic patients
- Poor prognosis

Thymic Carcinoid
- Neuroendocrine neoplasm; atypical carcinoid (necrosis / mitoses / invasion)
- Males > Females; 3:1; wide age range (average, 43 yrs)
- 50% functionally active
  - ➢ ACTH – Cushing syndrome (33-40%)
- MEN type 1 – (Wermer syndrome) (19-25%)
  - ➢ Hyperparathyroidism (90%), islet cell tumor of pancreas (80%) pituitary adenoma (65%)

Figure 1-16-11

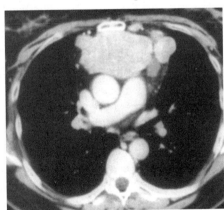

Thymic Carcinoma
- Male > Female; wide age range (mean: 5th decade)
- Cell types identical to those of primary lung cancer; R/O metastases
- WHO Type C thymoma

Thymic Carcinoid / Carcinoma: Imaging Features
[Figure 1-16-11]
- Large anterior mediastinal mass (R/O thymoma)
- R/O metastatic lung malignancy (histology)
- Lymphadenopathy
- Local invasion, pleural or pericardial effusion/implantation, metastases
- Carcinoid
  - ➢ Octreotide imaging for occult lesions (non-specific - metastases other neoplasms)

*Thymic carcinoid; lymphadenopathy [
History of clinical hormone syndrome
(MEN 1)]*

Thymolipoma
- Rare benign thymic neoplasm
- M=F; wide age range (average age, 28 yrs)
- Asymptomatic patients: 50%
- Symptoms with large tumors

Thymolipoma: Pathologic Features [Figure 1-16-12]
- Encapsulated, soft, lobular, yellow
- Mature adipose tissue and thymic tissue in variable proportions

Thymolipoma: Imaging Features [Figure 1-16-13]
- Well-defined anterior / inferior mediastinal mass
  - Unilateral or bilateral, slow growth
- May conform to shape of adjacent structures
  - R/o cardiac enlargement/diaphragmatic elevation
  - Positional change in shape
- Anatomic connection to the thymus (pedicle)
- Mixed fat and soft tissue attenuation/signal

Thymic Hyperplasia
- Rebound hyperplasia
  - After chemotherapy, treatment for Cushing syndrome, severe stress
  - Between 2 weeks and 14 months after therapy
- True hyperplasia
  - Autoimmune or systemic disorder
  - Graves disease, sarcoidosis
- Mediastinal widening, homogeneous soft tissue
- Maximal thickness
  - Under 20 years - 1.8 cm
  - Over 20 years - 1.3 cm
- Follicular thymic hyperplasia - Normal size

Germ Cell Neoplasms
- Most common in the gonad
- Extragonadal germ cell neoplasms; midline locations
  - Most commonly the mediastinum
- Postulated origin in multipotential primitive germ cells "misplaced" during embryogenesis
- Cell types:
  - Teratoma (mature, immature, "malignant")
  - Seminoma
  - Non-seminomatous germ cell neoplasms

Mature Teratoma
- 60-75% of mediastinal germ cell neoplasms
- Males=Females
  Children and young adults (< 40 yrs)
- Often asymptomatic
  Symptoms of compression or rupture

Mature Teratoma: Pathologic Features [Figures 1-16-14 and 1-16-15]
- More than one embryonic germ cell layer
  - Ectoderm – skin, dermal appendages
  - Mesoderm – bone, cartilage, muscle
  - Endoderm – GI, respiratory tissue, mucus glands
- Spherical, encapsulated, lobulated
- Multilocular or unilocular cyst
  - Oily, sebaceous, gelatinous material (lipid)
  - Focal solid areas: Hair, teeth, bone

Figure 1-16-12

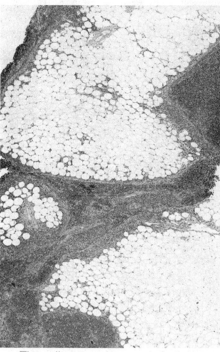

Thymolipoma; microscopic features

Figure 1-16-13

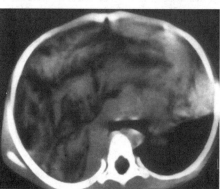

Thymolipoma; imaging features - Anterior mediastinal mass with fat and soft tissue elements and anatomic connection to thymus

Figure 1-16-14

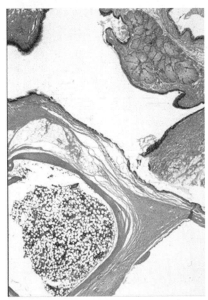

Mature teratoma; microscopic features

Figure 1-16-15

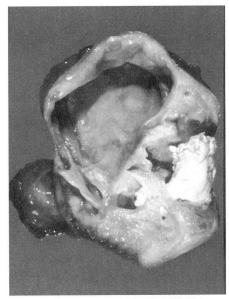

Mature teratoma; gross features

Figure 1-16-16

Mature Teratoma: Imaging Features [Figure 1-16-16]
- Unilateral anterior mediastinal mass
- Spherical, lobular contours, well-defined
- Multilocular cystic - 85%
- CT attenuation:
  - Fluid 89%, Fat 76%, Ca++ 53%
  - Fat fluid level - 11%
  - ST/FL/FAT/Ca++ - 39%
  - ST/FL/FAT - 24%
  - ST/FL - 15%

Mature Teratoma: Therapy and Prognosis
- Complete excision is curative
- Excellent prognosis
  - Near 100% five-year survival

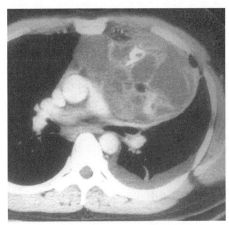

Mature teratoma; imaging features - Multilocular cystic anterior mediastinal mass with fluid, fat, soft tissue and calcium

Seminoma [Figure 1-16-17]
- 40% of malignant germ cell neoplasms of a single histology
- Caucasian males, third to fourth decade
- Most are symptomatic
- Homogeneous soft tissue mass
- Radiation therapy/Cisplatin-based chemotherapy
  - 60-80% long-term survival

Figure 1-16-17

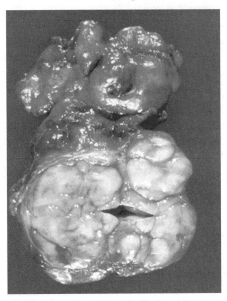

Seminoma; gross features

Seminoma: Imaging Features [Figure 1-16-18]
- Anterior mediastinal mass (both sides of midline)
  - ➤ Large, bulky, well-marginated, lobular, local invasion
- CT:
  - ➤ Homogeneous soft tissue mass
  - ➤ Mimics nodal coalescence
  - ➤ Slight homogeneous contrast-enhancement
  - ➤ Rarely necrosis/cystic change (8%)

Non-Seminomatous Malignant Germ Cell Neoplasms
- Yolk sac (endodermal sinus) tumor
  - ➤ Embryonal carcinoma
  - ➤ Choriocarcinoma
  - ➤ Mixed germ cell neoplasm
- Males, 90% symptomatic
  - ➤ Klinefelter syndrome (20%); concurrent hematologic malignancy
- Serology)
  - ➤ Alphafetoprotein (EST, EC)
  - ➤ β-human chorionic gonadotropin (HCG)
  - ➤ LDH (60%) tumor burden
- Large, unencapsulated
- Hemorrhage, necrosis, "cyst" formation
- Cisplatin-based chemotherapy; excision of residual tumor

Non-Seminomatous GCN: Imaging Features [Figure 1-16-19]
- Large, well or poorly-defined anterior mediastinal mass
  - ➤ Extends to both sides of midline
- Heterogeneous
  - ➤ Large areas of central low attenuation
  - ➤ Frond-like peripheral soft tissue
- Loss of tissue planes
  - ➤ Local invasion, lymphadenopathy

Mediastinal Lymphadenopathy
- Metastatic lymphadenopathy
  - ➤ Lung cancer, extrathoracic malignancy
- Lymphoma
- Granulomatous disease
  - ➤ Tuberculosis, fungal disease, sarcoidosis
- Castleman disease

Lymphoma
- Non-Hodgkin lymphoma - 75% of all cases
- 50-70% of mediastinal lymphoma is Hodgkin disease
  15-21% of mediastinal lymphoma is non-Hodgkin lymphoma
- Hodgkin – 66% intrathoracic at presentation
  Non-Hodgkin – 37% intrathoracic at presentation
- Treatment: Radiotherapy, chemotherapy

Lymphoma: Clinical Features
- Hodgkin Disease
  - ➤ Males=Females but NSHD, 2 X more common in females
  - ➤ Bimodal distribution: 2nd to 3rd and > 5 th decades
  - ➤ Lymphadenopathy: cervical, supraclavicular
  - ➤ 20-30%; chest pain, systemic complaints
- Non-Hodgkin lymphoma
  - ➤ Systemic disease with constitutional symptoms: lymphadenopathy, local invasion
  - ➤ Lymphoblastic - male children/adolescents
  - ➤ Diffuse large-B cell - young adult females

Figure 1-16-18

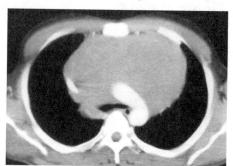

Seminoma; imaging features - Homogeneous locally invasive anterior mediastinal mass

Figure 1-16-19

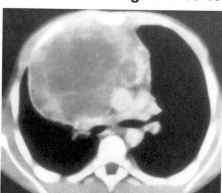

Non-seminomatous GCN; imaging features - Heterogeneous right anterior mediastinal mass

Lymphoma: Pathologic Features *[Figure 1-16-20]*
- Hodgkin Disease
  - ➤ Nodal cellular infiltrate, collagenous connective tissue (NS), Reed-Sternberg cell
  - ➤ Lymphadenopathy, nodal coalescence, primary thymic involvement, cystic change
  - ➤ Local invasion, hemorrhage, necrosis
- Non-Hodgkin Lymphoma
  - ➤ Lymphoblastic (precursor T-lymphoblastic) -lymphoblasts
  - ➤ Diffuse large B-cell (primary mediastinal [thymic] large B-cell) large cells, vesicular nuclei, prominent nucleoli
  - ➤ Large, infiltrative, locally invasive, necrosis

Lymphoma: Imaging Features *[Figures 1-16-21 and 1-16-22]*
- Lobulated diffuse mediastinal enlargement
- Hodgkin
  - ➤ Intrathoracic involvement in 85%
  - ➤ Lymphadenopathy; prevascular, paratracheal
  - ➤ Nodal coalescence (homogeneous or heterogeneous)
  - ➤ Ca++; 1% - 1 year post-therapy, rare pre-therapy
- Non-Hodgkin
  - ➤ Prevascular, paratracheal
  - ➤ Isolated involvement of other mediastinal nodes
  - ➤ Local invasion
  - ➤ Primary mediastinal involvement
  - ➤ High signal on T2 - active disease, inflammation, cystic change, immature fibrosis

Metastatic Lymphadenopathy
- Advanced lung cancer; small cell carcinoma
- Extrapulmonary malignancy; renal cell, testicular, head and neck

Mediastinal Fibrosis
- Young patients with signs and symptoms of obstruction
  - ➤ Trachea, bronchi, esophagus, vessels
- Mediastinal mass, circumscribed or locally invasive, calcification
- Systemic antifungal agents, excision, dilatation, bypass graft
- 30% mortality

Castleman Disease
- Angiofollicular or giant lymph node hyperplasia
- Hyaline vascular type (>90%) vs plasma cell variant
- Localized vs. systemic
- Adult females (M:F - 4:1) may be asymptomatic
- Imaging findings
  - ➤ Middle mediastinal / hilar mass
  - ➤ Solitary mass
  - ➤ Dominant mass with lymphadenopathy
  - ➤ Multiple enlarged lymph nodes
  - ➤ Enhancement, calcification (10%)

Bronchogenic Cyst
- Most common congenital cyst of the mediastinum
- Abnormal ventral foregut bud
- Failure to induce mesenchymal development to lung parenchyma

Figure 1-16-20

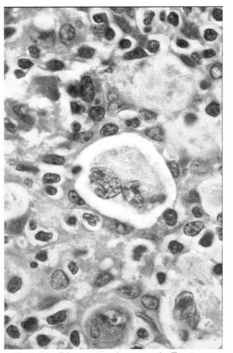

Hodgkin Disease; microscopic Features

Figure 1-16-21

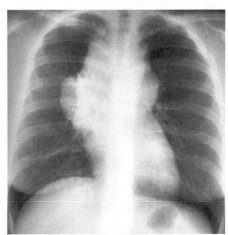

Hodgkin disease; imaging features - Diffuse anterior mediastinal enlargement

Figure 1-16-22

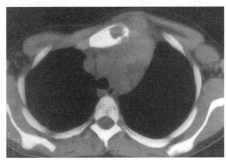

Hodgkin disease; imaging features - Locally invasive mediastinal lymphadenopathy, axillary lymphadenopathy

- Mediastinum (85%), pericardium, diaphragm, pleura and lung

Figure1-16-23

Bronchogenic Cyst: Clinical Features
- Rare in infants, infrequent in children
  - Young adults
- Asymptomatic – incidental finding
  - Symptomatic – chest pain, mass effect, obstruction, infection
- Excision, observation, drainage, sterile alcohol ablation

Bronchogenic Cyst : Pathologic Features
[Figures 1-16-23 to 1-16-25]
- Ciliated pseudostratified columnar epithelial lining (respiratory epithelium)
- Bronchial glands, cartilage plates, smooth muscle in the wall
- Closed connection to foregut structures (fibrous stalk)
- Middle mediastinum (posterior / anterior)
- Spherical, ovoid, unilocular
- Thin wall
- Fluid – clear, turbid, hemorrhagic, serous, viscous

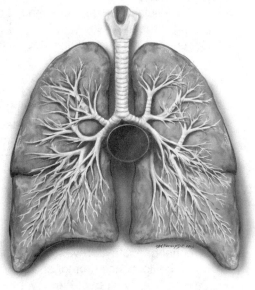

Mediastinal bronchogenic cyst

Figure 1-16-24

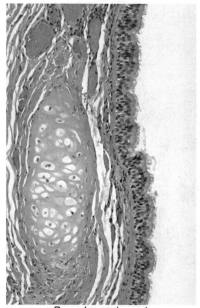

Bronchogenic cyst;
microscopic features

Figure 1-16-25

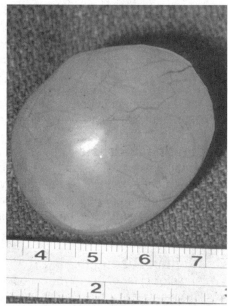

Bronchogenic cyst; gross features

Bronchogenic Cyst: Imaging Features *[Figures 1-16-26 and 1-16-27]*
- Well-defined, spherical, middle mediastinal mass
- Near trachea, carina, stem bronchi
- CT:
  - Well-defined, thin smooth wall (contrast enhancement)
  - Water (40%) or soft tissue (43%) attenuation
  - Homogeneous non-enhancing contents
- MR:
  - T-1; variable (most slightly hyperintense to skeletal muscle)
  - T-2; isointense or hyperintense to CSF
  - Symptomatic patients
- Thin-walled pulmonary cyst; air, fluid, air-fluid level

Figure 1-16-26

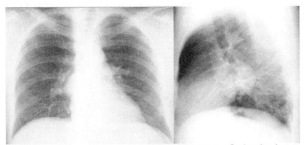

Bronchogenic cyst; imaging features - Spherical subcarinal soft tissue mass

Figure 1-16-27

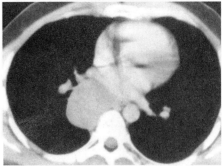

Bronchogenic cyst; imaging features - Spherical subcarinal non-enhancing mass of homogeneous soft tissue attenuation

Other Congenital Cysts

- Foregut cysts
- Esophageal - within the esophageal wall may contain ectopic gastric mucosa)
- Neuroenteric - Associated spinal anomaly
- Pericardial - Cardiophrenic angle, imperceptible wall, fluid attenuation (asymptomatic)

Thymic Cyst *[Figures 1-16-28 and 1-16-29]*

- Uncommon (3% of mediastinal masses)
- Congenital vs. Acquired
- Children / young adults
  - ➤ Association with neoplasia, AIDS
  - ➤ (DILS - diffuse infiltrative lymphocytosis syndrome)
  - ➤ Lymphocyte infiltration of parotid glands, lungs
  - ➤ Lacrimal glands, liver, stomach, kidney and thymus
- Epithelial lining and thymus in cyst wall
- Multilocular / unilocular
- R/O cystic neoplasm

Figure 1-16-28

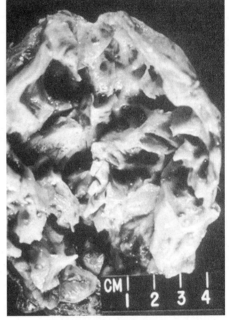

Thymic cyst; gross features

Figure 1-16-29

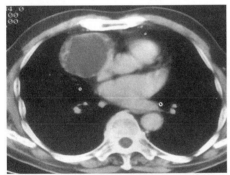

Thymic cyst; imaging features - Anterior mediastinal multilocular cyst with thin enhancing soft tissue septa

Neurogenic Neoplasms *[Figure 1-16-30]*

- 20% of primary mediastinal neoplasms
  - ➤ 35% in children
- 70–80% benign
- Peripheral nerves
  - ➤ Schwannoma, neurofibroma
  - ➤ Malignant peripheral nerve sheath tumor
- Sympathetic ganglia
  - ➤ Ganglioneuroma
  - ➤ Ganglioneuroblastoma
  - ➤ Neuroblastoma

Figure 1-16-30

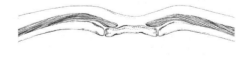

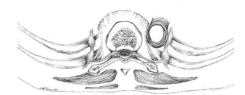

Neurogenic neoplasms

Schwannoma / Neurofibroma [Figure 1-16-31]
- Schwannoma – Most common mediastinal neurogenic neoplasm
  - Spherical, encapsulated
  - Cellular and less cellular areas (Antoni A and B)
  - Calcification, cystic change, hemorrhage
- Neurofibroma – second most common mediastinal neurogenic neoplasm
  - Spherical/fusiform, unencapsulated
- Neurofibromatosis (NF1)
  - Multiple neoplasms (including ganglioneuroma)
  - Plexiform neurofibroma
  - Vagus nerve, sympathetic chain, phrenic nerve
  - Diffuse enlargement of peripheral nerve
  - Multiple masses along a nerve
- Young adults; 3rd and 4th decade
  - Most (65%) asymptomatic
  - Symptoms and signs of compression

Schwannoma / Neurofibroma: Imaging Features
[Figures 1-16-32 and 1-16-33]
- Spherical, smooth or lobular, well-defined paravertebral mass
- Osseous findings (50%)
  - Pressure erosion/deformity of ribs/vertebrae
  - Expanded neuroforamen
- Homogeneous/heterogeneous
  - Heterogeneous enhancement
  - Ca++ in 10%
  - Growth into spinal canal 10%
- MR Imaging – R/O spinal involvement
  - T1 – Low-to-intermediate signal
  - T2 – Foci of high signal

Neurofibromatosis (NF1)
- Multiple neoplasms (ganglioneuroma)
- Plexiform neurofibroma
- Vagus, sympathetic chain, phrenic nerve
- Diffuse enlargement of peripheral nerve
- Multiple masses along a nerve

Malignant Peripheral Nerve Sheath Tumor
- Most frequent in the posterior mediastinum
  - Rare among neurogenic neoplasms
- Large (>5 cm) spherical mass
  - Central low attenuation – necrosis
  - Calcification
  - May exhibit local invasion

Thoracic Meningocele
- Intrathoracic extrusion of meninges and their fluid content
- Well-defined spherical paraspinal mass
- Enlarged neuroforamen, pressure erosion, sclerosis
- Homogeneous, fluid attenuation / signal

Peripheral Nerve Neoplasms: Therapy and Prognosis
- Excision
- Schwannoma/Neurofibroma
  - Excellent prognosis
- Malignant peripheral nerve sheath tumor
  - Solitary – 75% five-year survival
  - Neurofibromatosis – 30% five-year survival

Figure 1-16-31

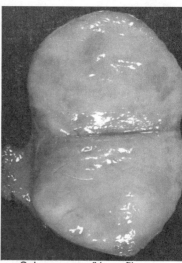

Schwannoma/Neurofibroma; gross features

Figure 1-16-32

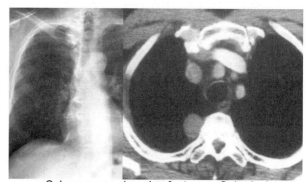

Schwannoma; imaging features - Spherical paravertebral soft tissue mass

Figure 1-16-33

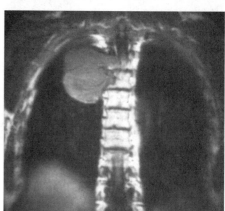

Schwannoma; imaging features - Spherical lobular paravertebral soft tissue mass with intraspinal growth

Ganglioneuroma [Figure 1-16-34]
- Children, adolescents, young adults
- Asymptomatic patients
- De novo; maturation of neuroblastoma
- Benign posterior mediastinal neoplasm
- Mature ganglion cells, Schwann cells, nerve fibers
- Encapsulated, elongate mass
  - ➢ Gray/yellow with lobular surface

Ganglioneuroma: Imaging Features [Figure 1-16-35]
- Well-defined, oblong posterior mediastinal mass
- Osseous erosion/displacement
- Homogeneous or heterogeneous
- Calcification in 25%
- MR: Homogeneous intermediate signal on T1 and T2
- R/O intraspinal extension

Ganglioneuroblastoma/Neuroblastoma
- Infants and young children
- Asymptomatic/chest wall pain
  - ➢ Paraplegia, Horner syndrome, diarrhea, hemothorax
- Elevation of urine catecholamines
- Elevation of urine/serum VMA (screening)
- Neuroblastoma
  - ➢ 50% < 2 years
  - ➢ 90% < 5 years
  - ➢ May be congenital

Ganglioneuroblastoma/Neuroblastoma: Pathologic Features
- Adrenal – most common location
  - ➢ Mediastinum – second most common location
- Ganglioneuroblastoma
  - ➢ Neuroblasts and ganglion cells
  - ➢ Well/poorly differentiated
- Neuroblastoma
  - ➢ Neuroblasts, Homer – Wright pseudorosettes
  - ➢ Well/poorly differentiated

Neuroblastoma: Imaging Features [Figure 1-16-36]
- Well-defined large elongate posterior mediastinal mass
- Radiographic evidence of Ca++ in 10%
- Osseous erosion
- R/O intraspinal growth
- Local soft tissue invasion

Sympathetic Ganglia Tumors: Prognosis
- Ganglioneuroma
  - ➢ Excision is curative
- Ganglioneuroblastoma
  - ➢ Five-year survival near 90%
- Neuroblastoma
  - ➢ Five-year survival – 30%
  - ➢ More favorable course with: Age < 2 yrs, mediastinal tumors, spontaneous maturation to ganglioneuroma

Figure 1-16-34

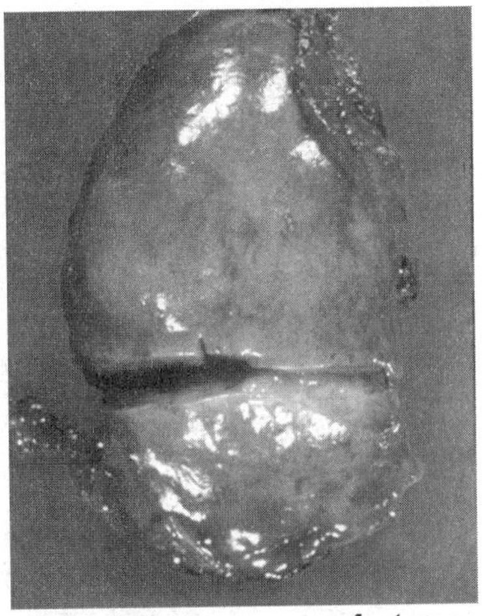

Ganglioneuroma; gross features

Figure 1-16-35

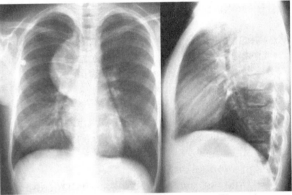

Ganglioneuroma; imaging features - Elongate paravertebral soft tissue mass with benign pressure erosion and displacement of adjacent rib

Figure 1-16-36

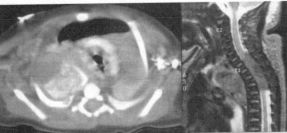

Neuroblastoma; imaging features - Elongate calcified paravertebral mass with extensive intraspinal growth

Paraganglioma

- Middle mediastinum – Aortopulmonary paraganglia
  - Paravertebral – aortico sympathetic paraganglia
  - Heart
- Adults (average age 30-40 yrs)
  - Males > Females; 2:1
  - Asymptomatic/excess catecholamines
- Well-defined spherical mass
  - Homogeneous/heterogeneous
- Marked contrast enhancement
  - 90% uptake of I^{131} or I^{123} MIBG

Mediastinal Goiter

- 20% of cervical goiters
- Asymptomatic females: incidental finding
  - May produce symptoms by mass effect
- Adenomatous goiter; rarely malignancy/thyroiditis
- Fibrous capsule; nodules composed of thyroid follicles
- Hemorrhage, calcification, cystic change

Mediastinal Masses: Surgical

- Thymoma
- Teratoma

Mediastinal Goiter: Imaging Features *[Figures 1-16-37 and 1-16-38]*

- Unilateral anterior mediastinal mass (80%), unilateral
  - Other compartments also affected, R>L
- Well-defined lobular borders
- Cervico-thoracic sign
  - Continuity with cervical thyroid
- Calcification - punctate, coarse, curvilinear
- Cystic change
- High attenuation
  - Intense, sustained contrast enhancement

Parathyroid Adenoma

- Ectopic parathyroid glands: superior pole of thymus (39%), mediastinum (2%)
- Primary hyperparathyroidism post-surgical parathyroidectomy
- MEN I
- Imaging
  - Tc99m/Tl201 subtraction imaging
  - T123/Tl201
  - Tc99m - Sestamibi (mitochondria)
  - Single radionuclide/Dual radionuclide
- CT/MRI correlation of mediastinal uptake

Lymphangioma

- Benign mesenchymal mediastinal tumor
- Proliferation of lymphatic vessels without communication with lymphatic tree
- Developmental vs. neoplasm vs. hamartoma
- Asymptomatic/symptoms of compression
- Mediastinal extension of cystic hygroma (10%), soft palpable mass
- 90% diagnosed in infancy
- Mediastinal mass in asymptomatic child / adult

Figure 1-16-37

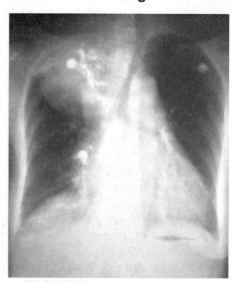

*Mediastinal goiter; imaging features -
Calcified soft tissue mass with
cervicothoracic extension*

Figure 1-16-38

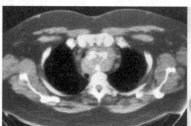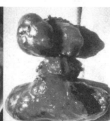

*Mediastinal goiter; imaging features and pathologic
correlation - High attenuation mediastinal mass with
dense internal calcification*

Lymphangioma: Pathologic Features [Figure 1-16-39]
- Intercommunicating vascular spaces of variable size lined by endothelial cells
- Soft, cystic mass
- Cystic hygroma - macroscopic vascular spaces

Figure 1-16-39

Lymphangioma: Imaging Features [Figure 1-16-40]
- Anterosuperior mediastinum; other compartments affected
- Cervical/axillary/chest wall mass with mediastinal extension
- Spherical, lobular, well-defined borders
- Circumscribed mass/infiltrative mass
- Multilocular, cystic, heterogeneous
  - Solid components, tissue septa

Hemangioma
- Rare vascular mediastinal tumor
- Neoplasm vs. developmental
- Young patients; 75% < 35 yrs.
- Asymptomatic; 1/3-1/2 /symptoms of compression
  - Rendu-Osler-Weber syndrome
- Communicating vascular spaces
  - Endothelial lining, organized thrombi, Ca++, phleboliths
- Anterior mediastinal mass (other compartments)
  - Spherical, well-defined
- Heterogeneous intense (central) contrast enhancement
  - Calcification: approx. 28%, punctate, phleboliths

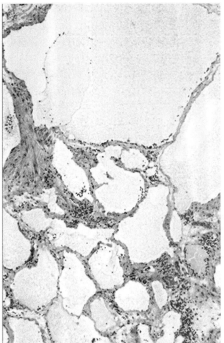

Lymphangioma; microscopic features

Mediastinal Masses: Pathognomonic
- Lateral thoracic meningocele
- Extramedullary hematopoiesis
- Aneurysm
- Esophageal varices
- Teratoma
- Lipomatosis
- Congenital cyst (bronchogenic/pericardial)
- Mediastinal goiter

Figure 1-16-40

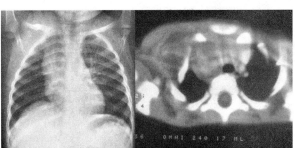

Paraesophageal Varices
- Supplied by left gastric vein, portosystemic collateral pathway in portal hypertension
- Outside esophageal wall; communicate with esophageal varices (mural)
- Drain into the systemic venous circulation
- Severe liver disease and portal hypertension
- Middle-posterior/ paravertebral lobular soft tissue mass
- Visible on radiography in less than 10%
- Dilated serpiginous masses with intense enhancement

Lymphangioma; imaging features; Multilocular cystic anterior/middle mediastinal mass with extension into the axilla

Hiatus Hernia
- Intrathoracic gastric herniation through enlarged esophageal hiatus
- Herniation of fat, abdominal fluid
- Increased intra-abdominal pressure
- Increased prevalence with increasing age
- Asymptomatic patients; symptoms of gastroesophageal reflux or bleeding
- Retrocardiac mass: homogeneous soft tissue, air-filled, air-fluid level (s)
- Foregut cyst **

Achalasia
- Absent peristalsis and incomplete relaxation of esophageal sphincter
- Primary: ganglion cell deficiency
  - Presentation between 30 and 50 years
  - Dysphagia, bad breath, recurrent pulmonary infection
- Secondary: malignancy or Chagas disease
  - Malignancy; presentation after age 60 years
  - Recent dysphagia, weight loss
- Esophageal dilatation; air-fluid level
- Poor visualization of stomach
- Associated pulmonary disease

Extramedullary Hematopoiesis
- Compensatory erythrocyte production
- Inadequate production, hemolysis
- Congenital hemolytic anemia, lymphoproliferative disorder, sickle cell disease
- Unilateral / bilateral paravertebral mass
- Between T6 and T12 (or along entire thoracic spine)
- Osseous marrow expansion, coarse trabeculation
- Homogeneous, fat attenuation

Mediastinal Masses: Cystic
- Thymoma (mural nodules)
- Congenital cysts (unilocular, middle mediastinum)
- Neurogenic neoplasm (Heterogeneous soft tissue mass, osseous erosion)
  - Lateral meningocele (neurofibromatosis, continuity with spinal canal)
- Mature teratoma (multilocular cyst w/fat)
- Lymphoma (cystic mass with lymphadenopathy)
- Lymphangioma (vascular channels)
- Esophageal enlargement
- Mediastinal goiter (high attenuation soft tissue elements)

Mediastinal Masses: Fat
- Lipomatosis (diffuse involvement)
- Lipoma
- Thymolipoma (fat/soft tissue mixture)
- Mature teratoma (multilocular cystic mass with fat content)
- Morgagni hernia (continuity with abdominal contents)

Mediastinal Masses: Intense Enhancement
- Mediastinal goiter (continuity with cervical thyroid)
- Hemangioma (phleboliths, follows vascular enhancement)
- Castleman disease (enhancing lymphadenopathy)
- Paraganglioma (catecholamine production)
- Aneurysm/Varices

Mediastinal Masses References

Aquino SL, Duncan G, Taber KH, Sharma A, Hayman LA. Reconciliation of the anatomic, surgical, and radiographic classifications of the mediastinum. J Comput Assist Tomogr 2001; 25: 489-492.

Felson B. Chest Roentgenology. Philadelphia: Saunders, 1973: 380-420.

Fraser RS, Müller NL, Colman N, Paré PD. Masses situated predominantly in the anterior mediastinal compartment. Masses situated predominantly in the middle-posterior mediastinal compartment. Masses situated predominantly in the paravertebral region. In: Fraser RS, Müller NL, Colman N, Paré PD, eds. Fraser and Paré's Diagnosis of Diseases of the Chest. 4th ed. Philadelphia, PA: W.B. Saunders 1999:2875-2983.

Kim M-J, Mitchell DG, Ito K. Portosystemic collaterals of the upper abdomen: Review of anatomy and demonstration on MR imaging. Abdom Imaging 2000; 25: 462-470.

McAdams HP, Rosado de Christenson ML, Moran CA. Mediastinal hemangioma: radiographic and CT features in 14 patients. Radiology 1994; 193:399-402.

McAdams HP, Rosado de Christenson ML, Fishback NF, Templeton PA. Castleman disease of the thorax: radiologic features with clinical and histopathologic correlation. Radiology 1998;209:221-228.

McAdams HP, Kirejczyk WM, Rosado de Christenson ML, Matsumoto S. Bronchogenic cyst: imaging features with clinical and histopathologic correlation. Radiology 2000; 217: 441-446.

Moeller KH, Rosado de Christenson ML, Templeton PA, Moran CA. Mediastinal mature teratoma: Imaging features. Am J Roentgenol 1997;169:985-990.

Rosado de Christenson ML, Galobardes J, Moran CA. Thymoma: Radiologic Pathologic Correlation. RadioGraphics 1992;12:1013-1030.

Rosado de Christenson ML, Templeton PA, Moran CA. Mediastinal germ cell tumors: Radiologic-pathologic correlation. RadioGraphics 1992;12:151-168.

Rosado de Christenson ML, Pugatch RD, Moran CA, Galobardes J. Thymolipoma: analysis of 27 cases. Radiology 1994;193:121-126.

Rosado de Christenson ML, Abbott GF, Kirejczyk WM, Galvin JR, Travis WD. Thoracic carcinoids: Radiologic-pathologic correlation. RadioGraphics 1999;19:7107-736 (730-733).

Rosado de Christenson ML, Pugatch RD, Moran CA, Galobardes J. Thymolipoma: analysis of 27 cases. Radiology 1994;193:121-126.

Rosado de Christenson ML, Abbott GF, Kirejczyk WM, Galvin JR, Travis WD. Thoracic carcinoids: Radiologic-pathologic correlation. RadioGraphics 1999;19:7107-736 (730-733).

Rosai J, Sobin LH. Histological Typing of Tumours of the Thymus. International Histological Classification of Tumours, Second edition. New York: Springer 1999.

Rossi SE, McAdams HP, Rosado-de-Christenson ML, Franks TJ, Galvin JR. Fibrosing mediastinitis. RadioGraphics 2001; 21:737-757.

Shaffer K, Rosado de Christenson ML, Patz EF Jr, Young S, Farver CF. Thoracic lymphangioma in adults: CT and MR imaging features. Am J Roentgenol 1994;162:283-289.

Shimosato Y, Mukai K. Tumors of the thymus and related lesions. In: Rosai J, ed. Atlas of Tumor Pathology: Tumors of the Mediastinum, fasc 21, ser 3. Washington, DC: American Registry of Pathology and Armed Forces Institute of Pathology, 1997: 33-247.

Strollo DC, Rosado de Christenson ML, Jett JR. Primary mediastinal tumors - Part 1, Tumors of the anterior mediastinum. Chest 1997;112:511-522.

Strollo DC, Rosado de Christenson ML. Tumors of the Thymus. J Thorac Imag 1999;14:152-171.

Strollo DC, Rosado-de-Christenson ML. Primary mediastinal malignant germ cell neoplasms: imaging features. Chest Surg Clin N Am 2003; 12: 645-658.

Thomas CR, Wright CD, Loehrer PJ, Sr. Thymoma: state of the art. J Clin Oncol 1999; 17: 2280-2289.

Tomiyama N, Müller NL, Ellis SJ, et al. Invasive and noninvasive thymoma: distinctive CT features. J Comput Assist Tomogr 2001; 25: 388-393.

Radiologic Pathology: Unknown Case Seminar: Where is the lesion?

Melissa L. Rosado de Christenson, MD, FACR

Clinical Professor of Radiology
The Ohio Sate University
Columbus, OH

Adjunct Professor of Radiology
Uniformed Services University
Bethesda, MD

Learning Objectives
- To review the radiologic features of thoracic radiologic abnormalities based on location
- To emphasize radiologic-pathologic correlation
- To enumerate the radiologic characteristics that allow lesion localization and the formulation of a focused radiologic differential diagnosis

Case1: 38-year-old female with cough
- Location
- Differential diagnosis
- Next best study
- Diagnosis:

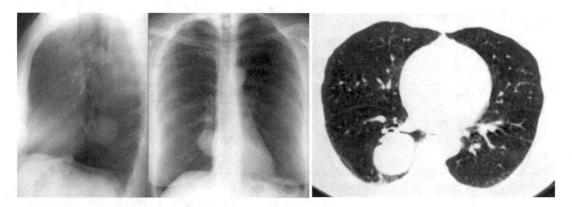

Solitary Lung Mass
- Lung cancer
  - ➢ Size / frequency
  - ➢ Stage ?
- Carcinoid tumor
  - ➢ Borders / bronchus
- Solitary metastasis
  - ➢ Location / shape
- Hamartoma / Infection
  - ➢ Borders

Solitary Lung Mass
- Young, relatively asymptomatic female
- Mass with well-defined lobular borders
- Lower lobe
- Abutting bronchus

Case 2: 16-year-old female with cough
- Location
- Differential diagnosis
- Next best study
- Diagnosis:

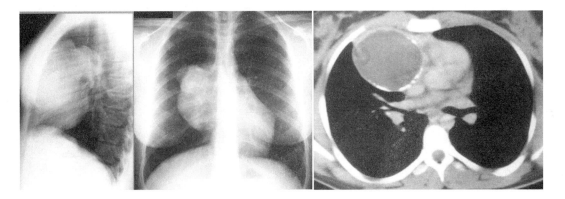

Anterior Mediastinal Mass
- Young, relatively asymptomatic female
- Well-defined, Ca++ lobular borders
- Non-enhancing low attenuation center
- Heterogeneous low attenuation areas

Anterior Mediastinal Mass
- Mature teratoma
  - Fluid / fat / Ca++
- Thymic cyst
  - Fluid
- Lymphoma
  - Age
- Thymoma
  - Fluid
- Other

Case 3: 58-year-old male with chest pain and hemoptysis
- Location
- Differential diagnosis
- Next best study
- Diagnosis:

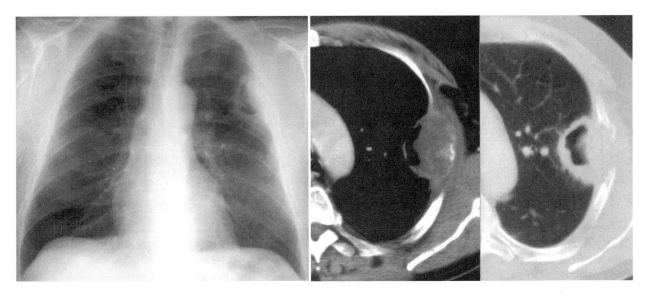

Chest Wall Involvement / Cavitation
- Symptomatic older male
- Chest wall invasion (rib destruction)
- Upper lobe
- Cavitation

Chest Wall Mass / Cavitation
- Bronchogenic CA
  - ➢ Chest wall invasion
  - ➢ Stage?
- Infection
  - ➢ Actinomycosis, TB, fungal
- Primary chest wall tumor
- Other

Case 4: Asymptomatic 40-year-old male Pre-operative chest radiograph
- Location
- Differential diagnosis
- Next best study
- Diagnosis:

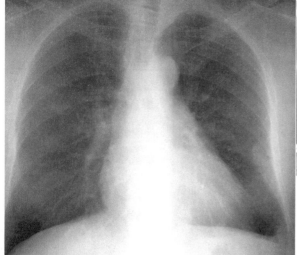
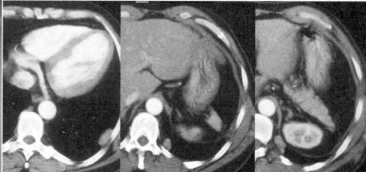

Multifocal Pleural Nodules
- Asymptomatic male
- No known malignancy
- Well-defined peripheral pleural-based nodules
- Associated findings
- Abdominal abnormalities?

Multifocal Pleural Nodules
- Splenosis
  - ➢ Where is the spleen?
- Metastases
- Malignant pleural mesothelioma
- Other

Splenosis
- Auto-transplantation of splenic tissue typically following splenic rupture
- Most common manifestation: Multiple peritoneal nodules
- Thoracic splenosis:
  - ➢ Multiple pleural-based nodules
  - ➢ May be missed on radiography
  - ➢ 99mTC-tagged heated RBC scintigraphy
  - ➢ Liver-spleen scan

Case 5: 34-year-old male with left chest pain for many years

- Location
- Differential diagnosis
- Next best study
- Diagnosis:

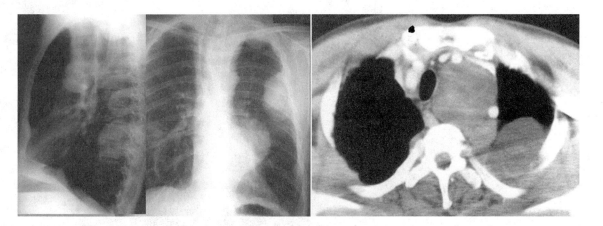

Multifocal Chest Wall and Mediastinal Masses

- Chronic lesions
  - ➢ Minimal symptoms
- Unilateral or bilateral?
- Benign pressure erosion
- Pulmonary disease
- Other chest wall involvement

Multifocal Chest Wall and Mediastinal Masses

- Neurofibromatosis
  - ➢ Malignant potential
- Vascular lesions
- Metastases
- Other

Radiologic Pathology: Unknown Case Seminar: Differential Diagnosis of Mediastinal Masses

Melissa L. Rosado de Christenson, MD, FACR
Clinical Professor of Radiology
The Ohio Sate University
Columbus, OH

Adjunct Professor of Radiology
Uniformed Services University
Bethesda, MD

Case 1: Elderly male with chest pain
- Location
- Characterization
- Next study
- Biopsy
- Differential diagnosis

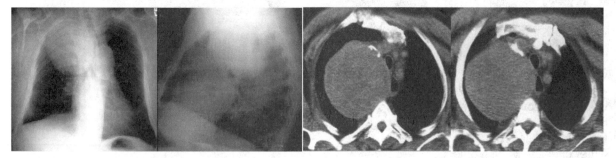

Heterogeneous Middle Mediastinal Mass; Rim CA++
- Neoplasia
  - ➢ Carcinoma
  - ➢ Lymphoma
- Congenital Cyst
- Vascular lesion
  - ➢ Aneurysm
- Other

Case 2: Asymptomatic 52-year-old male
- Differential diagnosis
- Next best study

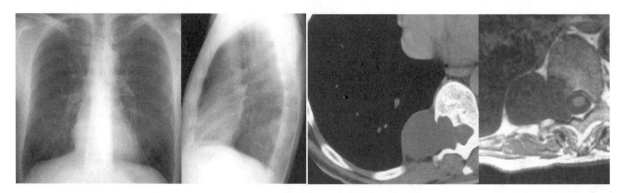

Spherical Posterior Mediastinal Mass with Pressure Erosion
- Neurogenic
  - ➢ Neoplasm
  - ➢ Next study?
- Lateral Thoracic Meningocele
  - ➢ History?
- Other

Case 3: 40-year-old female with difficulty swallowing
- Differential diagnosis
- Next best study

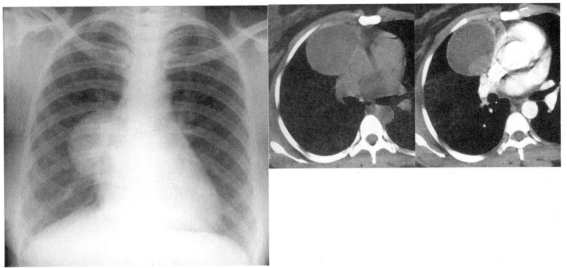

Unilateral Cystic Anterior Mediastinal Mass; Mural CA++
- Cystic Thymoma
- Cystic Teratoma
- Thymic Cyst
- Cystic Lymphoma
- Pericardial Cyst

Unilateral Cystic Anterior Mediastinal Mass; Mural CA++
- Symptomatic female
- Age over 40
- Pattern of enhancement

Case 4: 24-year-old male with abdominal discomfort for many years
- Differential diagnosis
- Diagnosis
- Should the lesion be excised?

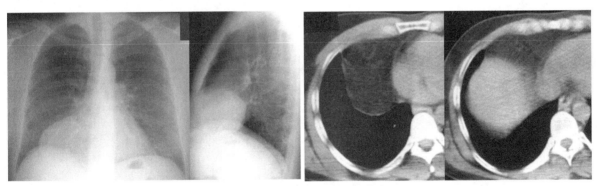

Right Cardiophrenic Angle Mass of Fat and Soft Tissue Attenuation
- Thymolipoma
  - ➢ Fat / soft tissue
- Lipoma
  - ➢ Fat / soft tissue
- Mature Teratoma
  - ➢ But...No fluid
- Morgagni Hernia
  - ➢ Continuity with abdominal fat

Case 5: 29-year-old female with fatigue and persistent cough
- Differential diagnosis
- Diagnosis
- Should the lesion be
  - excised?
  - biopsied?

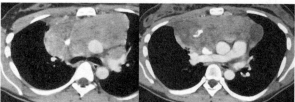

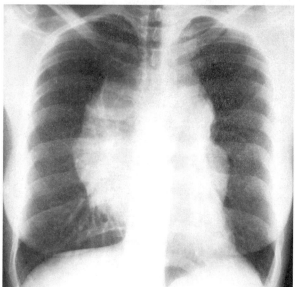

Anterior Mediastinal Mass
(Cystic change, Ca++)
- Lymphoma:
  - Gender
  - Age
  - Local invasion
  - Lymphadenopathy
  - Cystic change
  - Ca++ ?
- Thymoma
  - Cystic change
  - Ca++
  - But…lymphadenopathy

Anterior Mediastinal Mass
(Cystic change, Ca++)
- Teratoma
  - But…lymphadenopathy
- Malignant GCN
  - But…wrong gender

PNEUMONIA: Usual and Unusual Organisms

Rosita M. Shah, MD
Hospital of the University of Pennsylvania

Classification of Pulmonary Infection
- Community-acquired Pneumonia
  - S. pneumoniae LOBAR
  - Mycoplasma LOBULAR
  - Influenzae INTERSTITIAL
- Aspiration Pneumonia
- Nosocomial Pneumonia

Pulmonary Infection: Classification: Morphology
- 3 radiographic and pathologic patterns
  - Lobar
  - Lobular (bronchopneumonia)
  - Interstitial

Pulmonary Infection: Classification
- Lobar and lobular pneumonias both produce air space filling
- Significant differences include:
  - Site of initial inflammation
  - Degree of lobular opacification
  - Radiographic pattern
  - Etiologic agents

Alveolar Filling Pneumonias
- Site of initial infection varies
  - Lobar Pneumonia
  - Bronchopneumonia

Alveolar Filling Pneumonias
- Degree of opacification of secondary lobule is different
  - Lobar Pneumonia
  - Bronchopneumonia

Alveolar Filling Pneumonias
- Radiographic pattern will vary
  - Lobar Pneumonia
  - Bronchopneumonia

Alveolar Filling Pneumonias
- Etiologic agent may vary

Lobar Pneumonia	Bronchopneumonia
S.pneumoniae	Gram –'s, anaerobes
K.pneumoniae	Legionella
also seen with	Actinomycosis
Legionella	Nocardia
Mycoplasma	Mycoplasma
H.influenzae	Typical, atypical TB
	Parasites

Alveolar Filling Pneumonias
- Accurate pattern recognition depends on:
  - Early imaging
  - Normal lung structure
- Organisms may produce more than one pattern
- Basic pattern differentiation may be difficult
  - Interstitial vs bronchopneumonia

Community-acquired Pneumonia: Epidemiology
- 2–10 /1000 annual incidence
- 22-50% hospitalization rate
  - Outpatient mortality 1-5%
  - Inpatient mortality 25%

Community-acquired Pneumonia: Pathology
- Failure of normal defenses
  - Mucociliary clearance
  - Macrophage function
  - Humoral and cellular immunity

Community-acquired Pneumonia: Etiology
- In up to 50%, no definitive organism isolated
- Most common isolates:
  - S. pneumoniae
  - M. pneumoniae
  - K. pneumoniae
  - H. influenzae
  - L. pneumophila
  - Respiratory viruses

S. pneumoniae: Demographics
- S. pneumoniae most frequent isolate in CAP
  - 8-76% incidence
- Recognized risk factors
  - alcoholism, splenic dysfunction, viral pneumonia, congenital and acquired immune deficiencies

S. pneumoniae: Demographics
- 25% incidence of bacteremia
- 25-40% mortality, unchanged >30y
  - Age >65
  - CHF,DM
  - Alcoholism
  - Thrombocytopenia
  - Renal dysfunction
  - Number of lobes

Chest 1993; 103:1152-56

S. pneumoniae: Pathology
- Aspiration to peripheral air spaces
- Alveolus represents site of initial inflammatory lesion
- Spread occurs by contignous involvement of adjacent alveoli
- 3 pathologic stages

S. pneumoniae: Pathology
- ACUTE RESPONSE
  - ➢ Increased capillary permeability
  - ➢ Protein rich edema
  - ➢ Contiguous alveolar filling via Pores of Kohn and Canals of Lambert
- RED HEPATIZATION
  - ➢ PMN infiltration and intra-alveolar hemorrhage
- GRAY HEPATIZATION
  - ➢ Macrophage infiltration and uptake of blood products

S. pneumoniae: Radiology *[Figure 1-19-1]*

Figure 1-19-1

- Spread at alveolar level results in nonsegmental distributions characteristic of early lobar pneumonia
- Round pneumonia
  - ➢ Manifestation of nonsegmental distribution
  - ➢ Most common in pediatric infection with S.pneumoniae
- LOBAR pattern
  - ➢ Prominent air bronchograms
  - ➢ Preserved volume

S. pneumoniae: Radiology
- 48% of consecutive hospitalized pts demonstrated focal lobar patterns
- 16% lobular pattern
- Dominant pattern did not vary with immune status or disease severity

AJR 2000;175:1533

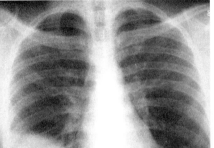

Lobar pattern in S.pneumoniae

S. pneumoniae: Radiology
- Small pleural effusions up to 60%
- Infrequent cavitation
  - ➢ Associated with serotype 3
- Most frequent organism in pulmonary gangrene
  - ➢ Vascular thrombosis from severe necrosis
  - ➢ Intracavitary mass (sloughed lung)

M. pneumoniae: Demographics
- 15-35% of CAP
  - ➢ 50% of CAP during summer months
- Peak age 5-25 yo
- Self limited
  - ➢ Few fatal cases associated with ARDS
  - ➢ Increased severity in sickle cell anemia
- Most frequent etiology in Atypical Pneumonia Syndrome
  - ➢ Atypical radiographic features
  - ➢ Prominent extrapulmonary complaints

M. pneumoniae: Pathology
- Eaton agent-1944
  - ➢ Gram -- filamentous rod
  - ➢ Absent cell wall
- Acute cellular bronchiolitis
  - ➢ Superficial inflammation involving luminal surface of bronchi, bronchioles
  - ➢ Associated interstitial infiltrates

M. pneumoniae: Radiology [Figure 1-19-3]

- LOBULAR pattern Bronchopneumonia
- Heterogeneous, patchy consolidation
  - ➢ Minimal exudate into centrilobular alveoli
- Segmental distribution
  - ➢ Spread at bronchiolar level
- Volume loss
- Minimal air bronchograms
  - ➢ Peribronchial thickening

M. pneumoniae: Radiology

CT Findings [Figure 1-19-3]

    86% centrilobular
    82% bronchovascular thickening
    59% consolidation with lobular distribution

Reittner, AJR 2000; 174:37

Respiratory Viruses

- Influenzae A,B,C
- Para-influenzae
- Respiratory syncytial virus
- Adenovirus
- Herpes viruses
- Hantavirus
- SARS

Influenzae A: Demographics

- 10-20% CAP
- 10,000-40,000 deaths/ influenzae epidemic
- Peak incidence
  - ➢ Pediatric population
- Highest mortality-adult and aged
  - ➢ Superinfection
  - ➢ S.aureus
  - ➢ S.pneumoniae

Influenzae A: Pathology

- St 1 infection of epithelial cells, proliferation and necrosis
- St 2 bronchial and alveolar wall edema,hemorrhage
- Ulceration, bacterial infection

Influenzae A: Radiology

- INTERSTITIAL pattern
  - ➢ Reticular
  - ➢ Nodular
  - ➢ Peribronchial thickening
  - ➢ Subpleural edema
  - ➢ Hilar haze

Influenzae A: Radiology

[Figure 1-19-4]

- Bilateral, parahilar, lower lobe
- Air trapping
- Prominent GGO

Figure 1-19-2

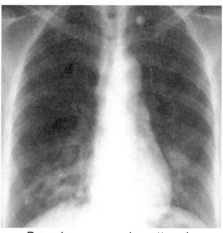

Bronchopneumonia pattern in Mycoplasma

Figure 1-19-3

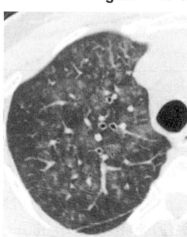

Prominent nodular pattern with centrilobular features and GGO in Mycoplasma

Figure 1-19-4

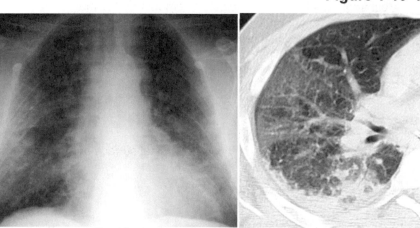

(left) reticular interstitial pattern in Influenzae
(right) extensive GGO and bronchovascular infiltration on corresponding HRCT

Influenzae A: Radiology
- Pleural effusions, cavitation uncommon without bacterial superinfection
- Rapid deterioration should suggest superinfection

Adenovirus
- Interstitial pneumonia with prominent necrotizing bronchiolitis
- Potential infection in immune competent and suppressed hosts with high mortality
  - Military epidemics
  - Transplant recipients
  - pediatric population
- Swyer James, Macleod's syndrome
  - Bronchiolitis obliterans following viral infection in early childhood

Respiratory Herpesviruses
- HSV-1, HSV-2, VZV, EBV, CMV
  - Primary infection, latency, reactivation
  - Up to 40% mortality
- Risk factors
  - Immune-suppression, lung transplantation, airway management, pregnancy

Varicella Pneumonia
- Complication of adult chickenpox
  - 5-50% incidence
- Prominent acinar opacities
  - 5-10mm nodules, coalescence
  - Patchy GGO

Kim AJR 1999;172:113
- May heal with miliary calcifications

Varicella Pneumonia *[Figure 1-19-5]*
- Prominent acinar opacities

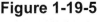
Figure 1-19-5

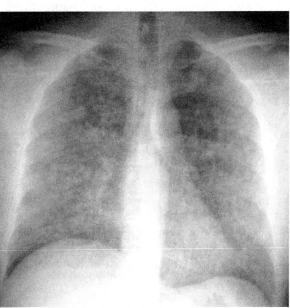

Acinar opacities in Varicella pneumonia

Severe Acute Respiratory Syndrome
- SARS-CoV (corona virus)
- Initial cases Nov 2002-June 2003, rapid spread from Asia
- 20-50% require mechanical ventilation
- 10% mortality, age dependant
- Severe DAD

Severe Acute Respiratory Syndrome
- Predominant consolidation 1-2weeks
  - Focal (39%), multifocal (28%), diffuse (14%)
- Ground glass opacity
- Reticulation
- Bronchiolar dilation
- Residual changes in 50% at 4wks

Ooi GC. Radiology 2004;230:836; Paul NS. AJR 2003;182:493

Hantavirus
- Incidental human transmission from rodent hosts
- North America strain first recognized 1993 in SW USA
  - Other recognized strains, including Korean hemorrhagic fever
- Normal young adults with rapid respiratory insufficiency and demise. 50% mortality

Duchin JS. NEJM 1994; 330:949

Hantavirus
- Diffuse alveolar consolidation
  - Manifestation of severe alveolar edema and hyaline membrane formation
  - Similar to SARS

Severe Community-acquired Pneumonia: Definition
- Impending respiratory failure
- Hemodynamic instability
- Radiographic assessment
  - Bilateral or multilobar involvemnt
  - 50% increase in size of opacity within 48hr

Severe Community-acquired Pneumonia: Etiology
- S. pneumoniae
- L. pneumophila
- Gram-negative bacilli in patients with chronic disease
- S. aureus
- P. aeruginosa in patients with bronchiectasis

L. pneumophila: Demographics
- 15% of CAP
  - Epidemic and sporadic forms
  - Legionnaire's disease= pneumonic form
  - Peak summer
- Aerobic Gram -- bacillus
- Proliferates in warm, humid environments

L. pneumophila: Pathology
- Bronchocentric inflammation

L. pneumophila: Demographics
- Acute onset
- Prominent extrapulmonary symptoms
  - Neurologic manifestations, diarrhea, renal insufficiency
- 10% mechanical ventilation
- 15% mortality in cases requiring hospitalization

L. pneumophila: Radiology [Figure 1-19-6]
- Bronchopneumonia pattern
- Pleural effusions in 2/3
- Bilateral and multifocal in 50%
- May produce lobar or mass-like consolidation
- Cavitation uncommon without immunosupression
- Delayed resolution

Figure 1-19-6

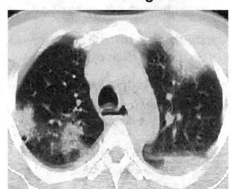

Bronchopneumonia pattern and pleural effusion in Legionella

K. pneumoniae: Demographics
- Nosocomial or community acquired
- 5-10% lobar pneumonias
- 25% bacteremic, 50% mortality
- Males, >60yo
- Risk factors: alcoholism, COPD, DM

K. pneumoniae: Pathology
- Gram -- bacillus
  - Abundant PMN infiltration of alveoli, edema
  - Lobar expansion - Friedlander's pneumonia
  - Massive necrosis
  - Common association with gangrene

K. pneumoniae: Radiology [Figure 1-19-7]
- Lobar pattern
  - ➢ Bulging fissures
- Abscess 30-50%
- Necrotizing pneumonia at CT
  - ➢ Low density areas with small cavities

Moon JCAT 1995;19:176

S.aureus: Demographics
- CAP associated with viral pneumonia
  - ➢ 50% follow influenza, 30% mortality
- Frequent cause of nosocomial infection
- Extremes of age
  - ➢ Nursing home population
- Risk factors
  - ➢ Debilitated states, mechanical ventilation, burns, indwelling catheters, IVDA

S. aureus: Radiology [Figure 1-19-8]
- Aerogenous infection
  - ➢ Multifocal Broncho-pneumonia
- Hematogenous infection
  - ➢ Multifocal, discrete nodular or wedge shaped abnormality with normal intervening lung
- Cavitation / abscess (25-75%)
- Pneumatoceles (60% ped infection)
- Pleural effusions / empyema (50%)

L. pneumophila: Pathology
- Aerobic Gram negative bacillus
- Aquatic environments, elevated temperatures
- Peribronchial inflammation

L. pneumophila: Radiology
- Bronchopneumonia pattern most common
  - ➢ May produce lobar or mass-like consolidation
- Bilateral and multifocal in 50%
- Pleural effusions in 2/3
- Cavitation uncommon without immunosuppression
- Slow resolution

The Practical Points
- S.pneumoniae and K.pneumoniae most commonly associated with lobar pattern and pulmonary gangrene
- M.pneumoniae, L.pneumophilus most commonly associated with broncho-pneumonia pattern and atypical pneumonia syndrome
- Viral pneumonias associated with interstitial pattern
- Pathologic in immune-competent and suppressed hosts

Aspiration Pneumonia
- 5-15% of CAP
  - ➢ 20% of nursing home pneumonias
  - ➢ 10% of drug OD
  - ➢ 10-30% of anesthesia-related deaths

Aspiration Pneumonia
- Community-acquired aspiration
  - ➢ S. pneumoniae
  - ➢ S. aureus
  - ➢ H. influenzae
- Anaerobic organisms identified in hospital-acquired and late aspiration

Figure 1-19-7

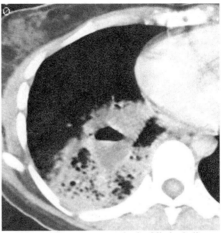

Necrotic pneumonia in Klebsiella

Figure 1-19-8

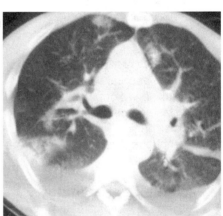

Septic emboli due to S.aureus

Aspiration Pneumonia: Radiology
- Dependant consolidation
  - Abscess / empyema

Aspiration Pneumonia: 18hr follow-up
Rapid clearing in aspiration pneumonitis

Aspiration Pneumonia: Radiology
Frequent bronchopneumonia pattern

Nosocomial Pneumonia
- Gram negative colonization of oropharynx
  - 22% at 24hr
  - 40% at 5 d
- Elevated gastric pH
- Mechanical ventilation

P. aeruginosa: Demographics
- Most common cause of nosocomial infection
  - Community acquired infection recognized in HIV, CF
- 60-80% mortality
- Risk factors
  - Mechanical ventilation, debilitated states, neutropenia, cystic fibrosis

P. aeruginosa: Pathology
- Gram -- bacillus
  Exotoxins - exotoxin A
  Elastase, phospholipase C
- Hemorrhage
- Microabscesses
- Necrotic vasculiti

P. aeruginosa: Radiology
- Bronchopneumonia pattern
  - Discrete nodules may be indicative of vasculitis
- Frequent cavitation
- Pleural effusions/empyema

P.aeruginosa sepsis, 1mo s/p BMT [Figure 1-19-9]

Community Acquired P.aeruginosa, advanced HIV

P. aeruginosa in Cystic Fibrosis [Figure 1-19-10]
- Chronic colonization with P. aeruginosa
  - Mucoid variant
  - ABX resistance
  - Elastase production
  - Bronchiectasis

Nodular or Mass-like Consolidations
- Nonsegmental distribution
  - 'round' pneumonia
- Granulomatous infection
  - M. tuberculosis
  - Fungi
  - Actinomycosis
  - Nocardia

Figure 1-19-9

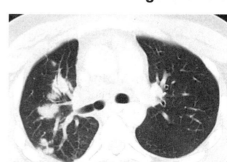
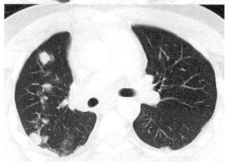

Prominent nodular pattern in P.aeruginosa in a patient following BMT

Figure 1-9-10

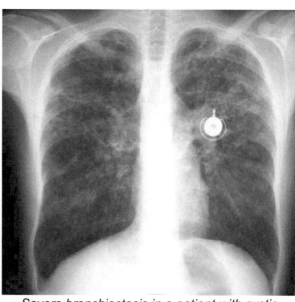

Severe bronchiectasis in a patient with cystic fibrosisand chronic colonization with P.aeruginosa

A. Israelii; Demographics
- Normal oral flora
- Sites of infection:
  - Cervicofacial   55%
  - Abdomen   20%
  - Pulmonary   25%

Smego RA. Clin Infec Dis 1998;26:1255

A. Israelii: Pathology
- Multifocal abscesses
- Interconnecting sinus tracts
- Sulphur granule
  - Spoke-wheel arrangement of neutrophils surrounding filamentous organism

A. Israelii: Radiology [Figure 1-19-11]
- Consolidation
  - Mass-like
  - Cavitary
- Pleural, chest wall and osseous involvement
  - Up to 50%

N. Asteroides: Demographics
- Ubiquitous distribution
- 50% of patients are immunocompetent
- Risk factors:
  - Neutropenia
    - Steroids, late HIV, hemetologic malignancy, alveolar proteinosis

N. Asteroides: Pathology
- Peribronchial abscesses, granulomatous inflammation
- Extensive necrosis
  - May mimic M.TB or fungal infection

N. Asteroides: Radiology [Figure 1-19-12]
- Extrapulmonary disease 50% with 40-90% mortality
  - CNS 25%
  - Skin and subcutaneous abscesses

N. Asteroides: Radiology
- Consolidation
  - Mass-like
  - Cavitary
- Pleural and chest wall involvement 30-50%
- Adenopathy 40%

Cavitary Pneumonia in AIDS
- N. asteroides

Alveolar Proteinosis and N. asteroides

Parasitic Infection
- Pulmonary involvement due to hypersensitivity or direct invasion
  - Echinococcosis
  - Paragonimiasis
  - Ascariasis
  - Strongyloidiasis

Figure 1-19-11

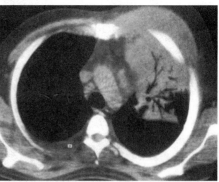

LUL consolidation with chest wall invasion due to Actinomycosis

Figure 1-19-12

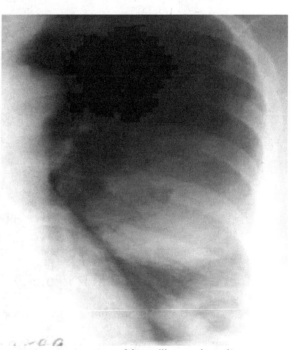

Mass-like and cavitary consolidations due to Nocardia

Parasitic Infection
- Radiographic findings may overlap with other infections
  - Fleeting, patchy infiltrates
  - Reticulonodular opacities
  - Bronchopneumonia
  - Atelectasis

Echinococcus granulosus
- Cestode (tapeworm), endemic to S.America, Australia, Middle East, Africa and Mediterranean
- Definitive host - dog,wolf
  Intermediate host - sheep, cow,deer, moose

Echinococcus granulosus
- Duodenum - portal venous system liver
  - 45-75% isolated liver involvement
  - 15-35% pulmonary involvement

Echinococcus granulosus [Figure 1-19-13]
- Pulmonary cysts acquired in childhood
- Diagnosis 30-40yo
- Intact cyst - asymptomatic
- Eosinophilia 25-40%

Echinococcus granulosus: Pathology
- Hydatid cyst consists of 3 layers
  - Pericyst – host inflammatory cells
  - Exocyst – acellular laminated membrane
  - Endocyst – fluid-filled germinal center, daughter cysts

Echinococcus granulosus: Radiology
- Intact cyst
  - Well demarcated, homogeneous mass
  - Spherical when central, ovoid when peripheral
  - Multiple 20-30%
  - Lower lobes 60%

Echinococcus granulosus: Radiology
- Impending Rupture
  - Crescent sign - air between pericyst and laminated membrane

Echinococcus granulosus: Radiology
- Ruptured cyst
  - Water lily sign – rupture of endocyst

Paragonimiasis westermani
- Trematode (lung fluke)
  - endemic to Asia
  - Contaminated freshwater crab
- Jejunum – peritoneal cavity – diaphragm – pleura – lung
- Chronic granulomatous reaction

Paragonimiasis westermani: Radiology
- Pulmonary findings dependant on stage of infection
  - PTX and pleural infection during pleural penetration by juvenile worms
  - Transient, patchy consolidation and linear tracts during larval migration
- Peribronchial cysts associated with mature worm

Figure 1-19-13

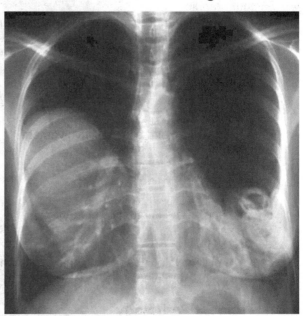

Intact(right) and ruptured(left) echinococcal cysts

Ascariasis lumbricoides
- Roundworm infection
- Most common parasitic infection
  - Endemic worldwide
  - 25-95% prevalence
  - Highest incidence in children

Ascariasis lumbricoides
- Large iingestion associated with pneumonitis
- Small bowel – systemic circulation – alveoli - trachea – small bowel

Strongyloides stercoralis
- Round worm
- Skin – systemic circulation – alveoli – trachea – small bowel

Ascariasis Strongyloides: Radiology
- Bronchopneumonia
- Patchy, transient consolidation
- Eosinophilic pneumonia

B. Anthracis: Anthrax
- Gram+ spore forming rod
  Dormant spores are virulent
- Infection typical in livestock
- Exotoxin production associated with hemorrhagic mediastinitis, edema and pleuritis

Earls Radiology:222:305, 2001

Complications of Pneumonia
- Pleural Infection
- Empyema
  - Purulent exudate
  - WBC>25,000
  - pH<7.0
  - + organisms

S.mitis Empyema in 51yo male with IVDA hx

Complications of Pneumonia
- Cavitation
  - Cavitary pneumonia
  - Lung abscess
  - Pneumatocele
  - Gangrene
  - DDX bronchopleural fitula

Complications of Pneumonia
- Pneumatocele
  - Ball-valve mechanism
  - Rapid evolution
  - No lung destruction
- Most common with S.aureus
  - 60% of peds infection

Complications of Pneumonia [Figure 1-19-14]
- Pulmonary Gangrene
  - Lung necrosis due to vascular thrombosis
- Most common with S.pneumoniae K.pneumoniae

Figure 1-19-14

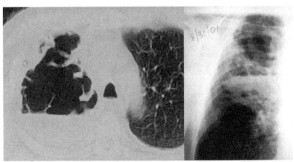

RUL pulmonary gangrene

Complichations of Pneumonia [Figure 1-19-15]

Figure 1-19-15

- Bronchiectasis
  - ➢ Irreversible dilation
    - ✧ Should not be diagnosed < 4 m of acute infection
  - ➢ Colonization with atypical TB, aspergillus

Complications of Pneumonia

- Bronchiectasis
  - ➢ Advanced course in HIV
  - ➢ +/- antecedant infection

A.fumigatus complicating post-infectious bronchiectasis

The Role of Imaging in Pneumonia

- Diagnosis of infection
  - ➢ Presence of centrilobular nodules in acute parenchymal disease favors pneumonia

    Tomiyama N. AJR 2000;174:1745

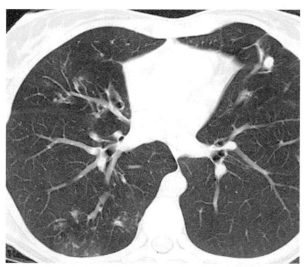

M. avium-intracellulare complex in a patient with RML bronchiectasis due to severe childhood pneumonia

- Thin section CT allows earlier diagnosis of pneumonia in immunosuppressed pts (5 days)

  Heussel CP. AJR 1997;169:1347

- Recognition of complications
  - ➢ Decreased enhancement in pneumonia indicates severe necrosis

    Donnelly LF. Radiology 1997;205:817

The Practical Points

- Organisms may produce more than one pattern
- Bacterial, viral and fungal pneumonia have similar CT findings post lung transplantation

  Collins AJR 2000;175:811
- Consider clinical setting

Uncommon Malignant Tumors of the Lung

Dr. Gerald F. Abbott
Brown University Medical School
Providence, Rhode Island

Uncommon Primary Malignant Neoplasms of the Lung:
- Bronchial Carcinoid
- Adenoid Cystic Carcinoma
- Mucoepidermoid Carcinoma
- Carcinosarcoma
- Pulmonary Blastoma

"Bronchial Adenoma"
- Term formerly referred to:
  - ➢ Bronchial Carcinoid
  - ➢ Adenoid Cystic Carcinoma
  - ➢ Mucoepidermoid Carcinoma
- A misnomer
- These tumors are not benign

"Carcinoid"
- Carcinoma-like neoplasm
- 1907 – Oberndorfer

Carcinoids
- Gastrointestinal tract (90%)
- Thymus
- Lung
- Biliary tract
- Ovarian teratomas

Bronchial Carcinoid
- Typical carcinoid
- Atypical carcinoid

Typical Carcinoid
- 0.6-2.4% of all pulmonary neoplasms
- Low grade malignancy
- Good prognosis
  - ➢ 95% five-year survival
- Not associated with smoking

Typical Carcinoid: Demographics
- Males = Females
- Wide age range
- Median age: 50 years
- Symptoms:
- cough, hemoptysis, dyspnea

Typical Carcinoid: Microscopy
- Cells form nests, ribbons, rosettes, trabeculae
- Stroma highly vascular
- May exhibit calcification / osseous metaplasia
- Polygonal cells, pale cytoplasm,stippled nuclear chromatin
- Rare mitoses
- Ultrastructure: neurosecretory granules

Neuroendocrine Tumors: World Health Organization criteria (1999)

- Typical carcinoid: <2 mitoses per 10 HPF
- Atypical carcinoid: 2-10 mitoses per 10 HPF
- Large cell neuroendocrine ca: 11 or more mitoses per 10 HPF (median 70)
- Small cell ca: 11 or more mitoses per 10 HPF (median 80)

Atypical Carcinoid: Microscopy

- Poor architectural organization
- Cellular pleomorphism
- Focal necrosis
- Increased mitotic activity

Arrigoni J Thorac Cardiovasc Surg 1972

Carcinoid: Relationship to Small Cell Carcinoma

- Similarities:
  - ➢ Neurosecretory granules
  - ➢ Rosette and trabecula formation
- Differences:
  - ➢ Carcinoid: no association with smoking
  - ➢ Fewer granules in Small Cell Carcinoma

Atypical Carcinoid

- Morphology intermediate between Typical Carcinoid and Small Cell Ca
- Larger, more invasive
- Tend to be peripheral
- Age: Decade older than Typical
- Symptoms: similar to Typical
- Imaging: similar to Typical

Atypical Carcinoid

- 10% of cases
- Peripheral
- Increased mitoses
- Aggressive behavior; early metastases
- Osteoblastic bone metastases
- DDx: Small Cell Carcinoma

Bronchial Carcinoid: Gross *[Figures 1-20-1, 1-20-2, 1-20-3]*

- Soft, fleshy, endobronchial mass
- Sessile, may be pedunculated
- Usually seen at bronchoscopy
- Often extends through bronchial wall

Figure 1-20-1

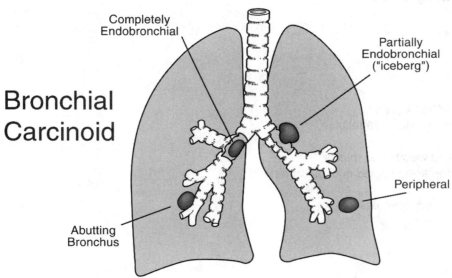

Bronchial Carcinoid

Completely Endobronchial

Partially Endobronchial ("iceberg")

Peripheral

Abutting Bronchus

Bronchial Carcinoid: Radiologic Findings
- Central tumors in 80% of patients
  - ➢ Lobar, segmental, subsegmental bronchi
- Endobronchial nodule / mass
- Adjacent to bronchus
- Peripheral nodule or mass
- Consolidation, atelectasis
- Pleural effusion

Bronchial Carcinoid: CT Features
- 83% associated with bronchus
- Partially endobronchial ("iceberg" tumor)
- Completely endobronchial
- Abutting a bronchus
- Sharply marginated lobulated mass
- May enhance or demonstrate Ca^{++}
- Atelectasis, consolidation, bronchiectasis, mucoid impaction
- Lymphadenopathy

Kirejczyk (AFIP), Radiology 1995 197(p);366.

Bronchial Gland Tumors
- Adenoid Cystic Carcinoma
- Mucoepidermoid Carcinoma
- Equivalent to salivary gland tumors of same name

Adenoid Cystic Carcinoma
- Synonym - Cylindroma
- 80% of bronchial gland tumors
- 20 to 35% of all tracheal tumors
- Second most common tracheal malignancy (most common = squamous cell carcinoma)

Adenoid Cystic Carcinoma
- Guarded prognosis
- Common local recurrence
- Occasional metastases to regional nodes
- Rarely extrathoracic spread

Adenoid Cystic Carcinoma: Demographics
- Males = Females
- Wide age range
- Average age: 40 - 50
- Symptomatic patients:
- Cough, wheezing, dyspnea, hemoptysis

Adenoid Cystic Carcinoma: Microscopy
- Mucin-containing cysts of varying caliber within larger tumor tubules
- Surrounds and invades nerves, encases vessels, infiltrates bronchi
- Few mitoses
- Pathology DDX: Adenocarcinoma

Adenoid Cystic Carcinoma: Gross [Figure 1-20-4]
- Rubbery firm mass
- Nodular vs. annular constricting lesion
- Bronchial mucosa intact over the tumor
- Growth along tracheobronchial walls
- Locally invasive

Figure 1-20-2

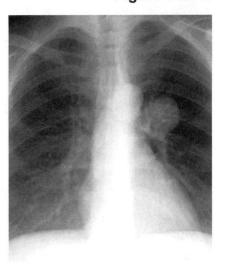

Figure 1-20-3

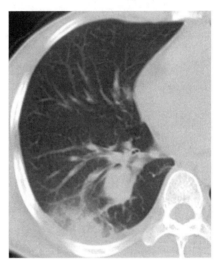

Figure 1-20-4

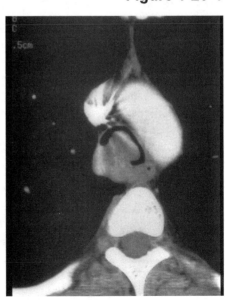

Adenoid Cystic Carcinoma: Radiologic Findings
- Central: trachea and main bronchi
- Intraluminal nodule or mass
- Constriction of tracheal/bronchial lumen
- 10 - 15% in lung periphery
- CT / MRI: length of involvement; mediastinal involvement

Mucoepidermoid Carcinoma: Demographics and Prognosis
- Slight male predominance
- Wide age range
- Symptomatic patients - cough, fever, hemoptysis, pneumonia, atelectasis
- Low grade tumors - excellent prognosis
- High grade tumors - prognosis still better than that of Bronchogenic Ca

Mucoepidermoid Carcinoma: Microscopy
- Low, moderate, and high grades
- Low grade: Abundant mucinous cysts and solid collections of squamous cells
- High grade: Solid tumor sheets with mitoses and necrosis
- Pathology DDX: Poorly diff. Squamous Cell Carcinoma, Adenosquamous Carcinoma

Mucoepidermoid Carcinoma: Gross
- Submucosal, smooth surfaced
- Endobronchial, exophytic, polypoid
- High grade tumors may have ragged invasive appearance

Mucoepidermoid Carcinoma: Radiologic Findings
- Central: most in bronchi, few in trachea
- Ill defined mass, atelectasis, pneumonia
- Solitary nodule or mass
  - most frequent finding in AFIP series

Yousem. Cancer 1987; 60:1346.

Mixed Tumors: Neoplasms with malignant epithelial and mesenchymal components
- Carcinosarcoma
- Pulmonary Blastoma

Carcinosarcoma
- Rare - 0.3% of all lung neoplasms
- Middle aged and elderly males
- Poor prognosis
- Aggressive: local invasion, widespread metastases, and rapid death

Carcinosarcoma: Microscopy
- Epithelial component:
- Squamous Cell Carcinoma
- Adenocarcinoma
- Undifferentiated Carcinoma

Carcinosarcoma: Microscopy
- Mesenchymal component:
- Spindle cell type - most common
- Chondrosarcoma, Osteosarcoma, Rhabdomyosarcoma
- Mesenchymal component usually dominant
- Pathology DDX: Spindle Cell variant of Squamous Cell Ca

Carcinosarcoma: Gross

- Peripheral
- Large mass; Average diameter 6 cms.
- Frequent central necrosis and hemorrhage
- Central
- Endobronchial growth
- May extend to adjacent parenchyma
- Tumor-distended bronchi may resemble mucus plugs

Carcinosarcoma: Radiologic Findings

- Peripheral
- Large, sharply circumscribed mass
- Central
- Atelectasis, pneumonia, "mucus plugs"
- Upper lobe predominance
- Direct extension to pleura, chest wall,or mediastinum may occur

Pulmonary Blastoma

- Primary lung tumor
- Mixture of blastomatous and immature epithelial and mesenchymal components
- Morphologic mimic of the embryonal lung
- Initially thought to be analogous to the renal nephroblastoma
- ? a variant of carcinosarcoma

Pulmonary Blastoma: Demographics and Prognosis

- Predominantly males
- Biphasic age distribution:
- First and seventh decades
- Symptoms: cough, hemoptysis, dyspnea, chest pain
- Poor survival

Pulmonary Blastoma: Microscopy

- Mixture of epithelial-lined tubules and primitive stroma
- Suggests recapitulation of early embryonal lung development
- Metastases can be mesenchymal, epithelial, or mixed
- Pathology DDX: Carcinosarcoma

Pulmonary Blastoma: Gross

- Large mass
- Unencapsulated and soft
- Abundant central necrosis and hemorrhage

Pulmonary Blastoma: Radiologic Findings

- Large peripheral mass
- Well-circumscribed
- May show pleural invasion
- May Metastasize

Benign Tumors of the Lung and Tumor-like Lesions

Dr. Gerald F. Abbott
Brown University Medical School
Providence, Rhode Island

Benign Tumors and Tumor-like lesions
- Hamartoma
- Papilloma / Papillomatosis
- Inflammatory pseudotumor
- Granuloma

"Hamartoma"
- Albrecht, 1904
- Tumor-like malformation
- Tissues normal to location
- In excess or disarray (disorganized)
- *"Adult", "Classic", "Local"* hamartoma

Hamartoma
- Most common benign tumor of lung
- 5 – 8% of SPNs
- 77% of benign lung tumors
- 3% of all lung tumors

Hamartoma
- Acquired lesion (although the term implies a congenital malformation)
- Disorganized growth of tissues normally found in lung
- Benign neoplastic proliferation
- Probably derived from bronchial wall mesenchymal cell
  ("benign mesenchymoma")

Hamartoma: Evidence of Acquired Lesion
- Onset in adult life
- Often adults with previously normal CXR
- Almost never seen in infants
- Histology: passive entrapement of epithelium
  - ➢ Cytogenetics: Chromosome 12: abnormal q13-q15 regions
    (as in other benign soft-tissue neoplasms)

Hamartoma: Demographics
- Age range: 30-70 years
- Peak incidence: 6th decade
- Female: Male = 3:2 (1:1 for endobronchial hamartoma)
- Asymptomatic in 90%
  < 8% obstructive symptoms

Hamartoma: Clinical
- Most are peripheral and asymptomatic
- If symptomatic: hemoptysis
- If bronchial obstruction: pneumonitis
- Fever, cough, expectoration, chest pain

Hamartoma: Microscopic
- Cartilage nests (lobules) in 95%
- Surrounded by fibrous tissue
- *Often:* collections of mature fat cells
- *Sometimes:* monotonous, without cartilage
  - ➢ Glandular component: traced from adjacent alveoli or bronchioles

Hamartoma: Gross
- Solitary (Rarely multiple: "Carney's Triad")
- 1 – 3 cm (rarely "Giant")
- Rounded, well-circumscribed, lobulated
- Firm lesions. Usually cartilaginous
- May see areas of fat
- Easily "shelled-out"

Hamartoma: Distribution
- Peripheral > Central
- 80 – 90 % Peripheral
- No lobar predilection

Hamartoma: Radiographic
- Sharply defined, often lobulated
- Often subpleural
- Most < 3 cm
- May see Ca^{++} on CXR (10-15%)
- Rarely see fat on CXR

Hamartoma: Calcification
- 10 – 15% speckled or "Popcorn"
- Smaller nodular growths within lesion
- Protrude in different directions
- "Popcorn" calcification less frequent than once thought
- Diagnostic when present

Hamartoma: CT
- Distinguishes fat and cartilage
- Most are 2.5 cm or less
- Smooth edge
- Fat: No fat / Focal fat alone / Fat with areas of calcification
- Cavitation: rare

Figure 1-21-1

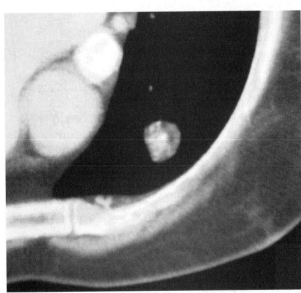

Hamartoma: CT *[Figure 1-21-1]*
- Thin sections (2mm)
- Smoothly contoured nodule
- = or < 2.5 cm diameter
- focal fat (-80 to –120 HU) in 8 voxels or more
- or fat alternating with calcification (>175 HU)

Siegelman. Radiology 1986; 160:313-317.

Hamartoma: CT
- 17/47 (36%) no fat or calcification
- 2/47 (4%)   diffuse calcification
- 18/47 (38%) areas of fat
- 10/47 (21%) calcium and fat
- Occasionally: focal Calcification, No fat

Siegelman. Radiology 1986; 160:313-317.

Hamartoma: Growth
- ➢ May enlarge on serial CXRs
- ➢ One study: 5 mm per year (diameter)
- ➢ Another study: 3.2 mm per year

"Carney's Triad" (1979)
- Epitheloid gastric smooth muscle tumor (leiomyomas, leiomyosarcomas)
- Functioning extra-adrenal paraganglioma
- Pulmonary chondroma
- Association unclear
- Young females < 20 years
- May have only 2/3 of the triad

Hamartoma: Endobronchial
- Morphologically identical to parenchymal
- Often polypoid
- Sessile or thin pedicle
- Manifest by airway obstruction
- Micro: Greater proportion of fat, lack clefts, cartilage scant or absent

Hamartoma: Treatment and Prognosis
- Benign
- Surgical excision = cure in vast majority
- Exceptional cases: additional hamartomas

Hamartoma: SPN
- Third most common cause of SPN
- Granuloma, Lung Cancer, Hamartoma

Papillomas
- Branching or coarsely lobulated tumor
- Arise from and project above an epithelial surface
- Rare pulmonary tumors
- Solitary (rare) or Multiple (papillomatosis)
- Proximal or peripheral

Solitary Papillomas
- Rare
- Usually found in adults
- Papillary exophytic growth
- Lobar or segmental bronchus, trachea
- Males >40 years of age
- Post-obstructive pneumonia, bronchiectasis

Juvenile Laryngeal Papillomatosis
- Larynx of children 18 months to 3 years of age
- Majority remain localized, disappear spontaneously
- May spread distally and cause complete or partial airway obstruction
- Most cases remain limited to trachea (5%)
- 1% develop lung disease (10 years after laryngeal disease) extension to bronchi, bronchioles, alveolar airspaces

Laryngeal Papillomatosis: Etiology
- Human papilloma virus types 6 and 11
- 0.1% of infants develop LP; predilection for first-born infants
- 50% of their mothers have genital tract involvement
- HPV spread transvaginally at birth
- Infects oropharyngeal secretions of child

Papillomas: Microscopic
- Bland non-keratinizing squamous cells
- Multilayered
- Form papillomatous projections
- Rarely glandular histology
- Sometimes mixed squamous and glandular epithelium

Papillomatosis: Gross
- Sessile or pedunculated; cauliflower-like excrescences
- Protrude into bronchial lumens
- May extend into parcenchyma as nodules or cavities
- Cavities lined by papillary growths or nodules
- Cavitation may be prominent feature

Papillomatosis: Pathogenesis of lower respiratory tract involvement:
- Implantation of inhaled fragments from larynx?
- Multifocal viral infection?
- Trauma-induced by tracheostomy for laryngeal disease?
- In children, multiple papillomas in bronchi and lung always associated with multiple papillomas of trachea or larynx

Laryngeal Papillomatosis: Radiology
- Multiple small well-defined round pulmonary nodules
- Frequent cavitation
- Polypoid lesions in airways

Figure 1-21-2

Papillomatosis in Lung: Imaging [Figure 1-21-2]
- Multiple, well-defined nodules
- Perihilar, Posterior half of thorax
- Grow to several centimeters
- Then cavitate, 2-3 mm thick walls
- Air-fluid levels may develop
- Cavities may represent:
  - ➢ Papillomatosis
  - ➢ Necrotic Squamous cell carcinoma
  - ➢ Abscess secondary to obstructive pneumonitis

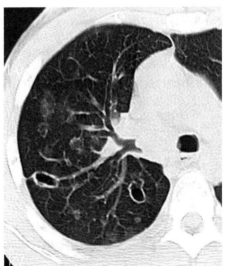

Papillomatosis: Treatment and Prognosis
- Multiple recurrences. Multiple excisions. Tracheostomy
- 37.5% mortality If spread to lungs
- Worse if malignant degeneration occurs
- Significant risk for Squamous cell carcinoma
- Associated risk factors:
  - ➢ Cigarette smoking
  - ➢ Radiation exposure
  - ➢ Other carcinogens

Inflammatory Pseudotumor: Synonyms
- Plasma cell granuloma
- Histiocytoma
- Fibroxanthoma, Xanthoma
- Myofibroblastic tumor
- Mast cell granuloma

Inflammatory Pseudotumor
- Uncommon. Non-neoplastic. Reactive process
- Occasionally aggressive
- Proliferative process
- May begin as organizing pneumonia
- Aggressive features may mimic neoplasia
  - ➢ Vascular invasion
  - ➢ Vertebral destruction
  - ➢ Recurrence

Inflammatory Pseudotumor: Demographics
- Males = Females
- Wide age range: 1 to 77 years. Average: 29.5 years
- 60% <40 years
- Children: peak age 6-7 years (most common 1° lung mass in children)
- 74% asymptomatic
- Many patients have history of respiratory infection
  - ➢ ? trigger for development of IP

Inflammatory Pseudotumor: Microscopic
- Variable.
- A continuum from plasma cell granuloma to fibrohistiocytic
- Mixture of collagen, fibroblasts, myofibroblasts, and chronic inflammatory cells (plasma cells, lymphocytes, foam cells, giant cells, macrophages)

Inflammatory Pseudotumor: Gross
- SPN or Mass
- Well-defined
- Firm
- Lobulated
- Cut-surface: whorled, heterogeneous
- 1-10cm, 4.4 cm mean diameter

Inflammatory Pseudotumor: Radiographic
- Solitary, well-defined nodule or mass - 70%
- Endobronchial lesions occur - 10%
- May extend into mediastinum –5%
- Calcification, cavitation infrequent
- Parenchymal consolidation – 6%
- May mimic malignant neoplasm
- Usually no or slow growth
- May regress

Inflammatory Pseudotumor: CT
- SPN or mass
- Sharply circumscribed
- Lobulated
- Heterogeneous or homogeneous
- Contrast enhancement: variable and nonspecific
- Calcification: variable

Inflammatory Pseudotumor: Therapy and Prognosis
- Dx and Rx: surgical excision
- Excellent prognosis after resection
- Recurrence in 5%

Granuloma
- Infectious
- Sarcoid (necrotizing granuolomatosis)
- Hypersensitivity pneumonitis

Infectious Granulomas
- Mycobacterial   64%
- Fungal   30%
- Parasitic   6%

Granuloma [Figure 1-21-3]
- Inflammatory
- Tuberculoma or Histoplasmoma
- Satellite lesions common
- Usually small, smooth
- Often calcified when healed

Granuloma – Well-defined pulmonary nodule
- TB
- Histoplasmosis
- Coccidioidomycosis
- Cryptococcosis
- Aspergillosis

Granulomas – Multiple ill-defined nodules
- TB
- Histoplasmosis
- Coccidioidomycosis
- Cryptococcosis
- Aspergillosis

Granulomas – Tiny nodules
- <5 mm, micronodular, military
- Histoplasmosis
- Blastomycosis
- Cryptococcosis
- Coccidioidomycosis

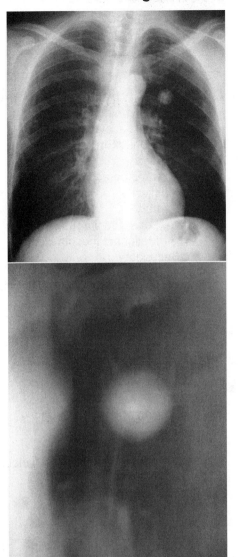

Figure 1-21-3

Solitary Pulmonary Nodule ("Coin Lesions") (n = 955)
- Malignant   49%
  - 1° carcinoma   38%
  - Metastases   9%
  - Other 1° malignancy   2%
- Benign   51%
  - Non-neoplastic lesion   37%
  - Tumor   14% (Hamartoma 8%)

Toomes H. The coin lesion of the lung. Cancer 1983.

SPN Patterns of Calcification
- Benign
  - Diffuse
  - Central
  - "Popcorn" (some Hamartomas)
  - Lamellated / concentric (Granuloma)
- Malignant (occurs in 7% of lung cancers)
  - Stippled
  - Eccentric

SPN – Cigarette smokers
- 35 years of age: increased likelihood of bronchogenic ca
- Even with known extrathoracic malignancy:
  - SPN more likely to be a primary

Pleural Disease I

Dr. Gerald F. Abbott
Brown University Medical School
Providence, Rhode Island

Outline of Pleural Disease I and II
- Pleural anatomy & physiology
- Non-neoplastic pleural disease
  - ➢ Effusions / Empyema
  - ➢ Fibrosis
  - ➢ Pneumothoraces
- Neoplastic pleural disease
  - ➢ Primary
    - ✧ Localized fibrous tumor
    - ✧ Malignant mesothelioma
  - ➢ Secondary
    - ✧ Pleural metastases
      - – Bronchogenic carcinoma
      - – Other carcinomas
      - – Lymphoma
      - – Invasive thymoma
- Chest wall disease

Pleural Anatomy
- Parietal Pleura
- Covers non-pulmonary surfaces
- Systemic supply/drainage
- Pain fibers
- Lymphatics communicate with pleural space
- Visceral Pleura
- Covers lung surface
- Dual supply/drainage
- Vagus nerve/sympathetic trunks
- Lymphatics do not communicate with pleural space

Pleural Imaging - Radiography / CT
- Inconspicuous
- Visceral + Parietal pleura = 0.2 mm
- CT thin-collimation - 1-2 mm thick line
- Intercostal regions
  - ➢ Visceral + Parietal pleura
  - ➢ Normal fluid
  - ➢ Endothoracic fascia
  - ➢ Innermost intercostal m.

Pleural Anatomy
- Junction Lines
  - ➢ Apposition of layers of pleura
    - ✧ Anterior junction line
    - ✧ Posterior junction line

Pleural Anatomy - Fissures
- Visceral pleura
- Variable depth into parenchyma
- Complete
- Incomplete
- Standard fissures - divide lung into lobes
- Accessory fissures - occur within lobe itself
  - ➢ 50% anatomic specimens

Major Fissure- Radiography
- Major (oblique) fissures
- Best seen on lateral CXR
- Originate at ~ T5 vertebra
- Parallel 6th rib
- Right fissure more oblique
- Courses further anterior and inferior

Major Fissure - CT
- 80-90% of standard CT
  - Lucent band, line, or dense band

Propeller-like morphology:
- Upper thorax, anterior concave, lateral-facing
- Inferior thorax, anterior convex, medial-facing

HRCT
- Usually conspicuous
  - Single line
  - Two parallel lines (motion artifact)
  - Dense band

Incomplete Major Fissure - CT [Figure 1-22-1]
- Fails to reach hilus/mediastinum
- 12-75% of CTs
- More frequent on the right
  - RUL / RLL - 70%
  - RML / RLL - 47%
  - LUL / LLL - 40%
  - Lingula / LLL - 46%

Standard Fissures - Radiography
- Minor (horizontal) fissure
  - 44 - 80% normal radiographs
  - Variable position
  - 2/3 level 4th intercostal space

Accessory Fissures
Radiography
- 10% CXR
- 20% CT
  - Azygos
  - Inferior
  - Superior
  - Left minor

Azygos (mesoazygos)
- Abnormal migration right posterior cardinal vein
- "Sling" of four pleural layers
- ~1% population
- 2M : 1F

Accessory Fissures - Inferior Accessory
[Figure 1-22-2]
- Separates medial basal segment from remaining basilar segments
- Most common
- 30 - 45% anatomic specimens
- 5 - 10% of frontal radiographs
- Right-sided - 80%
- 15% of CTs

Figure 1-22-1

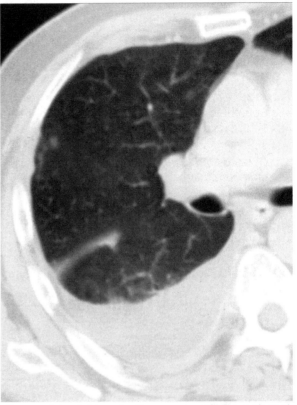

Incomplete right major fissure opacified by pleural effusion

Figure 1-22-2

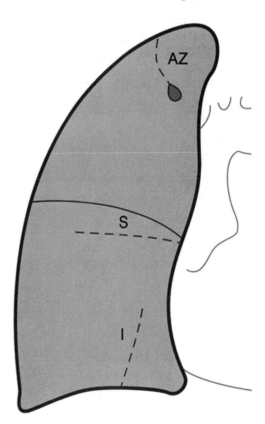

Accessory fissures of the right lung (coronal diagram): azygos (AZ), superior accessory (S), and inferior accessory (I)

Accessory Fissures - Superior Accessory
- Separation of superior segment from basilar segments
- 6% anatomic specimens
- Right > Left
- Horizontal course (Ømn. fissure)
- Superior Accessory aka "Dorsal lobe of Nelson"

Accessory Fissures - Left Minor Fissure
- Separates lingula from remainder of upper lobe
- 8-18% anatomic specimens
- ~ 1.5% of chest radiographs
- Oblique course
- More cephalad

Pulmonary Ligament
- Union at hilum of parietal and visceral pleura
- Courses posteriorly and inferiorly
- Adjacent to azygos vein and IVC, esophagus and aorta
- Contains bronchial veins, lymphatics and lymph nodes

Pulmonary Ligament - Imaging
- Not seen on radiography
- LPL - 60-70% CT scans
- RPL - 40-60% CT scans

Pleural Effusion
Cardiac Decompensation
- Most common cause
- >90% of transudative effusions
- Increased hydrostatic pressure
- Imaging
  - ➢ Bilateral (>80%)
  - ➢ Approximate equal volume
  - ➢ Unilateral - right-sided
  - ➢ Pseudotumor (minor fissure)

Pleural Effusion - Bacterial Pneumonia
- ~ 40% cases
- 2/3 aerobic / 1/3 "mixed"
- Exudative effusion
- Most parapneumonic effusions resolve with antibiotics
- ~10% require pleural drainage
- Loculate, enlarge despite Abx therapy
- >10 mm decubitus films

Empyema - CT [Figure 1-22-3]
- Empyema vs. lung abscess
- Lenticular shape
- Obtuse margins
- Compress lung
- "Split pleura" sign

Empyema - Treatment
- Requires prompt treatment
- Antibiotics
- Drainage
  - ➢ Tube(s)
  - ➢ Fibrinolytics
  - ➢ Open drainage (20%)

Figure 1-22-3

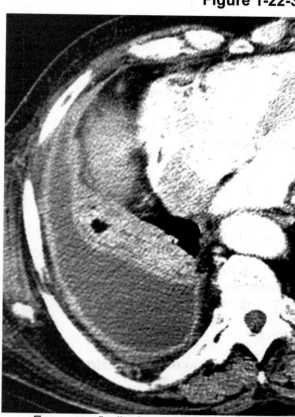

Empyema: "split-pleura sign" on contrast enhanced chest CT

Complications of Empyema
- Bronchopleural fistula
- Air-fluid level
- Varies in length on orthogonal radiographs
- Aids in differentiaton from lung abscess

Pleural Effusion - Tuberculosis
- Less common in "developed" countries
- Exudate
  - ↑ lymphocyte count
  - (>70% total wbc)
  - ↓ glucose level
- Unilateral
- Small to moderate

Pleural Effusion - Pulmonary Thromboembolic Disease
- 30-50% patients
- ~18% only finding
- 75% exudative
- 3rd most common exudate
- Bloody effusion - infarction
- Imaging: small, unilateral

Pleural Effusion - Pulmonary Thromboembolic Disease
- Enlarging effusion after treatment suggests:
  - Recurrent embolism
  - Anticoagulant-related hemorrage
  - Infection

Figure 1-22-4

Pleural Effusion - Subpulmonic
- Fluid accumulates between
- lung base and diaphragm
- Usually transudate
  - Cardiac decompensation
  - Renal failure
  - Cirrhosis with ascites

Pleural Effusion - Subpulmonic [Figure 1-22-4]
- Imaging
- Bilateral - not appreciated
- Unilateral "right-sided"
- Apparent elevation diaphragm
- Ill-defined costophrenic angle
- Diaphragmatic spur
- Mobile
- Displace gastric bubble

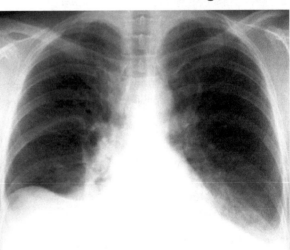

Right subpulmonic pleural effusion

Pleural Effusion vs. Ascites
- CT
  - Displaced crus sign
  - Bare area liver / spleen
  - Diaphragm sign

Pleural Effusion - Connective Tissue Disease
- Rheumatoid arthritis
- Effusion most common thoracic manifestation
- Middle aged males
- Antedates clinical disease
- Exudate / chyliform / low glucose
- Imaging
  - Unilateral
  - Chronic (months to years)
  - Transient / relapse
  - Fibrothorax / decortication

Pleural Effusion - Asbestos Exposure
- Diagnosis of exclusion
- Occupational exposure
- No malignancy within 3 yrs
- 1st 10 yrs post-exposure
- Exudate
- 1/3 patients have chest pain
- 15 - 30% recurrent effusions
- Imaging
  - 2 weeks to 6 months
  - Small (<500 ml)

Pleural Effusion - Asbestos Exposure
- Diffuse pleural thickening
- Rounded Atelectasis

Pleural Fibrosis
- 2nd most common pleural abnormality
- End result of many primary diseases of the pleura
- Potential complication of virtually any inflammatory disease
- Most cases localized to a single small area
- Less often diffuse / one / both pleural cavities
- (functional abnormalities)

Pleural Fibrosis - Focal
- Healed Pleuritis
- Sequela of bacterial pleuritis/trauma
- Imaging
  - Blunt posterior/lateral CP sulci
  - Rule-out small effusion

Pleural Fibrosis - Focal [Figure 1-22-5]
- Pleural Plaques
- Serpentine (chrysotile) asbestos
- Dense hyalinized collagen
- Parietal pleural surface
- Asbestos exposure
- Asymptomatic

Pleural Fibrosis - Focal [Figure 1-22-6]
- Pleural Plaques
- 50% of exposed individuals
- Visible plaques
  - 15 years non-calcified
  - 20 years calcified

Figure 1-22-5

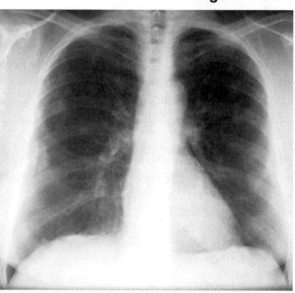

Pleural plaques on PA chest radi

Figure 1-22-6

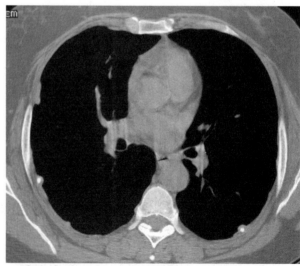

Calcified and non-calcified pleural plaques on chest CT

Pleural Fibrosis - Focal

- Imaging
- 80% bilateral
- Lateral chest wall
- B/w 4th and 8th ribs
- Spares apices and CPAs
- Tendinous hemidiaphragm
- En face "Holly leaf"

Pleural Fibrosis - Diffuse Fibrothorax

- Fibrous obliteration of normal pleural space
- Tuberculosis/bacterial empyema
- Hemothorax
- Asbestos-related pleural effusions
- Rheumatoid effusions
- Volume loss/restrictive disease

Pleural Fibrosis - Diffuse Fibrothorax

Figure 1-22-7]
- Radiographic definition
  - ➢ Smooth/uninterrupted thickening
  - ➢ At least 1/4 chest wall
  - ➢ +/- obliterate costophrenic suclus
  - ➢ ≤ 2.0 cm thickness
  - ➢ +/- calcification

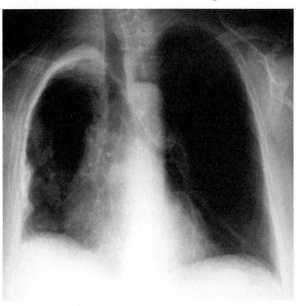

Right fibrothorax with extensive calcification

Pleural Fibrosis - Diffuse Fibrothorax

- Imaging CT
  - ➢ Extends > 8.0 cm cranio-caudal
  - ➢ Pleura > 3 mm thick
  - ➢ Extrapleural fat hypertrophy
  - ➢ +/- Pleural calcification
  - ➢ Mediastinal pleura spared

Pneumothorax

- Air within the pleural space
- Spontaneous
  - ➢ Primary
  - ➢ Secondary
- Traumatic

Pneumothorax - Primary Spontaneous

[Figure 1-22-8]
- 5M : 1F
- 3rd - 4th decade
- Right-sided predominance
- ~30% ipsilateral recurrence
- ~10% contralateral recurrence
- Rupture of apical bleb/bulla
  - ➢ Infrequent CXR
  - ➢ > 80% CT

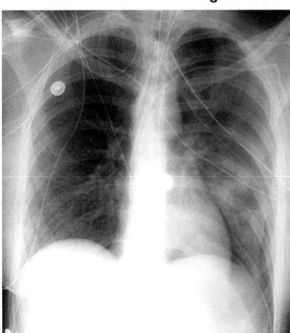

*Left pneumothorax with "deep sulcus sign"
in a supine patient*

Pneumothorax - Secondary Spontaneous

- "Predisposing" lung disease
- Subpleural cystic lesions

x

Pneumothorax - Secondary Spontaneous
- COPD
- Most common concurrent condition
- 0.5% per year
- 45-65 years of age
- Peripheral emphysematous lung
- Mortality rate ~3%

Pneumothorax - Secondary Spontaneous
- Pneumocystis Carinii Pneumonia (PCP)
- destruction alveolar septa → bulla
- subpleural necrosis → cystic degeneration / bulla

Pneumothorax - Secondary Spontaneous
- Pneumocystis Carinii Pneumonia (PCP)
- Complicates ~12% patients
- Persistent / refractory "air-leaks"
- Poor prognosis
- Death within 8 weeks (<57%)

Pneumothorax - Secondary Spontaneous
- Lymphangioleiomyomatosis (LAM)
- Women child-bearing age
- Proliferation of immature smooth muscle
- Bronchiolar obstruction → Cysts → PTX
- Recurrence ~40%

Pneumothorax - Secondary Spontaneous
- Langerhans Cell Histiocytosis
- Etiology/pathogenesis unclear
- Strong association w/ tobacco
- Rupture of subpleural cysts
- Recurrent ptx (25%)

Pleural Disease II and Chest Wall

Dr. Gerald F. Abbott
Brown University Medical School
Providence, Rhode Island

Neoplastic Pleural Disease

Malignant Pleural Effusion

Lung Cancer
- Malignant Effusion = T4

Breast Cancer
- Second most common
- 50% of patients with systemic disease
- Positive cytology in 66%
- Poor prognosis

Pleural Effusion in Malignancy - Pathogenesis
- Direct involvement of pleura
- Lymphatic obstruction
- Pneumonia / atelectasis
  - ➢ Central obstruction with parapneumonic effusion
- Severe hypoproteinemia

Malignant Pleural Effusion Diagnosis and Prognosis
- Combined pleural cytology and pleural biopsy
- Multiple thoracenteses / pleural biopsies
- Poor prognosis
- Bronchogenic Carcinoma - mean survival 2 to 3 months
- Breast Carcinoma - mean survival 7 to 15 months

Pleural / Chest Wall Mass – Imaging Features
- Discrepant margins
- Elliptical shapes
- Obtuse angles
- Cross boundaries

Incomplete Border Sign
= Extraparenchymal Lesion (Pleura or Chest wall)
- If border is tangential to beam: smooth, sharp on radiograph
- If border is En face to beam: fading / invisible
- Between those two orthogonal views, borders may appear incomplete
- Suggests pleural or chest wall origin

Pleural Neoplasms
- Focal pleural mass
- Multiple pleural masses
- Diffuse pleural thickening / nodularity

Pleural Neoplasms
- Primary
- Localized fibrous tumor
- Malignant mesothelioma
- Secondary
- Pleural metastases
  - ➢ Bronchogenic carcinoma
  - ➢ Other carcinomas
  - ➢ Lymphoma
  - ➢ Invasive thymoma

Localized Fibrous Tumor
- Rare (< 5% of pleural neoplasms)
- Not related to asbestos
- M=F
- Mean age: 50 years
- Symptoms in 54%
- Cough, chest pain, dyspnea
- HPO (up to 35% in some series)
- Hypoglycemia 4%

Localized Fibrous Tumor - Microscopic
- Variable patterns
- Disorderly arrangement
- Spindle cells and collagen
- High mitotic activity
  - ➢ suggests malignancy 20%

Localized Fibrous Tumor - Gross
- 2 - 40 cm
- 80% visceral / 20% parietal
- Lobular, encapsulated
- Pedicle: good prognosis
- Cut-surface: whorled, nodular, fibrous
- hemorrhage, necrosis, cysts

Localized Fibrous Tumor - CXR [Figure 1-23-1]
- Incidental finding
- Solitary rounded, lobular mass
- Mid to inferior thorax
- Large tumors: acute angles at interfaces
- Pedunculated tumors may demonstrate positional mobility
- (A pathognomonic feature)

Localized Fibrous Tumor - CT [Figure 1-23-2]
- Well-defined, smooth, lobular
- Abutting pleural surface
- Elongated, lenticular
- Heterogeneity:
  - ➢ hemorrhage, necrosis, cysts
- Contrast enhancement

Localized Fibrous Tumor
Therapy and Prognosis
- Treatment of choice: complete excision
- 90% cure rate
- Symptoms usually resolve post-op
- Recur with tumor recurrence
- Recurrence in 10% of patients

Malignant Mesothelioma
- Most common primary pleural neoplasm
- 2,000 to 3,000 cases / year in USA
- 10% of asbestos-exposed individuals
- Shipyards / asbestos plants
- Sixth to eighth decades
- Male : Female 3-6 : 1
- Asbestos: Amphibole form the most tumorigenic
- Latency: 30-40 years

Figure 1-23-1

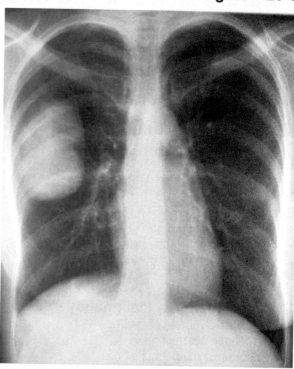

*Localized fibrous tumor of the pleura
on PA chest radiograph*

Figure 1-23-2

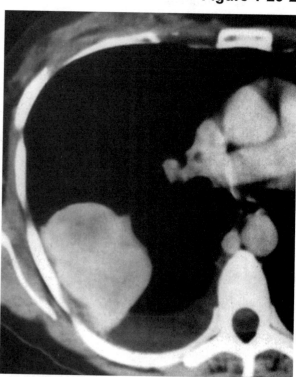

*Localized fibrous tumor of the pleura
on chest CT*

Malignant Mesothelioma - Clinical
- Insidious onset of symptoms
- 6-8 months prior to Dx
- Dyspnea, chest pain, cough, weight loss
- Rarely: SVC Syndrome, Horner Syndrome, dysphagia, vocal cord paralysis, HPO, clubbing, hypoglycemia

Malignant Mesothelioma - Microscopic
- Epithelioid   50 %
- Sarcomatous   15 %
- Biphasic   25 %
- Interobserver agreement   50%

Malignant Mesothelioma - Gross
- Sheets, plaques, masses
- Parietal > Visceral
- Bulk in inferior hemithorax
- Lung encasement
- Fissural growth
- Parenchymal involvement
- Mediastinal, chest wall, diaphragmatic invasion

Malignant Mesothelioma - Radiographic
- Pleural effusion
- Pleural masses
- Circumferential
- Mediastinal shift
- Pleural plaques 25%

Malignant Mesothelioma - CT [Figure 1-23-3]
- Pleural thickening   92%
- Fissural thickening   86%
- Pleural effusion   74%
- Ipsilateral ↓ volume 42%
- Pleural calcification   20%
- Ipsilateral ↑ volume   14%

Kawashima AJR 1990

Malignant Mesothelioma - DX
- Video-Assisted-Thoracoscopic-Surgery (VATS)
- VATS = procedure of choice (Sensitivity 98%)
  - ➤ Complication: tumor seeding along entry ports
- Open biopsy: when adhesions preclude VATS
- Cytology and FNA Bx of limited value

Malignant Mesothelioma - MR
- Used for Staging
- Comparable / superior to CT
- Tumor enhancement
- Increased signal intensity

Malignant Mesothelioma Treatment and Prognosis
- Median survival: 10 months
- Best prognosis:
  - ➤ 25-30% 5-year survival
  - ➤ Negative margins
  - ➤ Epithelial cell type
  - ➤ No metastases
- Surgery: Extrapleural pneumonectomy
  - ➤ High mortality / morbidity

Figure 1-23-3

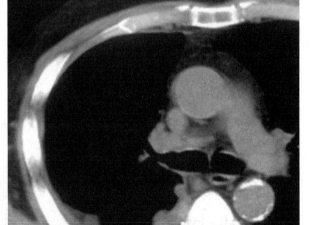

Mesothelioa with nodular and circumferential pleural thickening

Pleural Metastases
Most common pleural neoplasm
- Common:
  - ➤ Adenocarcinoma
    - ✧ Lung, breast, ovary, stomach
- Less common:
  - ➤ Lymphoma, Thymoma

Pleural Metastases
- Hematogenous / Lymphatic
- Direct extension (lung ca, breast ca)
- Drop metastases (invasive thymoma)
- May be bilateral
- Pleural Metastases - Imaging
- Pleural effusion
- Pleural masses
- Or both
- May mimic malignant mesothelioma

Pleural Thickening

CT Features suggesting malignancy
- Circumferential
- Nodular
- > 1 cm
- Mediastinal pleura

Leung et al AJR 1990

Chest Wall
- Congenital and developmental anomalies
- Inflammatory and infectious diseases
- Non-neoplastic conditions
- Neoplasia: benign and malignant

Chest Wall Congenital / Developmental Anomalies [Figure 1-23-4]
- Pectus deformities
- Anomalous ribs
- Cleidocranial dysostosis
- Poland syndrome

Chest Wall - Inflammatory / Infectious Diseases

Tuberculosis
- Uncommon
- Hematogenous spread
- Contiguous spread
- Abscess / sinus tract 25%
- Imaging:
- Bone / cartilage destruction
- Soft-tissue mass
- Calcification
- Peripheral enhancement

Figure 1-23-4

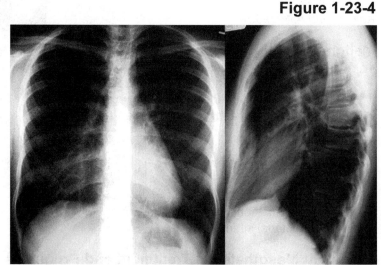

Pectus excavatum

Chest Wall - Inflammatory / Infectious Diseases

Actinomycosis

- *Actinomyces israelii*
- Anaerobic gram-positive
- Lung → Pleura → Chest Wall
- Proteolysis → Fistulas
- Diagnosis: anaerobic cultures
- Imaging: soft-tissue mass
- draining sinus, periostitis

Chest Wall Neoplasms - Adults

- Benign:
  - Lipoma
  - Other mesenchymal neoplasms
- Malignant:
  - Fibrosarcoma
  - Malignant fibrous histiocytoma
  - Other mesenchymal neoplasms
  - Lymphoma

Chest Wall Lipoma (aka "pleural lipoma")

[Figure 1-23-5]

- Common
- Subcutaneous
- Intrathoracic
- Both
- Diagnostic CT number

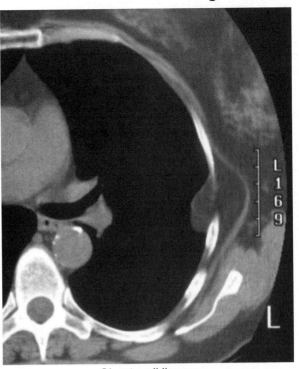

Figure 1-23-5

Chest wall lipoma

Desmoid (Fibromatosis)

- About the shoulder
- Soft tissue mass
- Low signal on MR
- High signal areas suggest greater biologic activity

Chest Wall Neoplasms - Osseous Involvement

- Rib expansion
  - Fibrous Dysplasia
  - Enchondroma
- Pressure erosion
  - Slow growth
- Rib destruction:
  - Secondary malignant neoplasia
  - Primary malignant neoplasia
  - Inflammatory
- Pressure erosion:
  - Slow growth (e.g.Neurogenic)

Chest Wall Neoplasms Osseous Destruction *[Figure 1-23-6]*

- Adult
  - Metastatic disease
  - Lung, Breast, Prostate
  - Multiple myeloma
  - Chondrosarcoma
- Child
  - Ewing sarcoma
  - Neuroblastoma
  - Lymphoma
  - Askin tumor (PPNET)

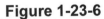

Figure 1-23-6

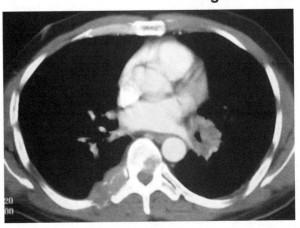

Chest wall metastases with bone destruction (right hemithorax) from primary lung cancer of left hilum

Myeloma

- Males > Females
- 5th - 7th decades
- Axial skeleton
- Multiple or solitary
- Imaging:
  - ➢ Osseous destruction
  - ➢ Soft-tissue mass

Chondrosarcoma

- Adults
- Painful, palpable mass
- Costochondral junction, rib, sternum
- Imaging:
- Expansile, destructive
- Chondroid calcification
- Soft-tissue mass

PNET "Askin Tumor"
Primitive Neuroectodermal Tumor

- Malignant small round cell tumor
- Children, adolescents
- Female: Male = 3:1
- Unilateral
- Rib destruction 2/3
- Pleural effusion
- Poor prognosis

Classic Breast Lesions

Leonard M. Glassman, M.D.FACR
Washington Radiology Associates, PC
Visiting Scientist
Armed Forces Institute of Pathology
Washington DC

Figure 1-24-1

Most Lesions are Non-specific [Figure 1-24-1]
- Differentials can be given
- High likelihood diagnoses can be made
- Is this a cyst or a solid mass?

Aunt Minnie Does Exist
- Who is Aunt Minnie and why do we care?

Aunt Minnie Does Exist
- No differential is needed
- Short interval follow-up unnecessary

Normal Variants
- Pectoralis major
- Lymph nodes

Pectoralis Major [Figure 1-24-2]

Sternalis [Figure 1-24-3]

Lymph Node
- Axillary
- Intramammary
- Lymphoma

Intramammary Lymph Nodes
- Normal finding
- 28% of breasts
- May enlarge and shrink in size
- Circumscribed with hilar notch or fatty hilum
- Usually less than 15 mm in size
- Not related to the usual lymphatic drainage patterns
- Usually upper outer quadrant

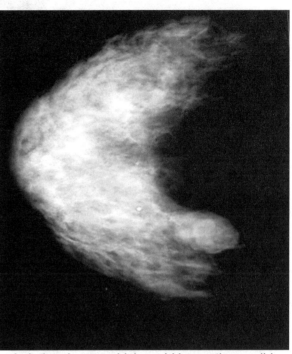

Lobulated mass which could be cystic or solid, benign or malignant

Figure 1-24-2

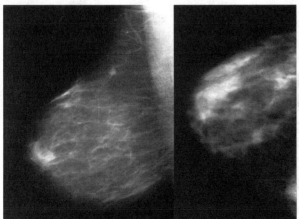

(left) Oblique view showing pectoralis major muscle; (right) Cc view showing the medial attachment of the pectoralis as a rounded "half mass".

Figure 1-24-3

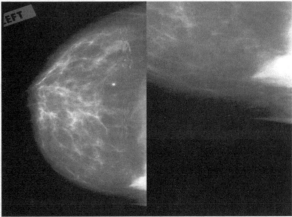

(left) Sharper narrower medial "half mass" is the sternalis muscle; (right) Close-up view

Intramammary Lymph Nodes *[Figure 1-24-4 and 1-24-5]*

Figure 1-24-4

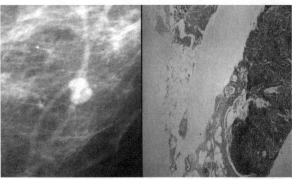

Hilar notch diagnostic of a lymph node

Figure 1-24-5

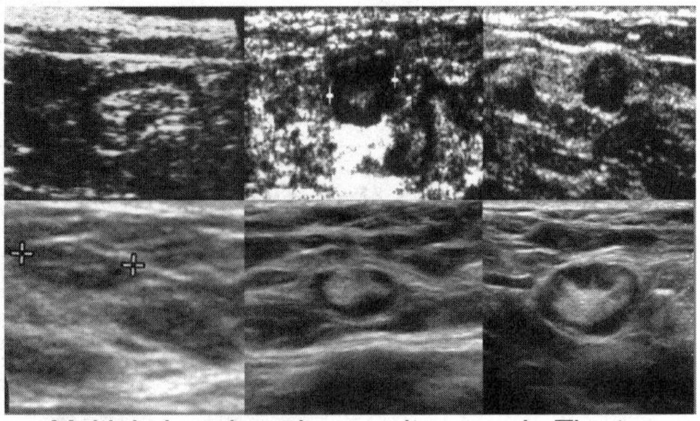

Multiple lymph nodes on ultrasound. The top three are seen on standard scanning and the bottom three on compound scanning. All show an echogenic hilum

Congenital Anomalies
- Polythelia
  - ➢ Accessory nipples
  - ➢ 2.4% of neonates
- Polymastia
  - ➢ 2-3% of women
  - ➢ Axillary breast tissue most common
  - ➢ Inframammary fold and labia next most common

Polythelia *[Figure 1-24-6]*

Polymastia *[Figure 1-24-7]*
- Can be palpable or visible

Benign Abnormalities
- Fatty lesions
- Gynecomastia
- Fibrocystic changes
- Foreign bodies

Fatty Lesions
- Hamartoma
- Lipoma
- Fat necrosis
- Galactocele

All Lesions that Contain Fat are Benign Except
- Very rare hamartomas
- 1 Phyllodes with liposarcoma

Figure 1-24-6

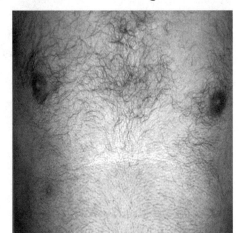

Accessory nipple on the right abdominal wall in this male patient

Figure 1-24-7

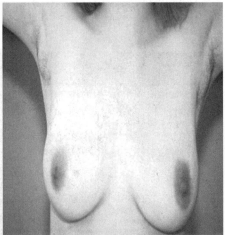

Bilateral palpable and visible axillary breast tissue

Figure 1-24-8

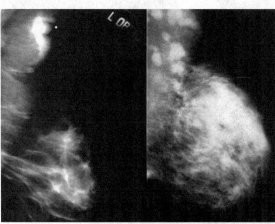

(left) Axillary breast tissue; (right) Axillary breast tissue with a spiculated carcinoma

Hamartoma [Figure 1-24-9]

- Fibroadenolipoma
- Palpable mass or mammographic finding
  - ➢ Can be large and not palpable
- Encapsulated normal breast elements

Lipoma [Figure 1-24-10]

- Benign tumor
- Usually not palpable because it is soft
- Liposarcoma usually water density

Liposarcoma [Figure 1-24-11]

Figure 1-24-9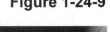

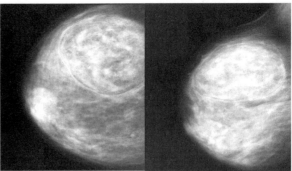

(left) CC view. Encapsulated mass containing fat, glandular elements and fibrous tissue; (right) Oblique view

Figure 1-24-10

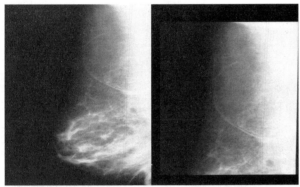

(left) Fatty mass in axillary tail; (right) Close-up

Figure 1-24-11

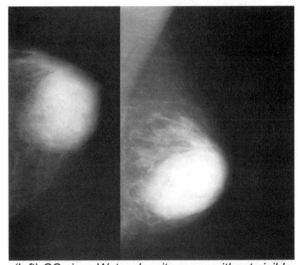

(left) CC view. Water density mass without visible fat; (right) Oblique view

Fat Necrosis [Figure 1-24-12]

- 50% have history of trauma
  - ➢ Including surgery & XRT
- Oil cyst
- Partially calcified lesion
- Can be spiculated
- Can progress from fatty to spiculated

Oil Cyst

Fat Necrosis - Progression [Figure 1-24-13]

Figure 1-24-13

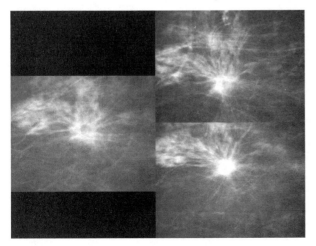

Figure 1-24-12

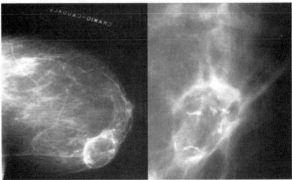

(left) Fatty lesion with irregular calcifications; (right) Close-up also showing some speculation

Three views, each one year apart, showing progression from fatty lesion to spiculated mass

Galactocele [Figure 1-24-14]
- Pregnant or breast feeding
- Cystic lesion
- Fat fluid level on horizontal beam film
- Aspiration usually curative

Gynecomastia [Figure 1-24-15]
- Potentially reversible enlargement of the male breast
- Proliferation of connective tissue and ducts
- Bilateral or unilateral palpable subareolar mass
- Occasionally diffuse enlargement

Gynecomastia is Caused by Hyperestrogenism
- Hormone imbalance
  - Puberty & senescence
  - Estrogen administration
- Drugs (partial list)
  - Digitalis
  - Reserpine
  - Dilantin
  - Cimetidine
  - Marijuana

Further Causes of Gynecomastia
- Hypogonadism
- Neoplasm
  - Pituitary
  - Hepatoma
  - Leydig cell
- Systemic disease
  - Hepatic
  - Renal
  - Hyperthyroidism

Gynecomastia [Figure 1-24-15]

Fibrocystic Changes [Figure 1-24-16 and 1-24-17]
- Exaggerated physiologic phenomenon
  - Cysts
  - Apocrine metaplasia and hyperplasia
  - Stromal alterations
  - Mild epithelial hyperplasia
  - Mild adenosis

Figure 1-24-14

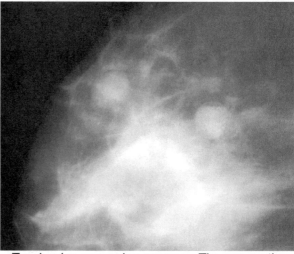

Two benign appearing masses. The one on the right shows a fat - fluid level in this lateral view

Figure 1-24-15

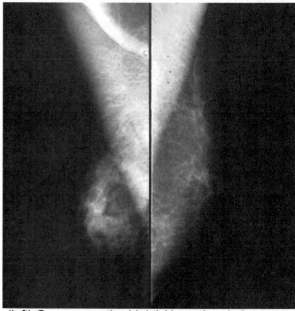

(left) Gynecomastia; (right) Normal male breast on the opposite side

Figure 1-24-16

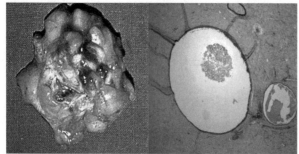

(left) Gross specimen showing multiple small cysts; (right) Histological view of cyst

Figure 1-24-17

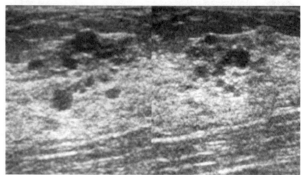

(left) Mixed pattern of small cystic spaces and hypoechoic nodularity; (right) Another view of the same lesion

Cyst [Figure 1-24-18]

- Cystic lobular involution
- Anechoic with sharp back wall
- Enhanced thru-transmission of sound
- 10% atypical

Pneumocystography

Cyst ?

Apocrine Metaplasia [Figure 1-24-19]

Foreign Body

- Silicone or paraffin
  - ➤ Free injection
  - ➤ Leakage from implants
- Surgical drain
- Wire fragments

Free Silicone (Implant Rupture) [Figure 1-24-20]

Free Silicone or Paraffin

Free Silicone [Figure 1-24-21]

Surgical Drain

Wire Fragment

Thickened Skin Pattern

- Edema
- Mastitis
- Inflammatory carcinoma
- Post-radiation change
- Obstruction to lymphatic drainage in the axilla or superior mediastinum
- Lymphoma

Figure 1-29-20

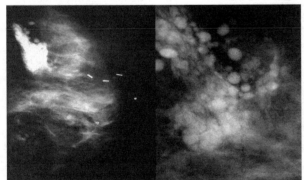

(left) Silicone in tissue from ruptured implant; (right) Close-up of silicone in tissue

Figure 1-24-18

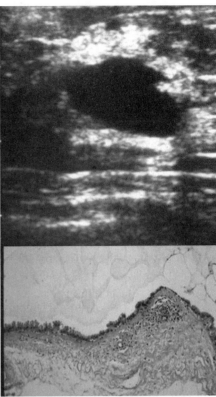

(top) Anechoic mass; (bottom) Biopsy specimen of cyst wall

Figure 1-24-19

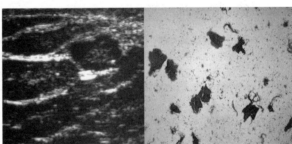

(left) Nodule with solid center and peripheral small cysts; (right) FNA specimen of lesion

Figure 1-24-21

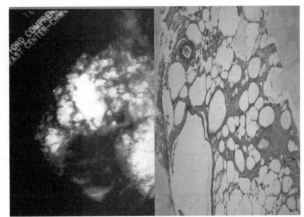

(left) Multiple silicone nodules from injection, not rupture; (right) Histological specimen showing many rounded spaces from the injected silicone

Thickened Skin Pattern – Mastitis

Thickened Skin Pattern – Radiation Therapy

Thickened Skin Pattern – Mediastinal Obstruction

Thickened Skin Pattern – Inflammatory Carcinoma [Figure 1-24-22]

Inflammatory Carcinoma [Figure 1-24-23]
- Clinical findings
  - ➢ Heavy firm breast
  - ➢ Red skin
  - ➢ Warm skin
  - ➢ Peau d'orange
- Can not differentiate from acute mastitis
- Far advanced local disease
  - ➢ Usually poorly differentiated ductal carcinoma
- Radiographic findings
  - ➢ Obstruction of dermal lymphatics
    - ◇ Can diagnose with a skin biopsy
  - ➢ Diffuse lymphatic invasion within the breast
  - ➢ Increased density
  - ➢ Trabecular thickening
- 50% five year survival
  - ➢ Pre-op chemo, mastectomy and radiation

Mammographic Findings
- Skin thickening
- Diffuse increased density
- Trabecular thickening
- Adenopathy
- Signs of carcinoma
  - ➢ Mass, calcification, asymmetry, distortion

Inflammatory Carcinoma
- Axillary nodes
- Supraclavicular node

Lymphoma

Classically Benign Calcifications
- Lobular
- Sutural
- Fibroadenoma
- Skin
- Vascular
- Secretory
- Lucent centered
- Egg shell

Lobular Calcifications
- Tightly clustered
- Round
- Fit together like a jigsaw puzzle

Sutural Calcifications [Figure 1-24-24]
- Look like sutures
- Usually post radiation therapy

Figure 1-24-22

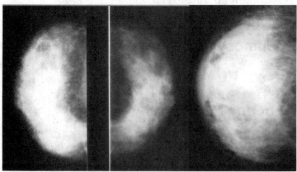

(left) CC views, one normal and one (on the left) showing increased density and indistinct Cooper's ligaments; (right) CC view with increased density and thickened Cooper's ligaments

Figure 1-24-23

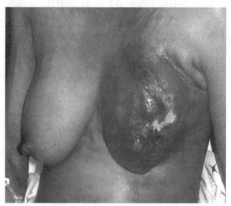

Large edematous breast with peau d'orange skin changes and skin breakdown

Figure 1-24-24

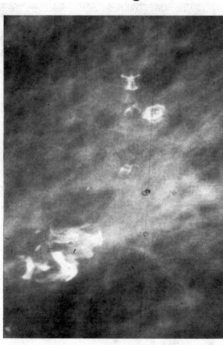

Dystrophic calcifications. Topmost calcification shows a typical suture shape

Calcified Fibroadenoma
- Coarse or "popcorn-like"
- Calcification generally peripheral

Peripheral Calcification

Calcified Fibroadenoma [Figure 1-24-25]

Skin Calcifications
- Faint peripheral clusters with lucent centers
- Tangent view

Dermal Localization

Vascular Calcifications
- Parallel tracks associated with blood vessels
- Calcifications are on the outside of the tube
- Diabetes ?
- Heart Disease ?

Vascular / Ductal

Vascular Calcification

Secretory Calcifications
- Large rods
  - Luminal calcifications
  - Oriented toward nipple
  - Relatively smooth surface
  - May branch

Osteosarcoma
- 27 to 89 years old
- Median 64.5 years
- Highly aggressive tumors

Primary Osteosarcoma [Figure 1-24-26]

National Flower of the Radiologist is the Hedge

Some Diagnoses Can be Made
- Make them when you can

Figure 1-24-25

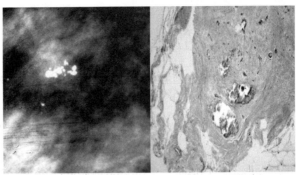

(left) Coarse irregular cluster of calcifications; (right) Fibrotic fibroadenoma with calcification

Figure 1-24-26

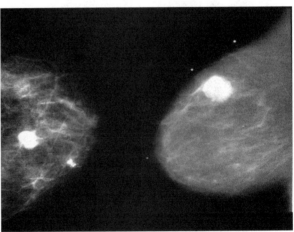

(left) Osteoid matrix in a mass; (right) Another patient with the same appearance

References

"Augmentation Mammoplasty: Normal and Abnormal Findings with Mammography and US." Ganott, MA. et. al. Radiographics 12:281-295, 1992.

"Breast Hamartomas: Variable Mammographic Appearance." Helvie, MA, et. al. Radiology 170:417-421, 1989.

"Calcification in Breast Disease--- Mammographic – Pathologic Correlation." Levitan, LH, et.al. Radiology 92:29-39, 1964.

"Calcified Suture Material in the Breast after Radiation Therapy." Stacey-Clear, A, et. al. Radiology 183:207-208, 1992.

"Cystic Lesions of the Breast: Sonographic – Pathologic Correlation." Berg, W, et.

al. Radiology 227:183-191, 2003.

"Fat Necrosis in the Breast: Sonographic Features." Scott, SM, et. al. Radiology 206:261-269 , 1998.

"In Situ and Infiltrating Ductal Carcinoma Arising in a Breast Hamartoma." Mester, Jolinda, et.al. AJR175:64-66, 2000.

"Inflammatory Breast Cancer, Current Imaging Perspectives." Whitman, G. et.al. Sem Breast Dis 4:122-131, 2001.

"Inflammatory Carcinoma of the Breast. A Pathologic Definition." Ellis, DL & Teitelbaum, SL. Cancer 33:1045-1047, 1974.

"Inflammatory Breast Carcinoma: Mammographic Findings." Dershaw, D, et. al. Radiology 190:831-834,1994.

"Mammographic – Pathologic Correlation of Apocrine Metaplasia Diagnosed Using Vacuum – Assisted Stereotactic Core – Needle Biopsy: Our 4- Year expericnce." Kushwaha, AC, et. al. AJR 180:795-798, 2003.

"Mammographic Spectrum of Traumatic Fat Necrosis: The Fallibility of "Pathognomonic Signs of Carcinoma." Bassett, L. et. al. AJR 130:119-122, 1987.

"Male Breast Carcinoma and Gynecomastia: Comparison of Mammography with Sonography." Jackson, VP & Gilmore, RL. Radiology 149: 533-536 , 1983.

"The Mammographic Spectrum of Fat Necrosis in the Breast."   Hogge, JP, et. al. Radiographics 15:1347-356 , 1995.

"Radiologic Appearance of Non-palpable Intramammary Lymph Nodes." Acta Radiologica 34:577-580, 1993.

Breast Pathology – What the Radiologist Needs to Know

Leonard M. Glassman, M.D. FACR
Washington Radiology Associates, PC
Visiting Scientist
Armed Forces Institute of Pathology
Washington DC

But First Some Philosophy

Mammography is the Easiest Study in Radiology

There are Two Diseases:
- Cancer and no Cancer

Cancer has Two Predominant Signs
- Mass and Calcification

You Have the Opposite Side for Comparison
- Anatomy is simple
- Physiology is almost irrelevant

What You Need to Remember
- 90% of cancers present as calcification, mass or both
- 10% present as
  - Asymmetric, developing or neodensities
  - Dilated duct
  - Thickened skin pattern
  - Architectural distortion
  - Paget's disease

Rad Path Correlation – What You Need to Remember
- The mass edge reflects the aggressiveness of the underlying abnormality
- Benign masses tend to be less aggressive than malignant masses

Rad Path Correlation – What You Need to Remember
- The shape of the calcification represents a cast of an underling anatomic or pathologic space

Normal Anatomy
- Skin
- Nipple and areola
- Subcutaneous fat
- Premammary fascia

Normal Anatomy
- Glandular cone
  - Breast disease occurs here
- Retromammary fascia
- Retromammary fat
- Muscle
- Ribs

Segmental Anatomy
- 15 - 20 lobes or segments

Normal Ducts *[Figure 1-25-1]*

Figure 1-25-1

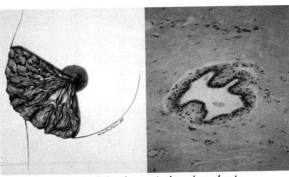

(left) Quadrant of the breast showing ducts, lobules and Cooper's ligaments;
(right) Histological section of a normal duct

Terminal Duct Lobular Unit (TDLU) [Figure 1-25-2]

- Short segment of terminal duct and a cluster of ductules (acini)
- Functional unit of the breast
- Ductal and lobular cancers begin here
- Explains mixed ductal & lobular features in the same neoplastic lesion

Embryology

- Milk ridges
  - ➢ Ventral ectodermal thickenings from the axillary to the inguinal region
  - ➢ Usually limited to the pectoral regions by the ninth week of embryonic life

Figure 1-25-2

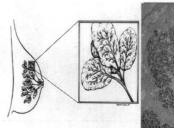
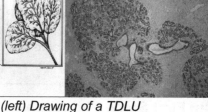

(left) Drawing of a TDLU

(right) Histological section of a TDLU

Congenital Anomalies

- Athelia
  - ➢ Rarest anomaly of the breast
  - ➢ Absence of the nipple
- Amastia
  - ➢ Agenesis of breast & nipple
  - ➢ Associated with hypoplasia of the ipsilateral pectoral muscles in 90%
  - ➢ Can be iatrogenic

Congenital Anomalies

- Polythelia
- Polymastia

Pregnancy Changes

- Increased estrogen & progesterone
  - ➢ Estrogen promotes ductal growth
  - ➢ Progesterone promotes lobular growth and breast secretion
- Hyperplasia and hypertrophy
- Extremely dense breast pattern
- Can still see calcifications on mammography
- Can see masses on sonography

Mastitis

- 3% of primary diagnoses at biopsy
- 2/3s of women under 50 years old at biopsy
- Many different types
  - ➢ Infection
  - ➢ Systemic
  - ➢ Antigen-antibody reaction
  - ➢ Idiopathic

Mastitis

- Acute mastitis
  - ➢ Usually in lactating women with a cracked nipple
  - ➢ Can go on to abscess
- Chronic mastitis

Granulomatous Mastitis

Most Common Benign Neoplasms

- Fibroadenoma
  - ➢ Biphasic tumor
- Intraductal papilloma
- Hamartoma

Biphasic Tumors

- Epithelial & stromal elements
  - Fibroadenoma
    - Benign epithelial and stromal elements
  - Phyllodes tumor
    - Benign epithelial & hyperplastic or sarcomatous stroma
  - Carcinosarcoma
    - Both elements malignant

Fibroadenoma *[Figure 1-25-3]*

- Begins in TDLU
- Response to unopposed estrogen in young women
- Oval or round circumscribed nodule
- May have coarse calcification, especially in periphery
- Growth pushes surrounding tissue without invasion

Fibroadenoma *[Figure 1-25-4; 1-25-5; 125-6]*

- Fibroadenoma
- Carcinoma

Carcinoma Arising in a Fibroadenoma

- Rare
- Most often lobular neoplasia (LCIS) or DCIS
- Invasive carcinoma very rare
  - Usually grows in from outside

Fibroadenoma Phyllodes

Figure 1-25-5

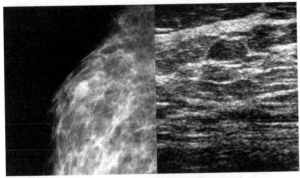

(left) Low to intermediate density oval mass.

(right) Ultrasound showing similar findings.

Figure 1-25-3

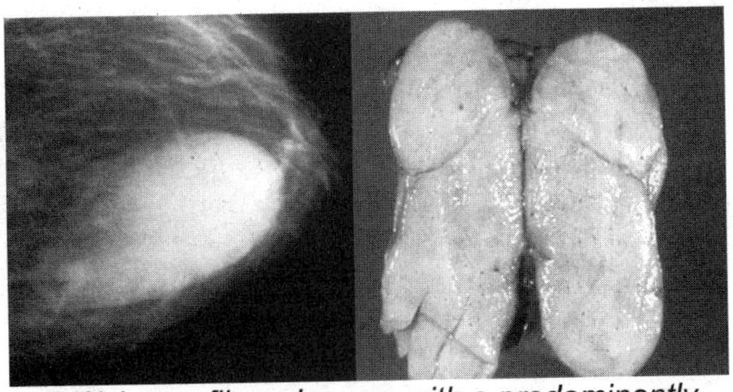

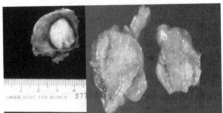

(left) Large fibroadenoma with a predominantly circumscribed border.
(right) Gross specimen of fibroadenoma showing a lack of involvement of surrounding tissue which explains the circumscribed border

Figure 1-25-4

(left) Fibroadenoma showing no invasion of surrounding tissue.
(right) Carcinoma showing invasion of surrounding tissue.

Figure 1-25-6

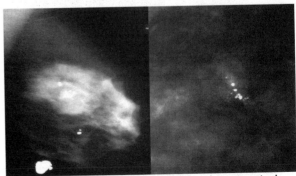

(left) Popcorn calcification of a degenerated fibroadenoma.
(right) Irregular calcification in a degenerated fibroadenoma.

Phyllodes Tumor [Figure 1-25-7 and 1-25-8]
- Benign epithelial elements and cellular spindle cell stroma
- Can act malignant
  - ➢ Local recurrence
  - ➢ Distant blood born metastases
  - ➢ Lymph node enlargement reactive usually
- Well circumscribed lobulated mass
- Similar appearance on sonography
  - ➢ May have cystic spaces

Carcinosarcoma

Papilloma [Figure 1-25-9 and 1-25-10]
- Papillary growth pattern supported by a fibrovascular stalk
  - ➢ Arises centrally
  - ➢ Usually solitary
- Papillomatosis
  - ➢ Arises peripherally in the TDLU
  - ➢ Usually multiple

Lobular Neoplasia
- No mammographic signs
- Incidental finding on biopsy
- Includes atypical lobular hyperplasia and LCIS

Lobular Neoplasia
- High incidence of bilaterality and multifocality
  - ➢ Consider it a bilateral disease
- High risk marker for the development of invasive carcinoma
  - ➢ Up to 15% in either breast equally within 20 years
  - ➢ Lobular or ductal features

Figure 1-25-7

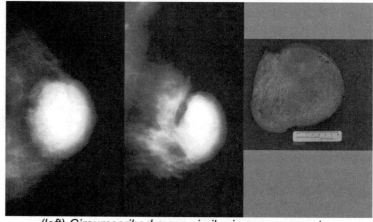

(left) Circumscribed mass similar in appearance to a fibroadenoma.
(middle) Mass without involvement of surrounding tissue.
(right) Note the clefts in the body of the specimen.

Figure 1-25-8

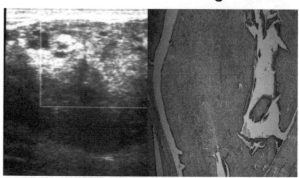

(left) Ultrasound of clefts.
(right) Histology of clefts.

Figure 1-25-9

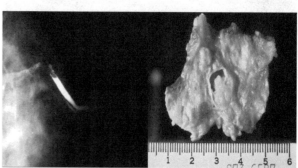

(left) Ductogram showing filling defect.

(right) Gross specimen of papilloma in dilated duct.

Figure 1-25-10

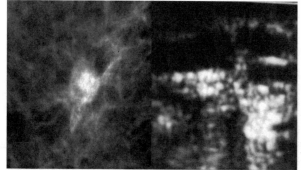

(left)Slightly indistinct mass was papilloma on biopsy. (right) Filling defect in duct on ultrasound

Invasive Ductal Cancer [Figure 1-25-11 to 1-25-14]

- NOS (not otherwise specified)
  - ➤ 50 to 75% of invasive cancers
- Medullary
- Papillary
- Colloid (Mucinous)
- Tubular
- Metaplastic
- Cribriform
- Adenoid cystic
- Paget's disease
- Inflammatory

Figure 1-25-11

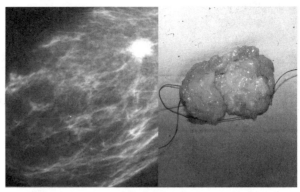

(left) Irregular spiculated mass.(right) Gross specimen showing invasion of surrounding tissues

Figure 1-25-12

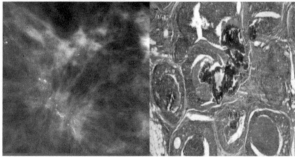

(left) Pleomorphic calcifications and spiculation (right) Irregular calcifications in ductal lumen and wall

Figure 1-25-13

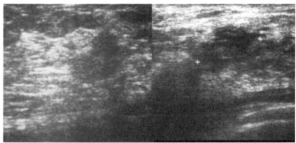

(left) Irregular mass on ultrasound.(right) Irregular mass showing acute angle border at the cursor on the right side of the image.

Figure 1-25-14

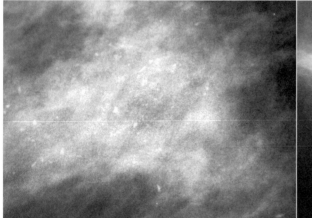

Pleomorphic calcifications

Paget's Disease [Figure 1-25-15 and 1-25-16]

- Red nipple and areola
- Scaling eczematoid reaction
- 50% have a palpable mass
- Must have Paget's cells in skin
- Usually has underlying carcinoma

Figure 1-25-15

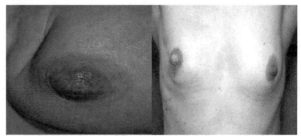

(left) Wet form of Paget's (right) Dry scaly form

Types of Invasive Ductal Carcinoma With Rounded Expansile Periphery
- Medullary
- Papillary
- Cribriform
- Colloid

Types of Invasive Ductal Carcinoma with Improved Prognosis
- Medullary
- Papillary
- Cribriform
- Colloid
- Tubular
- Adenoid cystic

Medullary Carcinoma [Figure 1-25-17]

Papillary Carcinoma

Tubular Carcinoma [Figure 1-25-18]
- Typically spiculated
- Must have 75 - 100% tubular formation
- Less than 75% acts like usual invasive carcinoma

Figure 1-25-18

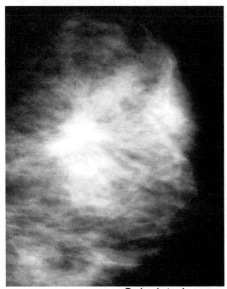

Spiculated mass

Adenoid Cystic Carcinoma [Figure 1-25-19]

Figure 1-25-16

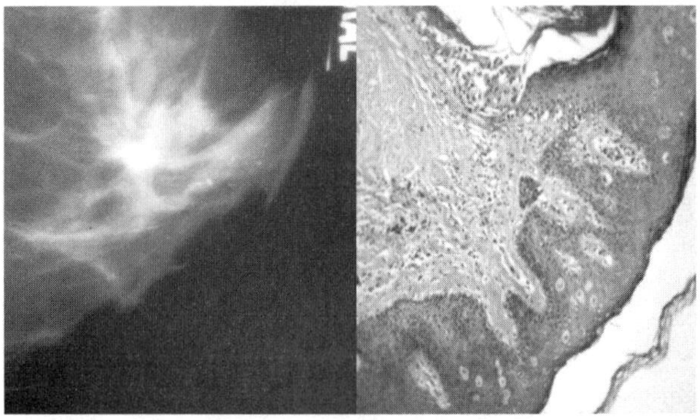

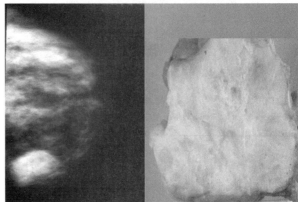

(left) Irregular calcifications from carcinoma. (right) Skin biopsy showing Paget's.

Figure 1-25-17

(left) Mostly circumscribed lobulated mass. (right) Gross specimen showing only minimal invasion of surrounding tissue

Figure 1-25-19

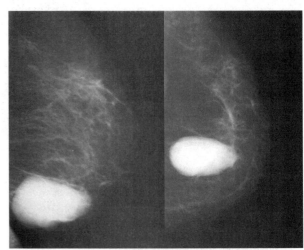

(left) Oblique view of circumscribed lobulated mass. (right) CC view.

Invasive Lobular Cancer
- Prognosis similar to invasive ductal cancer
- Most commonly a spiculated mass
- Some are more difficult to see as they are diffusely infiltrating
  - Present as asymmetric density

Invasive Lobular Cancer [Figure 1-25-20]
- Invasive lobular
- Invasive ductal

Sarcoma
- 1% of breast malignant tumors
- Breast contains fat, fibrous tissue, blood vessels, etc.
  - Angiosarcoma, malignant fibrous hystiocytoma, chondrosarcoma, rhabdomyosarcoma etc.
- Metaplasia can occur
- Malignant transformation can occur
- Often after chest or breast irradiation

Fibrosarcoma [Figure 1-25-21]

Spindle Cell Sarcoma [Figure 1-25-22]

Angiosarcoma [Figure 1-25-23]

What You Need to Remember
- The mass edge represents the aggressiveness of the underlying abnormality

What You Need to Remember
- The shape of the calcification represents a cast of an underling space

Figure 1-25-20

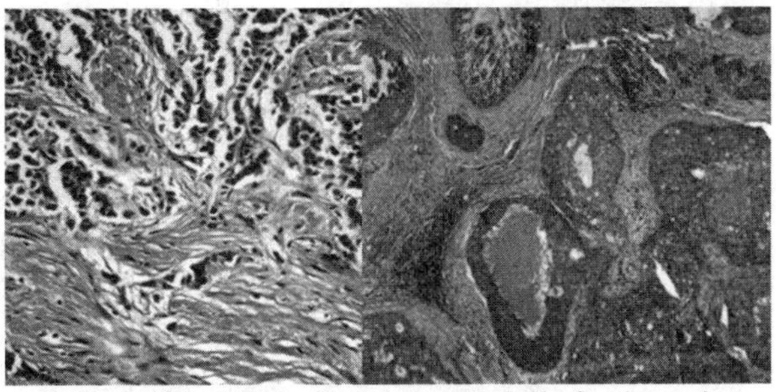

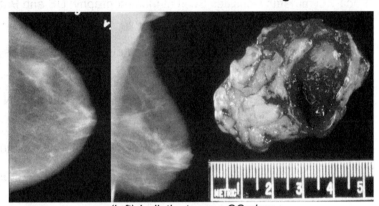

(left) Cell in single file characteristic for invasive lobular carcinoma.

(right) Cells forming thickened ductal walls in invasive ductal carcinoma.

Figure 1-25-21

(left) Indistinct mass CC view.
(middle) Indistinct mass oblique view.
(right) Gross specimen showing invasion

Figure 1-25-22

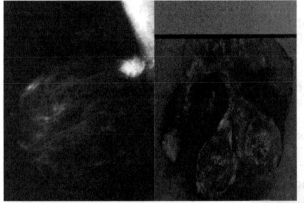

(left) Irregular mass with indistinct borders and spiculation.
(right) Gross specimen with invasion.

Figure 1-25-23

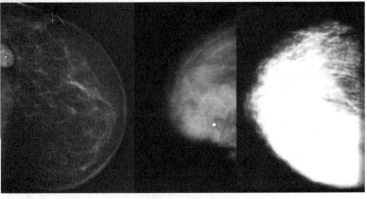

(left) Small circumscribed tumor.
(middle) Large diffuse tumor.
(right) White out from massive tumor

References

"Analysis of Sonographic Features for the Differentiation of Benign and Malignant Breast Tumors of Different Sizes." Chen, S-C, et.al. Ultrasound Obstst Gynecol 23:188-193, 2004.

"Comparison of the Performance of Screening Mammography, Physical Examination, and Breast US and Evaluation of Factors that Influence Them: An Analysis of 27,825 Patient Evaluations." Kolb, Thomas M., et.al. Radiology 225:165-175, 2002

"Digital Mammography, Sestamibi Breast Scintigraphy and Position Emission Tomography Breast Imaging." Etta D. Pisano et.al. Rad.Clin.NA 38: 861 - 870, July 2000.

"Ductography: How To and What If?" Slawson and Johnson. RadioGraphics 21: 133 – 150, 2001.

"Focal Asymmetric Densities Seen at Mammography: US and Pathologic Correlation." Samardar, Shaw de Paredes et. al. RadioGraphics 22:19-33, 2002.

"Imaging – Histologic Discordance at Percutaneous Breast Biopsy." Liberman, L, et.al. Cancer 89:2538-2546,2000.

"Imaging of Breast Massses." Bassett, Lawrence B. Rad. Clin. N.A. 38:669-700, 2000.

Pathology of the Breast 2nd Edition , Tavassoli, Fattaneh, Appleton & Lange 1999

"Papillary carcinoma of the Breast: Imaging Findings." Soo, MS. Et. al. AJR 164:321-326, 1995.

"Radial Scar of the Breast: Radiologic-Pathologic Correlation in 22 Cases." Alleva, D. Quentin, et.al. Radiographics19:27-35, 1999.

"Radiology – Pathology Correlation of Some Uncommon Breast Lesions." Cardenosa, G & Shaw, J. Sem Breast Dis 4:100-115, 2001.

"Short-term Follow-up Results in 795 Nonpalpable Probably Benign Lesions Detected at Screening Mammography." Vizcaino, I et.al. Radiology 219: 475-483, 2001.

"Solid Breast Nodules: Use of sonography to distinguish between benign and malignant lesions." Stavros, AT, et.al. Radiology 196:123-134, 1995.

"Sonography of the Breast." Jackson, Valerie P., et.al. Seminars in Ultrasound, CT, and MRI 17:460-475, 1996.

"The Use of Magnetic Resonance Imaging in Breast Cancer Screening." Lee, CH and Weinreb, JC. J Am Col Radiol 1:176-182, 2004.

"Tubular Carcinoma of the Breast: Mammographic and Sonographic Features." Sheppard, DG, et. al. AJR 174:253-257, 2000.

"Unusual Breast Lesions:Radiologic-Pathologic Correlation." Feder, Jay M., et.al. ,Radiographics:19, S11-S26, 1999.

Ductal Carcinoma in Situ (DCIS)

Leonard M. Glassman MD FACR
Visiting Scientist
Armed Forces Institute of Pathology
Washington DC
Washington Radiology Associates, PC
Washington DC
glassmanl@afip.osd.mil

Figure 1-26-1

Ductal Carcinoma in Situ (DCIS)
- Also called intraductal carcinoma
  - Not invasive ductal carcinoma
  - DCIS is "benign"
    - Disease is confined to the breast
    - Patients die from metastatic disease

Confined to the Duct [Figure 1-26-1]
- No spread to blood or lymph nodes
- Less than 1% positive axillary nodes
  - Probably unrecognized invasion
  - Most likely in large lesions and palpable lesions

The Problems
- How big is the problem?
- How do we classify the disease?
- How do we diagnose it?
- What is adequate treatment?

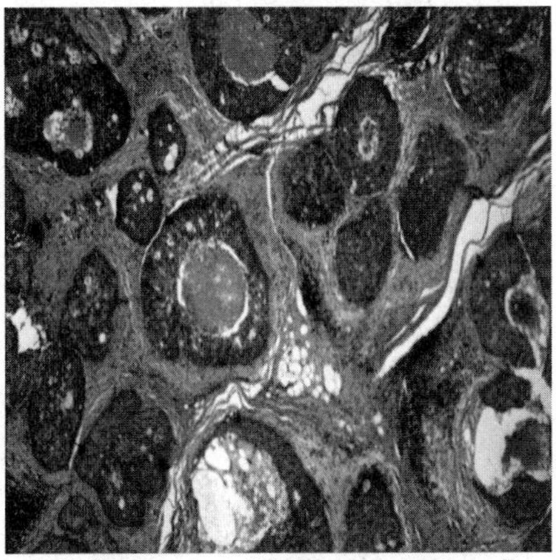

DCIS showing thickened duct walls with abnormal cells and eosinophilic secretion in the lumen

How Big is the Problem?
- USA data
  - 50% eligible women get screening annually after 40
  - 190,000 new breast cancers annually
    - Includes invasive and intraductal
- 1980 5% of new breast cancers were DCIS
  - Usually a palpable lump or nipple discharge
- 2000 20% of new breast cancers
  - Usually microcalcifications on mammography
- Age-adjusted incidence increasing
  - 2.4 per 100,000 in 1973
  - 15.8 per 100,000 in 1992

Is It Malignant?
- 30 to 60% of underdiagnosed DCIS becomes invasive cancer within 25 years
- Usually in the same breast and near the biopsy site

Invasive Cancer after DCIS
- NASBP B17 (790 women) at 5 years
  - Women treated with breast conservation
  - 115 cancers
    - 80% same breast
    - 15.7% opposite breast
    - 4.3% regional or distant metastases
  - 12.1% recurrence with lumpectomy + radiation (36% invasive)
  - 26.8% recurrence with lumpectomy alone (51% invasive)

Indicators of Recurrence after Conservative Treatment
- Tumor size
- Nuclear grade
- Necrosis
- Margin status
- Multifocality
- Lymphocytic infiltrate

Epidemiology
- Same risks as for invasive cancer
  - Increasing age
  - Early menarche
  - Family history
  - Previous breast biopsy
  - Nulliparity or late age at first birth

Pathologic Classification of DCIS
- No uniform agreement on single scheme
- Interobserver agreement between schemes is poor

Classifications of DCIS
- Architectural
  - Comedo
    - Needs comedonecrosis and high nuclear grade
  - Non-comedo
    - Cribriform
    - Micropapillary
    - Papillary
    - Solid
- Special type
  - Apocrine
  - Clear cell
  - Signet ring cell
  - Small cell
  - Endocrine
  - Spindle cell

Intraductal Carcinoma (DCIS)
- Histology may be abble to predict recurrence risk
  - High grade, large cell, comedo have higher recurrence
  - Low grade, small cell, noncomedo (cribriform, micropapillary)
- Poor correlation of calcification type and extent with grade and extent of tumor

Is DCIS One Disease?

	Low Grade	High Grade
ER	+++	+
PR	+++	+
HER-2/neu	+	+++
p53	+	++
bcl-2	+	−

Is DCIS One Disease?
- Associated invasive carcinoma shows marker phenotype like precursor DCIS
- Low grade DCIS yields low grade invasive tumors
- High grade DCIS yields high grade invasive tumors
- Theory: Low grade and high grade DCIS are different from the start

Classification of DCIS
- DIN (AFIP)
- European Commission Working Group
- Lagios
- Modified Lagios
- Nottingham
- UKNBCSP
- Van Nuys

Relative Risk of Invasive Carcinoma
- No increased risk
  - Mild intraductal hyperplasia (IDH)
- Slight increased risk
  - Moderate or florid IDH
- Mild to moderate increased risk
  - Atypical hyperplasia (ductal or lobular)
    - No family history
    - Postmenopausal
- High risk
  - Atypical hyperplasia (ductal or lobular)
    - Family history
    - Premenopausal
  - Ductal carcinoma in situ
  - Lobular carcinoma in situ

Pathologic Findings Needed in Any Report
- Nuclear grade
  - Low, intermediate or high
- Necrosis
  - Comedo or punctate
- Architectural pattern

Pathologic Findings Needed in Any Report
- Lesion size
- Margin assessment
- Specimen processing
  - Report should include
    - Presence of calcification
    - Correlation with specimen radiograph and/or mammogram

Diagnosis of DCIS
- Mass
- Mammographic calcifications
  - Can't distinguish from invasive carcinoma
  - Associated mass usually invasive disease

Mass
- Rare today
- Usually small

DCIS Mass Close-up [Figure 1-26-2]

DCIS Mass [Figure 1-26-3 and 1-26-4]

Intraductal Carcinoma
- Microcalcification usually without mass
- Particles < 1 mm
- Varying size shape and density
- Clustered
- May coexist with benign calcifications

Figure 1-26-2

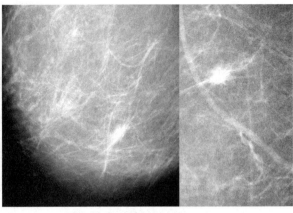

(left) Small irregular mass
(right) Close-up

Figure 1-26-3

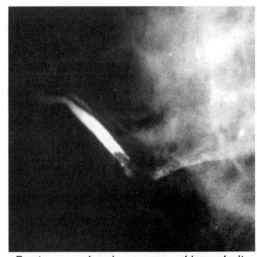

Ductogram showing mass and irregularity within the duct

Figure 1-26-4

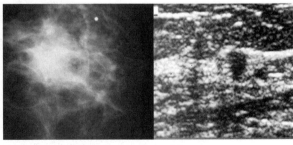

(left) Large palpable mass.
(right) Ultrasound of small mass

Calcification
- Size
- Number
- Distribution
- Shape
- Change over time

Size of Particles
- < 1 mm
  - ➤ Evaluate malignant potential by smallest particles in the abnormality

Size [Figure 1-26-5]
- Macro
- Micro

Number
- Cluster is 5 particles or more in 1 cubic cm.

Is 5 important?

Distribution
- Cluster
- Linear
  - ➤ DCIS involves a duct
  - ➤ Linear distribution toward nipple
  - ➤ High grade is continuous involvement
  - ➤ Low grade has skip areas
- Segmental
  - ➤ Involvement of an entire ductal system

Cluster / Linear

Intraductal Carcinoma [Figure 1-26-6]

Segmental [Figure 1-26-7]

Shape is Most Important
- Irregular
  - ➤ Not smooth round or hollow
- Heterogeneous or pleomorphic
  - ➤ Not all the same

Smooth / Round / Hollow

Figure 1-26-5

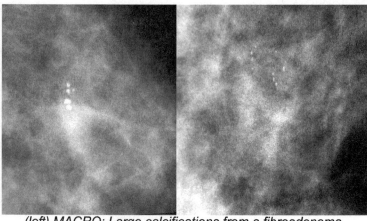

(left) MACRO: Large calcifications from a fibroadenoma.
(right) MICRO: Small calcifications from DCIS

Figure 1-26-6

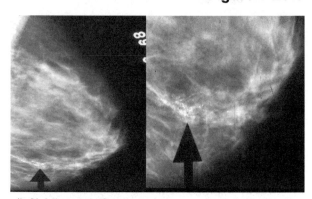

(left) Microcalcifications in a segmental distribution
(right) Close-up

Figure 1-26-7

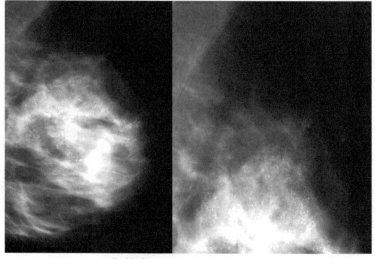

(left) Segmental distribution
(right) Close-up

Pleomorphic [Figure 1-26-8]

Figure 1-26-8

Calcifications represent the caste of a space
- Irregular duct
- Necrotic tissue space

Intraductal Carcinoma [Figure 1-26-9]

Irregular Duct [Figure 1-26-10]

Shapes of DCIS Calcification
- Granular
- Irregular rods
- Casting
- Irregular
  - ➤ Branching
  - ➤ Comma shaped
  - ➤ Arrow shaped or pointed

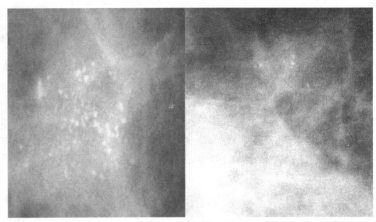

(left) Mixture of micro and macrocalcifications with varying shapes. (right) Small calcifications with varying irregular shapes.

Figure 1-26-9

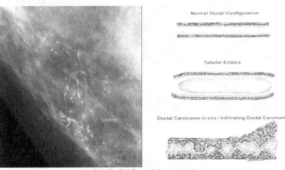

(left) DCIS with casting.
(right) Drawing showing ductal calcification shape as a function of wall irregularity

Figure 1-26-10

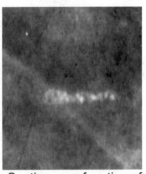

Casting as a function of irregular duct walls.close-up (lowest on drawing in Fig. 1-26-9)

Granular [Figure 1-26-11]
- Very small (<0.5 mm)
- Need magnifying glass to evaluate
- Too small to see true shape
- "Grains of sand"

Irregular Rods
- Made up of many tiny pieces on magnification
- Not solid large rods
  - ➤ Secretory disease
- Often branch

Rods [Figure 1-26-12]
- Regular
- Irregular

Figure 1-26-12

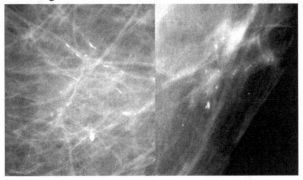

Figure 1-26-11

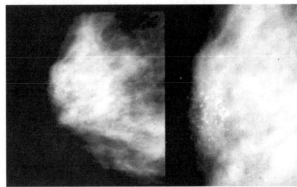

(left) Multiple subareolar calcifications. (right) Close-up shows many very small calcifications intermixed with larger pleomorphic ones.

(left) Benign ductal calcifications.(right) irregular broken rods secondary to an irregular wall contour.

Casting
- Granular calcifications filling the lumen of an irregular duct
- Often branch

Irregular
- Castes of necrotic spaces
- Branching
- Comma shaped
- Arrow shaped or pointed

Intraductal Carcinoma [Figure 1-26-13]

Irregular [Figure 1-26-14]

Intraductal Carcinoma [Figure 1-26-15]

Irregular

Change Over Time
- Benign processes can change
- Malignant processes almost always change within 3 years
- Short interval follow-up
  - ➢ Probably benign findings
  - ➢ 6 months unilateral, annual bilateral for 3 years
    - ❖ No scientific basis

Biopsy
- Imaging guided biopsy with specimen radiography
  - ➢ Usually stereotactic
- Wire guided excision with specimen radiography

Extent of Calcification Does Not Correspond to the Extent of the Tumor
- Best correlation is with comedo type but not good enough
  - ➢ Poor correlation with cribriform and micropapillary
- Must use histologic margins to define true extent

Treatment
- Simple mastectomy without axillary dissection
  - ➢ 25% of patients choose this option
  - ➢ Large lesions in small breasts
  - ➢ Multiple lesions
  - ➢ No radiation
    - ❖ Unavailability
    - ❖ Prior radiation
    - ❖ Collagen vascular disease
  - ➢ Patient preference
- Reconstruction

Figure 1-26-13

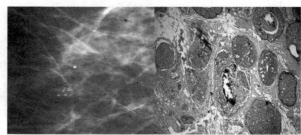

(left) Small cluster of irregular calcifications.
(right) Thickened duct walls with irregular calcifications.

Figure 1-26-14

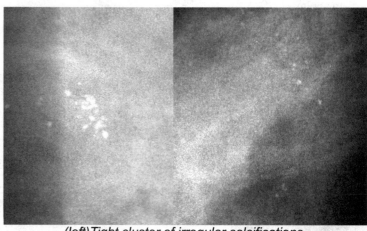

(left)Tight cluster of irregular calcifications.
(right) More scattered non-uniform calcifications

Figure 1-26-15

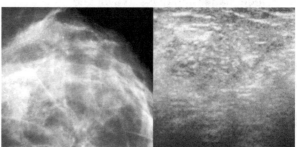

(left) Segmental granular calcifications.
(right) Ultrasound of same patient showing microcalcifications

Breast Conservation
- Wide local excision without axillary dissection
  - Sentinel node when large or palpable lesions
- Post -excision mammogram with magnification views of biopsy site
  - May be done 2 or 3 months after excision
  - Not necessary if specimen radiograph shows complete excision with 10 mm margin
- Radiation is standard
  - Helps in all patients
  - Benefit may be small in a subset of patients
    - ❖ Small lesions
    - ❖ Low grade histology
    - ❖ Wide clear margins
- Local excision alone
  - Controversial
  - Less than 2 - 3 cm lesion
  - Margins should be 10 mm or greater
  - Nuclear grade low or intermediate
- Recurrence risk 1% per year

What is a Clear Margin?
- Relative risk of recurrence after excision and radiation
  - 10 mm or greater   1.14
  - 1 – 9 mm   1.49
  - <1 mm   2.54

Radiation Therapy
- 1.8 to 2.0 Gy fractions Monday through Friday
- 45 to 50 Gy total dose
- Boost 10 to 20 Gy to surgical bed
- No axillary radiation

Chemotherapy
- No cytotoxic drugs
- Tamoxifen 20 mg daily for 5 years
  - Newer drugs possible with fewer side effects
  - Decreases invasive recurrences
  - No change in survival
    - ❖ Survival is over 90% without chemotherapy

Treatment of Recurrence
- DCIS
  - Mastectomy if radiation given previously
  - Mastectomy or wide excision with radiation
- Invasive carcinoma
  - Treat like any invasive cancer
  - Can not give radiation twice

Follow-up
- Lifetime
- Annual mammography
  - First exam 6 months after completion of treatment
  - Every 6 months for the first two years?
  - Use of magnification views common
    - ❖ Most common in first exam after treatment

Summary
- DCIS is carcinoma without the ability to spread YET
- It is detected on mammography as calcification
- Adequate detection and treatment decreases the incidence of invasive cancer and therefore death

References

"Chromosomal Alterations in Ductal Carcinomas in Situ and their in Situ Recurrences." Waldman, FM, et. al. J Nat Cancer Inst 92:313-320, 2000.

"Clinically Occult Ductal Carcinoma in Situ detected with Mammography: Analysis of 100 Cases with Radiologic – Pathologic Correlation." Stomper, PC et.al. Radiology 1989:172:235 – 241.

"Consensus Conference on the Classification of Ductal Carcinoma In Situ." Consensus Conference Committee: April 25- 28, 1997. Cancer 80:1798 -18021, 1997.

"High Detection Rate of Breast Ductal Carcinoma In Situ Calcifications on Mammographically Detected High Resolution Sonography." Hashimoto, B et.al. J Ultrasound Med 20:501-508, 2001.

"Mammographic Pattern of Microcalcifications in the Preoperative Diagnosis of Comedo Ductal Carcinoma in Situ: Histopathologic Correlation." Hermann, G, et.al. Can Assoc Radiol J 50:235-240, 1999.

"Microcalcifications Associated with Ductal Carcinoma in Situ:Mammographic-pathologic Correlation." Holland, R & Hendriks, JH, Sem Diag Pathol 11:181-192, 1994.

"Pathology and Clinical Evolution of Ductal Carcinoma in Situ (DCIS) of the Breast." Cancer Lett 86:1-4, 1994.

"Pathology of Ductal Carcinoma in Situ: Differential Diagnosis and Markers of Recurrence." Palazzo, Juan P . Seminars in Breast Disease 3: 2-7, 2000.

"Potential Role of Magnetic Resonance Imaging and Other modalities in Ductal Carcinoma in Situ Detection." Ikeda, Debra M., et.al. Seminars in Breast Disease 3: 50-60, 2000.

"The Consensus Conference on the Treatment of In Situ Ductal Carcinoma of the Breast," Schwartz, G. et. al. April 22 - 25, 1999. Seminars in Breast Disease 3:209 - 219, 2000
.

"The Influence of Margin Width on Local Control of Ductal Carcinoma in Situ of the Breast." Silverstein, MJ, et.al. NEJM 340:1455-1461, 1999.

"Ultrasound of Ductal Carcinoma in Situ." Moon, WK, et. al. Radiographics 22:269-281, 2002

Notes

Notes

Notes

Notes

Gastrointestinal Radiology

Hepatic Neoplasms: Radiologic–Pathologic Correlation

Angela D. Levy, LTC, MC, USA
Department of Radiologic Pathology
Armed Forces Institute of Pathology
Washington, DC

AFIP Classification - Tumors of the Liver and Intrahepatic Bile Ducts
- Hepatocellular origin
  - Hepatocellular adenoma, focal nodular hyperplasia, nodular regenerative hyperplasia
  - Hepatocellular carcinoma, fibrolamellar carcinoma, hepatoblastoma
- Cholangiocellular origin
  - Bile duct cyst, biliary cystadenoma, bile duct adenoma
  - Cholangiocarcinoma, biliary cystadenocarcinoma
- Mesenchymal origin
  - Hemangioma, angiomyolipoma, myelolipoma, mesenchymal hamartoma
  - Angiosarcoma, epithelioid hemangioendothelioma

Benign Hepatic Neoplasms - Objectives
- Benign neoplasms
  - Hemangioma
  - Focal nodular hyperplasia (FNH)
  - HCA
  - Biliary cystadenoma/carcinoma
  - Lipomatous tumors
- Surgical vs. nonsurgical neoplasms

Hemangioma
- Most common benign hepatic tumor
- 1% to 7% of the population
- More common in women, 5:1
  - Estrogen influences
  - May enlarge during pregnancy
- Symptoms
  - 85% asymptomatic
  - Pain
  - Palpable mass
  - Rupture

Hemangioma
- Kasabach-Merritt syndrome
  - Hemolytic anemia and consumptive coagulopathy
- Erythropoietin secretion
  - Erythrocytosis
- Associations
  - Focal nodular hyperplasia
  - Tuberous sclerosis

Hemangioma - Pathology
- Peripheral feeding vessels
- Blood filled spaces
- Endothelial lining
- Fibrosis from
  - Slow flowing blood
  - Thrombosis
  - Hyalinization
  - Scar formation

Hemangioma - Pathology
- Single or multiple
- Well-circumscribed
- Subcapsular
- Occasionally
  - Calcification
  - Cystic areas
  - Pedunculated

Figure 2-1-1

Hemangioma Sonography *[Figure 2-1-1]*
- Homogeneous, hyperechoic
- Minimal posterior acoustic enhancement
- Atypical features
  - Hypoechoic center
  - Echogenic border
  - Scalloped borders
  - Heterogeneous hypoechoic

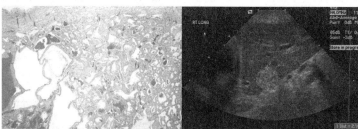

Hepatic hemangioma on sonography shows a well-defined mass that is homogenously hyperechoic

Hemangioma - Hypoechoic Foci

Hemangioma - Scalloped, echogenic border

Hemangioma - Heterogeneous, hypoechoic

Hemangioma - CT and MR
- Peripheral globular enhancement in arterial phase
- Slow centripetal filling during portal venous/equilibrium
- Rapid enhancement pattern
  - Capillary hemangiomas
  - "Flash fill" phenomenon
- MR
  - Homogenous hyperintense T2
  - Progressive hyperintensity as TE increases
  - "Light bulb" phenomenon

Figure 2-1-2

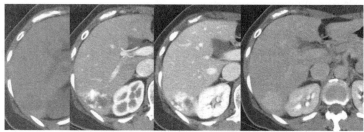

Hemangioma - CT *[Figure 2-1-2]*

Typical appearance of hemangioma on CT. There is nodular peripheral enhancement and gradual contrast filling in the lesion

Hemangioma - MR

Hemangioma - Pedunculated

Hemangioma - Edematous scar

Hemangioma - Heterogeneous with Fibrosis

Focal Nodular Hyperplasia
- Second most common benign liver neoplasm
- 80% to 95% occur in women
  - Peak age, 20 to 40 years
- 80% asymptomatic

Focal Nodular Hyperplasia
- Associations
  - Hepatic hemangiomas
  - Intracranial aneurysms
  - Dysplastic system arteries
  - Intracranial neoplasms: meningioma, astrocytoma

Focal Nodular Hyperplasia
- Pathogenesis
  - Hyperplastic response to a vascular malformation
  - Central artery
  - Central scar

Focal Nodular Hyperplasia
- Gross Pathology
  - Central scar
  - Nodular with fibrous septa
  - No hemorrhage or necrosis
  - No capsule

Focal Nodular Hyperplasia
- Histology
  - Fibrous septa
  - Large arteries
  - Normal hepatocytes
  - Kupffer cells
  - No portal tracts or central veins

Figure 2-1-3

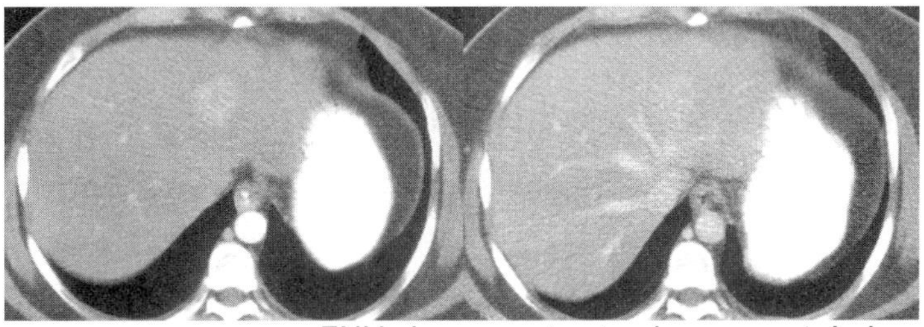

FNH shows contrast enhancement during the arterial phase and near isoattenuation during the portal venous phase

Focal Nodular Hyperplasia - Sonography
- Subtle
  - Similar texture to normal liver
- Scar is hypoechoic
- Doppler
  - Peripheral and central vessels

Focal Nodular Hyperplasia - CT
- Noncontrast
  - Iso- or hypodense
  - Hypodense scar
- Arterial
  - Rapid enhancement
  - Hypodense scar
- Portal venous
  - Iso- or hypo- or hyperdense
  - Delayed enhancement of scar
  - Peripheral capsule-like vessels

FNH *[Figures 2-1-3 and 2-1-4]*

Figure 2-1-4

FNH - Sulfur Colloid
Normal uptake 60%
Defect 30%
Increased uptake 10%

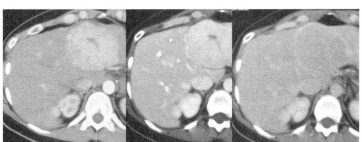

FNH on CT showing late enhancement of the central scar and peripheral vessels.

FNH - MR
Figure 2-1-5

- T1 isointense
  - ➢ Low signal scar
- T2 iso or slightly hyperintense
  - ➢ High signal scar
- Gd-DTPA
  - ➢ Rapid homogeneous enhancement
  - ➢ May have flash enhancement
  - ➢ Delayed enhancement of the scar
  - ➢ Rim-like enhancement late
- T2 with ferumoxide
  - ➢ Lesion decreases signal
  - ➢ Except scar

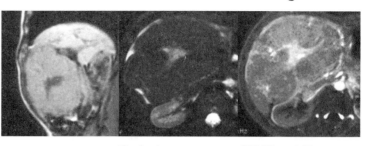

Typical appearance of FNH on MR

FNH *[Figure 2-1-5]*

FNH - Flash Enhancement

FNH - Ferumoxide-enhanced MR *Paley MR, & al. AJR 2000;175:1:159-63*

FNH Variants Controversial
- Telangiectatic FNH
  - ➢ Multiplicity
  - ➢ Lack of a central scar
  - ➢ Lesion heterogeneity
  - ➢ Persistent contrast enhancement
  - ➢ Hyperintensity on T1 and T2
- Mixed hyperplastic FNH
- Adenomatous FNH
- FNH with large cell change

Nguyen BN, et al. Am J Surg Path 1999; 23: 1441-54.

Attal P, et al. Radiology 2003

Atypical FNH - ?Telangiectatic FNH

Hepatocellular Adenoma
- Third most common benign liver tumor
- Composed of benign hepatocytes
- Almost always occur in women
  - ➢ Mean age, 30 years
  - ➢ History of oral contraceptive use
  - ➢ Declining incidence

Hepatocellular Adenoma
- Surgical resection
  - ➢ Risk of hemorrhage
  - ➢ Small risk of malignant transformation to HCC

Hepatocellular Adenoma
- Hepatocyte proliferation
  - ➢ Exogenous estrogens
  - ➢ Ovarian tumors
  - ➢ Anabolic steroids
  - ➢ Antiestrogens
  - ➢ Glycogenosis, type Ia and III
  - ➢ Hurler syndrome

Hepatocellular Adenoma - Clinical Features

- Acute abdominal pain 40%
  - Hemorrhage within tumor
  - I➤ ntraperitoneal hemorrhage
- Palpable mass 35%
- Incidental 10%

Hepatocellular Adenoma - Pathologic Features

- Histology
  - Benign hepatocytes
  - Rich in glycogen
  - Kupffer cells

Hepatocellular Adenoma - Pathologic Features

- Gross
  - Solitary
  - Multiple (up to 50%)
  - Capsule (25%)
  - Peripheral vessels
  - Central fat
  - Necrosis, infarcts, hemorrhage

Hepatocellular Adenoma

Figure 2-1-6

Hepatocellular Adenoma - CT and MR

- Capsule
- Heterogeneous
- Hemorrhage (25% to 50%)
  - Acute, high density on unenhanced CT
  - Chronic, hemosiderin rings on MR
- Focal fat
- Enhancement
  - Variable

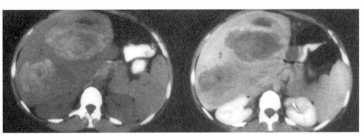

Hemorrhagic hepatocellular adenoma

Hepatocellular Adenoma

Figure 2-1-7

- Intracellular glycogen/fat
  - Diffuse low attenuation on CT
  - Loss of signal on out-of-phase MR

Hepatocellular Adenoma
Acute Hemorrhage [Figure 2-1-6]

Hepatocellular Adenoma
Hemosiderin Rings

Hepatocellular Adenoma
Focal Fat and Capsule

Hepatocellular Adenoma
Diffuse Low Attenuation [Figure 2-1-7]

Hepatocellular Adenoma
Out-of-Phase MR

Hepatocellular Adenoma
Fat Suppression

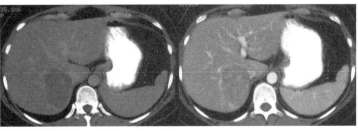

Diffuse low attenuation in hepatocellular adenoma due to intracellular glycogen

Hepatocellular Adenoma - Imaging Difficulties
- Nonhemorrhagic
- Fibrosis/scar formation
- Multiple
  - ➢ Glycogenosis
- Hepatocellular adenomatosis

Hepatocellular Adenoma

Hepatocellular Adenomatosis
- Affects men and women
- Unrelated to estrogens
- Abnormal LFT's
- Biopsy for diagnosis
- Treated symptomatically

Biliary Cystadenoma
- Benign tumor, but
  - ➢ May recur after excision
  - ➢ May develop into cystadenocarcinoma
- Middle-aged women
  - ➢ 42 - 55 years
  - ➢ Ovarian stroma histologically
- Cystic neoplasms
  - ➢ Unilocular or multilocular
  - ➢ Septations
  - ➢ Mural nodules
  - ➢ Calcification

Biliary Cystadenoma - Imaging Features
- Cystic neoplasms
  - ➢ Unilocular or multilocular
  - ➢ Cyst fluid variable composition
- Septations
- Mural nodules
  - ➢ May enhance
- Calcification
  - ➢ Punctate or linear
- May communicate or extend into biliary system

Figure 2-1-8

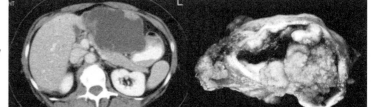

Biliary Cystadenoma *[Figure 2- 1-8]*

Biliary cystadenoma

Lipomatous Tumors
- Angiomyolipoma
  - ➢ Benign
  - ➢ Composed of adipose, smooth muscle, and blood vessels
  - ➢ Most cases sporadic
  - ➢ Tuberous sclerosis in 6%
- Myelolipoma
  - ➢ Rare
  - ➢ Benign
  - ➢ Composed of myeloid, adipose, and blood vessels

Angiomyolipoma

Myelolipoma

Summary - Benign Hepatic Neoplasms
- Nonsurgical lesions
  - Hemangioma
  - Focal nodular hyperplasia
- Surgical lesions
  - Hepatocellular adenoma
  - Biliary cystadenoma

Summary - Benign Hepatic Neoplasms
- If typical features present, firmly suggest diagnosis
- If atypical features present
  - MR
  - Nuclear medicine
  - If all fails, BIOPSY!

Summary - Hemangioma
- Sonography
  - Homogenous
  - Hyperechoic
- CT/MR
  - Peripheral nodular enhancement
- Tagged-RBC

Summary - FNH
- CT/MR
  - Rapid enhancement
  - Homogenous tumor
  - Hypodense/intense scar
  - Delayed scar enhancement
  - Delayed peripheral enhancement
- Sulfur colloid

Summary - HCA
- For imaging diagnosis
  - Female patient
  - Oral contraceptive use
  - Evidence of hemorrhage
- Suggest HCA
  - Diffuse low attenuation
  - Diffuse fat on MR
  - Appropriate patient
- BIOPSY!

Summary - Biliary Cystadenoma
- Cystic neoplasm
  - Septations
  - Nodules
  - Calcification
- Most common in middle-aged women

Malignant Hepatic Neoplasms - Objectives
- Malignant neoplasms
  - Hepatocellular carcinoma (HCC)
  - Fibrolamellar carcinoma (FLC)
  - Intrahepatic cholangiocarcinoma
  - Angiosarcoma
  - Epithelioid hemangioendothelioma
- Incidentally discovered hepatic mass

Hepatocellular Carcinoma
- Fifth most common cancer worldwide
- Neoplasm composed of malignant hepatocytes

Hepatocellular Carcinoma
- Strong association with chronic liver disease
  - Cirrhosis
  - Hepatitis B
  - Hepatitis C
- Other associations
  - Aflatoxins
  - Hereditary hemochromatosis (25%)
  - Hereditary tyrosinemia (20%)
  - Alpha-1-antitrypsin deficiency (15%)
  - Porphyria cutanea tarda
  - Anabolic steroids

Hepatocellular Carcinoma
- High incidence areas
  - Sub-Saharan Africa, Asia
  - 30 to 45 years old
  - Hepatitis B and C, aflatoxins
  - Aggressive
- Low incidence areas
  - Western hemisphere
  - 70 to 80 years old
  - Alcoholic cirrhosis, hepatitis C, hemochromatosis
  - Insidious

Hepatocellular Carcinoma - Clinical Features
- More common in men
  - 2:1 to 5:1
- Elevated alpha-fetoprotein (AFP)
- Paraneoplastic syndromes
  - Hypoglycemia
  - Erythrocytosis
  - Hypercholesterolemia
  - Rare, hypercalcemia, precocious puberty, gynecomastia, carcinoid syndrome, osteoporosis, hypertrophic pulmonary osteoarthropathy

Hepatocellular Carcinoma - Gross Pathology
- Morphology
  - Solitary
  - Multifocal
  - Infiltrating
- Important features
  - Capsule
  - Necrosis/hemorrhage
  - Vascular invasion
  - Macroscopic fat
  - No calcification
  - Underlying cirrhosis

Hepatocellular Carcinoma - Histologic Features
- Trabecular growth
- Occasional Kupffer cells
- Vascular invasion

Hepatocellular Carcinoma - CT and MR Features

- Small HCC
  - ➤ <2 cm
  - ➤ Do not differ, other than size
- Arterial phase
  - ➤ Rapid enhancement
- Portal venous phase
  - ➤ Heterogeneous, "mosaic pattern"
- Important features
  - ➤ Capsular enhancement
  - ➤ Fatty change
  - ➤ Cirrhosis

Figure 2-1-9

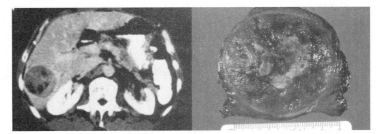

HCC with capsule and macroscopic fat

Figure 2-1-10

Hepatocellular Carcinoma - Enhancement

Hepatocellular Carcinoma Capsule and Macroscopic Fat
[Figure 2-1-9]

Hepatocellular Carcinoma Mosaic Pattern [Figure 2-1-10]

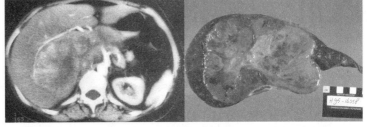

HCC with a mosaic pattern

Hepatocellular Carcinoma Fibrosis

Hepatocellular Carcinoma In Cirrhosis [Figure 2-1-11]

Hepatocellular Carcinoma Multifocal with Portal Vein Invasion
[Figure 2-1-12]

Figure 2-1-11

Figure 2-1-12

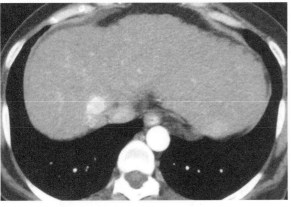

Hypervascular HCC in cirrhosis

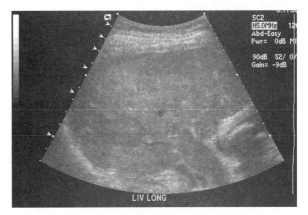

HCC with portal venous invasion

Hepatocellular Carcinoma - Utility of MR

Hepatocellular Carcinoma - Noncirrhotic Liver
- Large, solitary masses
- Heterogeneous
- Capsule
- Fat (10%)
- Calcification (25%)

Fibrolamellar Carcinoma
- Variant of HCC
  - Bands of fibrous lamellae
  - Tumor cells have "oncocytic" cytoplasm
- Young patients
  - Mean age, 23 years
  - No cirrhosis
  - AFP usually normal

Figure 2-1-13

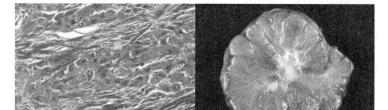

Fibrolamellar carcinoma

Fibrolamellar Carcinoma
Gross Pathology [Figure 2-1-13]
- Central scar
  - Radiating septa
  - Calcification
- Lobulated contour
- Bile staining

Figure 2-1-14

Fibrolamellar Carcinoma
CT Features [Figure 2-1-14]
- Lobulated, well defined margins
- Heterogeneous
- Arterial phase enhancement
  - Except scar
- Central scar
  - Hypodense
  - Calcification in 40%

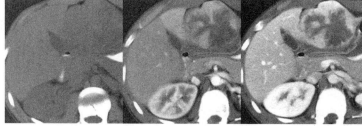

Fibrolamellar carcinoma

Fibrolamellar Carcinoma - MR Features
- Lobulated margins
- Heterogeneous signal
  - Dark T1
  - Bright T2
- Hypointense central scar
  - Dark T1
  - Dark T2
  - No enhancement

Fibrolamellar Carcinoma

How can I differentiate FLC from FNH?
- Tumor heterogeneous in FLC
  - Homogeneous in FNH
- Scar nonenhancing in FLC
  - Delayed
  - Enhancement in FNH
- Scar dark T2 signal in FLC
  - Scar bright T2 in FNH

Intrahepatic Cholangiocarcinoma (ICC)
- Adenocarcinoma arising from intrahepatic bile ducts
  - 10% of bile duct adenocarcinomas
- Synonyms
  - Peripheral cholangiocarcinoma, cholangiocellular carcinoma, intrahepatic bile duct carcinoma
- Geographic incidence variation
  - 10 times more common in Japan compared to U.S.

Intrahepatic Cholangiocarcinoma - Clinical Features
- Male predominance
- No cirrhosis
- Associations
  - Caroli disease/congenital hepatic fibrosis
  - Primary sclerosing cholangitis
  - Primary biliary cirrhosis
  - Recurrent pyogenic cholangitis
  - Lithiasis
  - Parasitic infection
  - Hepatitis B, C
  - Radiation therapy
  - ETOH abuse
  - Thorotrast

Intrahepatic Cholangiocarcinoma - Pathologic Features
- Morphology
  - Solitary
  - Multifocal
  - Diffuse
- Satellite nodules
- Marked fibrosis
- No capsule
- Rare, hemorrhage and necrosis
- Rare, calcification

Intrahepatic Cholangiocarcinoma - CT and MR Features
- Irregular borders
- Enhancement pattern
  - Due to fibrosis/hypovascularity
  - Delayed peripheral to central
- Biliary dilatation peripheral to the tumor
- Capsular contraction
- Vascular invasion

Figure 2-1-15

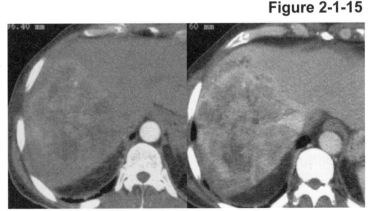

Intrahepatic cholangiocarcinoma

Intrahepatic Cholangiocarcinoma
[Figure 2-1-15]

How can I differentiate ICC from HCC?
- Difficult
  - HCC has variable morphology
  - HCC occurs more commonly
  - HCC associated with cirrhosis and hepatitis
  - But, HCC may occur in normal livers
- Ultimately
  - Biopsy is needed for diagnosis

How can I differentiate ICC from HCC?
- Enhancement
  - Delayed, peripheral to central favors ICC
  - Rapid filling favors HCC
  - Marked heterogeneity (mosaic) favors HCC
- Tumor margins
  - Lobulated, irregular favors ICC
  - Capsule favors HCC
- Capsular contraction
  - More common in ICC
- Biliary dilatation peripheral to the tumor
  - More common in ICC

Angiosarcoma

- Rare
  - ➤ But, most common hepatic sarcoma
- Malignant neoplasm of endothelial cells
- Etiologic associations
  - ➤ Vinyl chloride
  - ➤ Arsenical compounds
  - ➤ Radiation therapy
  - ➤ Anabolic steroids
  - ➤ Historically, Thorotrast
- More common in men, 3:1
- Clinical presentation
  - ➤ Variable
  - ➤ Hemoperitoneum
  - ➤ Metastasis in 60%, spleen, lung

Angiosarcoma - Imaging Features

- Solitary or multifocal
- Evidence of hemorrhage
- Enhancement
  - ➤ Peripheral or heterogeneous

Angiosarcoma [Figure 2- 1-16]

Epithelioid Hemangioendothelioma

- Rare malignancy of endothelial origin
- Fibrous stroma
- Imaging
  - ➤ Multifocal, lesions coalesce over time
  - ➤ Peripheral enhancement
  - ➤ Central fibrous stroma
  - ➤ Retracted liver capsule
  - ➤ May calcify

Incidentally discovered liver mass?

- Clinical history
- Contrast-enhanced MDCT
- Depending upon interpretation/clinical history
  - ➤ MR
  - ➤ Nuclear medicine
  - ➤ Biopsy
- If history of maligancy
  - ➤ Consider biopsy
- If otherwise normal patient and too small to biopsy
  - ➤ Consider periodic follow up

Summary Hepatocellular Carcinoma

- Most common primary hepatic malignancy
- Strong association with chronic liver disease
- Variable imaging features
  - ➤ Rapid enhancement
  - ➤ Capsule
  - ➤ Mosaic pattern
  - ➤ Focal fat
  - ➤ Vascular invasion

Figure 2-1-16

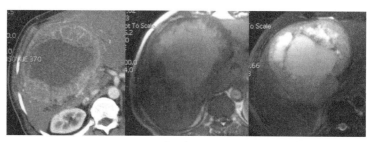

Angiosarcoma

Summary Fibrolamellar Carcinoma
- Variant of HCC
- Young patients
- Otherwise normal liver
- Key features
  - ➢ Lobular tumor
  - ➢ Central scar
  - ➢ Heterogeneous mass

Summary Intrahepatic Cholangiocarcinoma
- Arise from bile duct epithelium
- Uncommon
- Key features
  - ➢ Delayed central enhancement
  - ➢ Biliary dilatation peripheral to tumor
  - ➢ Capsular contraction

Imaging of Diffuse Liver Disease Radiologic-Pathologic Correlation

Angela D. Levy, LTC, MC, USA
Deparment of Radiologic Pathology
Armed Forces Institute of Pathology
Washington, DC

Diffuse Liver Disease
- Steatosis
- Cirrhosis
- Budd-Chiari
- Disorders of Iron Deposition
  - Hemosiderosis
  - Hemochromatosis

Steatosis
- Fatty infiltration
- Very common
- Pathogenesis unclear
  - Abnormal fatty acid metabolism
  - Insulin/glucagon imbalance
- Associations
  - Obesity, diabetes
  - ETOH
  - Malnutrition, TPN
  - Hepatitis, hepatotoxins, early cirrhosis chemotherapy, hyperlipidemia, drugs, CHF, jejunoileal bypass, idiopathic

Steatosis: Clinical Features
- Asymptomatic
- Mild RUQ pain
- Mild hepatomegaly and/or tenderness on exam
- Abnormal liver function tests (LFT's)

Fatty Infiltration: Pathology
- Steatosis
  - Hepatocyte accumulation of lipid
- Steatohepatitis
  - Alcoholic steatohepatitis
  - Nonalcoholic steatohepatitis (NASH)

Steatosis

Steatohepatitis

Fatty Infiltration: Sonography
[Figure 2-2-1]
- Diffuse
  - Echogenic parenchyma
  - Poor visualization hepatic vasculature
  - Absorption of sound
- Focal
  - Focal fat
  - Focal sparing

Figure 2-2-1

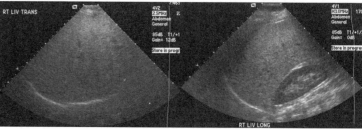

Diffuse fatty infiltration

Fatty Infiltration: CT
- Normal liver noncontrast CT
  - ➢ 30 to 60 HU
  - ➢ 8 to 10 HU > spleen
- Fatty liver noncontrast CT
  - ➢ 10 HU < spleen
- Fatty liver contrast CT
  - ➢ 25 HU < spleen

Fatty Infiltration: CT *[Figure 2-2-2]*
- Features of focal fat
  - ➢ No mass effect
  - ➢ Straight line margin
  - ➢ No contour abnormality
- Often transient
- Common locations
  - ➢ Falciform ligament
  - ➢ Subcapsular
  - ➢ Adjacent to porta hepatis
  - ➢ Adjacent to gallbladder fossa

Focal Fat: Common Locations

Focal Fat vs. Focal Sparing

Focal Sparing *[Figure 2-2-3]*

Focal Fat Transient

Fatty Infiltration: MR
- Conventional spin echo typically insensitive to fat deposition
- Chemical shift imaging
  - ➢ Fat and water signal additive in-phase
  - ➢ Fat signal subtracted from water signal out-of-phase

Fatty Infiltration 1.5T MR *[Figure 2-2-4]*

Fatty Infiltration MR *[Figure 2-2-5]*

Cirrhosis: Definition
- Histopathology features
  - ➢ Hepatocyte injury
  - ➢ Fibrosis
  - ➢ Nodule Formation
  - ➢ Architectural reorganization
- Gross pathology
  - ➢ Micronodular (<3mm)
  - ➢ Macronodular (>3mm)

Micronodular Cirrhosis: Pathology

Cirrhosis: Etiology
- Alcohol (60-70%)
- Postnecrotic: viral hepatitis (10%)
- Biliary cirrhosis
  - ➢ Primary and secondary (5-10%)
- Hemochromatosis (5%)
- Schistosomasis
- Hereditary

Figure 2-2-2

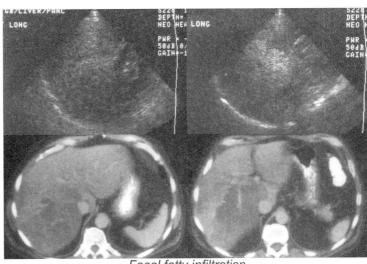

Focal fatty infiltration

Figure 2-2-3

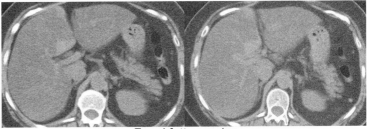

Focal fatty sparing

Figure 2-2-4

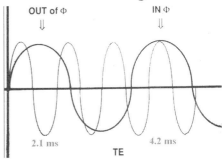

1.5 T MR fat and water proton signal intensity

OUT of Φ   IN Φ

2.1 ms   4.2 ms

TE

Figure 2-2-5

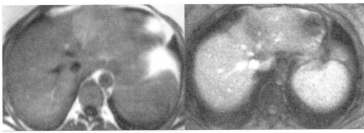

Focal fat on in-phase and out-of-phase images

- ➢ Glycogen storage disease
- ➢ Tyrosinemia
- Congestive
  - ➢ Veno-occlusive disease
  - ➢ Prolonged CHF

Cirrhosis: Sonography
- Fibrosis
  - ➢ Increased parenchymal echogenicity
  - ➢ Decreased penetration of the ultrasound beam
  - ➢ Poor visualization of hepatic vasculature
  - ➢ Loss of triphasic hepatic vein doppler
  - ➢ Increased pulsatility of portal vein doppler
- Nodules
- Morphologic changes
  - ➢ Atrophy
  - ➢ Compensatory hypertrophy

Cirrhosis: CT
- Morphologic changes
  - ➢ Volume redistribution
  - ➢ Atrophic right lobe and medial left lobe
  - ➢ Enlarged lateral segment left lobe and caudate lobe
- Nodules
- Fibrosis
  - ➢ Prominent porta and fissures
  - ➢ Focal confluent fibrosis
- Decreased parenchymal enhancement
- Mesenteric changes
  - ➢ Lymphadenopathy
  - ➢ Increased mesenteric attenuation

Figure 2-2-6

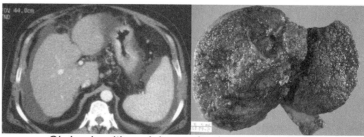

Cirrhosis: Volume redistribution and nodules [Figure 2-2-6]

Cirrhosis: Volume redistribution

Cirrhosis: Fibrosis, altered enhancement, nodules

Cirrhosis with nodules and volume redistribution

Cirrhosis: Mesenteric Changes, Adenopathy [Figure 2-2-7]

Figure 2-2-7

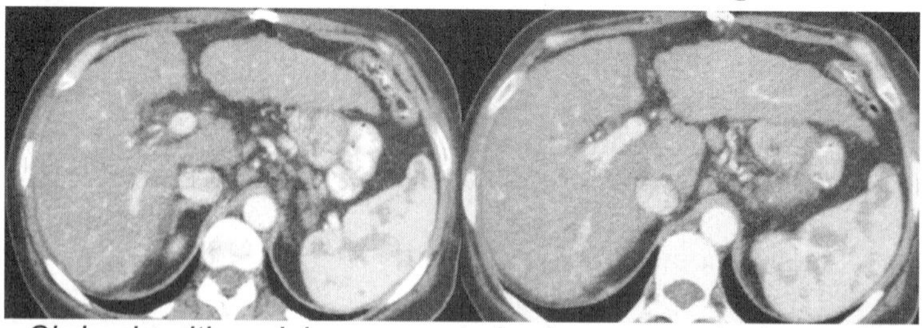

Cirrhosis: Nodules
- Regenerative nodule
  - ➢ Benign
  - ➢ Proliferation of hepatocytes
  - ➢ Precursor to dysplastic nodule and HCC
- Dysplastic nodule
  - ➢ Premalignant
- Hepatocellular carcinoma

Cirrhosis with nodules, mesenteric changes, and adenopathy

Cirrhosis: Regenerative Nodule
- Benign proliferation of hepatocytes
- Hemosiderin deposition
  - ➢ "Siderotic nodule"
- CT
  - ➢ Isodense with and without contrast
  - ➢ Hyperdense on noncontrast (siderotic nodule)
- MR
  - ➢ Dark T1, T2, gradient echo
  - ➢ Bright T1 (rare), Dark T2

Cirrhosis: Regenerative Nodules on CT [Figure 2-2-8]

Figure 2-2-8

Cirrhosis: Regenerative Nodules on MR

Cirrhosis: Dysplastic Nodule
- Premalignant nodule
  - Nodule with histologic evidence of dysplasia
- Very common in explanted livers
- Rarely seen on preoperative imaging
- CT
  - Most undetectable
- MR
  - Bright T1, dark T2
  - Variable appearance
- Malignant transformation
  - Nodule in a nodule
  - Bright T1 with central dark signal
  - Dark T2 with central high signal

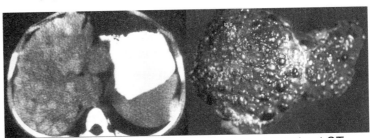

Cirrhosis with regenerating nodules on noncontrast CT

Cirrhosis: Hepatocellular Carcinoma
- CT or MR
  - Equally accurate
- Arterial phase imaging is important
- False positives
  - Focal confluent fibrosis--look for associated atrophy
  - Transient hepatic attenuation difference (THAD)
  - Enhancing regenerative nodule
  - Flash filling hemangioma

Cirrhosis: Focal Confluent Fibrosis
- Massive areas of fibrosis
  - Present in up to 30% of cirrhotic livers
- Typical location
  - Anterior segment right lobe
  - Medial segment left lobe
- Imaging
  - Focal mass
  - Wedge shape, radiating from porta hepatis
  - Capsular retraction
  - Low density on noncontrast CT
  - Isodense with contrast or irregular enhancement
  - MR: low signal T1, high signal T2

Portal Hypertension
- Classification
  - Pre-sinusoidal (Schistosomiasis)
  - Sinusoidal (Cirrhosis)
  - Post-sinusoidal (Budd-Chiari)
- Sonographic features
  - Portal vein enlargement (>13 mm)
  - Pulsatile portal vein
  - Hepatofugal flow (late feature)
  - Loss of normal triphasic hepatic vein waveform
  - Collateral veins
  - Splenomegaly

Cirrhosis: Collateral Pathways in Portal Hypertension

- Gastroesophageal
  - Coronary/short gastrics to systemic esophageal
  - Coronary vein >.7 cm correlates with severe portal hypertension
- Paraumbilical vein
  - Located in falciform ligament
  - Left portal vein to systemic epigastric veins
- Splenorenal and gastrorenal
  - Splenic, short gastrics, coronary to left adrenal or renal vein
- Retroperitoneal
  - Retroperitoneal GI tract veins anastomose with renal, phrenic, or lumbar veins
- Hemorrhoidal
  - Superior rectal to middle and inferior rectal

Cirrhosis: Coronary and Umbilical Vein Collaterals

Primary Biliary Cirrhosis

- Chronic cholestasis
- Unknown etiology
  - Probably immune mediated
- Middle-aged women
  - Median age 50
  - Female to male ratio 9:1

Primary Biliary Cirrhosis: CT *[Figure 2-2-9]*

- Global or segmental atrophy
- Nodules
- Fibrosis
  - Lace-like pattern
  - Segmental
  - Focal confluent
- Portal hypertension
  - Often present before morphologic changes
- HCC

Budd-Chiari Syndrome

- Hepatic venous outflow obstruction
- Primary
  - Membranous obstruction of hepatic veins
- Secondary
  - Hypercoaguable states, infections, neoplasms, trauma
- Pathology
  - Acute: hepatic enlargement, sinusoidal dilatation, hemorrhagic necrosis
  - Chronic: fibrosis, sinusoidal dilatation, cellular atrophy, nodular contour, caudate hypertrophy

Budd-Chiari Syndrome: Sonography

- Hepatic vein stenosis
- Intravascular thrombus
- Intrahepatic collaterals
- Hepatomegaly
- Chronic changes
  - Nonvisible hepatic veins
  - Narrowed IVC
  - Enlarged caudate lobe and left lobe
  - Atrophic right lobe
  - Ascites

Figure 2-2-9

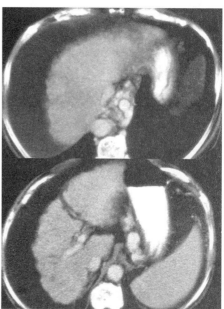

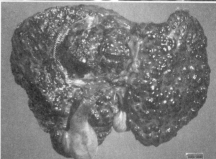

Primary biliary cirrhosis

Hepatic Venous Waveforms

Budd-Chiari Syndrome: CT

- Noncontrast
  - ➢ Hypodensity
    - ❖ Hepatic parenchymal congestion
  - ➢ hyperdense thrombi
- Contrast
  - ➢ Patchy enhancement
  - ➢ Normal central hepatic, left lobe, and caudate lobe enhancement
  - ➢ Late peripheral enhancement
    - ❖ Flip-flop pattern

Figure 2-2-10

Budd-Chiari Syndrome: Noncontrast CT

Budd-Chiari Syndrome: Contrast Enhanced CT

Budd-Chiari Syndrome: MR

- Absence of hepatic veins
- Thrombus in hepatic veins
- Narrowed intrahepatic IVC
- Intrahepatic collateral vessels

Budd-Chiari Syndrome: Angiography

[Figures 2-2-10 and 2-2-11]

- Narrowed intrahepatic IVC
- Hepatic vein occlusion
  - ➢ "Spider web" pattern on wedge hepatic venogram
  - ➢ Thrombi
  - ➢ Collaterals
  - ➢ Shunting to portal vein
- Celiac injection
  - ➢ Narrowed, stretched hepatic arteries
  - ➢ Prolonged hepatogram

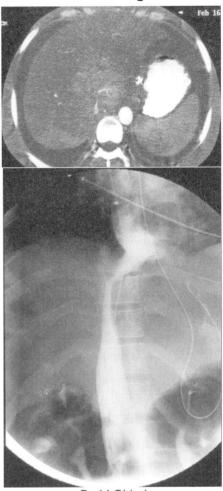

Budd-Chiari

Figure 2-2-11

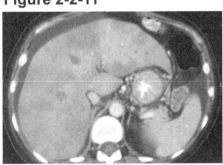

Budd-Chiari

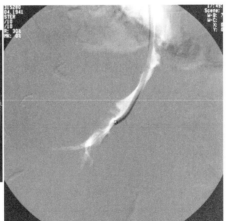

Disorders of Iron Deposition

- Hemosiderosis
  - ➢ Iron in the liver with <u>no</u> organ damage
  - ➢ Iron accumulation in the reticuloendothelial system
- Hemochromatosis
  - ➢ Iron in the liver with associated tissue damage
    - ❖ cirrhosis
  - ➢ Two types
    - ❖ Hereditary hemochromatosis
    - ❖ Secondary hemochromatosis

Hemosiderosis [Figure 2-2-12]

Figure 2-2-12

Hemochromatosis
- Hereditary hemochromatosis
  - Increased intestinal absorption of iron
  - Iron predominantly within hepatocytes
  - Highest incidence of cirrhosis and HCC (14%)
- Secondary hemochromatosis
  - Multiple transfusions
  - Iron predominantly in the reticuloendothelial system

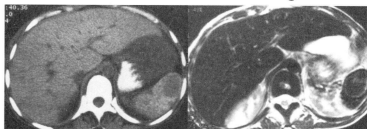

Hemosiderosis

Hereditary Hemochromatosis (HHC): Clinical Features
- Hyperpigmentation
- Diabetes mellitus (bronze diabetes)
- Hepatomegaly
- Chondrocalcinosis/osteoarthritis
- Cardiomyopathy

Hereditary Hemochromatosis (HHC): Pathology Features
- Iron accumulation
  - Hepatocytes
- Periportal fibrosis
- Micronodular cirrhosis

Hemochromatosis: Increased CT Attenuation (75-135 HU)

Hereditary Hemochromatosis

Hemochromatosis: MR
- Decrease signal on T2-weighted images
  - Hereditary
    - ❖ Iron in liver and pancreas
  - Secondary
    - ❖ Iron in liver and spleen
- T2*-gradient echo imaging is most sensitive
- Nodules or masses of bright signal should raise suspicion for HCC

Hereditary Hemochromatosis [Figure 2-2-13]

Figure 2-2-13

Secondary Hemochromatosis

Dense Liver on CT: Differential Diagnosis
- Iron deposition
- Glycogen storage disease
  - Type I, Von Gierke's disease
- Drugs
  - Amiodarone
  - Gold
- Wilson's disease
- Chronic arsenic poisoning

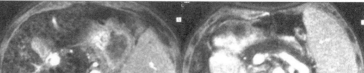

Hereditary Hemochromatosis

Amiodarone

Summary: Focal Fatty Infiltration
- No mass effect
- Straight line margins
- Typical Locations
  - ➢ Subcapsular
  - ➢ Falciform ligament
- Chemical shift MR
  - ➢ Signal loss on out-of-phase images

Summary: Cirrhosis
- Morphologic Changes
- Sonography
  - ➢ Portal hypertension
  - ➢ Portal-systemic collaterals
- MR
  - ➢ Regenerative nodule
  - ➢ Dysplastic nodule
  - ➢ HCC

Summary: Budd-Chiari Syndrome
- Hepatic venous outflow obstruction
- Sonography
- CT
  - ➢ Morphologic
  - ➢ Enhancement patterns
- MR

Summary: Disorders of Iron Overload
- Hemosiderosis
- Hemochromatosis
  - ➢ Hereditary
  - ➢ Secondary

Diffuse Liver Disease References

Steatosis/Fatty Infiltration
Brunt EM: Nonalcoholic steatohepatitis: definition and pathology. Semin Liver Dis 21:3, 2001

Debaere C, Rigauts H, Laukens P: Transient focal fatty liver infiltration mimicking liver metastasis. J Belge Radiol 81:174, 1998

Fukukura Y, Fujiyoshi F, Inoue H, et al: Focal fatty infiltration in the posterior aspect of hepatic segment IV: relationship to pancreaticoduodenal venous drainage. Am J Gastroenterol 95:3590, 2000

Grossholz M, Terrier F, Rubbia L, et al: Focal sparing in the fatty liver as a sign of an adjacent space-occupying lesion. AJR Am J Roentgenol 171:1391, 1998

Kawamori Y, Matsui O, Takahashi S, et al: Focal hepatic fatty infiltration in the posterior edge of the medial segment associated with aberrant gastric venous drainage: CT, US, and MR findings. J Comput Assist Tomogr 20:356, 1996

Kroncke TJ, Taupitz M, Kivelitz D, et al: Multifocal nodular fatty infiltration of the liver mimicking metastatic disease on CT: imaging findings and diagnosis using MR imaging. Eur Radiol 10:1095, 2000

Lee RG: Alcoholic and nonalcoholic steatohepatitis pathology. In Bloomer JR, Goodman ZD, Ishak KG (eds): Clinical and pathologic correlations in liver disease: approaching the next millennium. Washington, DC: Armed Forces Institute of Pathology, 1998

Loh YH, Dunn GD: Diffuse fatty infiltration of the liver: pitfalls in computed tomography diagnosis. Australas Radiol 41:383, 1997

Thu HD, Mathieu D, Thu NT, et al: Value of MR imaging in evaluating focal fatty infiltration of the liver: preliminary study. Radiographics 11:1003, 1991

Wang SS, Chiang JH, Tsai YT, et al: Focal hepatic fatty infiltration as a cause of pseudotumors: ultrasonographic patterns and clinical differentiation. J Clin Ultrasound 18:401, 1990

Yoshikawa J, Matsui O, Takashima T, et al: Focal fatty change of the liver adjacent to the falciform ligament: CT and sonographic findings in five surgically confirmed cases. AJR Am J Roentgenol 149:491, 1987

Cirrhosis

Baron RL, Gore RM: Diffuse Liver Disease. In Gore RM, Levine MS (eds): Textbook of gastrointestinal radiology, ed 2nd. Philadelphia: W.B. Saunders, 2000, Vol 2, pp 1590

Dodd GD, 3rd, Baron RL, Oliver JH, 3rd, et al: Spectrum of imaging findings of the liver in end-stage cirrhosis: Part II, focal abnormalities. AJR Am J Roentgenol 173:1185, 1999

Miller WJ, Baron RL, Dodd GD, 3rd, et al: Malignancies in patients with cirrhosis: CT sensitivity and specificity in 200 consecutive transplant patients. Radiology 193:645, 1994

Mitchell DG, Rubin R, Siegelman ES, et al: Hepatocellular carcinoma within siderotic regenerative nodules: appearance as a nodule within a nodule on MR images. Radiology 178:101, 1991

Mortele KJ, Ros PR: MR imaging in chronic hepatitis and cirrhosis. Semin Ultrasound CT MR 23:79, 2002

Ohtomo K, Baron RL, Dodd GD, 3rd, et al: Confluent hepatic fibrosis in advanced cirrhosis: appearance at CT. Radiology 188:31, 1993

Ohtomo K, Itai Y, Ohtomo Y, et al: Regenerating nodules of liver cirrhosis: MR imaging with pathologic correlation. AJR Am J Roentgenol 154:505, 1990

Valls C, Andia E, Roca Y, et al: CT in hepatic cirrhosis and chronic hepatitis. Semin Ultrasound CT MR 23:37, 2002

Disorders of Iron Deposition

Bonkovsky HL: Disorders of iron overload. In Bloomer JR, Goodman ZD, Ishak KG (eds): Clinical and pathologoical correlations in liver disease: approaching the next millennium. Washington, DC: Armed Forces Institute of Pathology, 1998

Gandon Y: Iron, liver, and MRI. http://www.radio.univ-rennes1.fr/Sources/EN/Hemo.html, 2001

Siegelman ES, Mitchell DG, Semelka RC: Abdominal iron deposition: metabolism, MR findings, and clinical importance. Radiology 199:13, 1996

Budd-Chiari Syndrome

Mergo PJ, Ros PR, Buetow PC, et al: Diffuse disease of the liver: radiologic-pathologic correlation. Radiographics 14:1291, 1994

Stanley P: Budd-Chiari syndrome. Radiology 170:625, 1989

Hepatic Infections: Radiologic Pathologic Correlation

Angela D. Levy, LTC, MC, USA
Department of Radiologic Pathology
Armed Forces Institute of Pathology
Washington, DC

Hepatic Infections
- Pyogenic Abscess
- Amebic Abscess
- Echinococcal Infections
- Schistosomiasis
- Clonorchiasis
- Infections in the Immunocompromised host
  - Candidasis
  - Pneumocystis

Pyogenic Hepatic Abscess
- Polymicrobial infections
- Variable clinical presentation
  - Septicemia, pain, fever, indolent symptoms
  - Tender hepatomegaly
- Mortality rate <10%
- Effectively treated with percutaneous drainage
  - 8% failure rate
  - 8% recurrence rate

Pyogenic Hepatic Abscess: Pathogenesis
- Biliary
  - MOST COMMON ETIOLOGY
  - Cholangitis, biliary obstruction
  - Multiple and bilateral
- Portal vein
  - Pylephlebitis
  - Solitary, 65% right lobe
- Hepatic artery
- Direct extension
- Traumatic-blunt or penetrating trauma
- Necrotic tumor

Pyogenic Hepatic Abscess: Sonography
- Variable echogenicity
  - Anechoic (50%)
  - Hyperechoic (25%)
  - Hypoechoic (25%)
- Ill-defined margins
- Internal character
  - Irregular wall
  - Septations
  - Fluid-fluid levels
  - Debris
  - Reverberation artifact if air is present
- Posterior acoustic enhancement

Pyogenic Hepatic Abscess: Sonography

Pyogenic Hepatic Abscess: CT
- Singe best imaging method
- Sensitivity 97%

Figure 2-3-1

- Intravenous contrast essential
- Hypodense
  - 0 to 45 H.U.
- Helpful features
  - Rim-enhancement
  - Transition zone
  - Cluster sign
  - Gas (<20%)
  - Air/fluid or debris/fluid level
    - ❖ Suspect GI communication

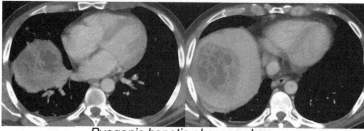

Pyogenic hepatic abscess shows cluster sign and transition zone

Pyogenic Hepatic Abscess CT

Pyogenic Hepatic Abscess: Cluster Sign

Pyogenic Hepatic Abscess: Cluster Sign/ Transition zone
[Figure 2-3-1]

Pyogenic Hepatic Abscess: Intrahepatic Gas

Pyogenic Hepatic Abscess: Imaging Guided Drainage
- Unilocular and liquefied
- Multilocular or multiple
  - Multiple catheters
- Multiple, small (<1 cm)
  - Aspiration for diagnosis
  - Treatment: antibiotics or aspiration + antibiotics

Amebic Liver Abscess
- Most common extra-intestinal manifestation of amebiasis
- 3 to 7% of patients with amebic infection
- Route of spread
  - Portal venous (most common)
  - Lymphatic
  - Direct extension from colon
- Clinical presentation: fever, pain
- 85% solitary
- 72% right lobe

Amebic Abscess: Sonography
- Round or oval shape
- Absent wall echoes
- Homogenous low level internal echoes
- Location
  - Near or touching the liver capsule
- Enhanced through transmission

Amebic Abscess

Figure 2-3-2

Amebic Abscess: CT *[Figure 2-3-2]*
- Round
  - Smooth or irregular margins
- Low attenuation/complex fluid
  - Septations
  - Fluid/debris level
- Enhancing wall (3-15 mm)
- Peripheral zone of edema
- Extrahepatic extension

Amebic Abscess

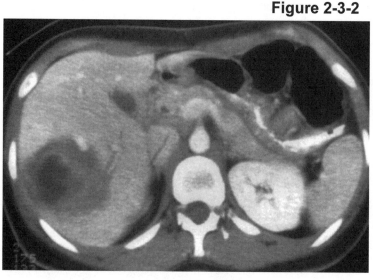

Amebic abscess

Amebic vs. Pyogenic Abscess
- Cannot be reliably differentiated by imaging
- Patients with amebic abscess
  - More likely to have hepatomegaly and diarrhea
  - History of recent travel or inhabitant of high prevalence areas
  - Serologic tests positive in >90%

Amebic Abscess: Therapy
- Medical therapy
- Percutaneous biopsy of abscess wall
  - If serology does not confirm diagnosis and clinical suspicion is high
- Percutaneous drainage if
  - Large, >5 cm abscess
  - Left lobe
  - Biliary communication
  - Pregnancy
  - Perforation
  - Poor response to drug therapy

Echinococcus: *E. granulosus* and *E. multilocularis*
- Endemic worldwide
- Humans accidental host
- Infection usually acquired during childhood

E. granulosus [Figure 2-3-3]

E. multilocularis [Figure 2-3-4]

Echinococcus *E. granulosus* and *E. multilocularis*
- Symptoms occur during adulthood
  - Cyst enlargement
  - Erosion of cyst into peritoneal or pleural cavity
  - Development of biliary communication
- Serology confirms diagnosis
  - Positive >80% of cases

Echinococcus [Figure 2-3-5]

Echinococcus: *E. granulosus*

Echinococcus: *E. multilocularis*

E. granulosus: Imaging Features
- Unilocular or multilocular cyst
  - Calcification in cyst wall
  - Internal debris (hydatid sand)
- Complex cyst
  - Internal daughter cysts
  - Undulating membrane (water lily sign)

Figure 2-3-3

Worldwide distribution of E. granulosus

Figure 2-3-4

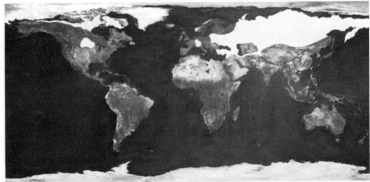

Worldwide distribution of E. multilocularis

Figure 2-3-5

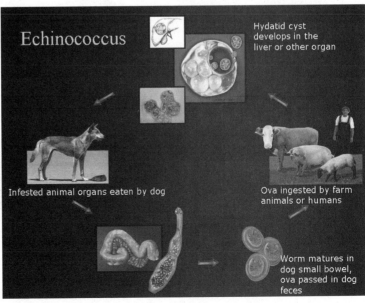

Echinococcus lifecycle

E. granulosus

E. granulosus:
Daughter cysts [Figure 2-3-6]

E. granulosus:
Water Lily Sign [Figures 2-3-7 and 2-3-8]

E. granulosus:
Complications and Treatment
- Cyst rupture
  - ➢ Anaphylaxis
  - ➢ Biliary tract, peritoneal cavity
  - ➢ Pleural, pericardial cavity
- Treatment
  - ➢ Surgical excision
  - ➢ Laparoscopic excision
  - ➢ Percutaneous drainage
    + sclerosing scolicidal agents

E. multilocularis:
Pathologic Features
- Alveolar hydatid disease
- Propagation by external budding
- Invade surrounding tissue
  - ➢ Infiltrative mass
  - ➢ No limiting host tissue
  - ➢ Resembles neoplasm

E. multilocularis:
Imaging Features
- Ultrasound
  - ➢ Echogenic
  - ➢ Single or multiple
  - ➢ Ill-defined walls
  - ➢ Partially calcified
- CT
  - ➢ Geographic
  - ➢ Infiltrating lesions
  - ➢ Amorphous calcification

E. multilocularis [Figure 2-3-9]

Schistosomasis
S. japonicum, S. mansoni, S. hematobium
- Bilharziasis
- Trematode (fluke)
- Humans are definitive host
- Mature in the portal venules
- Migrate to deposit eggs
  - ➢ Intestine (S. japonicum, S. mansoni)
  - ➢ Bladder (S. hematobium)

Figure 2-3-6

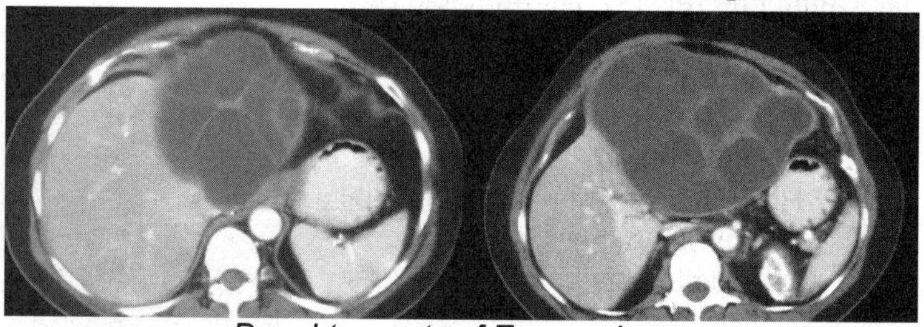

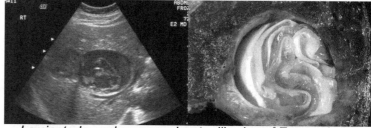

Daughter cysts of E. granulosus

Figure 2-3-7

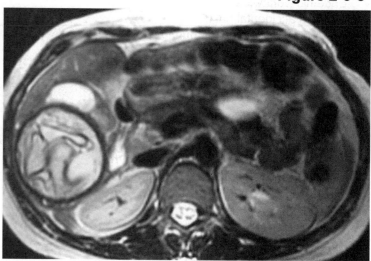

Laminated membranes and water lily sign of E. granulosus

Figure 2-3-8

Water lily sign of E. granulosus

Figure 2-3-9

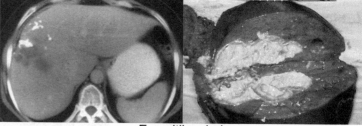

E. multilocularis

Schistosomasis: *S. japonicum*

Schistosomasis: *S. mansoni*

Schistosomasis: *S. hematobium*

Schistosomasis [Figure 2-3-10]

Schistosomasis [Figure 2-3-11]
- Granulomatous inflammation
- Fibrosis
  - ➢ Symmers' fibrosis
  - ➢ Turtle back liver
- Progressive portal vein occlusion
- Presinusoidal portal hypertension

Figure 2-3-10

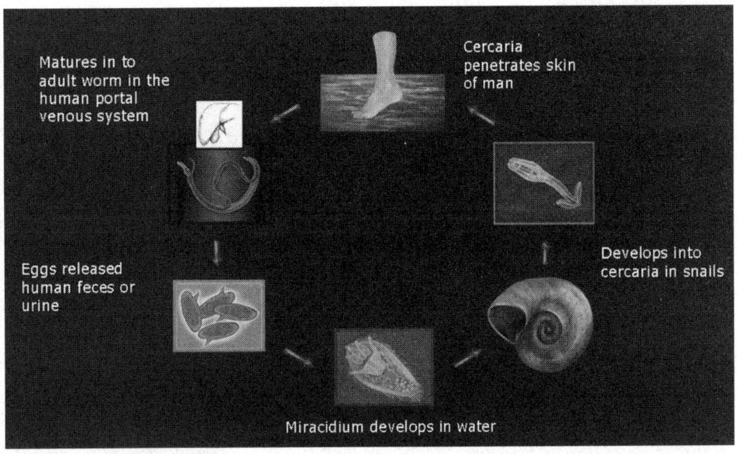

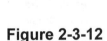

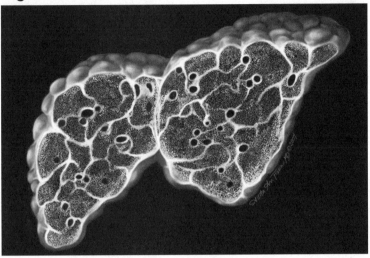

Lifecycle of Schistosomiasis

Figure 2-3-11

Symmers' fibrosis

Schistosomasis: Imaging Features
- *S. japonicum*
  - ➢ Hepatic calcification
  - ➢ "Turtle back" configuration
- *S. mansoni*
  - ➢ Low attenuation, rounded foci
  - ➢ Low attenuation, linear branching bands

Figure 2-3-12

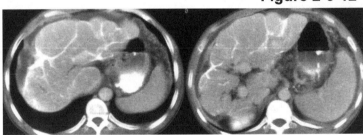

Schistosomiasis japonicum

Schistosomiasis japonicum
[Figure 2-3-12]

Biliary Parasites
- Parasites that invade bile ducts
  - ➢ Trematodes
    - ❖ Clonorchis sinensis
    - ❖ Fasciola gigantica, Fasciola hepatica
    - ❖ Opisthorchis viverrini
    - ❖ Opisthorchis felineus
  - ➢ Nematodes
    - ❖ Ascariasis lumbricoides
  - ➢ Cestodes
    - ❖ Taenia saginata

Clonorchis sinensis [Figures 2-3-13 and 2-3-14]

- Peripheral intrahepatic bile ducts
  - ➢ Dilatation of small intrahepatic ducts
  - ➢ Periductal fibrosis
- Complications
  - ➢ Cholangitis
  - ➢ Cholangiohepatitis
  - ➢ Liver abscess
  - ➢ Cholangiocarcinoma

Figure 2-3-13

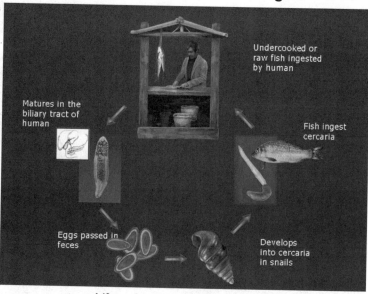

Lifecycle of Clonorchis sinensis

Figure 2-3-14

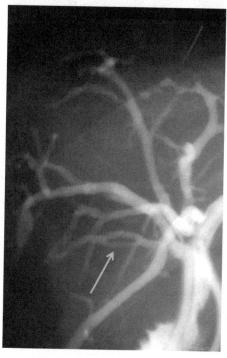

Cholangiogram shows a filling defect, peripheral intrahepatic strictures, and dilatation due to infestation of Clonorchis sinensis

Hepatic Infections in the Immunocompromised Host

- Candidiasis
- Pneumocystis Carinii
- Herpes Simplex Virus
- Liver Abscess
  - ➢ Pyogenic
  - ➢ Multiorganism

Disseminated Candidiasis

- Synonym: hepatosplenic candidiasis
- Pathogenesis
  - ➢ Prolonged neutropenia
  - ➢ Mucosal damage to the GI tract
  - ➢ Local invasion of candida with entry into the hepatosplenic circulation
- Clinical manifestations
  - ➢ Neutropenic with fever
  - ➢ Return of neutrophil count
- Organ Involvement
  - ➢ Spleen 94%, liver 75%, kidney 69%

Hepatosplenic Candidiasis: Pathology

- Necrosis with minimal inflammation
- Microabscesses with severe inflammation
- Collagen formation/fibrosis
- Granuloma formation

Hepatosplenic Candidiasis: Sonography [Figures 2-3-15]

- Type 1 lesion
  - ➢ "wheel-within-a-wheel"
- Type 2 lesion
  - ➢ "bull's-eye"
- Type 3 lesion-most common
  - ➢ hypoechoic nodule
- Type 4 lesion
  - ➢ hyperechoic nodule

Figure 2-3-15

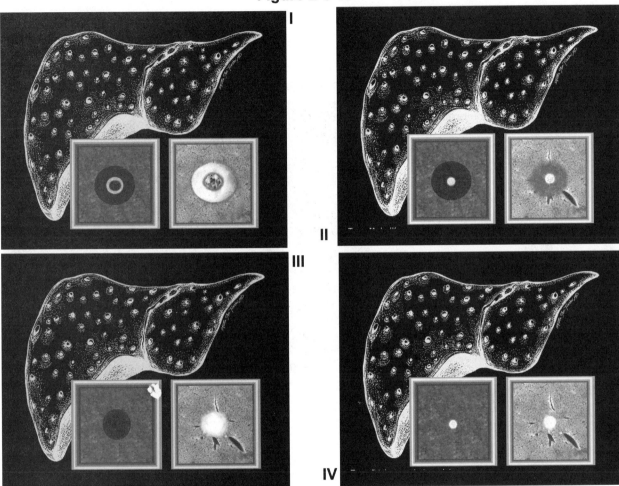

Hepatosplenic Candidiasis

[Figure 2-3-16]

- CT features
  - ➢ Concentric rings
  - ➢ Hypodense nodules
  - ➢ Punctate calcification

Hepatosplenic Candidiasis: MR Features

- Low T1, high T2
- Fat-suppressed T2 improves detection
- Gd-FLASH most sensitive
- Splenic gamna-gandy bodies false positive T1

Figure 2-3-16

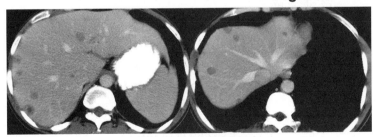

Hepatic candidiasis

Hepatosplenic Candidiasis: Imaging Management
- High index of suspicion
- Imaging during neutropenia is often negative
  - Follow up studies if clinical suspicion high and prophylactic therapy contraindicated
- Prophylactic therapy
- Biopsy
- Lesions change morphology with healing

Pneumocystis jiroveci
- Previously classified as Pneumocystis carinii
- Now considered a fungus
- Opportunistic infection
  - AIDS
  - Organ transplant recipients

Pneumocystis jiroveci (carinii): Imaging Features Figure 2-3-17]

Figure 2-3-17

- Sonography
  - Nonshadowing hyperechoic nodules
  - Shadowing echogenic clumps of calcification
- CT scan
  - Hypodense nodules with progressive calcification
  - Renal and lymph node calcification

Summary: Pyogenic Abscess
- Transition zone
- Cluster sign
- Percutaneous drainage

Summary: Amebic Abscess
- Cannot reliably distinguish from pyogenic abscess on imaging
- Percutaneous biopsy if necessary
- Viable organisms in wall
- Drainage if necessary

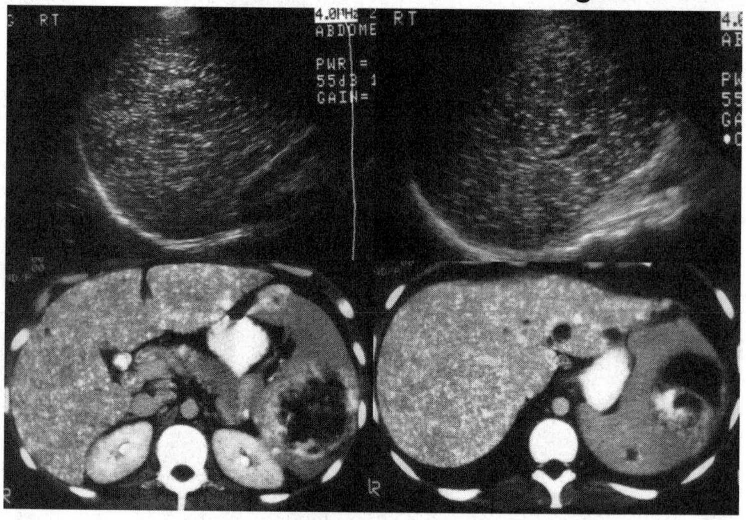

Sonogram and CT of disseminated pneumocystis

Summary Echinococcus
- E. granulosus
  - Daughter cysts
  - Water-lily sign
  - Calcification
- E. multilocularis
  - Infiltrating mass
  - Calcification

Summary: Immunocompromised Hosts
- Candidiasis
  - Neutropenics
  - Imaging negative during neutropenia
  - Imaging positive during WBC rebound

Summary: Immunocompromised Hosts
- Pneumocystis carinii
  - Hyperechoic nodules
  - +/- shadowing
  - Hypodense on CT with progressive calcification
  - Renal and lymph node calcification

Benign Biliary Disease

Angela D. Levy, LTC, MC, USA
Department of Radiologic Pathology
Armed Forces Institute of Pathology
Washington, DC

Objectives
- Congenital Disorders
  - Caroli disease
  - Choledochal cyst
  - Polycystic Liver Disease
- Inflammatory Disorders
  - Primary sclerosing cholangitis
  - AIDS-related cholangiopathy
  - Recurrent Pyogenic Cholangitis
  - Acute Pyogenic Cholangitis

Differential Diagnosis
- Obstructive biliary dilatation
- Caroli disease
- Choledochal cyst
- Polycystic liver disease
- Cholangitis
  - RPC, ascending

Obstructive Biliary Dilatation
- Tubular dilatation
- Diffuse dilatation proximal to the obstruction
- Abrupt termination at level of obstruction

Congenital Disorders
- Caroli disease
- Choledochal cyst
- Polycystic liver disease

Caroli Disease
- Autosomal recessive
- Secondary to ductal plate malformation (DPM)
- Associated with renal disorders
  - ARPCKD, ADPCKD
  - Medullary sponge kidney
  - Medullary cystic disease
- Complications
  - Recurrent biliary stones
  - Recurrent cholangitis
  - Liver failure
  - Increased incidence of carcinoma

41-year-old male with history of renal stones and diagnosis of medullary sponge kidney presents with abdominal pain, sepsis, elevated LFTs *[Figure 2-4-1]*

Figure 2-4-1

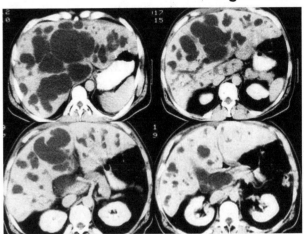

Saccular and fusiform biliary dilatation in Caroli disease

Ductal Plate - Embryologic precursor of intrahepatic bile ducts

Ductal Plate Malformation
- Abnormal development of intrahepatic bile ducts
- Lack of ductal plate remodeling
  - Persistence of embryonic structures (DPM)
  - Segmental dilatation
  - Destructive inflammation/fibrosis
- Spectrum of diseases
  - Small interlobular ducts: Congenital hepatic fibrosis (CHF)
  - Large intrahepatic ducts: Caroli disease
  - All ducts: Caroli syndrome (CHF and Caroli disease)

Intrahepatic Duct Embryology: Ductal Plate

[Figures 2-4-2 and 2-4-3]

Figure 2-4-2

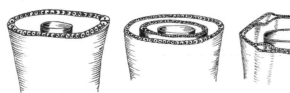

Normal ductal plate development of the intrahepatic bile ducts

Caroli Disease: Clinical Features

- Presentation at any age (mean age 37 years)
- Pain, fever, jaundice
- Recurrent bouts of cholangitis/stone formation
- Liver failure

Caroli Disease: Radiologic Features

- Intrahepatic duct dilatation
  - Segmental (83%)
  - Diffuse (17%)
  - Saccular (76%) or fusiform (24%)
- Extrahepatic dilatation (53%)
- "Central-dot" sign
- Strictures
- Complications
  - Stones
  - Abscess
  - Malignancy (7%)

Caroli Disease: "Central Dot Sign" *[Figure 2-4-4]*

Caroli Syndrome Cirrhosis, Portal Hypertension

Caroli Disease Cholangiography
[Figure 2-54]

Caroli Disease

Caroli Disease with Hepatic Abscess

Caroli Disease with Intrahepatic Lithiasis

Caroli Disease with Intraductal Adenocarcinoma

Caroli Disease Complicating Adenocarcinoma

- Enhancing intraductal masses
- Focal strictures
  - Irregular margins
  - Shoulders
  - Irregular tapering
- Infiltrating masses

Figure 2-4-3

NORMAL PORTAL TRACT

DUCTAL PLATE MALFORMATION

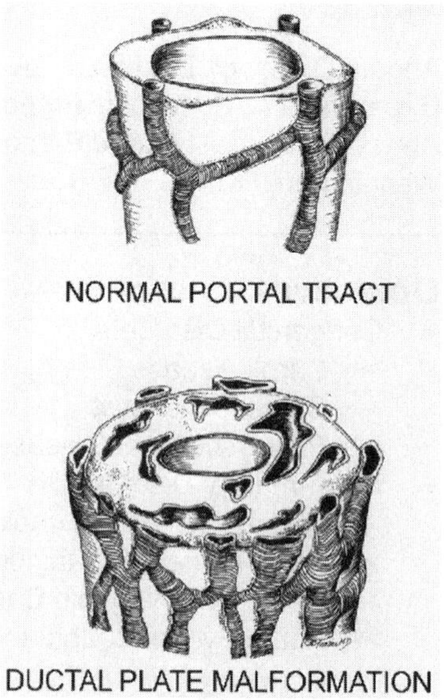

Normal ductal plate remodeling results in intercommunicating intrahepatic bile ducts surrounding a normal portal tract. Ductal plate malformation results in biliary duct ectasia and fibrosis surrounding the portal tract

Figure 2-4-4

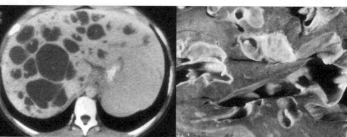

Caroli disease showing saccular biliary dilatation and the central dot sign

Figure 2-4-5

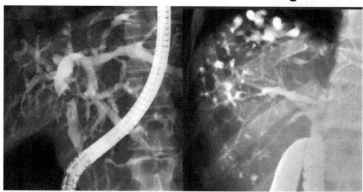

Caroli disease in two different patients showing diffuse fusiform and saccular dilatation

Choledochal Cyst

- Congenital dilatation of the bile ducts
- Association with anomalous pancreatico-biliary junction (APBJ)
  - Reflux of pancreatic enzymes into bile duct
- Todani Classification

Choledochal Cyst: Todani Classification [Figure 2-4-6]

Figure 2-4-6

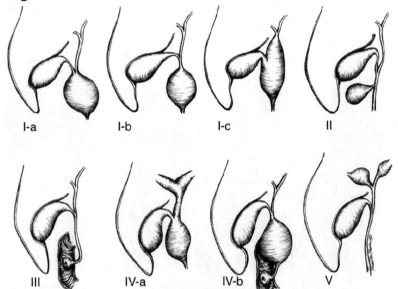

I-a   I-b   I-c   II

III   IV-a   IV-b   V

Todani classification of choledochal cysts

Choledochal Cyst: Etiology [Figures 2-56 and 2-57]

- Normal Pancreaticobiliary Junction
  - Sphincter complex encircles distal CBD and PD
  - 80% to 90% have a common channel (4-5 mm
- Anomalous Junction (APBJ)
  - Union of CBD and PD outside of duodenum and sphincter complex
  - Reflux of pancreatic enzymes into CBD)

Figure 2-4-7

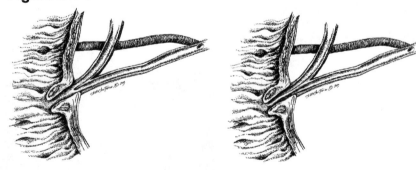

Normal pancreaticobiliary junction showing union of the ducts in the sphincter complex, which is located in the duodenal wall. There may be a common channel (ampulla) or not

Figure 2-4-8

Choledochal Cyst: Clinical Features

- Presentation at any age (mean, 17 years)
- F > M
- Pain, jaundice, palpable mass
- Complications
  - Stones
  - Cholangitis
  - Malignancy

Anomalous pancreaticobiliary junction showing union of the common bile duct and pancreatic duct proximal to the duodenal wall and sphincter complex

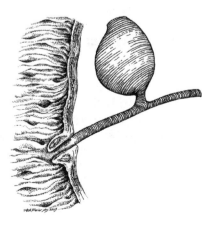

Choledochal Cyst: Pathologic Features
- Extrahepatic duct dilatation
- Mural thickening
- Normal epithelium

Todani Type I

Todani Type II: Diverticulum

Todani Type III: Choledochocele

Tubulovillous Adenoma

Todani Type IV [Figure 2-4-9]

Todani Type V: Caroli Disease

Choledochal Cyst vs. Caroli Disease
- Choledochal cyst
  - ➢ Congenital, not inherited
  - ➢ Extrahepatic bile duct dilatation with varying degrees of proximal dilatation
  - ➢ Surgical therapy with biliary reconstruction
- Caroli disease
  - ➢ Congenital, inherited
  - ➢ Intrahepatic +/- extrahepatic dilatation
  - ➢ Liver biopsy shows DPM
  - ➢ Medical therapy (surgery for complications)

Polycystic Liver Disease
- ADPCKD or isolated
- Bile duct cysts
  - ➢ Secondary to von Meyenberg complexes
  - ➢ Von Meyenberg complex is DPM at the lowest level

Polycystic Liver Disease: Radiologic Features
- Multiple liver cysts
- May have internal hemorrhage
- Rim-like calcification
- Normal bile ducts
- Associated feature of ADPCKD
  - ➢ Renal cysts
  - ➢ Pancreatic cysts
  - ➢ Thyroid cysts
  - ➢ Seminal vesicle cysts in males

Polycystic Liver Disease

Polycystic Liver Disease in ADPCKD [Figure 2-4-10]

41-year-old male with history of renal stones and diagnosis of medullary sponge kidney presents with abdominal pain, sepsis, elevated LFT's

Figure 2-4-9

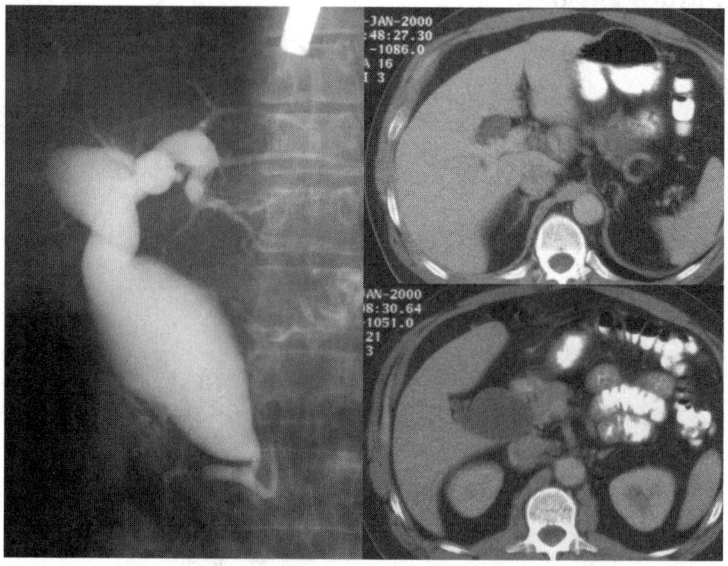

Todani Type IV choledochal cyst showing central intrahepatic and extrahepatic duct dilatation on CT. The cholangiogram shows an anomalous pancreaticobiliary junction as well as the extent of duct dilatation

Figure 2-4-10

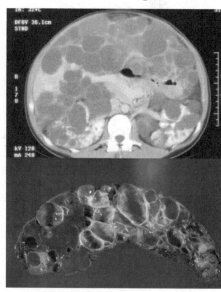

Polycystic liver disease occurring in ADPCKD

Differential Diagnosis
- Obstructive biliary dilatation
- Caroli disease
- Choledochal cyst
- Polycystic liver disease
- Cholangitis
  - RPC, Pyogenic

Caroli Disease

Summary: Congenital Disorders
- Exclude obstructive dilatation
- Congenital disorders
  - Caroli disease
    - ❖ Intrahepatic
  - Choledochal cyst
    - ❖ Extrahepatic
  - Polycystic liver disease
    - ❖ Noncommunicating cysts

40-year-old woman with elevated LFT's
[Figure 2-4-11]

Differential Diagnosis
- Cholangitis
  - Primary sclerosing
  - AIDS-related
  - Recurrent pyogenic
  - Acute pyogenic cholangitis
- Neoplasm

Inflammatory Disorders
- Primary sclerosing cholangitis
- AIDS-related cholangiopathy
- Recurrent pyogenic cholangitis
- Acute cholangitis

Primary Sclerosing Cholangitis [Figure 2-4-12]
- Cholestatic liver disease
- Unknown etiology
- Fibrosing inflammation
- Diagnosis
  - Liver biopsy
  - Cholangiogram

PSC: Imaging
- Thickened duct wall
  - Asymmetric or circumferential
  - 2 to 5 mm
- Hepatic parenchymal changes
  - Cirrhosis
  - Periportal fibrosis
  - Discontinuous duct dilatation
  - Portal hypertension
- Hepatic parenchymal changes
  - Cirrhosis
  - Periportal fibrosis
  - Discontinuous duct dilatation
  - Portal hypertension

Figure 2-4-11

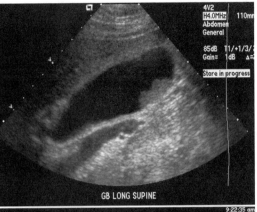
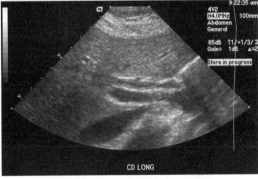

Primary sclerosing cholangitis

Figure 2-4-12

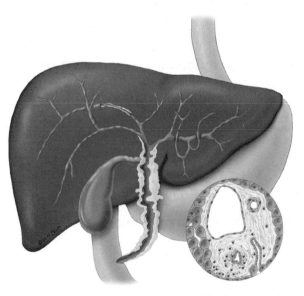

Illustration showing disease distribution, mural thickening, and inflammatory changes of primary sclerosing cholangitis

- Other features
  - Gallbladder disease (40%)
  - Ductal stones (8%)
  - Adenopathy
  - Neoplasm

PSC: Sonographic Features

PSC: CT Features [Figure 2-4-13]

PSC: Cholangiography [Figure 2-4-14]
- Beading
- Pruned-tree
- Mural irregularity
- Diverticula

PSC: Cholangiocarcinoma
- Stricture (90%)
  - Long strictures (>1cm)
  - Completely obstructing strictures
  - Associated mass
- Multicentric (10%)
- Polypoid mass

AIDS Cholangiopathy [Figure 2-4-15]
- Group of disorders
  - Sclerosing cholangitis
  - Papillary stenosis
  - Acalculous cholecystitis
- Opportunistic infection
  - Cryptosporidium
  - Cytomegalovirus
- Declining incidence
  - HAART therapy

AIDS Cholangiopathy
- Cholangiographic features
  - Beading
  - Pruning
  - Mural irregularity
  - Filling defects (granulation tissue)
  - Papillary stenosis (papillitis)
  - No EHD stenosis or diverticula

AIDS Cholangiopathy
- Sonographic features
  - Gallbladder wall thickening
    - ❖ Acalculous cholecystitis
  - Bile duct wall thickening
  - Hyperechoic nodule in distal CBD (papillitis)

AIDS Cholangiopathy: Acalculous cholecystitis

Recurrent Pyogenic Cholangitis (RPC)
- Clinical syndrome
  - Pigmented stones
  - Recurrent infection
- Unknown etiology
  - Biliary parasites
- Complications
  - Biliary cirrhosis
  - Cholangiocarcinoma

Figure 2-4-13

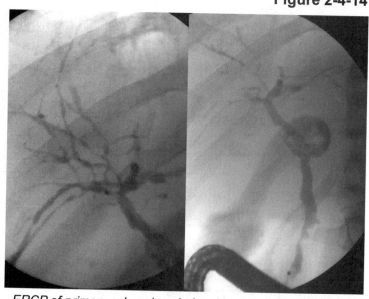

CT of primary sclerosing cholangitis showing discontinuous bile duct dilatation, mural thickening of the common hepatic duct, and hepatoduodenal ligament adenopathy

Figure 2-4-14

ERCP of primary sclerosing cholangitis showing beading and pruning of the intrahepatic bile ducts. The extrahepatic bile duct shows mural irregularity with focal stricture formation

Figure 2-4-15

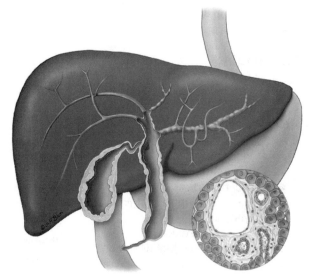

Illustration of AIDS cholangiopathy showing disease distribution

RPC: Imaging [Figure 2-4-16]
- Stones, sludge
- Duct dilatation
- Left lobe predominant
- Parenchymal changes
  - ➤ Atrophy
  - ➤ Fatty change
  - ➤ Altered enhancement
  - ➤ Abscess

Figure 2-4-16

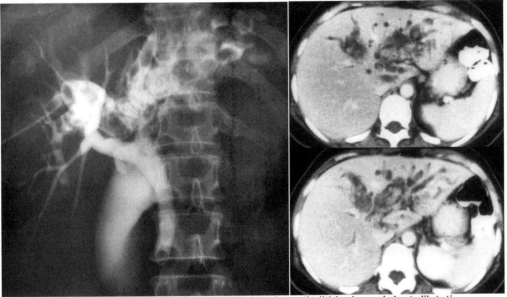

Recurrent pyogenic cholangitis with intrahepatic lithiasis and duct dilatation

Acute Pyogenic Cholangitis
- Almost always post-obstructive
- Polymicrobial
- Etiology
  - ➤ Stones
  - ➤ Anastomotic stricture
  - ➤ Papillary stenosis
  - ➤ carcinoma
  - ➤ Underlying biliary disease

Acute Pyogenic Cholangitis
- Imaging Features
  - ➤ Duct dilatation
  - ➤ Obstructive lesion
  - ➤ Echogenic bile
  - ➤ Mural irregularity
  - ➤ Hepatic abscess

Acute Pyogenic Cholangitis with Microabscesses

40-year-old woman with elevated LFT's

Differential Diagnosis
- Cholangitis
  - ➤ Primary sclerosing
  - ➤ AIDS-related
  - ➤ Recurrent pyogenic
  - ➤ Acute pyogenic cholangitis
- Neoplasm

Primary Sclerosing Cholangitis

Summary
- PSC
  - ➢ Fibrosis
- AIDS cholangiopathy
  - ➢ Papillary stenosis
  - ➢ Acalculous cholecystitis
- RPC
  - ➢ Stones
  - ➢ Focal dilatation
- Pyogenic cholangitis
  - ➢ Obstruction

Benign Biliary Disease References

Caroli Disease
Choi BI, Yeon KM, Kim SH, et al: Caroli disease: central dot sign in CT. Radiology 174:161, 1990

Desmet VJ: Ludwig symposium on biliary disorders—part I. Pathogenesis of ductal plate abnormalities. Mayo Clinic Proceedings 73:80, 1998

Krause D, Cercueil JP, Dranssart M, et al: MRI for evaluating congenital bile duct abnormalities. J Comput Assist Tomogr 26:541, 2002

Levy AD, Rohrmann CA, Jr., Murakata LA, et al: Caroli's disease: radiologic spectrum with pathologic correlation. AJR 179:1053, 2002

Marchal GJ, Desmet VJ, Proesmans WC, et al: Caroli disease: high-frequency US and pathologic findings. Radiology 158:507, 1986

Miller WJ, Sechtin AG, Campbell WL, et al: Imaging findings in Caroli's disease. AJR 165:333, 1995

Pavone P, Laghi A, Catalano C, et al: Caroli's disease: evaluation with MR cholangiopancreatography (MRCP). Abdom Imaging 21:117, 1996

Pavone P, Laghi A, Catalano C, et al: Caroli's disease: evaluation with MR cholangiography. AJR 166:216, 1996

Choledochal Cyst
Alexander MC, Haaga JR: MR imaging of a choledochal cyst. J Comput Assist Tomogr 9:357, 1985

Babbitt DP, Starshak RJ, Clemett AR: Choledochal cyst: a concept of etiology. AJR 119:57, 1973

De Vries JS, De Vries S, Aronson DC, et al: Choledochal cysts: Age of presentation, symptoms, and late complications related to Todani's classification. J Pediatr Surg 37:1568, 2002

Govil S, Justus A, Korah I, et al: Choledochal cysts: evaluation with MR cholangiography. Abdom Imaging 23:616, 1998

Lam WW, Lam TP, Saing H, et al: MR cholangiography and CT cholangiography of pediatric patients with choledochal cysts. AJR 173:401, 1999

Liu CL, Fan ST, Lo CM, et al: Choledochal cysts in adults. Arch Surg 137:465, 2002

Miyano T, Yamataka A: Choledochal cysts. Curr Opin Pediatr 9:283, 1997

O'Neill JA, Jr.: Choledochal cyst. Curr Probl Surg 29:361, 1992

Savader SJ, Benenati JF, Venbrux AC, et al: Choledochal cysts: classification and cholangiographic appearance. AJR 156:327, 1991

Savader SJ, Venbrux AC, Benenati JF, et al: Choledochal cysts: role of noninvasive imaging, percutaneous transhepatic cholangiography, and percutaneous biliary drainage in diagnosis and treatment. J Vasc Interv Radiol 2:379, 1991

Todani T, Watanabe Y, Fujii T, et al: Anomalous arrangement of the pancreatobiliary ductal system in patients with a choledochal cyst. Am J Surg 147:672, 1984

Todani T, Watanabe Y, Narusue M, et al: Congenital bile duct cysts: Classification, operative procedures, and review of thirty-seven cases including cancer arising from choledochal cyst. Am J Surg 134:263, 1977

Todani T, Watanabe Y, Toki A, et al: Co-existing biliary anomalies and anatomical variants in choledochal cyst. Br J Surg 85:760, 1998

Wearn FG, Wiot JF: Choledochocele: not a form of choledochal cyst. J Can Assoc Radiol 33:110, 1982

Polycystic Liver Disease

Dranssart M, Cognet F, Mousson C, et al: MR cholangiography in the evaluation of hepatic and biliary abnormalities in autosomal dominant polycystic kidney disease: study of 93 patients. J Comput Assist Tomogr 26:237, 2002

Grunfeld JP, Albouze G, Jungers P, et al: Liver changes and complications in adult polycystic kidney disease. Adv Nephrol Necker Hosp 14:1, 1985

Gupta S, Seith A, Dhiman RK, et al: CT of liver cysts in patients with autosomal dominant polycystic kidney disease. Acta Radiol 40:444, 1999

Itai Y, Ebihara R, Eguchi N, et al: Hepatobiliary cysts in patients with autosomal dominant polycystic kidney disease: prevalence and CT findings. AJR 164:339, 1995

Pirson Y, Lannoy N, Peters D, et al: Isolated polycystic liver disease as a distinct genetic disease, unlinked to polycystic kidney disease 1 and polycystic kidney disease 2. Hepatology 23:249, 1996

Segal AJ, Spataro RF: Computed tomography of adult polycystic disease. J Comput Assist Tomogr 6:777, 1982

Primary Sclerosing Cholangitis

Ament AE, Haaga JR, Wiedenmann SD, et al: Primary sclerosing cholangitis: CT findings. J Comput Assist Tomogr 7:795, 1983

Brandt DJ, MacCarty RL, Charboneau JW, et al: Gallbladder disease in patients with primary sclerosing cholangitis. AJR Am J Roentgenol 150:571, 1988

Campbell WL, Ferris JV, Holbert BL, et al: Biliary tract carcinoma complicating primary sclerosing cholangitis: evaluation with CT, cholangiography, US, and MR imaging. Radiology 207:41, 1998

Campbell WL, Peterson MS, Federle MP, et al: Using CT and cholangiography to diagnose biliary tract carcinoma complicating primary sclerosing cholangitis. AJR Am J Roentgenol 177:1095, 2001

Dodd GD, 3rd, Baron RL, Oliver JH, 3rd, et al: End-stage primary sclerosing cholangitis: CT findings of hepatic morphology in 36 patients. Radiology 211:357, 1999

Fulcher AS, Turner MA, Franklin KJ, et al: Primary sclerosing cholangitis: evaluation with MR cholangiography-a case-control study. Radiology 215:71, 2000

Gulliver DJ, Baker ME, Putnam W, et al: Bile duct diverticula and webs: nonspecific cholangiographic features of primary sclerosing cholangitis. AJR Am J Roentgenol 157:281, 1991

Ito K, Mitchell DG, Outwater EK, et al: Primary sclerosing cholangitis: MR imaging features. AJR Am J Roentgenol 172:1527, 1999

Lumsden AB, Alspaugh JP: Cholangiocarcinoma complicating primary sclerosing cholangitis: cholangiographic appearances. Radiology 158:856, 1986

MacCarty RL, LaRusso NF, Wiesner RH, et al: Primary sclerosing cholangitis: findings on cholangiography and pancreatography. Radiology 149:39, 1983

Majoie CB, Smits NJ, Phoa SS, et al: Primary sclerosing cholangitis: sonographic findings. Abdom Imaging 20:109, 1995

May GR, Bender CE, LaRusso NF, et al: Nonoperative dilatation of dominant strictures in primary sclerosing cholangitis. AJR Am J Roentgenol 145:1061, 1985

Olsson R, Danielsson A, Jarnerot G, et al: Prevalence of primary sclerosing cholangitis in patients with ulcerative colitis. Gastroenterology 100:1319, 1991

Teefey SA, Baron RL, Rohrmann CA, et al: Sclerosing cholangitis: CT findings. Radiology 169:635, 1988

Teefey SA, Baron RL, Schulte SJ, et al: Patterns of intrahepatic bile duct dilatation at CT: correlation with obstructive disease processes. Radiology 182:139, 1992

Williams SM, Harned RK: Hepatobiliary complications of inflammatory bowel disease. Radiol Clin North Am 25:175, 1987

AIDS Cholangiopathy

Collins CD, Forbes A, Harcourt-Webster JN, et al: Radiological and pathological features of AIDS-related polypoid cholangitis. Clin Radiol 48:307, 1993

Da Silva F, Boudghene F, Lecomte I, et al: Sonography in AIDS-related cholangitis: prevalence and cause of an echogenic nodule in the distal end of the common bile duct. AJR Am J Roentgenol 160:1205, 1993

Dolmatch BL, Laing FC, Ferderle MP, et al: AIDS-related cholangitis: radiographic findings in nine patients. Radiology 163:313, 1987

Farman J, Brunetti J, Baer JW, et al: AIDS-related cholangiopancreatographic changes. Abdom Imaging 19:417, 1994

Forbes A, Blanshard C, Gazzard B: Natural history of AIDS related sclerosing cholangitis: a study of 20 cases. Gut 34:116, 1993

Keaveny AP, Karasik MS: Hepatobiliary and pancreatic infections in AIDS: Part II. AIDS Patient Care STDS 12:451, 1998

Sherlock S: Pathogenesis of sclerosing cholangitis: the role of nonimmune factors. Semin Liver Dis 11:5, 1991

Teixidor HS, Godwin TA, Ramirez EA: Cryptosporidiosis of the biliary tract in AIDS. Radiology 180:51, 1991

Recurrent Pyogenic Cholangitis

Chan FL, Man SW, Leong LL, et al: Evaluation of recurrent pyogenic cholangitis with CT: analysis of 50 patients. Radiology 170:165, 1989

Chau EM, Leong LL, Chan FL: Recurrent pyogenic cholangitis: ultrasound evaluation compared with endoscopic retrograde cholangiopancreatography. Clin Radiol 38:79, 1987

Fan ST, Choi TK, Wong J: Recurrent pyogenic cholangitis: current management. World J Surg 15:248, 1991

Federle MP, Cello JP, Laing FC, et al: Recurrent pyogenic cholangitis in Asian immigrants. Use of ultrasonography, computed tomography, and cholangiography. Radiology 143:151, 1982

Kim MJ, Cha SW, Mitchell DG, et al: MR imaging findings in recurrent pyogenic cholangitis. AJR Am J Roentgenol 173:1545, 1999

Lim JH: Radiologic findings of clonorchiasis. AJR Am J Roentgenol 155:1001, 1990

Okuno WT, Whitman GJ, Chew FS: Recurrent pyogenic cholangiohepatitis. AJR Am J Roentgenol 167:484, 1996

Park MS, Yu JS, Kim KW, et al: Recurrent pyogenic cholangitis: comparison between MR cholangiography and direct cholangiography. Radiology 220:677, 2001

Gallbladder and Biliary Neoplasms

Angela D. Levy, LTC, MC, USA
Department of Radiologic Pathology
Armed Forces Institute of Pathology
Washington

Objectives
- Gallbladder adenocarcinoma
  - ➢ Benign disease mimicking carcinoma
    - ❖ Cholesterol polyp
    - ❖ Gallbladder adenoma
    - ❖ Adenomyomatous Hyperplasia
    - ❖ Xanthogranulomatous cholecystitis
- Biliary Adenocarcinoma
  - ➢ Benign disease mimicking carcinoma
    - ❖ Post-inflammatory strictures
    - ❖ Inflammatory cholangitis
    - ❖ Benign bile duct tumors

83-year-old woman with 5 week history of RUQ pain and 10-pound weight loss

Gallbladder Adenocarcinoma

Gallbladder Carcinoma
- Sixth most common GI tract malignancy
  - ➢ Worldwide: stomach, colorectal, liver, esophagus, pancreas, gallbladder
  - ➢ US: colorectal, pancreas, stomach, liver, esophagus, gallbladder
- More common in women (3:1), mean age 72 years

Gallbladder Carcinoma
- Etiology
  - ➢ Chronic inflammation
- Associations
  - ➢ Cholelithiasis (74% – 92%)
  - ➢ Low insertion of the cystic duct
  - ➢ Anomalous pancreaticobiliary junction (APBJ)
  - ➢ Choledochal cyst
  - ➢ Primary sclerosing cholangitis

Gallbladder Carcinoma: Anatomic Factors
- Gallbladder lacks a continuous muscular layer
  - ➢ No proper muscularis mucosa
  - ➢ No true submucosa
  - ➢ No muscularis propria
- Hepatic surface lacks serosa

Gallbladder Carcinoma: Pathology
- Epithelial malignancies (98%)
  - ➢ Adenocarcinoma (90%)
  - ➢ Squamous cell
  - ➢ Adenosquamous
  - ➢ Small cell carcinoma
- Other (2%)
  - ➢ Sarcomas
  - ➢ Lymphomas
  - ➢ Carcinoid
  - ➢ Metastases
    - ❖ Bronchogenic carcinoma, renal cell, melanoma

Gallbladder Carcinoma

- Gross Pathology
  - ➢ Diffusely infiltrating (68%)
  - ➢ Polypoid (32%)
- Radiology
  - ➢ Intraluminal polypoid mass (15% to 25%)
  - ➢ Focal or diffuse wall thickening (20% to 30%)
  - ➢ Mass replacing the gallbladder (40% to 65%)

Adenocarcinoma Diffuse Wall Thickening [Figure 2-5-1]

Figure 2-5-1

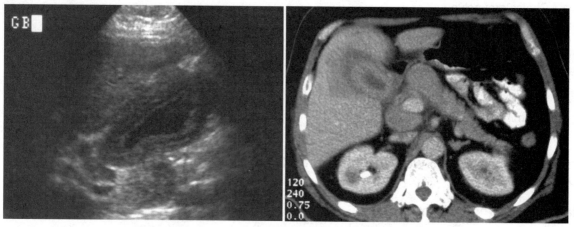

Gallbladder adenocarcinoma manifesting as diffuse wall thickening

Papillary Adenocarcinoma: Polypoid Mass [Figure 2-5-2]

Figure 2-5-2

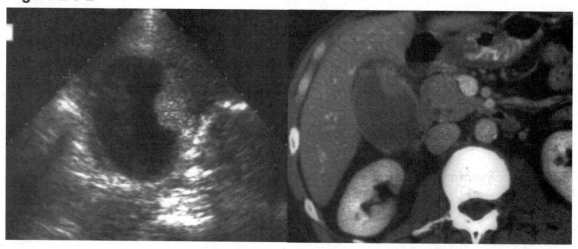

Gallbladder adenocarcinoma manifesting as a focal polypoid mass

Papillary Adenocarcinoma

Adenocarcinoma:
Mass Replacing the Gallbladder Fossa [Figure 2-5-3]

Figure 2-5-3

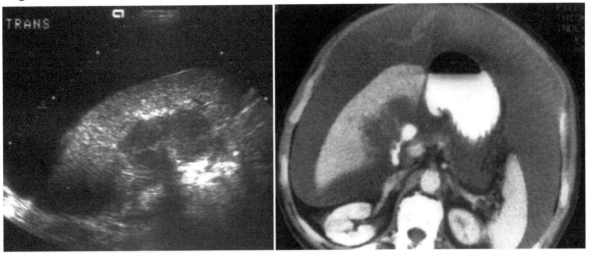

Gallbladder adenocarcinoma as a mass replacing the gallbladder

Gallbladder Adenocarcinoma: Direct Extension to Liver

Gallbladder Adenocarcinoma: Direct Extension to Transverse Colon

Gallbladder Adenocarcinoma: Direct Extension to Hepatoduodenal Ligament [Figure 2-5-4]

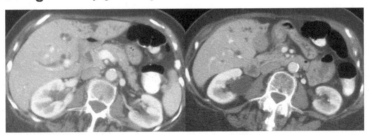

Figure 2-5-4

CT showing gallbladder carcinoma extension to the hepatoduodenal ligament

Gallbladder Adenocarcinoma: Role of MR [Figures 2-5-5]
Figure 2-5-5

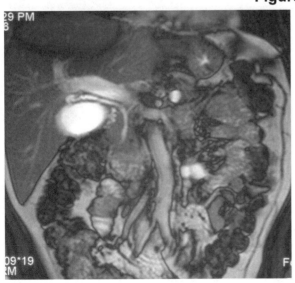
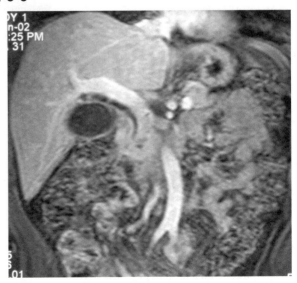

MR showing gallbladder carcinoma extension to the hepatoduodenal ligament

Gallbladder Carcinoma: Differential Diagnosis
- Gallbladder Wall Thickening
  - Cardiac, liver, renal failure
  - Hepatitis
  - Hypoalbuminemia
  - Cholecystitis
  - Xanthogranulomatous cholecystitis
  - Adenomyomatous hyperplasia
- Gallbladder polyp
  - Cholesterol polyp
  - Gallbladder adenoma
  - Adenomyomatous hyperplasia (adenomyomatosis)
  - Carcinoid
  - Metastatic disease
- Mass Replacing the gallbladder
  - Hepatocellular carcinoma
  - Cholangiocarcinoma
  - Metastatic disease

Benign Disease Mimicking Carcinoma
- Gallbladder polyps
  - Cholesterol polyp
  - Gallbladder adenoma
- Gallbladder Wall Thickening
  - Xanthogranulomatous cholecystitis
  - Adenomyomatous hyperplasia

Cholesterol Polyp [Figure 2-5-6]
- 50% of polypoid lesions in the gallbladder
- More common in women, 3:1
- Histology
  - Lipid-laden macrophages
  - Normal gallbladder epithelium
- Ultrasound
  - Small echogenic nodules
  - Hypoechoic nodules with multiple internal echogenic foci
  - Usually <10 mm

Gallbladder Adenoma
- Uncommon tumors
- Increase incidence
  - FAP
  - Peutz-Jeghers
- Histology
  - Tubular, papillary, or tubulopapillary
- Ultrasound
  - Echogenic intraluminal masses
  - Gallstones

Figure 2-5-6

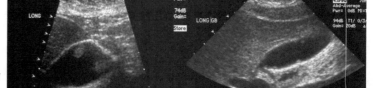

Cholesterol polyp

Management of Gallbladder Polyps
- Size < 5 mm
  - Do nothing
- Size 5 to 10 mm
  - Follow
- Size >10 mm
  - Remove
- Features suggesting malignancy
  - Adjacent gallbladder wall thickening
  - Abnormal gallbladder/liver interface
  - Abnormal liver parenchyma
  - Hepatoduodenal ligament adenopathy

Adenomyomatous Hyperplasia
- Common
  - 9% of cholecystectomy specimens
- Other nomenclature
  - Adenomyomatosis
  - Adenomyoma
- More common in women
- 90% have gallstones
- Three types
  - Segmental
  - Diffuse
  - Localized (fundal)

Adenomyomatous Hyperplasia: Imaging
- Sonography
  - "Comet-tail" reverberation artifact
  - Wall thickening
  - Narrowed gallbladder lumen
  - Fundal mass
- MR/MRCP
  - Visualization of Rokitansky-Aschoff sinuses
  - "Pearl necklace sign"

Figure 2-5-7

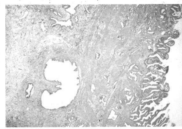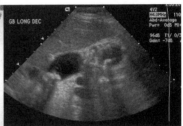

Adenomyomatous hyperplasia

Adenomyomatous Hyperplasia

Segmental Adenomyomatous Hyperplasia [Figure 2-5-7]

Adenomyomatous Hyperplasia "Pearl Necklace Sign"

Diffuse Adenomyomatous Hyperplasia

Fundal Adenomyomatous Hyperplasia "Adenomyoma"

Xanthogranulomatous Cholecystitis
- Aggressive inflammatory process
- Etiology
  - Intermittent cystic duct obstruction
  - Bile enters gallbladder wall
- Association with gallbladder carcinoma
- Clinical presentation
  - RUQ pain, fever, tenderness

Xanthogranulomatous Cholecystitis: Pathology
- Histology
  - Foamy histiocytes
  - Inflammatory cells
- Gross pathology
  - Infiltrative mass
  - Extension to adjacent liver and soft tissues

Xanthogranulomatous Cholecystitis: Imaging

Figure 2-5-8

[Figure 2-5-8]
- Wall thickening
- Mural nodules or bands
  - Hypoechoic on sonography
  - Low-attenuation on CT
- Stones
- Pericholecystic fluid
- Adjacent organ involvement
- Lymphadenopathy

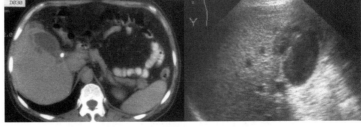

Xanthogranulomatous cholecystitis

Adenocarcinoma of the Bile Ducts [Figure 2-5-9]

- Extrahepatic bile duct
  - EHBD
- Hilar
  - Klatskin tumor
- Peripheral
  - Intrahepatic cholangiocarcinoma
- Hepatic duct
  - Intraductal

Figure 2-5-9

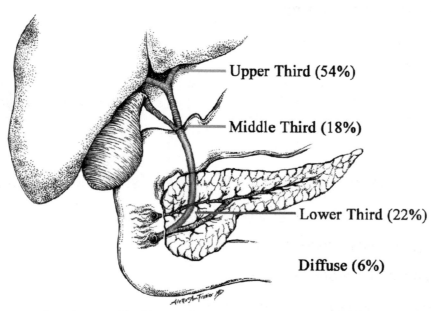

Locations and incidence of extrahepatic duct adenocarcinoma

EHBD Adenocarcinoma

- One-half as common as gallbladder carcinoma
- More common in men
  - Mean age 68 years
- Risk factors
  - Inflammatory bowel disease
  - Primary sclerosing cholangitis
  - Choledochal cyst
  - Anomalous pancreaticobiliary junction
  - Familial polyposis
  - Neurofibromatosis
  - Clonorchis sinensis

EHBD Adenocarcinoma: Clinical Features

- Presentation
  - Jaundice from obstruction
  - Pain
  - Fever if secondary cholangitis
- Early
  - Hepatomegaly
- Late
  - Secondary biliary cirrhosis

EHBD Adenocarcinoma

- Histology
  - ➢ Adenocarcinomas
- Gross Pathology [Figure 2-5-10]
  - ➢ Diffusely infiltrating [A]
  - ➢ Polypoid [B]
  - ➢ Nodular [C]
  - ➢ Constricting (scirrhous) [D]

Figure 2-5-10   *Morphology of extrahepatic duct adenocarcinoma*

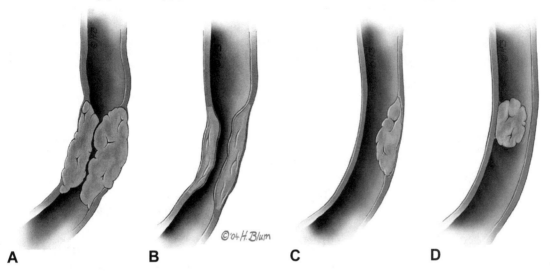

A   B   C   D

EHBD Adenocarcinoma: Imaging

- Obstruction
- Tumor
  - ➢ Intraluminal mass
  - ➢ Stenosis
  - ➢ Complete obstruction

EHBD Adenocarcinoma vs. Benign Stricture Cholangiography vs. CT

Figure 2-5-11

- Malignant
  - ➢ Duct abruptly terminates at stricture
- Benign
  - ➢ Duct tapers to stricture
- Extrinsic mass
  - ➢ Duct is displaced

Baron, RL. Radiol Clin N Am 1991. 29:1237.

Malignant Stricture [Figure 2-5-11]

EHBD Adenocarcinoma

Benign Stricture
[Figure 2-5-12 / next page]

Pancreatitis with Stricture

Extrinsic Compression

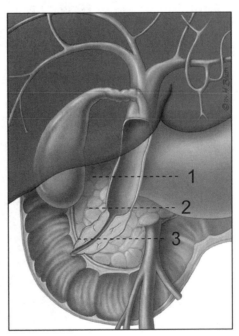

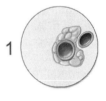

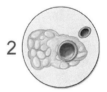

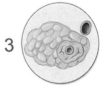

Cholangiographic and CT features of a malignant stricture

Figure 2-5-12

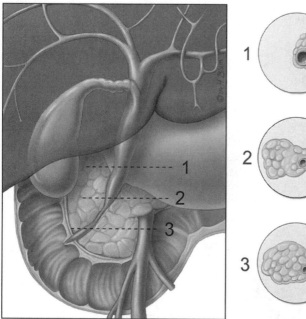

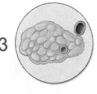

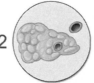

Cholangiographic and CT features of a benign stricture

Hilar Cholangiocarcinoma: Klatskin Tumor

- Aggressive histology
  - ➢ Adenocarcinoma
  - ➢ Pathologically identical to metastatic adenocarcinoma
- Risk factors
  - ➢ Inflammatory bowel disease, primary sclerosing cholangitis, biliary parasites, Thorotrast exposure
- Clinical presentation
  - ➢ Jaundice, pain

Hilar Cholangiocarcinoma: Sonography

- Duct dilatation
  - ➢ Discontinuous dilatation
- Ill-defined mass
- Lobar atrophy
- May have portal vein thrombus

Hilar Cholangiocarcinoma: Computed Tomography [Figure 2-5-13]

- Dilated ducts
  - ➢ Discontinuous ducts
- Poorly defined mass
  - ➢ Poor visibility of tumor mass
  - ➢ Minimal tumor enhancement (50% of cases)
  - ➢ Vascular encasement or invasion
  - ➢ Parenchymal invasion (segment IV) 30% of cases
- Atrophy
  - ➢ Segmental or lobar
  - ➢ Due to vascular compromise

Figure 2-5-13

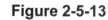

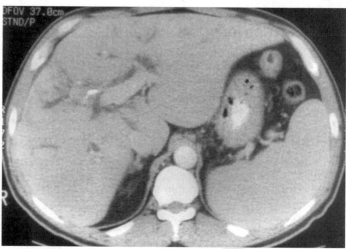

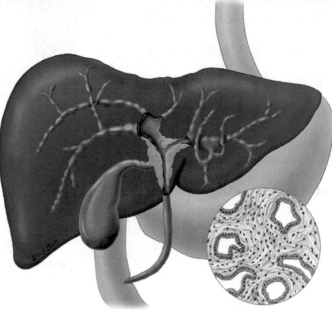

Hilar cholangiocarcinoma

Hilar Cholangiocarcinoma: Cholangiographic Features [Figure 2-5-14]
- Stenosis
- Shoulders
  - ➤ Evidence of mass
- Irregular tapering
- Complete obstruction

Benign Disease Mimicking Carcinoma
- Benign Strictures
  - ➤ Pancreatitis
- Inflammatory cholangitis
  - ➤ Primary sclerosing cholangitis
  - ➤ AIDS cholangiopathy
  - ➤ Recurrent pzogenic cholangitis
  - ➤ Biliary parasites
- Benign neoplasms
  - ➤ Granular cell tumor
  - ➤ Biliary papillomatosis

Primary Sclerosing Cholangitis
- Primary disease features
  - ➤ Strictures
    - ❖ Short, < 1-cm
  - ➤ Beading
  - ➤ Pruned-tree
  - ➤ Diverticula
  - ➤ Mural irregularity

PSC with Cholangiocarcinoma
- Stricture (90%)
  - ➤ Long strictures (>1cm)
  - ➤ Completely obstructing
  - ➤ Associated mass
- Polypoid mass
- Multicentric (10%)

Klatskin / PSC

Klatskin / PSC with Cholangiocarcinoma

Granular Cell Tumor
- Benign tumors of Schwann cell origin
- 90% of patients are females, mean age 34 years
- Location:
  - ➤ CBD (50%)
  - ➤ Cystic duct (37%)
  - ➤ CHD (11%)
  - ➤ Gallbladder (4%)
  - ➤ Intrahepatic ducts (4%)
- Infiltrative lesions that produce short annular strictures

Biliary Papillomatosis
- Multiple and recurrent adenomas of the biliary tract
- Men and women in the 6th and 7th decades
- Clinical presentation: biliary obstruction, cholangitis
- Local recurrence and malignant transformation common

Figure 2-5-14

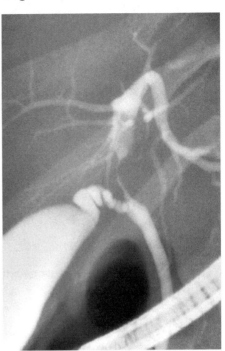

Granular cell tumor

Summary: Polypoid GB Masses
- Cholesterol polyp
- Adenoma
- Adenocarcinoma
  - ➢ Adjacent wall thickening
  - ➢ Adjacent liver abnormality
  - ➢ Adenopathy

Summary: Gallbladder Wall Thickening
- Adenomyomatous hyperplasia
  - ➢ "Comet tail" US
  - ➢ "Pearl necklace" MR
- Xanthogranulomatous cholecystitis
  - ➢ Nodules in GB wall
- Adenocarcinoma
  - ➢ Direct extension
  - ➢ Adenopathy

Summary: EHBD Adenocarcinoma
- Malignant stricture
  - ➢ Abrupt change
- Benign stricture
  - ➢ Tapering

Klatskin / PSC

Summary: Granular Cell Tumor
- Benign Neoplasm
  - ➢ Young, women
  - ➢ True mimic for carcinoma

Tumors of the Gallbladder and Biliary Ducts References

Gallbladder Carcinoma

Campbell WL, Ferris JV, Holbert BL, et al: Biliary tract carcinoma complicating primary sclerosing cholangitis: evaluation with CT, cholangiography, US, and MR imaging. Radiology 207:41, 1998

Kumar A, Aggarwal S: Carcinoma of the gallbladder: CT findings in 50 cases. Abdom Imaging 19:304, 1994

Levy AD, Murakata LA, Rohrmann CA, Jr.: Gallbladder carcinoma: radiologic-pathologic correlation. Radiographics 21:295, 2001

Ohtani T, Shirai Y, Tsukada K, et al: Carcinoma of the gallbladder: CT evaluation of lymphatic spread. Radiology 189:875, 1993

Ohtani T, Shirai Y, Tsukada K, et al: Spread of gallbladder carcinoma: CT evaluation with pathologic correlation. Abdom Imaging 21:195, 1996

Rossmann MD, Friedman AC, Radecki PD, et al: MR imaging of gallbladder carcinoma. AJR Am J Roentgenol 148:143, 1987

Sagoh T, Itoh K, Togashi K, et al: Gallbladder carcinoma: evaluation with MR imaging. Radiology 174:131, 1990

Tsuchiya Y: Early carcinoma of the gallbladder: macroscopic features and US findings. Radiology 179:171, 1991

Wada K, Tanaka M, Yamaguchi K: Carcinoma and polyps of the gallbladder associated with Peutz-Jeghers syndrome. Dig Dis Sci 32:943, 1987

Walsh N, Qizilbash A, Banerjee R, et al: Biliary neoplasia in Gardner's syndrome. Arch Pathol Lab Med 111:76, 1987

Yoshida H, Itai Y, Minami M, et al: Biliary malignancies occurring in choledochal cysts. Radiology 173:389, 1989

Cholesterol Polyp

Furukawa H, Takayasu K, Mukai K, et al: CT evaluation of small polypoid lesions of the gallbladder. Hepatogastroenterology 42:800, 1995

Jones-Monahan KS, Gruenberg JC, Finger JE, et al: Isolated small gallbladder polyps: an indication for cholecystectomy in symptomatic patients. Am Surg 66:716, 2000

Koga A, Watanabe K, Fukuyama T, et al: Diagnosis and operative indications for polypoid lesions of the gallbladder. Arch Surg 123:26, 1988

Mainprize KS, Gould SW, Gilbert JM: Surgical management of polypoid lesions of the gallbladder. Br J Surg 87:414, 2000

Majeski JA: Polyps of the gallbladder. J Surg Oncol 32:16, 1986

Sugiyama M, Atomi Y, Kuroda A, et al: Large cholesterol polyps of the gallbladder: diagnosis by means of US and endoscopic US. Radiology 196:493, 1995

Terzi C, Sokmen S, Seckin S, et al: Polypoid lesions of the gallbladder: report of 100 cases with special reference to operative indications. Surgery 127:622, 2000

Gallbladder and Bile Duct Adenoma

Albores-Saavedra J, Vardaman CJ, Vuitch F: Non-neoplastic polypoid lesions and adenomas of the gallbladder. Pathol Annu 28 Pt 1:145, 1993

Inagaki M, Ishizaki A, Kino S, et al: Papillary adenoma of the distal common bile duct. J Gastroenterol 34:535, 1999

Kawakatsu M, Vilgrain V, Zins M, et al: Radiologic features of papillary adenoma and papillomatosis of the biliary tract. Abdom Imaging 22:87, 1997

Levy AD, Murakata LA, Abbott RM, et al: From the archives of the AFIP. Benign tumors and tumorlike lesions of the gallbladder and extrahepatic bile ducts: radiologic-pathologic correlation. Armed Forces Institute of Pathology. Radiographics 22:387, 2002

Ponette E, Biebau G, Gelin J, et al: Imaging of polypoid endoluminal growing bile duct tumors. J Belge Radiol 77:157, 1994

Saxe J, Lucas C, Ledgerwood AM, et al: Villous adenoma of the common bile duct. Arch Surg 123:96, 1988

Tantachamrun T, Borvonsombat S, Theetranont C: Gardner's syndrome associated with adenomatous polyp of gall bladder: report of a case. J Med Assoc Thai 62:441, 1979

Terzi C, Sokmen S, Seckin S, et al: Polypoid lesions of the gallbladder: report of 100 cases with special reference to operative indications. Surgery 127:622, 2000

Walsh N, Qizilbash A, Banerjee R, et al: Biliary neoplasia in Gardner's syndrome. Arch Pathol Lab Med 111:76, 1987

Adenomatous Hyperplasia

Berk RN, van dVJH, Lichtenstein JE: The hyperplastic cholecystoses: cholesterolosis and adenomyomatosis. Radiology 146:593, 1983

Gerard PS, Berman D, Zafaranloo S: CT and ultrasound of gallbladder adenomyomatosis mimicking carcinoma. J Comput Assist Tomogr 14:490, 1990

Hwang JI, Chou YH, Tsay SH, et al: Radiologic and pathologic correlation of adenomyomatosis of the gallbladder. Abdom Imaging 23:73, 1998

Raghavendra BN, Subramanyam BR, Balthazar EJ, et al: Sonography of adenomyomatosis of the gallbladder: radiologic-pathologic correlation. Radiology 146:747, 1983

Sasatomi E, Miyazaki K, Mori M, et al: Polypoid adenomyoma of the gallbladder. J Gastroenterol 32:704, 1997

Yoshimitsu K, Honda H, Jimi M, et al: MR diagnosis of adenomyomatosis of the gallbladder and differentiation from gallbladder carcinoma: importance of showing Rokitansky-Aschoff sinuses. AJR Am J Roentgenol 172:1535, 1999

Xanthogranulomatous Cholecystitis

Casas D, Perez-Andres R, Jimenez JA, et al: Xanthogranulomatous cholecystitis: a radiological study of 12 cases and a review of the literature. Abdom Imaging 21:456, 1996

Chun KA, Ha HK, Yu ES, et al: Xanthogranulomatous cholecystitis: CT features with emphasis on differentiation from gallbladder carcinoma [see comments]. Radiology 203:93, 1997

Goodman ZD, et al.: Xanthogranulomatous cholecystitis. Am J Surg Pathol. 5:653, 1981

Kim PN, Ha HK, Kim YH, et al: US findings of xanthogranulomatous cholecystitis.

Clin Radiol 53:290, 1998

Kim PN, Lee SH, Gong GY, et al: Xanthogranulomatous cholecystitis: radiologic findings with histologic correlation that focuses on intramural nodules. AJR Am J Roentgenol 172:949, 1999

Levy AD, Murakata LA, Abbott RM, et al: From the archives of the AFIP. Benign tumors and tumorlike lesions of the gallbladder and extrahepatic bile ducts: radiologic-pathologic correlation. Armed Forces Institute of Pathology. Radiographics 22:387, 2002

Maeda T, Shimada M, Matsumata T, et al: Xanthogranulomatous cholecystitis masquerading as gallbladder carcinoma. Am J Gastroenterol 89:628, 1994

Parra JA, Acinas O, Bueno J, et al: Xanthogranulomatous cholecystitis: clinical, sonographic, and CT findings in 26 patients. AJR Am J Roentgenol 174:979, 2000

Reed A, Ryan C, Schwartz SI: Xanthogranulomatous cholecystitis. J Am Coll Surg 179:249, 1994

Ros PR, Goodman ZD: Xanthogranulomatous cholecystitis versus gallbladder carcinoma [editorial; comment]. Radiology 203:10, 1997

Hilar Cholangiocarcinoma

Campbell WL, Ferris JV, Holbert BL, et al: Biliary tract carcinoma complicating primary sclerosing cholangitis: evaluation with CT, cholangiography, US, and MR imaging. Radiology 207:41, 1998

Campbell WL, Peterson MS, Federle MP, et al: Using CT and cholangiography to diagnose biliary tract carcinoma complicating primary sclerosing cholangitis. AJR Am J Roentgenol 177:1095, 2001

Engels JT, Balfe DM, Lee JK: Biliary carcinoma: CT evaluation of extrahepatic spread. Radiology 172:35, 1989

Fulcher AS, Turner MA: HASTE MR cholangiography in the evaluation of hilar cholangiocarcinoma. AJR Am J Roentgenol 169:1501, 1997

Han JK, Choi BI, Kim AY, et al: Cholangiocarcinoma: pictorial essay of CT and cholangiographic findings. Radiographics 22:173, 2002

Han JK, Choi BI, Kim TK, et al: Hilar cholangiocarcinoma: thin-section spiral CT findings with cholangiographic correlation. Radiographics 17:1475, 1997

Hann LE, Greatrex KV, Bach AM, et al: Cholangiocarcinoma at the hepatic hilus: sonographic findings. AJR Am J Roentgenol 168:985, 1997

Keogan MT, Seabourn JT, Paulson EK, et al: Contrast-enhanced CT of intrahepatic and hilar cholangiocarcinoma: delay time for optimal imaging. AJR Am J Roentgenol 169:1493, 1997

Ponette E, Biebau G, Gelin J, et al: Imaging of polypoid endoluminal growing bile duct tumors. J Belge Radiol 77:157, 1994

Rosen CB, Nagorney DM: Cholangiocarcinoma complicating primary sclerosing cholangitis. Semin Liver Dis 11:26, 1991

Soyer P, Bluemke DA, Reichle R, et al: Imaging of intrahepatic cholangiocarcinoma: 2. Hilar cholangiocarcinoma. AJR Am J Roentgenol 165:1433, 1995

Tillich M, Mischinger HJ, Preisegger KH, et al: Multiphasic helical CT in diagnosis and staging of hilar cholangiocarcinoma. AJR Am J Roentgenol 171:651, 1998

Pancreatic Neoplasms
Radiologic-Pathologic Correlation

Angela D. Levy, LTC, MC, USA
Department of Radiologic Pathology
Armed Forces Institute of Pathology
Washington, DC

Classification of Pancreatic Tumors
- Tumors of the Exocrine Pancreas
  - Ductal adenocarcinoma
  - Acinar cell carcinoma
  - Solid-pseudopapillary neoplasm
  - Intraductal papillary mucinous neoplasm
  - Mucinous cystic neoplasm
  - Microcystic adenoma
  - Pancreatoblastoma
  - Mature cystic teratoma
- Tumors of the Endocrine Pancreas
  - Islet cell tumors (neuroendocrine tumors)
  - Small cell carcinoma
- Non-epithelial tumors
  - Soft tissue tumors
  - Lymphoma
- Secondary Tumors
- Tumor like lesions
  - Pancreatitis
  - Lymphoepithelial cyst
  - Pseudocyst

Objectives
- Adenocarcinoma
  - Ductal adenocarcinoma
  - Mucinous noncystic adenocarcinoma
- Intraductal papillary mucinous neoplasm
- Mucinous cystic neoplasm
- Solid and pseudopapillary epithelial neoplasm
- Microcystic adenoma
- Islet cell tumor
- Metastasis

Pancreatic Adenocarcinoma: Epidemiology
- 85 to 90% of pancreatic neoplasms
- 2004 U.S. statistics
  - 9th most common cancer in women, 10th in men
  - 4th leading cause of cancer death in men, 5th in women
- Second most common GI tract malignancy in the U.S.
  - US: colorectal, pancreas, stomach, liver, esophagus, gallbladder
  - Worldwide: stomach, colorectal, liver, esophagus, pancreas, gallbladder

Pancreatic Adenocarcinoma: Epidemiology
- Death:incidence ratio of .99
  - 31,860 new cases in 2004
  - 31,270 deaths in 2004
- 5-year survival 4%, overall
- 5-year survival 17%, early stage
- More common in men than women
- 80% of cases occur between 60 to 80 years of age

Pancreatic Adenocarcinoma: Risk Factors
- Cigarette smoking (2-3 fold relative risk)
- Hereditary risk factors
  - Hereditary nonpolyposis colon cancer (HNPCC)
  - Familial breast cancer (BRCA2)
  - Familial adenomatous polyposis
  - Peutz-Jeghers
  - Ataxia telangiectasia
  - Familial atypical multiple mole-melanoma
  - Familial pancreatitis

Pancreatic Adenocarcinoma: Clinical Features
- Pain is the most common symptom
- Unexplained weight loss
- Jaundice in 50% tumors in the head of the pancreas
- Diabetes occurs in 25 to 50%
- Distribution
  - 60% head
  - 20% body
  - 10% tail
  - 5% to 10% entire gland

Figure 2-6-1

Pancreatic Adenocarcinoma: Pathology *[Figure 2-6-1]*
- Microscopy
  - Moderately to well differentiated
  - Desmoplastic stromal reaction
- Gross Pathology
  - Fibrotic
  - Infiltration and invasion of adjacent structures
  - Hemorrhage and necrosis uncommon

Pancreatic Adenocarcinoma: Barium Studies
- Antral padding
- Inverted "3"
- Spiculation of duodenal folds
- Mucosal ulceration
- Left sided mass effect at the ligament of Treitz

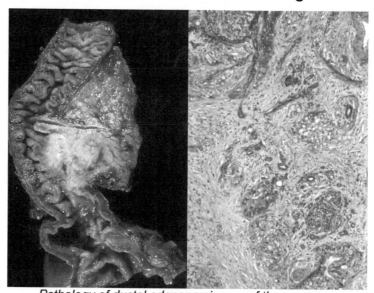

Pathology of ductal adenocarcinoma of the pancreas

Figure 2-6-2

"Inverted 3" *[Figure 2-6-2]*

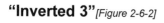

Pancreatic Adenocarcinoma: Ultrasound
- Echogenicity
  - Hypoechoic 55%
  - Heterogeneous 40%
  - Hyperechoic 3%
  - Isoechoic 2%
- Diffuse enlargement in 10%
- Biliary and pancreatic duct dilatation
- Liver metastasis
- Adenopathy
- Vascular encasement

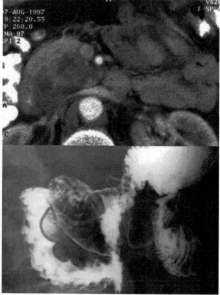

Ductal adenocarcinoma of the pancreas showing the "inverted 3" sign on barium examination

Hypoechoic Mass, Head of Pancreas

Hypoechoic Mass, Body of Pancreas

Pancreatic Adenocarcinoma: CT
- Dual Phase Technique
  - ➢ Multidetector CT, 1.25 mm
  - ➢ Rapid bolus, 3 ml/sec
  - ➢ Pancreatic phase, 40 sec after injection
  - ➢ Portal venous phase

Pancreatic Adenocarcinoma: CT
- CT features
  - ➢ Pancreatic and CBD duct dilatation
    - ❖ "Double duct sign"
    - ❖ Abrupt tapering of the CBD
  - ➢ Focal soft tissue density in a fatty gland
  - ➢ Spherical enlargement of the pancreatic head
  - ➢ Rounded borders of the uncinate process
  - ➢ Atrophy of the distal gland
  - ➢ Extension to adjacent organs
  - ➢ Vascular encasement

Figure 2-6-3

Double Duct Sign [Figure 2-6-3]

Spherical Enlargement of the Pancreatic Head

Rounded Borders of the Uncinate Process
[Figure 2-6-4]

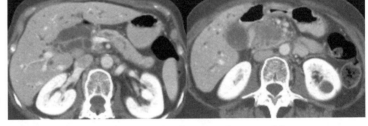

Double duct sign of ductal adenocarcinoma of the pancreas

Figure 2-6-4

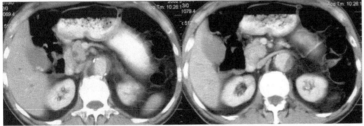

Ductal adenocarcinoma of the pancreas showing a rounded contour to the uncinate process

Atrophic Changes in the Distal Pancreas
[Figure 2-6-5]

Figure 2-6-5

Nonresectability
- Invasion of adjacent organs, except duodenum
- Tumor diameter > 5 cm
- Encasement or occlusion of vessels
  - ➢ SMA, SMV, portal vein
  - ➢ Celiac trunk and major branches
  - ➢ +/- isolated focal involvement of PV or SMV
  - ➢ Accuracy of CT 88%-90%
  - ➢ 3D CT angiography
- Distant nodal metastasis
- Liver metastasis

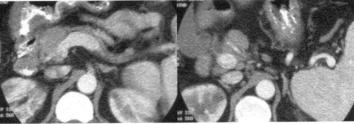

Ductal adenocarcinoma of the pancreas showing atrophy of the distal pancreas

Resectable? No, stomach and vascular invasion

Resectable? No, SMA Encasement

Resectable? No, SMA Encasement and Liver Mets

Resectable? YES

Mucinous Noncystic Adenocarcinoma (Infiltrating Colloid Carcinoma)
- Rare variant of adenocarcinoma
- Marked extracellular mucin
- Signet rings cells
- Imaging
  - ➢ Large tumors
  - ➢ Well-defined hypoattenuating mass
  - ➢ May have calcification

Intraductal Papillary Mucinous Neoplasm (IPMN)
- Mucin producing intraductal papillary neoplasm
- Low-grade malignancy/malignant potential
- Synonyms
  - ➢ Intraductal mucin-hypersecreting neoplasm
  - ➢ Ductectatic type of pancreatic ductal carcinoma
  - ➢ Mucinous ductal ectasia
  - ➢ Mucin-producing tumor (or carcinoma)
  - ➢ Mucin-hypersecreting tumor

Intraductal Papillary Mucinous Neoplasm (IPMN)
- Most common in men, 7th decade
- Clinical symptoms similar to chronic pancreatitis
  - ➢ Pain
  - ➢ Malabsorption
  - ➢ Diabetes
  - ➢ Prior episodes of pancreatitis

IPMN: Pathology [Figure 2-6-6]
- Papillary epithelium
- Mucin production
- Duct dilatation

IPMN: Imaging [Figure 2-6-7]
- Main duct or side branch
  - ➢ Duct dilatation
  - ➢ Cyst
- Intraductal masses
- Bulging duodenal papilla
- Glandular atrophy

Main Duct IMPN [Figure 2-6-8]

Figure 2-6-8

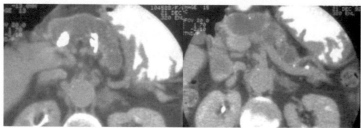
Main duct IPMN

Figure 2-6-6

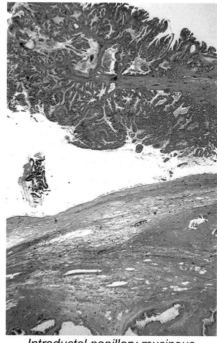
Intraductal papillary mucinous neoplasm

Figure 2-6-7

A
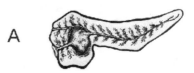

B
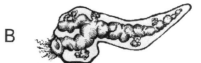

C
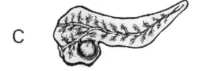

D
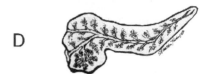

Patterns of duct dilatation in IPMN

Side Branch IPMN [Figure 2-6-9]

Bulging Papilla [Figure 2-6-10]

IPMN: Diagnostic Difficulties
- Chronic pancreatitis
- Side branch variant may mimic
  - ➢ Pseudocyst
  - ➢ Mucinous cystic neoplasm
  - ➢ Microcystic adenoma
- ERCP
  - ➢ Definitive imaging technique

Mucinous Cystic Neoplasm (MCN)
- Mucin-secreting cystic neoplasm
- 80% occur in women
- Mean age 49 years
- Rarely occurs in men
  - ➢ Older age, mean 70 years

Mucinous Cystic Neoplasm (MCN)
- Clinical presentation depends on tumor size
- Jaundice and CBD obstruction are rare
- Potentially malignant
  - ➢ Mucinous cystadenoma
  - ➢ Mucinous cystadenocarcinoma

MCN: Histopathology
- Columnar cell lining
- May have ovarian-type stroma
- Mucin
- Hemorrhage
- Calcification

Mucinous Cystic Neoplasm: Gross Pathology
- 70 to 95% in tail of pancreas
- Average size 6 to 10 cm
- Multilocular cysts
  - ➢ Unilocular, rare
- Septations
- Solid papillary nodules
- Occasional calcifications

MCN: Imaging
- Cannot differentiate benign from malignant
- Most common in the tail of the pancreas
- Multilocular or unilocular cyst
  - ➢ Septations
  - ➢ Mural nodules
- Septations and nodules may enhance
- Variable CT attenuation/MR signal intensity
  - ➢ Mucin
  - ➢ Hemorrhage
  - ➢ Proteinaceous fluid

Mucinous Cystic Neoplasm [Figure 2-6-11]

Figure 2-6-9

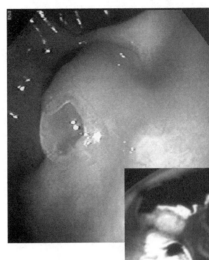

Side branch IPMN

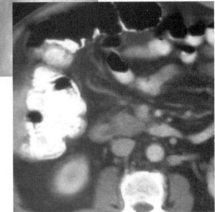

Figure 2-6-10

Bulging papilla in IPMN

Figure 2-6-11

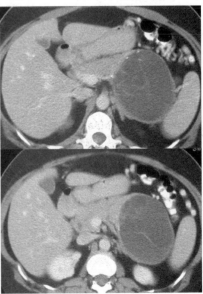

Mucinous cystic neoplasm

MCN: Diagnostic Difficulties
- Small lesions
- Lesions located in the head of the pancreas
- Lesions without septations and mural nodules
- Differential diagnosis
  - Pseudocyst
  - Oligocystic adenoma
  - Rare, congenital cysts

Solid and Pseudopapillary Epithelial Neoplasm (SPEN)
- Benign or low-grade malignancy
- Good prognosis
- Young women, mean age 24 years
- Synonyms
  - Solid-cystic tumor
  - Papillary cystic tumor
  - Solid and pseudopapillary tumor

SPEN: Clinical Features
- Usually incidentally discovered
- Abdominal discomfort, pain
- Jaundice is rare

SPEN: Pathology Features
- Pathogenesis unknown
- Gross Pathology
  - Hemorrhage, necrosis, cystic areas
  - Solid areas
  - Capsule
  - May contain calcification

SPEN: Pathology Features
- Histopathology
  - Highly cellular areas
  - Pseudopapillary areas
  - Hemorrhage
  - Sclerosis

SPEN: Imaging Features *[Figure 2-6-12]*
- Circumscribed
- Capsule
- Cystic change
  - Hemorrhage
  - Fluid-fluid levels
- Calcification
- MR/CT
  - Early peripheral enhancement
- Rare features
  - Biliary/pancreatic duct dilatation
  - Adjacent organ invasion

SPEN: Diagnostic Difficulties
- Older patient age
- May mimic other cystic lesions
  - Pancreatic pseudocyst
  - Mucinous cystic neoplasm
  - Oligocystic adenoma
- MR helpful
  - Evidence of capsule
  - Evidence of blood products

Figure 2-6-12

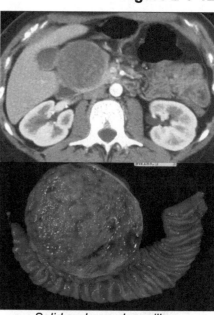

*Solid and pseudopapillary
epithelial neoplasm*

Microcystic Adenoma
- Benign
- Small cysts arranged around a central scar
- Synonyms
  - Serous cystadenoma
  - Glycogen-rich cystadenoma
- Variants
  - Oligocystic adenoma

Microcystic Adenoma
- 70% in women
- Mean age, 66 years
- Variable clinical presentation
  - Incidental
  - Pain, nausea, vomiting, weight loss
  - Jaundice is unusual

Microcystic Adenoma: Pathology
- 50% in body and tail
- "Honeycomb" or "sponge" appearance
- Thin fibrous septae
- Central stellate scar
- Occasional hemorrhage

Microcystic Adenoma: Pathology
- Histology
  - Small cysts
  - Cuboidal cells
  - High glycogen content

Microcystic Adenoma: Imaging features [Figure 2-6-13]
- Circumscribed margins
  - Lobular
- Honeycomb appearance
  - Multiple small cysts
- Central scar
  - +/- calcification
- Occasionally, evidence of hemorrhage on MR

Oligocystic Adenoma
- Uncommon variant of microcystic adenoma
- Few, very large cysts
- ? association with von Hippel Lindau syndrome
- Synonyms
  - Macrocystic serous cystadenoma
  - Serous oligocystic adenoma

Microcystic Adenoma: Diagnostic Difficulties
- Oligocystic variant
  - Differential diagnosis
    - ❖ Mucinous cystic neoplasm
    - ❖ Pseudocyst
- Small lesions
  - Difficult to identify central scar/septations

Islet Cell Tumors (Neuroendocrine Tumors)
- Tumors of the pancreatic islets
- Occur in all age groups
- Benign or malignant
- Functioning (65% to 85%)
- Nonfunctioning (15% to 35%)

Figure 2-6-13

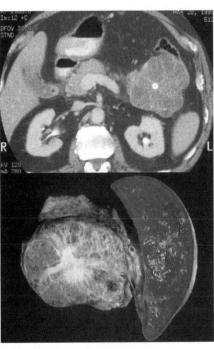

Microcystic adenoma

22-year-old woman complains of fainting spells

Insulinoma
- Most common functioning islet cell tumor
- Clinical-"Whipple's Triad"
  - Symptoms during fast or exercise
  - Symptoms relieved with glucose
  - Serum glucose <40
- Usually solitary, <2cm
- 10% occur with MEN I
- Usually benign biologic behavior

Insulinoma
- Hypoechoic on ultrasound
- Intense, transient enhancement on CT and MR
  - Arterial phase imaging!
- High signal on T2 MR
- Octreotide scans positive

55-year-old male complains of skin rash
Glucagonoma (DM-Dermatitis Syndrome)
- Third most common functioning tumor
- Clinical symptoms
  - Diabetes mellitus
  - Necrolytic migratory erythema
  - Weight loss
  - Anemia
- Most common in tail of pancreas
- Variable biologic behavior

Functioning Islet Cell Tumors
- Insulinoma
- Gastrinoma
  - Zollinger Ellison syndrome
  - 70% malignant
  - Ectopic locations: duodenum, nodes
  - MEN I
- Glucagonoma
- VIPoma
  - Werner Morrison syndrome, watery diarrhea, hypokalemia, acholorhydria
- Somatostatinoma
- Pancreatic polypeptide tumors

52-year-old male with abdominal pain
MEN I Syndrome (Wermer's Syndrome)
- 3P's
  - Pituitary
  - Pancreas
  - Parathyroid
  - Other: thymus, thyroid, adrenal gland, GI tract
- Autosomal dominant
  - Long arm chromosome 11

Non-functioning Islet Cell Tumors
- Occur at any age
- Typically large at time of diagnosis
  - Range, 6 to 20 cm
- Necrosis and cystic degeneration common
- 25% calcify
- Liver metastases are common

Metastatic Disease [Figure 2-6-14]

- Mets to pancreas
  - ➤ Lung, breast
  - ➤ Melanoma
  - ➤ Renal cell
  - ➤ Lymphoma-adjacent nodal disease
- Mimic primary pancreatic neoplasms
  - ➤ Ductal adenocarcinoma
  - ➤ Islet cell
- Biliary obstruction in 30%

Summary: Adenocarcinoma

- Most common pancreatic neoplasm
- CT technique important
  - ➤ Thin collimation
  - ➤ Dual phase
  - ➤ CT angiography
- RESECTABLILITY
  - ➤ Vascular encasement
  - ➤ Adjacent organ invasion
  - ➤ Liver mets

Summary: IMPN

- High index of suspicion
- Main duct or side branch
- Imaging
  - ➤ Focal or diffuse duct dilatation
  - ➤ Bulging papilla
- ERCP

Summary: Cystic Neoplasms

- SPEN
  - ➤ Young women
  - ➤ Hemorrhage
  - ➤ Capsule
- Microcystic Adenoma
  - ➤ Older women
  - ➤ Central scar
  - ➤ Honeycomb-like cysts
- Mucinous Cystic Neoplasm
  - ➤ Middle-aged women
  - ➤ Tail of the pancreas
  - ➤ Complex, large septated cyst

Figure 2-6-14

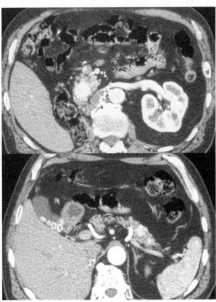

Renal cell metastatic to the pancreas

Pancreatic Neoplasms References

Adenocarcinoma

1. Fletcher JG, Wiersema MJ, Farrell MA, et al: Pancreatic malignancy: value of arterial, pancreatic, and hepatic phase imaging with multi-detector row CT. Radiology 229:81, 2003
2. Horton KM, Fishman EK: Adenocarcinoma of the pancreas: CT imaging. Radiol Clin North Am 40:1263, 2002
3. Hough TJ, Raptopoulos V, Siewert B, et al: Teardrop superior mesenteric vein: CT sign for unresectable carcinoma of the pancreas. AJR Am J Roentgenol 173:1509, 1999
4. Imbriaco M, Megibow AJ, Camera L, et al: Dual-phase versus single-phase helical CT to detect and assess resectability of pancreatic carcinoma. AJR Am J Roentgenol 178:1473, 2002
5. Keogan MT, Tyler D, Clark L, et al: Diagnosis of pancreatic carcinoma: role of FDG PET. AJR Am J Roentgenol 171:1565, 1998
6. Lu DS, Reber HA, Krasny RM, et al: Local staging of pancreatic cancer: criteria

for unresectability of major vessels as revealed by pancreatic-phase, thin-section helical CT. AJR Am J Roentgenol 168:1439, 1997

7. Lu DS, Vedantham S, Krasny RM, et al: Two-phase helical CT for pancreatic tumors: pancreatic versus hepatic phase enhancement of tumor, pancreas, and vascular structures. Radiology 199:697, 1996

8. McNulty NJ, Francis IR, Platt JF, et al: Multi--detector row helical CT of the pancreas: effect of contrast-enhanced multiphasic imaging on enhancement of the pancreas, peripancreatic vasculature, and pancreatic adenocarcinoma. Radiology 220:97, 2001

9. Megibow AJ: Pancreatic adenocarcinoma: designing the examination to evaluate the clinical questions. Radiology 183:297, 1992

10. Megibow AJ, Zhou XH, Rotterdam H, et al: Pancreatic adenocarcinoma: CT versus MR imaging in the evaluation of resectability--report of the Radiology Diagnostic Oncology Group. Radiology 195:327, 1995

11. O'Malley ME, Boland GW, Wood BJ, et al: Adenocarcinoma of the head of the pancreas: determination of surgical unresectability with thin-section pancreatic-phase helical CT. AJR Am J Roentgenol 173:1513, 1999

12. Prokesch RW, Chow LC, Beaulieu CF, et al: Isoattenuating pancreatic adenocarcinoma at multi-detector row CT: secondary signs. Radiology 224:764, 2002

13. Prokesch RW, Chow LC, Beaulieu CF, et al: Local staging of pancreatic carcinoma with multi-detector row CT: use of curved planar reformations initial experience. Radiology 225:759, 2002

14. Raptopoulos V, Steer ML, Sheiman RG, et al: The use of helical CT and CT angiography to predict vascular involvement from pancreatic cancer: correlation with findings at surgery. AJR Am J Roentgenol 168:971, 1997

15. Roche CJ, Hughes ML, Garvey CJ, et al: CT and pathologic assessment of prospective nodal staging in patients with ductal adenocarcinoma of the head of the pancreas. AJR Am J Roentgenol 180:475, 2003

16. Tabuchi T, Itoh K, Ohshio G, et al: Tumor staging of pancreatic adenocarcinoma using early- and late-phase helical CT. AJR Am J Roentgenol 173:375, 1999

17. Vargas R, Nino-Murcia M, Trueblood W, et al: MDCT in Pancreatic adenocarcinoma: prediction of vascular invasion and resectability using a multiphasic technique with curved planar reformations. AJR Am J Roentgenol 182:419, 2004

18. Zeman RK, Cooper C, Zeiberg AS, et al: TNM staging of pancreatic carcinoma using helical CT. AJR Am J Roentgenol 169:459, 1997

Intraductal Papillary Mucinous Neoplasm

1. Cellier C, Cuillerier E, Palazzo L, et al: Intraductal papillary and mucinous tumors of the pancreas: accuracy of preoperative computed tomography, endoscopic retrograde pancreatography and endoscopic ultrasonography, and long-term outcome in a large surgical series. Gastrointest Endosc 47:42, 1998

2. Fukukura Y, Fujiyoshi F, Sasaki M, et al: Intraductal papillary mucinous tumors of the pancreas: thin-section helical CT findings. AJR Am J Roentgenol 174:441, 2000

3. Itai Y, Kokubo T, Atomi Y, et al: Mucin-hypersecreting carcinoma of the pancreas. Radiology 165:51, 1987

4. Lim JH, Lee G, Oh YL: Radiologic spectrum of intraductal papillary mucinous tumor of the pancreas. Radiographics 21:323, 2001

5. Prasad SR, Sahani D, Nasser S, et al: Intraductal papillary mucinous tumors of the pancreas. Abdom Imaging 28:357, 2003

6. Procacci C, Graziani R, Bicego E, et al: Intraductal mucin-producing tumors of the pancreas: imaging findings. Radiology 198:249, 1996

7. Procacci C, Megibow AJ, Carbognin G, et al: Intraductal papillary mucinous tumor of the pancreas: a pictorial essay. Radiographics 19:1447, 1999

8. Taouli B, Vilgrain V, Vullierme MP, et al: Intraductal papillary mucinous tumors of the pancreas: helical CT with histopathologic correlation. Radiology 217:757, 2000

Mucinous Cystic Neoplasm

1. Buetow PC, Rao P, Thompson LD: From the Archives of the AFIP. Mucinous cystic neoplasms of the pancreas: radiologic-pathologic correlation. Radiographics 18:433, 1998
2. Procacci C, Carbognin G, Accordini S, et al: CT features of malignant mucinous cystic tumors of the pancreas. Eur Radiol 11:1626, 2001
3. Thompson LD, Becker RC, Przygodzki RM, et al: Mucinous cystic neoplasm (mucinous cystadenocarcinoma of low-grade malignant potential) of the pancreas: a clinicopathologic study of 130 cases. Am J Surg Pathol 23:1, 1999

Solid and Pseudopapillary Epithelial Neoplasm

1. Buetow PC, Buck JL, Pantongrag-Brown L, et al: Solid and papillary epithelial neoplasm of the pancreas: imaging-pathologic correlation on 56 cases. Radiology 199:707, 1996
2. Cantisani V, Mortele KJ, Levy AD, et al: MR imaging features of solid pseudopapillary tumor of the pancreas in adult and pediatric patients. AJR Am J Roentgenol 181:395, 2003
3. Coleman KM, Doherty MC, Bigler SA: Solid-pseudopapillary tumor of the pancreas. Radiographics 23:1644, 2003
4. Friedman AC, Lichtenstein JE, Fishman EK, et al: Solid and papillary epithelial neoplasm of the pancreas. Radiology 154:333, 1985

Microcystic Adenoma

1. Buck JL, Hayes WS: From the Archives of the AFIP. Microcystic adenoma of the pancreas. Radiographics 10:313, 1990
2. Healy JC, Davies SE, Reznek RH: CT of microcystic (serous) pancreatic adenoma. J Comput Assist Tomogr 18:146, 1994
3. Hough DM, Stephens DH, Johnson CD, et al: Pancreatic lesions in von Hippel-Lindau disease: prevalence, clinical significance, and CT findings. AJR Am J Roentgenol 162:1091, 1994
4. Itai Y, Ohhashi K, Furui S, et al: Microcystic adenoma of the pancreas: spectrum of computed tomographic findings. J Comput Assist Tomogr 12:797, 1988
5. Khurana B, Mortele KJ, Glickman J, et al: Macrocystic serous adenoma of the pancreas: radiologic-pathologic correlation. AJR Am J Roentgenol 181:119, 2003
6. Minami M, Itai Y, Ohtomo K, et al: Cystic neoplasms of the pancreas: comparison of MR imaging with CT. Radiology 171:53, 1989
7. Yeh HC, Stancato-Pasik A, Shapiro RS: Microcystic features at US: a nonspecific sign for microcystic adenomas of the pancreas. Radiographics 21:1455, 2001

Islet Cell Tumors

1. Buetow PC, Miller DL, Parrino TV, et al: Islet cell tumors of the pancreas: clinical, radiologic, and pathologic correlation in diagnosis and localization. Radiographics 17:453, 1997
2. Buetow PC, Parrino TV, Buck JL, et al: Islet cell tumors of the pancreas: pathologic-imaging correlation among size, necrosis and cysts, calcification, malignant behavior, and functional status. AJR Am J Roentgenol 165:1175, 1995
3. Ichikawa T, Peterson MS, Federle MP, et al: Islet cell tumor of the pancreas: biphasic CT versus MR imaging in tumor detection. Radiology 216:163, 2000
4. Semelka RC, Cumming MJ, Shoenut JP, et al: Islet cell tumors: comparison of dynamic contrast-enhanced CT and MR imaging with dynamic gadolinium enhancement and fat suppression. Radiology 186:799, 1993
5. Sheth S, Hruban RK, Fishman EK: Helical CT of islet cell tumors of the pancreas: typical and atypical manifestations. AJR Am J Roentgenol 179:725, 2002
6. Stafford Johnson DB, Francis IR, Eckhauser FE, et al: Dual-phase helical CT of nonfunctioning islet cell tumors. J Comput Assist Tomogr 22:59, 1998
7. Van Hoe L, Gryspeerdt S, Marchal G, et al: Helical CT for the preoperative localization of islet cell tumors of the pancreas: value of arterial and parenchymal phase images. AJR Am J Roentgenol 165:1437, 1995

Metastases

1. Chambers TP, Fishman EK, Hruban RH: Pancreatic metastases from renal cell carcinoma in von Hippel-Lindau disease. Clin Imaging 21:40, 1997
2. Klein KA, Stephens DH, Welch TJ: CT characteristics of metastatic disease of the pancreas. Radiographics 18:369, 1998
3. Ng CS, Loyer EM, Iyer RB, et al: Metastases to the pancreas from renal cell carcinoma: findings on three-phase contrast-enhanced helical CT. AJR Am J Roentgenol 172:1555, 1999

Gastric Malignancies: Radiologic–Pathologic Correlation

Angela D. Levy, LTC, MC, USA
Department of Radiologic Pathology
Armed Forces Institute of Pathology
Washington

Gastric Malignancies
- Adenocarcinoma
- Lymphoma
- Gastrointestinal Stromal Tumors
- Carcinoid
- Kaposi Sarcoma
- Metastases

Gastric Adenocarcinoma
- Fourth most common cancer worldwide[1]
  - Lung, breast, colorectum, stomach, liver
- Disease of poverty
- Majority of cases occur in China, Japan, South America, Eastern Europe
- Lowest rates are in North America and Northern Africa
- Gastric Carcinoma in the U.S.
  - Decreasing incidence in the U.S.
  - Shift from distal tumors to proximal tumors

[1]Steward BW and Kleihues P (eds). World Cancer Report. IARC Press. Lyon 2003.

Gastric Adenocarcinoma
- Peak incidence 50 to 70 years of age
- More common in men, 2:1
- Usually asymptomatic until disease is advanced
- Most common presenting symptoms:
  - epigastric pain, bloating, nausea
  - early satiety, anorexia, vomiting
  - upper GI bleeding

Gastric Adenocarcinoma: Etiology [Figure 2-7-1]
- Atrophic Gastritis
  - Helicobacter pylori (80% of cases)
  - Pernicious Anemia
  - Partial Gastrectomy
- Adenomatous Polyps
  - Polyposis syndromes
- HNPCC-Hereditary Nonpolyposis Colon Cancer Syndromes (Lynch Syndromes)

Figure 2-7-1

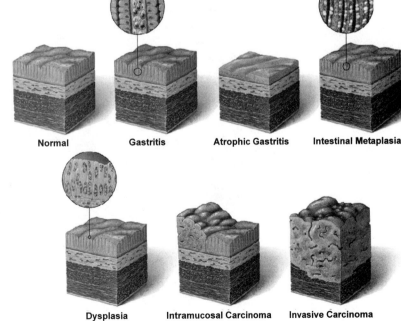

Normal   Gastritis   Atrophic Gastritis   Intestinal Metaplasia

Dysplasia   Intramucosal Carcinoma   Invasive Carcinoma

Pathogenesis of gastric adenocarcinoma

WHO Classification of Gastric Adenocarcinoma

- Signet Ring *[Figure 2-7-2]*
- Papillary *[Figure 2-7-3]*
- Mucinous *[Figure 2-7-4]*
- Tubular (Intestinal)

Figure 2-7-2

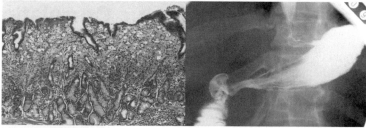

Signet ring cell adenocarcinoma produces "linitis plastica"

Figure 2-7-3

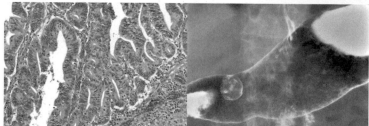

Papillary adenocarcinoma produces intraluminal polypoid masses

Early Gastric Carcinoma

[Figure 2-7-5]

- Japanese Research Society for Gastric Carcinoma
- Carcinoma limited to the mucosa and submucosa, irrespective of nodal metastases

Figure 2-7-4

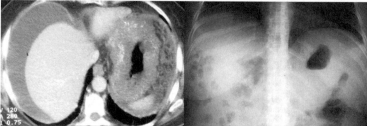

Mucinous adenocarcinoma produces tumor calcifications

Early Gastric Carcinoma Type I

Early Gastric Carcinoma Type II A

Early Gastric Carcinoma Type III

Advanced Gastric Carcinoma *[Figure 2-7-6]*

- Tumor penetrating the muscularis propria
- Symptomatic patients
- Most commonly seen gastric cancer in the U.S.
- Bormann Classification

Figure 2-7-6

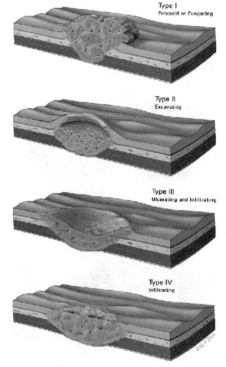

Advanced gastric carcinoma (Borrmann) classification

Figure 2-7-5

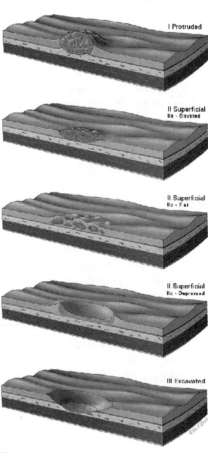

Early gastric carcinoma classification

Polypoid Masses

Polypoid Growth:
- Lobulated or fungating masses protruding into the gastric lumen

Ulcerated - Bulk of tumor mass has been replaced by ulceration

Ulcerated Carcinoma - Lesser Curvature

Carmen Meniscus Sign [Figure 2- 7-7]

Infiltrating: irregular narrowing of the stomach with nodality and spiculation

Scirrhous Carcinoma [Figure 2-7-8]
- Infiltrating tumors with desmoplasia
- Signet ring cell carcinomas
- Radiologic Features
  - Irregular narrowing
  - Decreased gastric capacity
  - Rigidity, "linitis plastica"
  - Most common in the antrum
  - Rarely-nodular,distorted folds when the tumor is proximal

Carcinoma of the Cardia
- One-third of all gastric carcinomas in the U.S.
- Compared to other gastric carcinomas:
  - male predominance, 6:1
  - 40% associated with hiatal hernia
  - Atrophic gastritis and signet ring cell types are uncommon
  - association with smoking and alcohol
- Early lesions are difficult to detect
- Difficult to differentiate from Barrett's adenocarcinoma
- Pseudoachalasia
- Pitfalls on CT:
  - GE junction pseudomass
  - hiatal hernias

Normal Gastric Cardia

Carcinoma of the Cardia [Figure 2-7-9]

Figure 2-7-7

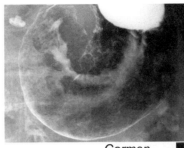
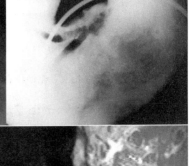

Carmen meniscus sign

Figure 2-7-8

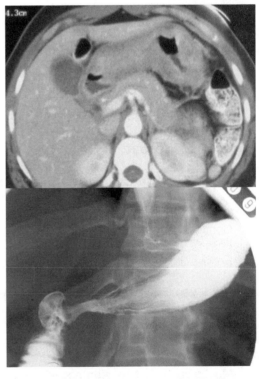

Figure 2-7-9

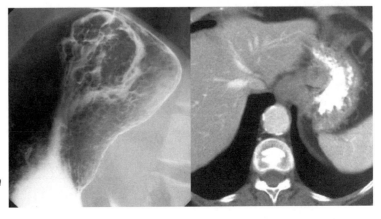

Carcinoma of the cardia

Staging
- Endoscopic Ultrasound
  - Depth of tumor invasion
    - ❖ T stage accuracy 85%
  - Perigastric nodes
    - ❖ Sensitivity for malignant node detection 55%-80%
- CT
  - Presence and extent of extragastric spread

Staging - Extragastric Spread [Figure 2-7-10]
- Anatomic Pathways
  - Lesser omentum (gastrohepatic and gastroduodenal ligament)
  - Gastrosplenic ligament
  - Greater omentum
  - Gastrocolic ligament
  - Lesser sac
  - Lower esophagus
- CT features
  - Soft tissue stranding
  - Soft tissue nodules

Pathways of Spread
- Lymphatic Spread
  - 90% of advanced cancers at diagnosis
  - 15% have left supraclavicular nodes (Virchow's node)
- Hematogenous Metastases
  - Liver
  - Lung
  - Adrenal
- Peritoneal Seeding
  Ovary (Krukenberg tumors) 10%

Lymphatic Spread

Krukenberg Tumor (Ovarian Metastasis)

Adjacent Organ Invasion
- Contiguous tumor
- Loss of fat planes
- Focal enlargement of the adjacent organ

Direct Extension and Adjacent Organ Invasion

Gastric Lymphoma
- Increasing incidence
- Up to 10% of gastric malignancies
- Most common site of extranodal lymphoma
- Most common site of GI lymphomas
- Clinical symptoms
  - Low grade: dyspepsia, nausea, vomiting
  - High grade: bleeding, pain, early satiety, weight loss

Mucosa-Associated Lymphoid Tissue (MALT)
- Organized lymphoid tissue located in mucosal sites
- Native MALT
  - intraepithelial lymphocytes
  - plasma cells, B and T lymphocytes in the lamina propria
  - Mesenteric lymph nodes
  - Peyer's patches

Figure 2-7-10

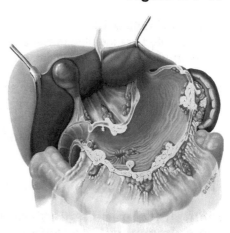

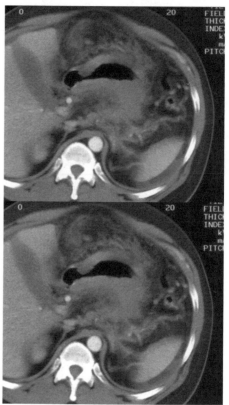

Routes of extragastric spread of carcinoma

Figure 2-7-11

- Acquired MALT
  - ➢ Arises as a result of antigenic stimulation (*H. pylori* infection)
  - ➢ Accumulates before the development of B cell lymphomas

Gastric MALT Lymphoma [Figure 2-7-11]

- Arises from acquired MALT
- *H. pylori* is invariably present
- Majority located in the antrum
- Good clinical prognosis
  - ➢ Rarely disseminated at the time of diagnosis
  - ➢ Long survival
  - ➢ 75% respond to antibiotic eradication of H. pylori

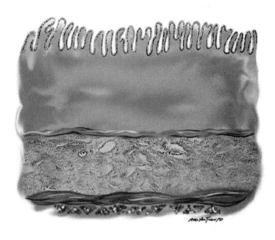

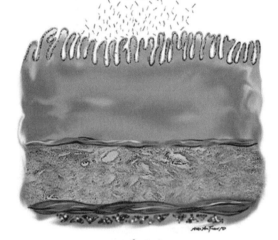

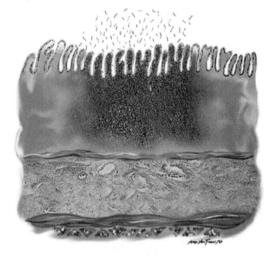

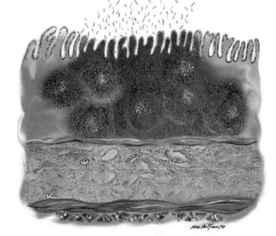

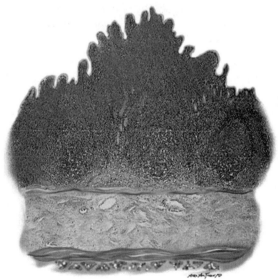

Evolution of gastric lymphoma:

normal mucosa,

H. pylori infection,

H. pylori gastritis,

formation of acquired MALT,

low-grade MALT lymphoma,

high-grade B-cell lymphoma

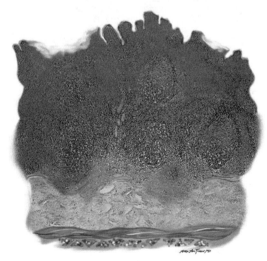

Gastric MALT Lymphoma
- Gross Pathologic features
  - ➢ Ill-defined inflammation
  - ➢ Mural thickening
  - ➢ Superficial erosions, ulcers
- Radiologic features
  - ➢ Shallow or deep ulcers
  - ➢ Mucosal nodularity
  - ➢ Thickened areae gastricae
  - ➢ Enlarged rugae
  - ➢ Multifocal

Low Grade MALT Lymphoma [Figure 2-7-12]

CT features of Gastric Lymphoma
- Wall thickening[1]
  - ➢ Tends to be greater (mean, 4 cm) than that of adenocarcinoma
  - ➢ Tends to be homogeneous attenuation
- Ulceration
- Polypoid masses
- Regional adenopathy

[1]Buy J, Moss A. AJR 138:859-865, 1982

Gastric Lymphoma

Figure 2-7-12

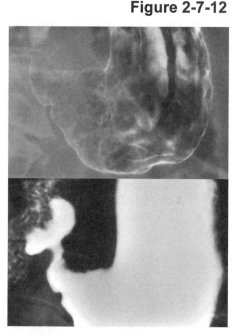

Low-grade MALT lymphoma

CT features differentiating Gastric Adenocarcinoma and Lymphoma
- Gastric wall thickening in lymphoma (mean 4 cm) is typically more impressive than adenocarcinoma (mean 1.8 cm)
- Wall thickening is more homogeneous in lymphoma
- Perigastric fat is more likely to be preserved in lymphoma
- Regional adenopathy is common in both
- Adenopathy in lymphoma tends to be bulky and may extend below the level of the renal veins

Buy J, Moss A. AJR 138:859-865, 1982
Fork FT, Haglund U, Hogstrom H. Endoscopy 17:5-7, 1985

Gastric Lymphoma [Figure 2-7-13]

Figure 2-7-13

Mesenchymal Neoplasm of the Stomach
- Gastrointestinal Stromal Tumor
- Leiomyoma
- Leiomyosarcoma
- Schwannoma
- Neurofibroma
- Ganglioneuroma
- Paraganglioma
- Granular cell tumor
- Lipoma, liposarcoma
- Fibrous lesions
- Tumors of blood vessels

Gastric lymphoma

Gastrointestinal Stromal Tumors (GISTs)
- Most common mesenchymal neoplasm of the GI tract
- Arise from the muscularis propria
- Cellular origin
  - ➢ Primitive "stem cell" like cell
  - ➢ Interstitial cell of Cajal (gut pacemaker cell)

GIST - Clinical Features
- Uncommon tumors
- Prevalence in the U.S.
  - ➢ 5000 to 6000 new cases per year[1]
- Increased incidence
  - ➢ Neurofibromatosis (NF-1)
  - ➢ KIT germline mutations

[1]Fletcher CD, Berman JJ, Corless C, et al. Diagnosis of gastrointestinal stromal tumors: A consensus approach. Hum Pathol 2002. 33:459-465

GIST - Clinical Features
- Median age 50-60 years
- 60% occur in the stomach
- Benign and malignant
- Defined by KIT expression
  - ➢ Initial diagnosis
  - ➢ Therapy (Gleevac)

What is KIT?
- *KIT*-tyrosine kinase growth factor
- KIT-tyrosine kinase growth factor receptor
- CD117 binds to KIT receptors
- Normally expressed
  - ➢ Hematopoietic stem cells
  - ➢ Germ cells
  - ➢ Interstitial cell of Cajal (gut pacemaker cell)
- KIT-inhibitor therapy
  - ➢ STI-571, Imatinib [Gleevac]

What Happened to Leiomyomas and Leiomyosarcomas?
- Very rare
- Except,
  - ➢ Leiomyomas are the most common benign tumor of the ESOPHAGUS
  - ➢ Leiomyosarcomas of the RETROPERITONEUM

GIST - CD117 (KIT) Positive

Gastrointestinal Stromal Tumor [Figure 2-7-14]

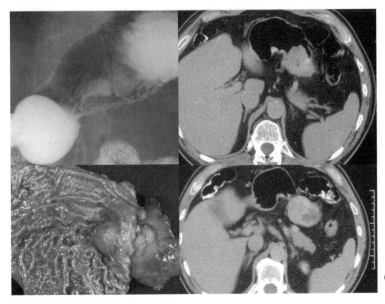

Figure 2-7-14

Gastrointestinal stromal tumor

GIST - Internal Hemorrhage and Necrosis

Figure 2-7-15

GIST - Cyst Formation

GIST - Cavity Formation

GIST - Calcification

Differential Diagnosis
Gastric GIST vs. Adenocarcinoma
[Figure 2-7-15]

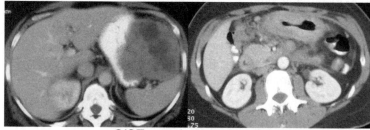

GIST vs. adenocarcinoma

Figure 2-7-16

Differential Diagnosis
Gastric GIST vs. Lymphoma
[Figure 2- 7-16]

GIST vs. lymphoma

Gastric Carcinoid
- Type I: autoimmune chronic atrophic gastritis
  - ➢ Hypergastrinemia
  - ➢ Multiple, small
  - ➢ Benign biologic behavior
- Type II: MEN I and Zollinger Ellison syndrome
  - ➢ Hypergastrinemia
  - ➢ Multiple, small
  - ➢ Benign biologic behavior
- Type III: sporadic
  - ➢ Single
  - ➢ Aggressive biologic behavior

Carcinoid: Imaging Features
- Submucosal mass
- Central ulceration-"bull's eye"
- Pedunculated polypoid lesions, rarely
- Large ulcerative masses
- Thick, rugal folds if hypergastrinemia is present

Carcinoid: "Bull's Eye Lesion"

Carcinoid: Pedunculated Polyps

Kaposi Sarcoma
- AIDS patients
- Cutaneous KS usually
- Stomach, duodenum, and small bowel most common gi locations
- Radiologic features
  - ➢ Submucosal masses
  - ➢ "Bull's-eye"appearance
  - ➢ Polypoid masses
  - ➢ Infiltrating variant, rare

Metastases
- Melanoma, breast, lung
- Radiologic features
  - ➢ Ulcerating masses
  - ➢ Polyps
  - ➢ Infiltrating
  - ➢ "Linitis Plastica"

Summary: Adenocarcinoma

- *H. pylori*
- Chronic atrophic gastritis
- Primary tumor morphology
  - ➢ Polypoid
  - ➢ Ulcerating
  - ➢ Infiltrating
  - ➢ Schirrous
- CT: extragastric spread

Summary: Lymphoma

- *H. pylori*
- Low grade MALT to high grade B cell
- Compared to adenocarcinoma
  - ➢ Greater wall thickening
  - ➢ Bulky, more extensive adenopathy

Summary: GIST

- Most common mesenchymal neoplasm
- KIT reactivity
  - ➢ Diagnosis
  - ➢ Gleevac therapy
- Classic mural masses on barium
- May have extensive extragastric growth

Summary: Bull's Eye Lesions

- Carcinoid
- Metastasis
  - ➢ (Breast, Lung, Melanoma)
- Kaposi's Sarcoma
- Lymphoma
- Adenocarcinoma
- Ectopic Pancreas

Gastric Malignancies References

Gastric Carcinoma

Balthazar EJ, Siegel SE, Megibow AJ, et al: CT in patients with scirrhous carcinoma of the GI tract: imaging findings and value for tumor detection and staging. AJR 165:839, 1995

Gore RM: Gastric cancer. Clinical and pathologic features. Radiol Clin North Am 35:295, 1997

Gore RM, Levine MS, Ghahremani GG, et al: Gastric cancer. Radiologic diagnosis. Radiol Clin North Am 35:311, 1997

Levine MS, Kong V, Rubesin SE, et al: Scirrhous carcinoma of the stomach: radiologic and endoscopic diagnosis. Radiology 175:151, 1990

Longmire WP, Jr.: A current view of gastric cancer in the US. Ann Surg 218:579, 1993

Miller FH, Kochman ML, Talamonti MS, et al: Gastric cancer. Radiologic staging. Radiol Clin North Am 35:331, 1997

Morales TG: Adenocarcinoma of the gastric cardia. Dig Dis 15:346, 1997

Parsonnet J: Helicobacter pylori and gastric cancer. Gastroenterol Clin North Am 22:89, 1993

Parsonnet J, Friedman GD, Vandersteen DP, et al: Helicobacter pylori infection and the risk of gastric carcinoma. N Engl J Med 325:1127, 1991

Sipponen P, Marshall BJ: Gastritis and gastric cancer. Western countries. Gastroenterol Clin North Am 29:579, 2000

Gastric Lymphoma

An SK, Han JK, Kim YH, et al: Gastric mucosa-associated lymphoid tissue lymphoma: spectrum of findings at double-contrast gastrointestinal examination with pathologic correlation. Radiographics 21:1491, 2001

Buy JN, Moss AA: Computed tomography of gastric lymphoma. AJR 138:859, 1982

Choi D, Lim HK, Lee SJ, et al: Gastric mucosa-associated lymphoid tissue lymphoma: helical CT findings and pathologic correlation. AJR 178:1117, 2002

Jaffe ES, Harris NL, Stein H, et al (eds): World Health Organization Classification of Tumours: Pathology and Genetics of Tumours of Haematopoietic and Lymphoid Tissues), Lyon: IARC Press, 2001

Kim YH, Lim HK, Han JK, et al: Low-grade gastric mucosa-associated lymphoid tissue lymphoma: correlation of radiographic and pathologic findings. Radiology 212:241, 1999

Levine MS, Elmas N, Furth EE, et al: Helicobacter pylori and gastric MALT lymphoma. AJR Am J Roentgenol 166:85, 1996

Levine MS, Rubesin SE, Pantongrag-Brown L, et al: Non-Hodgkin's lymphoma of the gastrointestinal tract: radiographic findings. AJR Am J Roentgenol 168:165, 1997

Megibow AJ, Balthazar EJ, Naidich DP, et al: Computed tomography of gastrointestinal lymphoma. AJR 141:541, 1983

Parsonnet J, Hansen S, Rodriguez L, et al: Helicobacter pylori infection and gastric lymphoma. N Engl J Med 330:1267, 1994

Wotherspoon AC, Doglioni C, de Boni M, et al: Antibiotic treatment for low-grade gastric MALT lymphoma. Lancet 343:1503, 1994

Yoo CC, Levine MS, Furth EE, et al: Gastric mucosa-associated lymphoid tissue lymphoma: radiographic findings in six patients. Radiology 208:239, 1998

Gastrointestinal Stromal Tumor (GIST)

Burkill GJ, Badran M, Al-Muderis O, et al: Malignant gastrointestinal stromal tumor: distribution, imaging features, and pattern of metastatic spread. Radiology 226:527, 2003

Chen MY, Bechtold RE, Savage PD: Cystic changes in hepatic metastases from gastrointestinal stromal tumors (GISTs) treated with Gleevec (imatinib mesylate). AJR 179:1059, 2002

Dematteo RP, Heinrich MC, El-Rifai WM, et al: Clinical management of gastrointestinal stromal tumors: before and after STI-571. Hum Pathol 33:466, 2002

Fletcher CD: Clinicopathologic correlations in gastrointestinal stromal tumors. Hum Pathol 33:455, 2002

Fletcher CD, Berman JJ, Corless C, et al: Diagnosis of gastrointestinal stromal tumors: A consensus approach. Hum Pathol 33:459, 2002

Levy AD, Remotti HE, Thompson WM, et al: From the Archives of the AFIP: Gastrointestinal Stromal Tumors: Radiologic Features with Pathologic Correlation. RadioGraphics 23:283, 2003

Miettinen M, El-Rifai W, Sobin LH, et al: Evaluation of malignancy and prognosis of gastrointestinal stromal tumors: a review. Hum Pathol 33:478, 2002

Miettinen M, Lasota J: Gastrointestinal stromal tumors—definition, clinical, histological, immunohistochemical, and molecular genetic features and differential diagnosis. Virchows Arch 438:1, 2001

Nishida T, Kumano S, Sugiura T, et al: Multidetector CT of high-risk patients with occult gastrointestinal stromal tumors. AJR Am J Roentgenol 180:185, 2003

Sharp RM, Ansel HJ, Keel SB: Best cases from the AFIP: gastrointestinal stromal tumor. Armed Forces Institute of Pathology. RadioGraphics 21:1557, 2001

Gastric Carcinoid

Balthazar EJ, Megibow A, Bryk D, et al: Gastric carcinoid tumors: radiographic features in eight cases. AJR Am J Roentgenol 139:1123, 1982

Berger MW, Stephens DH: Gastric carcinoid tumors associated with chronic hypergastrinemia in a patient with Zollinger-Ellison syndrome. Radiology 201:371, 1996

Binstock AJ, Johnson CD, Stephens DH, et al: Carcinoid tumors of the stomach: a clinical and radiographic study. AJR 176:947, 2001

Borch K, Renvall H, Kullman E, et al: Gastric carcinoid associated with the syndrome of hypergastrinemic atrophic gastritis. A prospective analysis of 11 cases. Am J Surg Pathol 11:435, 1987

Ho AC, Horton KM, Fishman EK: Gastric carcinoid tumors as a consequence of chronic hypergastrinemia: spiral CT findings. Clin Imaging 24:200, 2000

Abdominal Non Hodgkin Lymphoma: Radiologic–Pathologic Correlation

Angela D. Levy, LTC, MC, USA
Department of Radiologic Pathology
Armed Forces Institute of Pathology
Washington

Objectives
- Definition
- Patterns of disease
  - NHL Adenopathy
  - Gastrointestinal Lymphoma
- Immunodeficiency-related lymphomas
  - Post-transplantation Lymphoproliferative Disorder (PTLD)
  - AIDS-related Lymphomas

Lymphoid Neoplams
- 2001 WHO classification of Hematological Malignancies
- Three major categories
  - B cell, T and NK (natural killer) cell, Hodgkin lymphoma
- NHL
  - Large group of diverse diseases

Non-Hodgkin Lymphoma (NHL)
- 4% of all cancers
- 4 times more common than Hodgkin lymphoma in the U.S.
- More common in men, 1.3 to 1
- Median age 55 years
- Third most common cancer mortality in children under age 15

Non-Hodgkin Lymphoma
- Rising incidence
  - True increase in incidence
  - Improved identification and understanding
  - HIV infection
  - Organ transplants
- Immunodeficiency increases risk
  - Wiskott-Aldrich syndrome
  - Ataxia telangiectasia
  - Long-term immunosuppressive therapy

Role of Imaging in Newly Diagnosed NHL
- Clinical Staging:
  - Ann Arbor Staging Classification
  - Tumor bulk has important prognostic significance in intermediate and high grade NHL
- Identification of nodal and extranodal sites
  - Mesenteric adenopathy
  - GI tract
  - Liver
  - Spleen

NHL: Abdomimal Adenopathy
- Retroperitoneum
- Mesentery
- CT attenuation
  - Homogeneous in most cases
  - Heterogeneous in cases with aggressive histology

- Radiologic Patterns
  - Discrete rounded nodes
  - Confluent nodes
  - Ill-defined masses
  - Mesenteric caking
  - Stellate mesentery

NHL: Discrete Nodes [Figure 2-8-1]

NHL: Sandwich Sign [Figure 2-8-2]

NHL: Confluent Nodes [Figure 2-8-3]

NHL: Mesenteric Caking

Differential Diagnosis: Mesenteric Masses
- Lymphoma
- Castleman
- Fibromatosis
- Gastrointestinal Stromal Tumor (GIST)
- Metastasis
- Carcinoid
- Tuberculosis
- Histoplasmosis
- Sarcoid
- Inflammatory Pseudotumor

Castleman Disease

Mesenteric Fibromatosis (Desmoid Tumor)

Mesenteric Gastrointestinal Stromal Tumor (GIST)

Carcinoid

Gastrointestinal Lymphoma
- Lymphoma that presents with GI disease and no other major site of involvement
- Most common extranodal site of NHL
  - 4.4% of all lymphomas
  - 25% of all extranodal lymphomas

Gastrointestinal Lymphoma
- Almost exclusively NHL
- Stomach is the most common site in US and Western Europe
- Small bowel is the most common site in the Mediterranean, Northern Africa, Middle East
- Clinical Features
  - More common in men, 2:1
  - Presenting signs and symptoms dependent on anatomic location and tumor morphology

Gastrointestinal Lymphoma
- B-cell lymphomas
  - MALT lymphomas
    - ❖ Immunoproliferative small intestinal disease, "alpha-heavy chain disease"
  - Mantle cell lymphoma (multiple lymphomatous polyposis)
  - Burkitt and Burkitt-type lymphoma
  - Nodal equivalents (diffuse large B-cell lymphomas, follicular, etc)

Figure 2-8-1

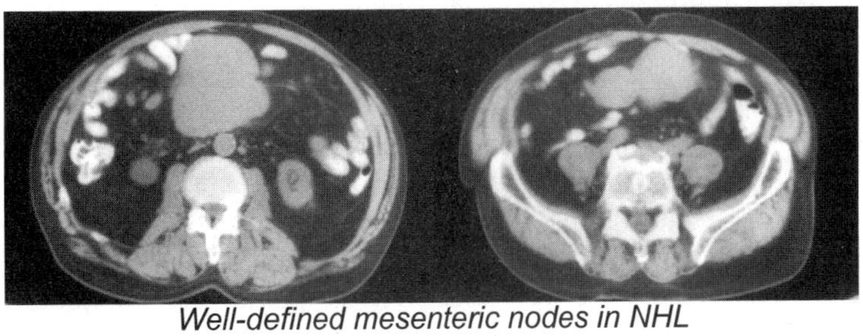

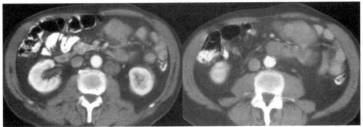

Well-defined mesenteric nodes in NHL

Figure 2-8-2

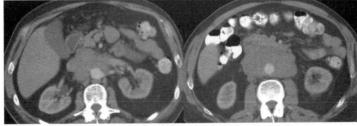

Sandwich sign of the mesentery in NHL

Figure 2-8-3

Confluent retroperitoneal nodes in NHL

- T-cell lymphoma
  - ➤ Enteropathy-type T-cell lymphoma (ETTL)

NHL: Small Intestine
- Approximately 25% of all primary small bowel malignancies
- Male predominance, mean age 60 years
- Clinical presentation:
  - ➤ Weight loss, pain, bleeding
  - ➤ Intussusception, obstruction, perforation
- Ileum most common location and duodenum least common
- Multiple lesions in 10 to 25% of cases

NHL Small Bowel Lymphoma: Radiologic Patterns
- Mural infiltration
  - ➤ Fold thickening
  - ➤ Circumferential wall thickening
  - ➤ Luminal dilatation
- Polypoid nodules
  - ➤ Solitary
  - ➤ Multiple (lymphomatous polyposis)
- Cavities
- Mesenteric disease

NHL Small Intestine: Tumor Morphology [Figure 2-8-4]

NHL Small Intestine: Mural Infiltration [Figure 2-8-5]

NHL Small Intestine: Cavitary Mass [Figure 2-8-6]

Figure 2-8-4

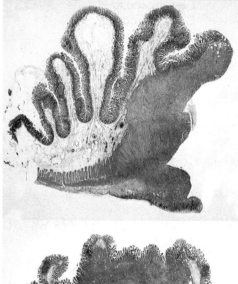

Lymphoma histology shows tumor extension from mucosa to serosa

Figure 2-8-6

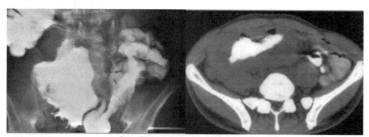

Cavitary mass

NHL Small Intestine: Adjacent Mesenteric Disease
[Figure 2-8-7]

Figure 2-8-7

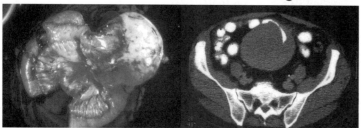

Mesenteric mass engulfing small intestine

Figure 2-8-5

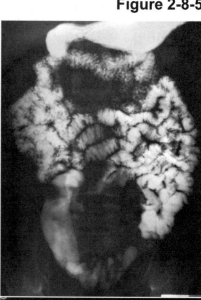

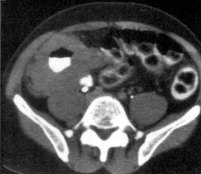

Mural infiltration with luminal dilatation

Burkitt Lymphoma
- High grade B-cell lymphoma
- More common in males
- Endemic
  - ➢ African Burkitt, related to EBV
  - ➢ Head and neck disease
- Sporadic
  - ➢ Western countries, non related to EBV
  - ➢ ileocecal region of children (not EBV-related)
- Clinical presentation
  - ➢ intestinal obstruction
  - ➢ intussusception

Figure 2-8-8

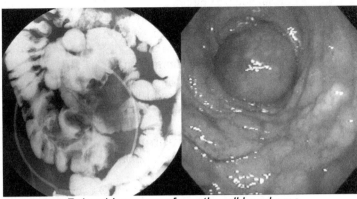

Polypoid masses of mantle cell lymphoma

Mantle Cell Lymphoma [Figure 2-8-8]

Mantle Cell Lymphoma (Multiple Lymphomatous Polyposis)
- Histologically resembles the mantle zone of the lymph follicle
- Median age 65, male predominance
- Presentation: abdominal pain and bloody stools
- Multiple polyps, 0.5 to 2.0 cm, or solitary
- Most common in the ileocecal region

Enteropathy-Type T-cell Lymphoma (ETTL) [Figure 2-8-9]
- Celiac disease (Sprue)
- Sixth to seventh decade of life
- Most common site jejunum
- Gross pathology: ulcerated plaques or strictures in the proximal small bowel
- Poor prognosis

NHL Small Intestine: Differential Diagnosis
- Adenocarcinoma
- GIST
- Carcinoid
- Metastases
- Crohn disease
- Tuberculosis
- Mesenteric fibromatosis
- Causes of fold thickening
  - ➢ Sprue
  - ➢ Hemorrhage
  - ➢ Edema
  - ➢ Ischemia

Figure 2-8-9

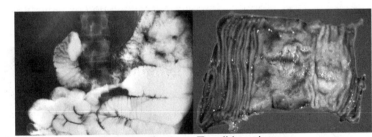

Enteropathy type T-cell lymphoma

Malignant Melanoma Metastases

Gastrointestinal Stromal Tumor

Jejunal Adenocarcinoma

Tuberculosis / Lymphoma

Post-transplantation Lymphoproliferative Disorder (PTLD)
- Spectrum of benign and malignant disorders
- Variable incidence
  - ➢ 1% renal transplants
  - ➢ 10% combined heart/lung
  - ➢ 10% of patients on cyclosporine and OKT3
- Association with EBV infection
- Lung, GI tract

PTLD *[Figures 2- 8-10 and 2-8-11]*
- Pathologic Features
  - ➤ Driven by Epstein-Barr Virus infection
  - ➤ Diffuse polyclonal expansion
  - ➤ Reduced T-cell control
  - ➤ Malignant transformation
- Clinical
  - ➤ May respond to reducing immunosuppression, anti-virals, surgery

AIDS-Related Lymphoma
- Second most common neoplasm in HIV infection
- AIDS defining illness
- Incidence is 4 to 10% in the AIDS population
- Three categories
  - ➤ Systemic (nodal and/or extranodal)
  - ➤ Primary CNS
  - ➤ Body cavity-based (primary effusion) lymphomas
- Major histologic subtypes
  - ➤ Burkitt lymphoma
  - ➤ Burkitt-like lymphoma
  - ➤ Large cell lymphoma
  - ➤ Large cell immunoblastic lymphoma

AIDS-Related Lymphoma
- 25% have GI tract disease
- Higher incidence of mesenteric disease than non-AIDS lymphomas
- Aggressive histology and biologic behavior
  - ➤ Atypical radiologic features
  - ➤ Hemorrhage
  - ➤ Necrosis
- Unique cavity-based lymphoma
  - ➤ Kaposi's sarcoma-associated herpes virus (KSHV)
- Anorectal lymphoma is unique to AIDS

Primary Peritoneal Lymphoma
[Figure 2-8-12]

Colonic Lymphoma

Anorectal Lymphoma

Summary
- Spectrum of Adenopathy
- ➤ GI lymphomas are predominantly NHL
  - ➤ Unique subtypes involve the bowel
  - ➤ Various patterns: infiltrating masses, luminal dilatation, polyps, cavitary masses, mesenteric masses
- AIDS-related
  - ➤ Aggressive behavior
  - ➤ Unusual sites, unusual manifestations
- PTLD
  - ➤ Colon, liver

Figure 2-8-10

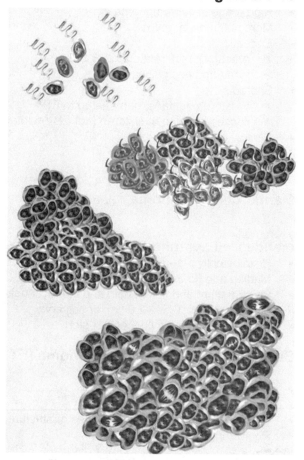

Pathogenesis of post-transplantation lymphoproliferative disorder

Figure 2-8-11

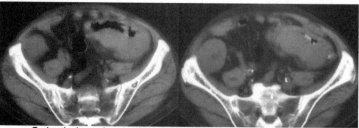

Colonic lymphoma in a patient with a renal transplant

Figure 2-8-12

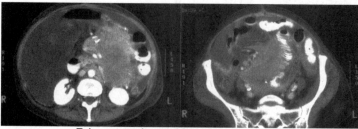

Primary peritoneal lymphoma in AIDS

Patterns of Adenopathy

Patterns of Small Bowel Disease

Mural Infiltration

Polyps

Cavitary Masses

Mesenteric Masses

AIDS-Related Lymphomas

Post Transplantation Lymphoproliferative Disorder (PTLD)

Lymphoma References

Ann Arbor Staging of Gastrointestinal Lymphomas

Stage IE: Confined to the wall of the stomach or bowel
Stage II1E: Regional lymph nodes contiguous to primary site
Stage II2E: Regional lymph nodes not contiguous to primary site
Stage III: Lymph nodes on both sides of the diaphragm, spleen (IIIS), or
   both (IIIE&S)
Stage IV: Bone marrow or other non-hematolymphoid organ

Lymphoma Classification

Harris NL, Jaffe ES, Diebold J, et al: The World Health Organization classification of
   neoplasms of the hematopoietic and lymphoid tissues: report of the Clinical
   Advisory Committee meeting--Airlie House, Virginia, November, 1997. Hematol
   J 1:53, 2000
Jaffe ES, Harris NL, Stein H, et al (eds): World Health Organization
   Classification of Tumours: Pathology and Genetics of Tumours of
   Haematopoietic and Lymphoid Tissues), Lyon: IARC Press, 2001

Imaging of non Hodgkin lymphoma

Byun JH, Ha HK, Kim AY, et al: CT Findings in Peripheral T-Cell Lymphoma Involving
   the Gastrointestinal Tract. Radiology 227:59, 2003
Choi D, Lim HK, Lee SJ, et al: Gastric mucosa-associated lymphoid tissue lymphoma:
   helical CT findings and pathologic correlation. AJR 178:1117, 2002
Crump M, Gospodarowicz M, Shepherd FA: Lymphoma of the gastrointestinal tract.
   Semin Oncol 26:324, 1999
Gossios K, Katsimbri P, Tsianos E: CT features of gastric lymphoma. Eur Radiol
   10:425, 2000
Isaacson PG: Gastrointestinal lymphoma. Hum Pathol 25:1020, 1994
Isaacson PG: Gastrointestinal lymphomas of T- and B-cell types. Mod Pathol 12:151,
   1999
Isaacson PG: Intestinal lymphoma and enteropathy. J Pathol 177:111, 1995
Isaacson PG: Mucosa-associated lymphoid tissue lymphoma. Semin Hematol 36:139,
   1999
Isaacson PG, MacLennan KA, Subbuswamy SG: Multiple lymphomatous polyposis of
   the gastrointestinal tract. Histopathology 8:641, 1984
Kessar P, Norton A, Rohatiner AZ, et al: CT appearances of mucosa-associated
   lymphoid tissue (MALT) lymphoma. Eur Radiol 9:693, 1999
Levine MS, Elmas N, Furth EE, et al: Helicobacter pylori and gastric MALT lymphoma.
   AJR Am J Roentgenol 166:85, 1996

Levine MS, Rubesin SE, Pantongrag-Brown L, et al: Non-Hodgkin's lymphoma of the gastrointestinal tract: radiographic findings. AJR Am J Roentgenol 168:165, 1997

Megibow AJ, Balthazar EJ, Naidich DP, et al: Computed tomography of gastrointestinal lymphoma. AJR 141:541, 1983

Park MS, Kim KW, Yu JS, et al: Radiographic findings of primary B-cell lymphoma of the stomach: low-grade versus high-grade malignancy in relation to the mucosa-associated lymphoid tissue concept. AJR 179:1297, 2002

Rodallec M, Guermazi A, Brice P, et al: Imaging of MALT lymphomas. Eur Radiol 12:348, 2002

Sheth S, Horton KM, Garland MR, et al: Mesenteric Neoplasms: CT Appearances of Primary and Secondary Tumors and Differential Diagnosis. Radiographics 23:457, 2003

AIDS-related lymphomas

Albin J, Lewis E, Eftekhari F, et al: Computed tomography of rectal and perirectal disease in AIDS patients. Gastrointest Radiol 12:67, 1987

Brar HS, Gottesman L, Surawicz C: Anorectal pathology in AIDS. Gastrointest Endosc Clin N Am 8:913, 1998

Burkes RL, Meyer PR, Gill PS, et al: Rectal lymphoma in homosexual men. Arch Intern Med 146:913, 1986

Ferrozzi F, Tognini G, Mulonzia NW, et al: Primary effusion lymphomas in AIDS: CT findings in two cases. Eur Radiol 11:623, 2001

Gottlieb CA, Meiri E, Maeda KM: Rectal non-Hodgkin's lymphoma: a clinicopathologic study and review. Henry Ford Hosp Med J 38:255, 1990

Ioachimm HL, Antonescu C, Giancotti F, et al: EBV-associated anorectal lymphomas in patients with acquired immune deficiency syndrome. Am J Surg Pathol 21:997, 1997?

Munn S: Imaging HIV/AIDS. Burkitt's lymphoma. AIDS Patient Care STDS 16:395, 2002

Post-transplantation lymphoproliferative disorder

Meador TL, Krebs TL, Cheong JJ, et al: Imaging features of posttransplantation lymphoproliferative disorder in pancreas transplant recipients. AJR Am J Roentgenol 174:121, 2000

Pickhardt PJ, Siegel MJ: Abdominal manifestations of posttransplantation lymphoproliferative disorder. AJR Am J Roentgenol 171:1007, 1998

Pickhardt PJ, Siegel MJ: Posttransplantation lymphoproliferative disorder of the abdomen: CT evaluation in 51 patients. Radiology 213:73, 1999

Pickhardt PJ, Siegel MJ, Hayashi RJ, et al: Posttransplantation lymphoproliferative disorder in children: clinical, histopathologic, and imaging features. Radiology 217:16, 2000

Tubman DE, Frick MP, Hanto DW: Lymphoma after organ transplantation: radiologic manifestations in the central nervous system, thorax, and abdomen. Radiology 149:625, 1983

Vrachliotis TG, Vaswani KK, Davies EA, et al: CT findings in posttransplantation lymphoproliferative disorder of renal transplants. AJR Am J Roentgenol 175:183, 2000

Wu L, Rappaport DC, Hanbidge A, et al: Lymphoproliferative disorders after liver transplantation: imaging features. Abdom Imaging 26:200, 2001

Small Intestinal Neoplasms
Radiologic-Pathologic Correlation

Angela D. Levy, LTC, MC, USA
Department of Radiologic Pathology
Armed Forces Institute of Pathology
Washington, DC

Small Intestinal Neoplasms
Case Based Approach
- Benign tumors and tumor-like lesions
  - Brunner gland lesions
  - Adenoma
  - Heterotopia
- Malignant neoplasms
  - Adenocarcinoma
  - Carcinoid
  - Lymphoma
  - Gastrointestinal stromal tumor
  - Metastatic disease

38-year-old HIV+ man with recent onset of abdominal pain
[Figure 2-9-1]

Differential Diagnosis Duodenal Polyp

Figure 2-9-1

- Nonneoplastic
  - Brunner gland hamartoma
  - Heterotopia
  - Prolapsed antral mucosa
- Neoplastic
  - Adenoma
  - Adenocarcinoma
  - GIST
  - Prolapsed gastric neoplasm

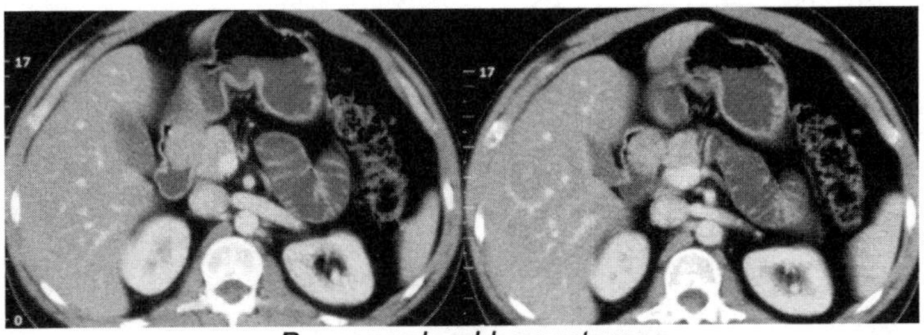

Brunner gland hamartoma

Brunner Gland Hamartoma
- Solitary hamartoma
  - Brunner glands, muscular, and fatty elements
  - Heterotopic pancreatic acini and ducts
- Synonym: Brunner gland adenoma
- Most common in duodenal bulb
- Patients
  - 4th to 6th decade
  - Incidental lesions
  - Rarely, obstruction, bleeding
- Treatment
  - Resection

Brunner Gland Hyperplasia
- Hyperplasia of Brunner gland tissue
- Associations
  - Duodenal ulcers
  - Gastric hypersecretory states
- Treatment
  - None

Brunner Gland Hyperplasia [Figure 2-9-2]

Figure 2-9-2

- Differential diagnosis
  - ➢ Brunner gland hyperplasia
  - ➢ Lymphoid hyperplasia
  - ➢ Duodenitis
  - ➢ Polyposis syndromes
  - ➢ Heterotopia

68-year-old woman with recurrent pancreatitis
[Figure 2-9-3]

Figure 2-9-3

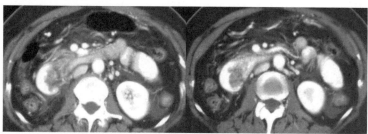

Periampullary tubulovillous adenoma

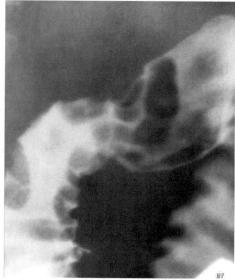

Brunner gland hyperplasia

Differential Diagnosis: Periampullary Duodenal Mass

- Adenoma
  - ➢ Villous adenoma
  - ➢ Polyposis syndromes
- Adenocarcinoma
  - ➢ Periampullary
  - ➢ Ampullary
  - ➢ Pancreatic
- Carcinoid
  - ➢ Neurofibromatosis (NF-1)
- GIST
- Mets
- Choledochocele
- Duplication cyst

Tubulovillous Adenoma

Adenoma

Figure 2-9-4

- Benign intraepithelial neoplasm composed of dysplastic cells
  - ➢ Tubular, villous, or tubulovillous histology
  - ➢ May progress to adenocarcinoma
- Uncommon
  - ➢ 30% of benign small bowel tumors
- Locations
  - ➢ 80% are periampullary
- Increased incidence
  - ➢ Familial adenomatous polyposis, FAP
  - ➢ Hereditary nonpolyposis colon carcinoma, HNPCC

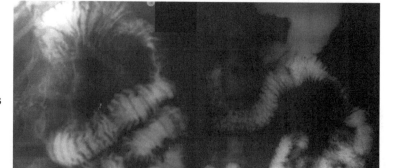

Pancreatic heterotopia

42-year-old woman with abdominal pain [Figure 2-9-4]

Differential Diagnosis
- Nonneoplastic
  - Pancreatitis
  - Diverticulitis
  - Crohn disease
  - Celiac disease
  - Parasitic infection
  - Cryptosporidiosis
  - Hemorrhage
- Neoplastic
  - Adenocarcinoma
  - Lymphoma
  - Metastasis

Pancreatic Heterotopia

Heterotopia
- Ectopic tissue
  - Pancreatic and gastric most common
- Term *myoepithelial hamartoma*
  - Composed of pancreatic ducts and muscle only

Heterotopia
- Small bowel most common site
  - Duodenum most common location in small bowel
  - Stomach most common symptomatic site
  - Meckel diverticulum
- Imaging features
  - Tumor-like nodule
  - Mural thickening
  - Inflammation

71-year-old woman with jaundice *[Figures 2-9-5]*

Figure 2-9-5

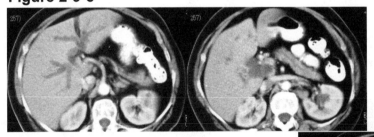

Periampullary adenocarcinoma

Differential Diagnosis
- Villous adenoma
- Adenocarcinoma
  - Pancreatic
  - Ampullary
  - Periampullary
- Carcinoid
- GIST
- Metastasis

Periampullary Adenocarcinoma

75-year-old woman with epigastric pain and nausea for 4 months

Intussuscepting Mass

Differential Diagnosis: Intussuscepting Mass
- Malignant
  - Adenocarcinoma
  - Carcinoid
  - Lymphoma
  - GIST
  - Metastasis

Differential Diagnosis: Intussuscepting Mass
- Benign
  - Adenoma
  - Peutz Jegher polyp
  - Lipoma
  - Uncommon
    - ❖ Neurofibroma
    - ❖ Schwannoma
    - ❖ Inflammatory fibroid polyp
    - ❖ Heterotopia

Adenocarcinoma Arising in a Villous Adenoma

Small Intestine: Malignant Neoplasms
- Uncommon
  - True incidence unclear
- SEER data
  - Annual incidence 9.9 per million
- Frequency
  - Adenocarcinoma
  - Carcinoid
  - Lymphoma
  - Gastrointestinal stromal tumor

Adenocarcinoma
- More common in proximal small intestine *
  - 55% periampullary/ampullary
  - 10% duodenum
  - 25% jejunum
  - 10% ileum
- Duodenal adenocarcinoma associated with colonic adenocarcinoma
  - APC gene
  - Mismatch repair gene

Riddel RH, Petras RE, Williams GT, Sobin LH. Atlas of Tumor Pathology:Tumors of the Intestines. AFIP 2003

Adenocarcinoma
- Most patients between 50 and 60 years
  - Mean age, 55 years
- Clinical presentation
  - Obstruction, intussusception, bleeding, jaundice

Adenocarcinoma
- Most patients have no predisposing condition
- Predisposing conditions
  - Familial adenomatous polyposis (FAP)
  - Hereditary nonpolyposis colon carcinoma (HNPCC)
  - Peutz-Jeghers syndrome
  - Crohn disease
  - Celiac disease
  - Duplication
  - Ileostomy sites
  - Ileal pouches
  - Bypassed bowel

Adenocarcinoma: Pathology
- Polypoid or infiltrative
  - Ampulla/periampullary
  - Duodenum
- Annular constricting
  - Jejunum
  - Ileum
- Ulcerating
- Linitis plastica
  - Rare

Adenocarcinoma Duodenum Periampullary

Adenocarcinoma Jejunum [Figure 2-9-6]

Crohn Disease and Adenocarcinoma
- Incidence 3 to 18x normal
- Cancer features
  - Male predominance, 3:1
  - Dysplasia to carcinoma sequence
  - Occur in the distribution of Crohn disease
  - Incidental finding in resected fistulas and fissures
- Distribution
  - Small intestine 25%
  - Colon 70%
  - Other sites 5% (fissure, fistula, stoma, bypassed bowel)

Crohn Disease and Adenocarcinoma [Figure 2-9-7]
- Difficult preoperative diagnosis
- Increase suspicion
  - New symptoms in quiescent disease
  - Development of mass, stricture, or obstruction

Differential Diagnosis: Jejunal or Ileal Stricture
- Neoplastic
  - Adenocarcinoma
  - Carcinoid
  - Lymphoma
  - Metastasis

Differential Diagnosis: Jejunal or Ileal Stricture
- Nonneoplastic
  - Crohn disease
  - Tuberculosis
  - Celiac
  - NSAID
  - Ischemia
  - Heterotopia
  - Radiation

Figure 2-9-6

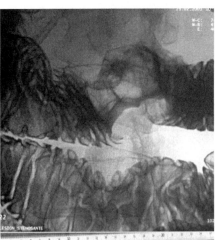
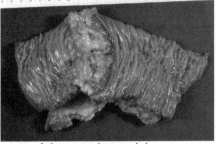

Adenocarcinoma jejunum

Figure 2-9-7

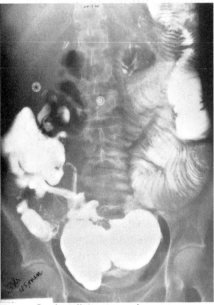

Crohn disease and adenocarcinoma

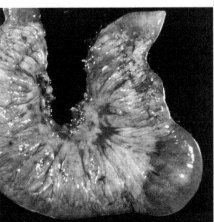

50-year-old man with abdominal pain and diarrhea [Figures 2-9-8]

Figure 2-9-8

Carcinoid
- Well-differentiated endocrine neoplasms
- All have malignant potential
- Classification
  - ➢ Foregut
    - ❖ Stomach and proximal duodenum
  - ➢ Midgut
    - ❖ Distal duodenum, small bowel, ascending colon, proximal transverse colon
  - ➢ Hindgut
    - ❖ Distal transverse colon, descending colon, rectum
- 60% to 80% carcinoids are midgut

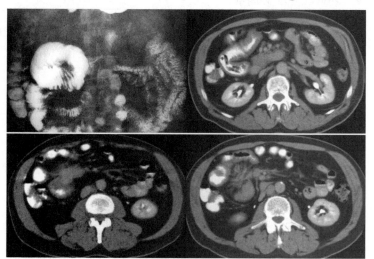

Carcinoid

Duodenal Carcinoid
- Most common in first and second portion
- Low-grade malignancies
- Associations
  - ➢ Zollinger-Ellison syndrome
  - ➢ Multiple endocrine neoplasia (MEN 1)
  - ➢ Neurofibromatosis

Duodenal Carcinoid: Imaging Features
- Sessile polyp
  - ➢ < 1 cm
  - ➢ Duodenal bulb
- Multiple polyps
  - ➢ Rare
- Intramural mass
  - ➢ May have ulceration
  - ➢ Periampullary region

Duodenal Carcinoid in NF-1

Jejunal and Ileal Carcinoid
- Second most common location after appendix
- Aggressive biologic behavior
- Serotonin production
- Associated desmoplasia
  - ➢ Wall of the bowel
  - ➢ Adjacent mesentery
  - ➢ Blood vessels, "elastic vascular sclerosis"

Carcinoid Pathology

Carcinoid Desmoplasia

Jejunal and Ileal Carcinoid: Imaging Features
- Local nodal metastasis most prominent feature
  - ➢ Spiculated, fibrotic mass adjacent to bowel
  - ➢ Sunburst pattern of vessels on angiogram
  - ➢ May calcify
- Extensive wall abnormalities
  - ➢ Luminal narrowing
  - ➢ Thick, spiculated folds
- Discrete mass in wall of bowel
  - ➢ Mural mass

- ➢ Polypoid mass
- ➢ Multiple masses, less common

Carcinoid Ileum

Jejunal and Ileal Carcinoid: Key Imaging Features
- Calcified mesenteric mass
- Radiating strands
- Adjacent bowel wall thickening

Carcinoid Syndrome
- 10% of patients with carcinoids
- Most common with ileal carcinoids
- Usually hepatic metastasis are present
  - ➢ Serotonin and metabolites in systemic circulation
- Classic syndrome
  - ➢ Paroxysms of sweating, flushing, cyanosis, wheezing, abdominal colic, right-sided heart failure, diarrhea
  - ➢ Symptoms precipitated by ETOH intake, stress, exercise
- Carcinoid heart disease

77-year-old asymptomatic man [Figure 2-9-9]

Figure 2-9-9

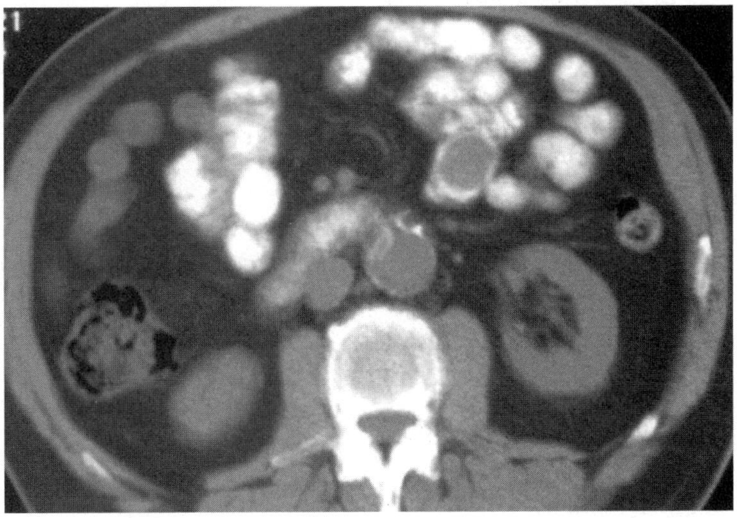

Differential Diagnosis: Small Bowel Polypoid Mass
- Benign
  - ➢ Adenoma
  - ➢ Peutz Jegher polyp
  - ➢ Inflammatory fibroid polyp
- Malignant
  - ➢ Adenocarcinoma
  - ➢ Lymphoma
  - ➢ GIST
  - ➢ Metastatic disease

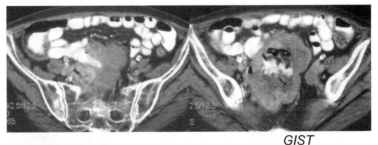

Gastrointestinal Stromal Tumor (GIST)
- Most common mesenchymal neoplasm
- Variable biologic behavior
  - ➢ Benign or malignant
  - ➢ Size, mitotic rate
- Pathology
  - ➢ Spindle or epithelioid cells
  - ➢ Skeinoid fibers present in small intestinal GISTs
  - ➢ KIT (CD 117) positive

Figure 2-9-10

GIST: Small Intestine
[Figures 2-9-10 and 2-9-11]

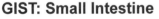

GIST

Figure 2-9-11

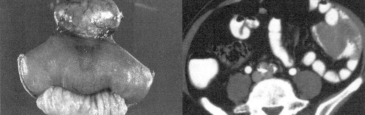

GIST

52-year-old man with NF-1 complains of abdominal pain

Gastrointestinal Neoplasms in NF-1
- Carcinoid
  - Duodenum
- Gastrointestinal stromal tumors
  - Small intestine, multiple
- Neurofibroma
- Ganglioneuroma
- Leiomyoma, leiomyosarcoma
- Adenocarcinoma

Metastatic Disease
- Intraperitoneal spread
- Hematogenous spread
  - Melanoma
  - Bronchogenic carcinoma
  - Breast
- Direct extension
- Lymphatic spread

Summary: Brunner Gland Lesions
- Brunner gland hamartoma
  - Solitary mass
  - Proximal duodenum
- Brunner gland hyperplasia
  - Multiple nodules
  - Proximal duodenum

Summary: Adenoma
- Uncommon
- Most periampullary
- Association
  - FAP
  - HNPCC

Summary: Heterotopia
- Ectopic normal tissue
- Most common in small bowel
- Imaging
  - Focal nodular mass
  - Mural thickening
  - Localized inflammation

Summary: Adenocarcinoma
- Periampullary location most common
- Morphology
  - Polypoid
  - Infiltrating
  - Annular
  - Ulcerating

Summary: Carcinoid
- Endocrine neoplasms
- Midgut most common
- Serotonin production
- Key imaging features
  - Mesenteric mass
  - Radiating strands
  - Bowel wall thickening

Summary: GIST

- Most common mesenchymal neoplasm
- KIT positive
- Mural masses
  - Intraluminal polyp
  - Exophytic component
  - Hemorrhage
  - Cyst formation
  - Cavitation

Colorectal Carcinoma
Radiologic-Pathologic Correlation

Angela D. Levy, LTC, MC, USA
Department of Radiologic Pathology
Armed Forces Institute of Pathology
Washington, DC

Colorectal Carcinoma: Objectives
- Epidemiology/pathogenesis
- Screening
- Detection
  - Preoperative assessment

Colorectal Carcinoma
- Third most frequent cancer in the U.S.
  - 147,000 new cases in 2003
  - 57,000 deaths in 2004
  - 11% of cancers in men and women
  - 10% of cancer deaths
  - Mortality rate is declining over the past 15 years, 1.7% per year

Colorectal Carcinoma
Risk Factors
- Lifetime risk 6%
- Incidence increases after age 50
- Familial risk
  - 2 to 4 fold increase risk with a single first degree relative
  - 3 to 6 fold increase risk with two first degree relatives
- Increased risk
  - Familial adenomatous polyposis syndrome (FAP)
  - Hereditary nonpolyposis colon cancer (HNPCC)
  - Inflammatory bowel disease

Colorectal Carcinoma
Pathogenesis
- Adenoma-Carcinoma Sequence
  - Slow evolution to cancer, average 10 years
  - Adenoma detection and removal = cure
- Exception to adenoma-carcinoma sequence
  - Carcinomas in inflammatory bowel disease
  - Hereditary nonpolyposis colon cancer (HNPCC)

Adenoma-Carcinoma Sequence
[Figures 2-10-1]

Colorectal Carcinoma: Role of Radiology
- Screening
  - ACBE
  - CT colonography
- Detection
  - Symptomatic patients
- Preoperative screening
  - Primary disease complications
  - Preoperative staging
- Recurrent disease

Figure 2-10-1

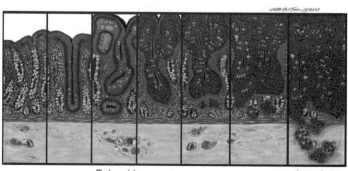

Polypoid Adenoma   Invasive Carcinoma

Adenoma to carcinoma sequence progressive from normal mucosa, unicryptal adenoma, polypoid adenoma, dysplasia, high-grade dysplasia, carcinoma in-situ, to invasive carcinoma

Colorectal Carcinoma: Screening

- Current ACS screening recommendations
  - ➢ FOBT annual, starting at age 50 and
  - ➢ Flex Sig, every 5 years starting at age 50, or
  - ➢ DCBE, every 5 years starting at age 50, or
  - ➢ Colonoscopy, every 10 years starting at age 50
- ACG Polyp guidelines[1]
  - ➢ Colonoscopy every 3 years, high risk for metachronous adenomas (>2, >1cm, villous histology or high-grade dysplasia)
  - ➢ Colonoscopy every 5 years, low risk for metachronous adenomas (1-2 tubular adenomas, no family history)

[1]*Bond JH. Am J Gastroenterology 2000. 95(11): 3053-3063*

Colorectal Carcinoma: Screening

- Air contrast barium enema
  - ➢ Accuracy 90% for polyps >1 cm
  - ➢ Pitfalls
    - ❖ Anatomic difficulties (overlapping segments)
    - ❖ Diverticular disease
    - ❖ Perceptive errors
- Colonoscopy
  - ➢ Accuracy 90%
  - ➢ Invasive, requiring sedation
  - ➢ Perforation rate .1% to .5%
  - ➢ Pitfalls
    - ❖ Failure to reach cecum
    - ❖ Blind spots

Colorectal Carcinoma: Screening

- Virtual colonography
  - ➢ Sensitivity 73% to 93% for >10mm polyps
  - ➢ Prone and supine imaging improves sensitivity
  - ➢ Difficult lesions
    - ❖ Poor bowel preparation
    - ❖ Flat adenomas
    - ❖ Adenomas on folds
    - ❖ Adenomas seen in only one position

Colorectal Polyps: Histologic Spectrum

- Hyperplastic
  - ➢ Most common
  - ➢ Usually <5 mm, descending colon and rectum
  - ➢ NOT neoplastic
- Adenoma
  - ➢ Tubular, 75% are <1 cm, most pedunculated
  - ➢ Villous, 60% are > 2 cm, most sessile
  - ➢ Mixed
- Juvenile
- Peutz-Jeghers
- Inflammatory/post-inflammatory

Tubular Adenoma

Villous Adenoma

Adenoma

- Size
  - ➢ < 5 mm, benign
  - ➢ 5 mm to 1 cm, 1% are carcinoma
  - ➢ 1 - 2 cm, 10% are carcinoma
  - ➢ > 2 cm, 30% to 50% are carcinoma

- Synchronous adenomas
  - ➢ 40% to 50%
- Recurrence
  - ➢ 20% to 60% recurrence rate
  - ➢ Majority recur within 2 years

Adenoma: Radiologic Features
- Filling defect in barium pool
- Protrusion into the lumen
  - ➢ "Innies not Outies"
  - ➢ Bowler hat sign
  - ➢ Sessile or pedunculated
- Carpet lesions
  - ➢ Sessile lesions
  - ➢ Bubbly or nodular contour
  - ➢ Villous change

Bowler Hat Sign [Figures 2-10-2 and 2-10-3]

Figure 2-10-3

Figure 2-10-2

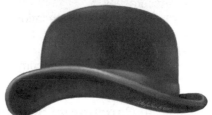

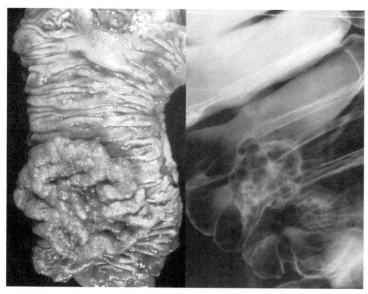

Villous adenoma showing a bubbly, carpet-like appearance

Sessile adenomatous polyp showing the Bowler Hat sign

Virtual Colonography

Colonic Adenocarcinoma

Colorectal Carcinoma: Distribution [Figure 2-10-4]

Colorectal Carcinoma: Clinical Presentation
- Minimal or absent symptoms in up to 12% of patients
- Bleeding
  - ➢ Initial complaint in 50%
- Weight loss, malaise
- Pain
- Change in bowel habits
- Right vs. left sided lesions
- Symptoms from complications
  - ➢ Obstruction, ischemia, perforation, peritonitis, fistula

Figure 2-10-4

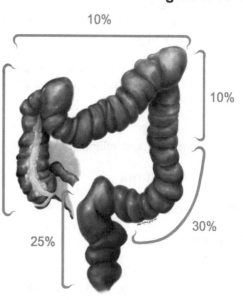

Distribution of colorectal carcinoma

Colorectal Carcinoma: Morphologic Patterns
- Polypoid
  - Intraluminal masses
  - Bulky, fungating masses in cecum and ascending colon
- Infiltrating/annular constricting
  - Transverse, descending, and sigmoid colon
  - Encircle the bowel
  - "Apple core"
  - Diffuse infiltration (linitis plastica) uncommon
- Ulcerating
  - Deeply invade colonic wall
  - Edge of tumor slightly elevated above normal mucosa
- Flat plaques
  - Arise from flat adenomas
  - Inflammatory bowel disease

Colorectal Carcinoma: Computed Tomography
- Primary Tumor
  - Discrete mass
  - Mural thickening
- Extension beyond the bowel
  - Irregular outer margin
  - Soft-tissue stranding in pericolonic fat
- Adjacent organ/muscle invasion
  - Loss of fat planes
  - Tumor mass in adjacent organ or muscle
- Liver metastasis
- Lymph node metastasis

Figure 2-10-5

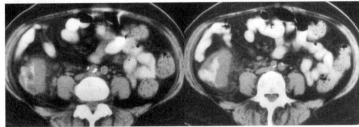

Polypoid adenocarcinoma of the cecum

Polypoid Adenocarcinoma
[Figure 2-10-5]

Annular Adenocarcinoma
[Figure 2-10-6]

Figure 2-10-6

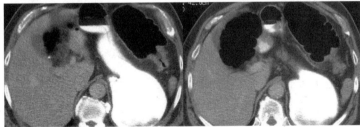

Annular adenocarcinoma of the distal transverse colon

Infiltrating Adenocarcinoma

Asymmetric Mural Thickening, Pericolonic Extension, Pericolonic Adenopathy

Adjacent Organ Invasion

Carcinoma with Fistula
- Direct extension
  - Contiguous soft tissue thickening
- Air in contrast in adjacent organ
  - Identify fistulous tract

Multiple Carcinomas
- Synchronous carcinomas
  - Diagnosed within 6 months of each other
  - Incidence 1.5% to 12%
  - Most are >5 cm away from each other
- Metachronous carcinomas
  - Incidence 0.6% to 9.1%
  - Time interval to second lesion discovery
    - 64% within 5 years
    - 45% within 3 years
    - 20% within 1 year
- 8% to 20% of patients with colorectal carcinomas have malignancies in other organs

Synchronous Carcinomas [Figure 2-10-7]

Adenocarcinoma in Inflammatory Bowel Disease [Figure 2-10-8]

- Ulcerative colitis
  - ➤ Highest incidence
- Crohn disease
  - ➤ Large and small intestinal adenocarcinoma
- Features of carcinoma in IBD
  - ➤ Typically do not arise in pre-existing adenomas
  - ➤ Arise in flat mucosa
  - ➤ Carcinomas may be long and flat

Adenocarcinoma in Ulcerative Colitis

Colorectal Carcinoma: Complications

- Bleeding
  - ➤ Occult
  - ➤ Chronic anemia
  - ➤ Massive bleeding, unusual
- Obstruction
  - ➤ Occlusion of the colonic lumen
  - ➤ Colocolic intussusception
- Perforation
  - ➤ Abscess
  - ➤ Fistula
  - ➤ Differential diagnosis, diverticulitis

CT of Obstructing Colon Carcinomas

- IV contrast
- Read from bottom up
- Identify obstructing lesion
  - ➤ Infiltration of adjacent fat
  - ➤ Adjacent organ invasion
- Evaluate bowel integrity
  - ➤ Obstructive colitis (1% to 7%)
  - ➤ Ischemic changes
  - ➤ Pneumatosis
- Stage
  - ➤ Lymph node mets
  - ➤ Liver mets

CT of Obstructing Colon Carcinomas

Ischemia in Obstructive Colitis [Figure 2-10-9]

Carcinoma with Perforation and Pericolonic Abscess

Carcinoma vs. Diverticulitis

- Wall thickening
  - ➤ Mild circumferential thickening in diverticulitis (4 to 5 mm)
  - ➤ Carcinoma usually > 2 cm
- Zone of transition
  - ➤ Abrupt change in lumen caliber favors carcinoma
  - ➤ Lobulated soft-tissue favors carcinoma
  - ➤ Tethered lumen favors diverticulitis
- Inflammatory changes

Figure 2-10-7

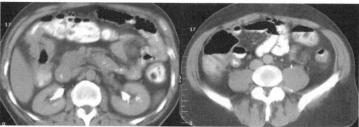

Synchronous adenocarcinomas of the hepatic flexure and descending colon

Figure 2-10-8

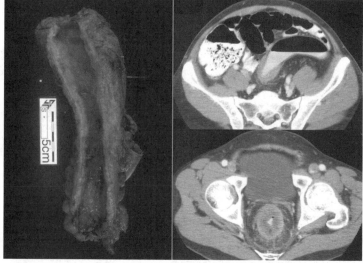

Adenocarcinoma in ulcerative colitis

Figure 2-10-9

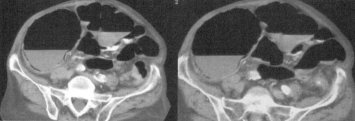

Colonic ischemia in an obstructing carcinoma of the descending colon

➢ Favors diverticulitis
- Regional adenopathy
  ➢ Favors carcinoma

Carcinoma vs. Diverticulitis

Carcinoma

Carcinoma vs. Diverticulitis

Diverticulitis

Carcinoma vs. Diverticulitis

Diverticulitis

Differential Diagnosis
- Adenocarcinoma
- Other colon primary
  ➢ Lipoma
  ➢ Lymphoma
  ➢ GIST
- Focal Colitis
  ➢ Crohn disease
  ➢ Post-radiation
  ➢ Ameboma
  ➢ Tuberculoma
- Diverticulosis
- Endometriosis
- Adjacent inflammation
  ➢ Pancreatitis

Crohn Disease

Colorectal Carcinoma Staging [Figure 2-10-10]
- TNM Classification
- Depth of invasion, T
  ➢ CT sensitivity 53% - 77%
  ➢ Endoscopic ultrasound
  ➢ Endorectal MR
- Nodes, N
  ➢ CT sensitivity 22% - 73%
  ➢ PET
- Distant mets, M
  ➢ CT
  ➢ PET

Colorectal Carcinoma: Preoperative CT
- Patients with clinical evidence of advanced disease
- Local tumor extension
  ➢ Adjacent organ invasion
- Liver metastasis
  ➢ Early rim enhancement, followed by hyperdensity
  ➢ Hypodense in the portal venous phase
  ➢ Isodense in the equilibrium phase
- Lymphatic Spread

Figure 2-10-10

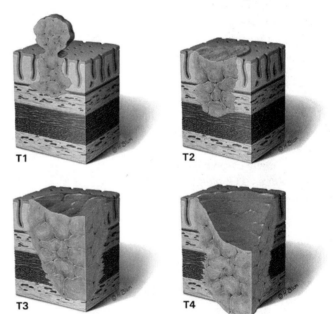

TNM Staging for colorectal carcinoma

Colorectal Carcinoma: Lymphatic Spread [Figure 2-10-11]

Figure 2-10-11

- Pericolonic nodes
  - ➤ Paracolic
  - ➤ Epiploic
- Mesenteric Nodes
  - ➤ Intermediate nodes
- Principal nodes
  - ➤ SMA
  - ➤ IMA

Pericolonic Nodes

Intermediate

Principal

Summary: Adenoma
- 40% - 50% synchronous
- 20% - 60% recur
- BE features
  - ➤ Filling defect
  - ➤ Bowler hat
  - ➤ Sessile
  - ➤ Pedunculated
  - ➤ Bubbly, villous change

Summary: Detection of Primary Tumor
- Morphology
  - ➤ Polypoid
  - ➤ Infiltrating/annular
  - ➤ Ulcerating
  - ➤ Flat plaques
- Synchronous carcinomas
- CT
  - ➤ Local extent
  - ➤ Adjacent organ invasion

Summary: Complications
- Bleeding
  - ➤ Usually chronic blood loss
  - ➤ Massive GI bleed, unusual
- Obstruction
  - ➤ CT
  - ➤ Identify lesion and bowel wall integrity
- Perforation
  - ➤ Abscess
  - ➤ Fistula
  - ➤ Differential diagnosis inflammatory disorders

Summary: Carcinoma vs. Diverticulitis
- Features of Carcinoma
  - ➤ Mural thickening > 2cm
  - ➤ Lobulated soft tissue
  - ➤ Abrupt change in lumen caliber
  - ➤ Regional adenopathy
- Features of Diverticulitis
  - ➤ Mild circumferential thickening
  - ➤ Tethering of the lumen
  - ➤ Pericolonic inflammation

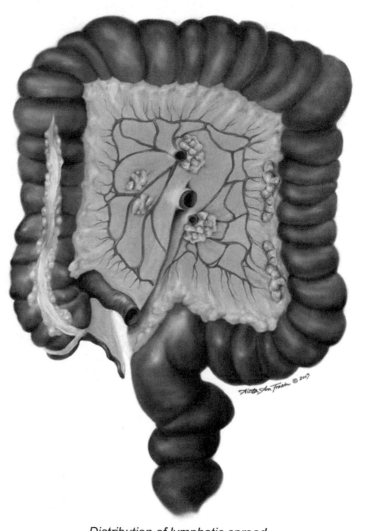

Distribution of lymphatic spread

Summary: Role of Imaging

- Preoperative CT
  - ➤ Local tumor extent
  - ➤ Liver metastasis
  - ➤ Lymphatic spread

Virtual Colonography Selected References:

Fidler JL, Johnson CD, MacCarty RL, et al: Detection of flat lesions in the colon with CT colonography. Abdom Imaging 27:292, 2002

Fletcher JG, Johnson CD, MacCarty RL, et al: CT colonography: potential pitfalls and problem-solving techniques. AJR Am J Roentgenol 172:1271, 1999

Fletcher JG, Johnson CD, Welch TJ, et al: Optimization of CT colonography technique: prospective trial in 180 patients. Radiology 216:704, 20

Gluecker TM, Fletcher JG, Welch TJ, et al: Characterization of Lesions Missed on Interpretation of CT Colonography Using a 2D Search Method. AJR Am J Roentgenol 182:881, 2004

Gluecker TM, Johnson CD, Harmsen WS, et al: Colorectal cancer screening with CT colonography, colonoscopy, and double-contrast barium enema examination: prospective assessment of patient perceptions and preferences. Radiology 227:378, 2003

Johnson CD, Ahlquist DA: Computed tomography colonography (virtual colonoscopy): a new method for colorectal screening. Gut 44:301, 1999

Johnson CD, Harmsen WS, Wilson LA, et al: Prospective blinded evaluation of computed tomographic colonography for screen detection of colorectal polyps. Gastroenterology 125:311, 2003

Johnson CD, Toledano AY, Herman BA, et al: Computerized tomographic colonography: performance evaluation in a retrospective multicenter setting. Gastroenterology 125:688, 2003

Macari M: Virtual colonoscopy: clinical results. Semin Ultrasound CT MR 22:432, 2001

Pescatore P, Glucker T, Delarive J, et al: Diagnostic accuracy and interobserver agreement of CT colonography (virtual colonoscopy). Gut 47:126, 2000

Pickhardt PJ: Three-dimensional endoluminal CT colonography (virtual colonoscopy): comparison of three commercially available systems. AJR Am J Roentgenol 181:1599, 2003

Pickhardt PJ, Choi JR, Hwang I, et al: Computed tomographic virtual colonoscopy to screen for colorectal neoplasia in asymptomatic adults. N Engl J Med 349:2191, 2003

Royster AP, Fenlon HM, Clarke PD, et al: CT colonoscopy of colorectal neoplasms: two-dimensional and three-dimensional virtual-reality techniques with colonoscopic correlation. AJR Am J Roentgenol 169:1237, 1997

Spinzi G, Belloni G, Martegani A, et al: Computed tomographic colonography and conventional colonoscopy for colon diseases: a prospective, blinded study. Am J Gastroenterol 96:394, 2001

Taylor SA, Halligan S, Bartram CI: CT colonography: methods, pathology and pitfalls. Clin Radiol 58:179, 2003

Taylor SA, Halligan S, Bartram CI, et al: Multi-detector row CT colonography: effect of collimation, pitch, and orientation on polyp detection in a human colectomy specimen. Radiology 229:109, 2003

Taylor SA, Halligan S, Goh V, et al: Optimizing bowel preparation for multidetector row CT colonography: effect of Citramag and Picolax. Clin Radiol 58:723, 2003

Taylor SA, Halligan S, Goh V, et al: Optimizing colonic distention for multi-detector row CT colonography: effect of hyoscine butylbromide and rectal balloon catheter. Radiology 229:99, 2003

Imaging of Anorectal Disease

Angela D. Levy, LTC, MC, USA
Department of Radiologic Pathology
Armed Forces Institute of Pathology
Washington, DC

Figure 2-11-1

Objectives

- Anatomy
- Neoplastic diseases
  - ➢ Villous adenoma
  - ➢ Adenocarcinoma
  - ➢ GIST
  - ➢ Anal canal tumors
- Nonneoplastic disorders
  - ➢ Retrorectal cyst
  - ➢ Mucosal prolapse syndromes

Anatomy [Figures 2-11-1, 2-11-2, 2-11-3]

- Extraperitoneal
- Rectosigmoid junction at S3
- Transverse rectal folds (valves)
  - ➢ Plicae transversales
- Dentate line (or pectinate line)
- Anal verge
- Levator Ani
  - ➢ Pubococcygeus
  - ➢ Puborectalis
  - ➢ Iliococcygeus
- External sphincter

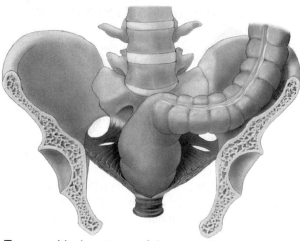

Topographical anatomy of the pelvic floor and rectum showing the relationship of the levator ani muscle complex to the rectum

Figure 2-11-3

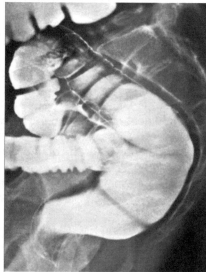

Figure 2-11-2

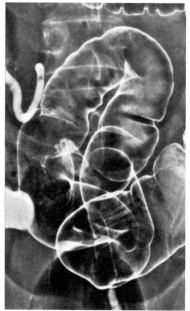
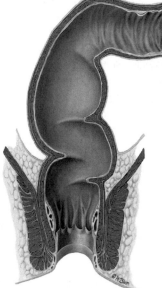

Coronal anatomy of the rectum, anus, and levator ani complex

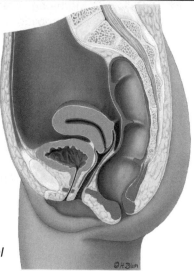

Lateral view of the rectum and sagittal anatomy of the peritoneal reflections in a female patient

Vascular Supply
- Arterial Supply
  - Superior rectal artery
    - Branch of IMA
  - Middle rectal artery
    - Branch of internal iliac
  - Inferior rectal artery
    - Branch of internal pudendal
- Venous drainage
  - Portal venous
    - Superior rectal vein
  - Systemic
    - Inferior and middle rectal vein

Lymphatic drainage [Figure 2-11-4]
- Pararectal nodes
- Internal iliac nodes
  - Above dentate line
- Inguinal nodes
  - Below dentate line

Neoplastic Diseases
- Villous adenoma
- Rectal adenocarcinoma
- Gastrointestinal stromal tumors (GISTs)
- Malignant Melanoma
- Anal canal tumors

Villous Adenoma
- Higher rate of malignancy
- Recurrence rate 9.3%
- Three types
  - Flat, carpet-like
  - Sessile, lobulated
  - Pedunculated
- Histology
  - Nonbranching finger-like fronds

Villous Adenoma: Pathology

Villous Adenoma: CT Features
- Soft tissue attenuation mass
  - Sessile
  - Eccentric
  - Stalk
- Expands rectal lumen
- Irregular luminal margin
  - Low attenuation luminal margin
  - High mucin content

Villous Adenoma [Figure 2-11-5]

Rectal Adenocarcinoma: Preoperative Imaging
- EUS/CT/MR/PET
  - Site and extent of disease
  - Tumor response to therapy
  - Post operative recurrence

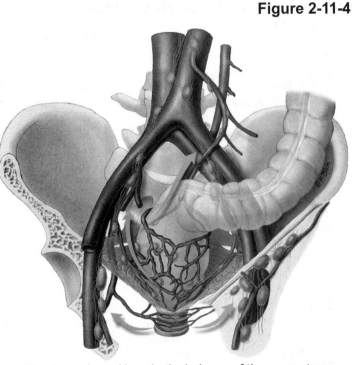

Figure 2-11-4

Blood supply and lymphatic drainage of the anorectum

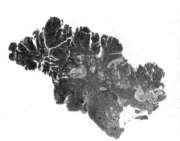
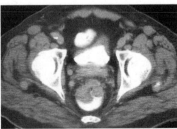

Figure 2-11-5

Villous adenoma of the rectum

Rectal Adenocarcinoma: Management
- High T1 or T2 lesion
  - ➢ Lesions 5 to 6 cm above dentate line or at peritoneal reflection
  - ➢ Primary resection and anastomosis (LAR)
- Low T1 or T2 lesion
  - ➢ APR (Miles procedure), LAR, coloanal anastomosis with J-pouch, local or transanal excision, total mesorectal excision, posterior proctotomy
- T3 or T4
  - ➢ Downstage with preoperative XRT?
  - ➢ APR and post operative XRT, chemotherapy

Local Staging
- CT
  - ➢ T stage accuracy 60 to 80%
- Endoscopic Ultrasound (EUS)[1]
  - ➢ 360 degree probe
  - ➢ Normal 5-layer rectal wall
  - ➢ T stage accuracy 80% to 90%
  - ➢ Nodal accuracy 70% to 80%
- Endorectal MRI[2]
  - ➢ Prone imaging, 1 mg glucagon, endorectal coil, +/- phased array pelvic coil
  - ➢ Sagittal T1 scout, SE T1, FSE T2
  - ➢ Normal 3-layer rectal wall
  - ➢ T stage accuracy 70% to 90%

[1]Wolfman NT, Ott DJ. Endoscopic Ultrasonography. Semin Roentgenol 1996. 31(2): 154-161.

[2]Zagoria RJ, Wolfman NT. Magnetic resonance imaging of colorectal cancer. Semin Roentgenol 1996. 31(2): 162-5.

TNM Staging [Figure 2-11-6]
- T-Primary tumor
  - ➢ T1 invades submucosa
  - ➢ T2 invades muscularis propria
  - ➢ <u>T3 through muscularis propria or into nonperitonealized pericolic fat</u>
  - ➢ T4 perforates visceral peritoneum or directly invades adjacent organs or structures
- N-Regional nodes
- M-Distant metastasis

Figure 2-11-6

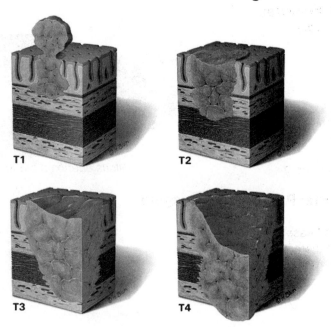

T1   T2

T3   T4

TNM staging of rectal adenocarcinoma

EUS Anatomy of the Rectum [Figure 2-11-7]

Figure 2-11-7

Layer1: Hyperechoic superficial mucosa

Layer 2: Hypoechoic deep mucosa

Layer 3: hyperechoic submucosa

Layer 4: Hypoechoic muscularis propria

Layer 5: Hyperechoic perirectal fat

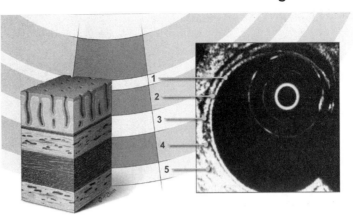

EUS anatomy of the rectum

Endorectal MR [Figure 2-11-8]

Figure 2-11-8

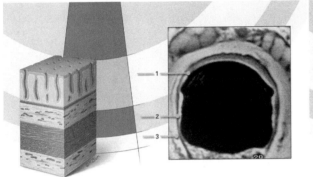
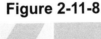
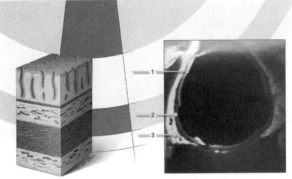

Endorectal MR anatomy of the rectum

Figure 2-11-9

T1 N0 M0

T2 N0 M0

T3 N2 M0 [Figure 2-11-9]

T3 N10 M0

T3 N8 M1

T4

T4: Extension to pelvic side wall

T4: Extension to labia

Gastrointestinal Stromal Tumors (GIST)
- Mesenchymal neoplasms
  - ➢ KIT (C117) positive
- Anorectum is the 3rd most common site
  - ➢ following stomach and small bowel
- CT features
  - ➢ Well-circumscribed
  - ➢ Evidence of hemorrhage
  - ➢ Intraluminal, mural, and/or exophytic
  - ➢ No adenopathy

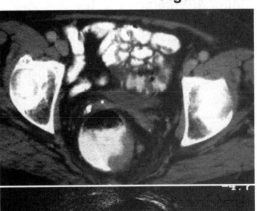
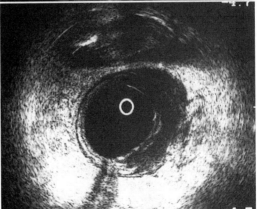

T3 rectal adenocarcinoma

GIST: Mural Mass

GIST: Exophytic Growth

Figure 2-11-10

GIST [Figure 2-11-10]

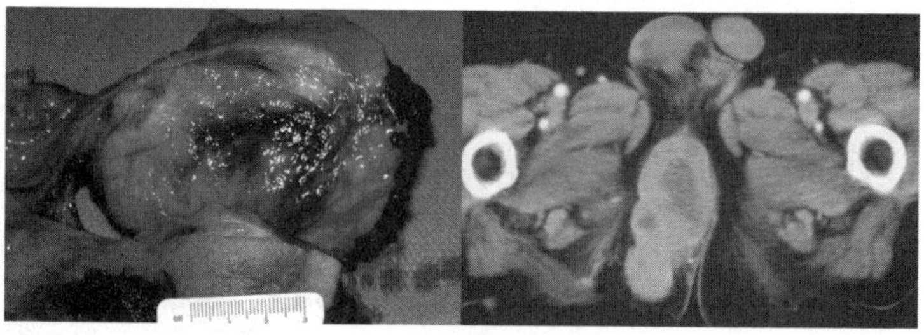

Differential Features
- GIST
  - ➢ Smooth margins
  - ➢ Evidence of hemorrhage
  - ➢ Adenopathy is not typically present
- Adenocarcinoma
  - ➢ Irregular margins
  - ➢ Soft-tissue stranding
  - ➢ Perirectal adenopathy common

Anorectal GIST

Anorectal GIST vs. Adenocarcinoma

Malignant Anal Canal Tumors
- Melanoma
- Squamous cell
- Basaloid carcinoma
- Mucoepidermoid carcinoma
- Anal duct carcinoma
- Small cell carcinoma
- Transitional cell carcinoma
- Colorectal type carcinoma

Malignant Anal Canal Tumors
- Role of imaging
  - ➢ Extent of disease
  - ➢ Tumor recurrence

Malignant Melanoma

Malignant Melanoma Recurrence

Anal Duct Carcinoma

Nonneoplastic Disorders
- Retrorectal cysts
- Mucosal prolapse syndromes

Retrorectal Cysts
- Developmental Cysts
  - ➢ Epidermoid cyst
  - ➢ Dermoid cysts
  - ➢ Enteric cysts
    - ❖ Tailgut cysts
    - ❖ Cystic rectal duplication
  - ➢ Neuroenteric cysts

Retrorectal Cysts
- Clinical presentation
  - ➢ Asymptomatic
  - ➢ Constipation
  - ➢ Rectal fullness, pain
- Complications
  - ➢ Infection
  - ➢ Fistulization
  - ➢ Malignant degeneration (7%)

Epidermoid Cyst [Figure 2-11-11]
- Epidermoid
  - Unilocular
  - Filled with clear fluid
  - Stratified squamous lining
- Dermoid
  - Contain skin appendages
  - Filled with fatty material
  - Stratified squamous lining

Tailgut Cyst
- Remnant of the embryonic hindgut
- Synonym: retrorectal cystic hamartoma
- Various epithelial linings
  - Mucin-secreting columnar, transitional, squamous

Tailgut Cyst [Figure 2-11-12]
- Most often found in middle aged women
- Malignant transformation occurs
- Imaging
  - Extrinsic retrorectal mass
  - Epicenter posterior to rectum
  - Sharply marginated
  - Complex cyst
  - Features of malignant transformation
    - Loss of sharp margins
    - Irregular wall thickening

Differential Diagnosis: Retrorectal Cystic Mass
- Pyogenic abscess
- Developmental cyst
- Anal duct or gland cyst
- Sacral Lesions
  - Cystic sacrococcygeal teratoma
  - Anterior sacral meningocele
  - Neurogenic cyst
  - Sarcoma chordoma
- Cystic lymphangiomas

Pyogenic Perirectal Abscess
[Figure 2-11-13]

Crohn Disease with Perirectal Abscess

Cystic Sacrococcygeal Teratoma

Mucosal Prolapse Syndromes
- Rectal prolapse
- Rectal intussusception
- Solitary rectal ulcer syndrome
- Proctitis cystica profunda

Rectal prolapse/occult intussusception
- Concentric invagination
- Rectal valve invaginates toward anal canal
- All layers of rectal wall involved
  - Evacuation proctography/MR
  - Location
- Anterior 62%
- Annular 32%
- Posterior 6%

Figure 2-11-11

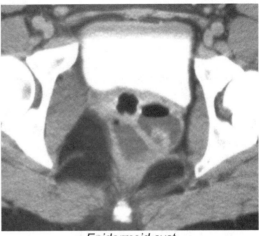

Epidermoid cyst

Figure 2-11-12

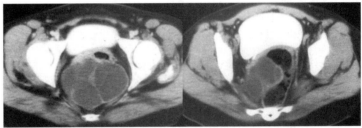

Tailgut cyst

Figure 2-11-13

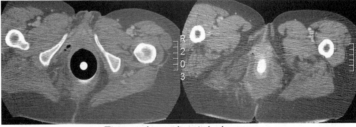

Pyogenic perirectal abscess

Solitary Rectal Ulcer Syndrome

- Evacuation disorder
  - ➢ Occult intussusception in 45% to 80%
  - ➢ Straining against an immobile pelvic floor
- Ulceration of rectal mucosa
  - ➢ Anterior or anterolateral rectal wall
- Mucosa regenerates
  - ➢ Development of polypoid mass

Solitary Rectal Ulcer Syndrome: Imaging Features

[Figures 2-11-14]

- Ulceration
- Stricture
- Thick rectal valves
- Nodular mucosa
- Polypoid mass
- Thickening of external sphincter

Summary: Villous Adenoma

- Carpet lesions
- Expand rectal lumen
- Low attenuation on luminal side of tumor

Summary: Rectal Adenocarcinoma

- Preoperative staging
  - ➢ EUS and CT
- T3 lesions
  - ➢ Through muscularis propria
  - ➢ Spiculated outer margin on CT
  - ➢ Perirectal adenopathy

Summary: Gastrointestinal Stromal Tumors

- Well-defined margins
- Central low attenuation
- Exophytic growth potential
- No adenopathy

Summary: Tail Gut Cyst

- Remnant of embryonic hindgut
- Epicenter posterior to rectum
- Malignant potential
- Must be differentiated from perirectal abscess

Summary: Mucosal Prolapse Syndromes

- Evacuation disorders
- Continuum
  - ➢ Prolapse/intussusception
  - ➢ Solitary rectal ulcer syndrome
  - ➢ Proctitis cystica profunda
- Radiologic features
  - ➢ Ulcer
  - ➢ Stricture
  - ➢ Polyp
  - ➢ Mural thickening

Figure 2-11-14

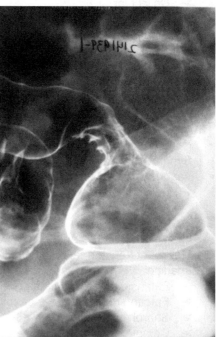

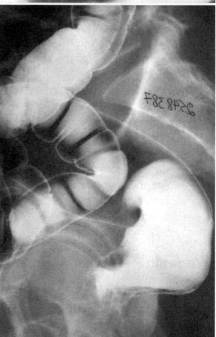

Solitary rectal ulcer syndrome

Imaging of Anorectal Disease References

Staging of Rectal Adenocarcinoma

Berlin JW, Gore RM, Yaghmai V, et al: Staging of colorectal cancer. Semin Roentgenol 35:370, 2000

de Lange EE: Staging rectal carcinoma with endorectal imaging: how much detail do we really need? Radiology 190:633, 1994

de Lange EE, Fechner RE, Edge SB, et al: Preoperative staging of rectal carcinoma with MR imaging: surgical and histopathologic correlation. Radiology 176:623, 1990

Hundt W, Braunschweig R, Reiser M: Evaluation of spiral CT in staging of colon and rectum carcinoma. Eur Radiol 9:78, 1999

Moss AA, Thoeni RF, Schnyder P, et al: Value of computed tomography in the detection and staging of recurrent rectal carcinomas. J Comput Assist Tomogr 5:870, 1981

Niederhuber JE: Colon and rectum cancer. Patterns of spread and implications for workup. Cancer 71:4187, 1993

Rifkin MD, Marks GJ: Transrectal US as an adjunct in the diagnosis of rectal and extrarectal tumors. Radiology 157:499, 1985

Rotte KH, Kluhs L, Kleinau H, et al: Computed tomography and endosonography in the preoperative staging of rectal carcinoma. Eur J Radiol 9:187, 1989

Vogl TJ, Pegios W, Mack MG, et al: Accuracy of staging rectal tumors with contrast-enhanced transrectal MR imaging. AJR Am J Roentgenol 168:1427, 1997

Zerhouni EA, Rutter C, Hamilton SR, et al: CT and MR imaging in the staging of colorectal carcinoma: report of the Radiology Diagnostic Oncology Group II. Radiology 200:443, 1996

Retrorectal Cysts

Dahan H, Arrive L, Wendum D, et al: Retrorectal developmental cysts in adults: clinical and radiologic-histopathologic review, differential diagnosis, and treatment. Radiographics 21:575, 2001

Lim KE, Hsu WC, Wang CR: Tailgut cyst with malignancy: MR imaging findings. AJR Am J Roentgenol 170:1488, 1998

Marco V, Autonell J, Farre J, et al: Retrorectal cyst-hamartomas. Report of two cases with adenocarcinoma developing in one. Am J Surg Pathol 6:707, 1982

Moulopoulos LA, Karvouni E, Kehagias D, et al: MR imaging of complex tail-gut cysts. Clin Radiol 54:118, 1999

Ottery FD, Carlson RA, Gould H, et al: Retrorectal cyst-hamartomas: CT diagnosis. J Comput Assist Tomogr 10:260, 1986

Scullion DA, Zwirewich CV, McGregor G: Retrorectal cystic hamartoma: diagnosis using endorectal ultrasound. Clin Radiol 54:338, 1999

Mucosal Prolapse Syndromes

Goei R, Baeten C, Arends JW: Solitary rectal ulcer syndrome: findings at barium enema study and defecography. Radiology 168:303, 1988

Goei R, Baeten C, Janevski B, et al: The solitary rectal ulcer syndrome: diagnosis with defecography. AJR Am J Roentgenol 149:933, 1987

Halligan S: Solitary rectal ulcer syndrome. Radiology 193:879, 1994

Halligan S, Nicholls RJ, Bartram CI: Evacuation proctography in patients with solitary rectal ulcer syndrome: anatomic abnormalities and frequency of impaired emptying and prolapse. AJR Am J Roentgenol 164:91, 1995

Hizawa K, Iida M, Suekane H, et al: Mucosal prolapse syndrome: diagnosis with endoscopic US. Radiology 191:527, 1994

Karasick S, Karasick D, Karasick SR: Functional disorders of the anus and rectum: findings on defecography. AJR Am J Roentgenol 160:777, 1993

Malde HM, Chadha D: Solitary rectal ulcer syndrome: transrectal sonographic findings. AJR Am J Roentgenol 160:1361, 1993

Appendicitis and Beyond

Angela D. Levy, LTC, MC, USA
Department of Radiologic Pathology
Armed Forces Institute of Pathology
Washington, DC

Objectives
- Appendiceal anatomy
- Appendicitis
- Neoplastic lesions of the appendix
- Differential diagnosis and case review

Normal Anatomy *[Figures 2-12-1, 2-12-2, 2-12-3]*
- Posteromedial cecum at the convergence of the taenia coli
- 8 to 10 cm long
  - ➢ Range 4 to 25 cm
- Mesoappendix
  - ➢ Appendiceal artery, vein
  - ➢ Lymphatics

Figure 2-12-1

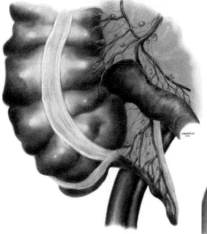

Normal anatomy. Appendiceal artery, vein, and lymphatics located in the mesoappendix

Figure 2-12-2

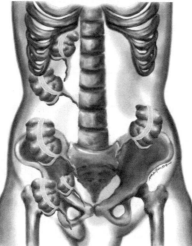

Normal positional variants of the cecum and appendix

Figure 2-12-3

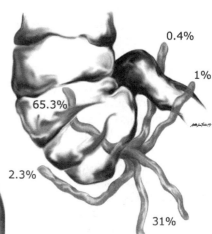

Normal positional variants of the appendix relative to the cecum

Acute Appendicitis
- Most common surgical emergency
- More common in western cultures
  - ➢ Low fiber diet
- Peak incidence second and third decades of perforation 20%
- Periappendiceal abscess or phlegmon 5%

Acute Appendicitis *[Figures 2-12-4 and 2-12-5]*
- Pathogenesis = luminal obstruction
  - ➢ Stones, food, mucus, adhesions, parasites
  - ➢ Tumors, endometriosis
  - ➢ Foreign objects
  - ➢ Lymphoid hyperplasia
- Appendicolith
  - ➢ 7–12% adults
  - ➢ 50% children

Figure 2-12-4

Normal appendix histology (left), Appendicitis (right)

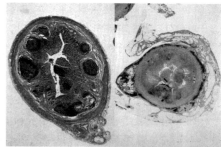

Figure 2-12-5

Gross pathology of acute appendicitis showing mural thickening

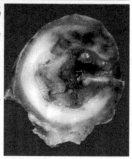

Acute Appendicitis: Abdominal Radiography [Figures 2-12-6 and 2-12-7]

- Abnormality in 80 %
- Appendicolith
- Ileus
  - Cecal ileus
  - RLQ fluid levels
- Distortion of the flank stripe
- Loss of the psoas margin
- Cecal changes
  - Mural thickening
  - Mass effect on cecal margins
- Scoliosis
- Mottled gas collection in the RLQ
- Mottled gas collection in RLQ

Appendicitis: Sonography versus CT

- Ultrasound
  - Advantage: no radiation, inexpensive
  - Limitations: requires experienced sonographers, obesity and overlying bowel gas limit visibility
  - Children, women of child-bearing age, pregnant women
- Computed Tomography
  - Advantage: complications, other pathology
  - limitations: radiation exposure, poor technique
- CT vs. US[1]
  - Sensitivity: 96% vs. 76%
  - Accuracy: 94% vs. 83%
  - PPV: 95% vs. 76%

[1]Balthazar EJ, et al. Radiology 190: 31-35, 1994.

Figure 2-12-6

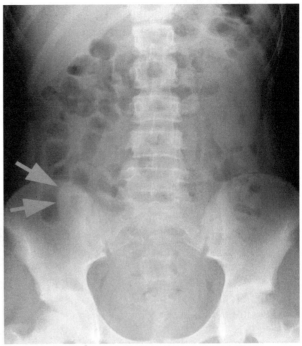

Acute appendicitis shows mass effect on the medial cecal margin

Figure 2-12-7

Acute Appendicitis: Sonography

[Figure 2-12-8]

- Non-compressible
- Diameter > 6 mm
- Inflamed perienteric fat
- Pericecal fluid collection
- Appendicolith
- Perforation
  - Loculated fluid
  - Abscess
- False positive
  - Terminal ileum
  - Other causes of mural thickening

Acute Appendicitis: CT

- Technique
  - 5 mm collimation, pitch 1.5
  - Reconstruction at 4 mm intervals
  - IV contrast 150cc at 2 to 3 ml/s
  - Oral vs. rectal contrast
- CT diagnosis
  - distended, fluid filled
  - 0.5 to 1.5-2 cm
  - diameter usually rarely exceeds 2 cm

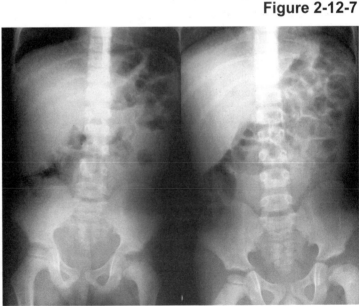

Acute appendicitis shows localized cecal ileus

Figure 2-12-8

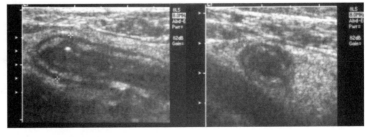

Sonographic appearance of acute appendicitis

Acute Appendicitis: CT Diagnosis
- Probably benign
  - ➢ > 6 mm, no inflammation, no wall thickening
  - ➢ Observation, follow up imaging
- Intermediate for appendicitis
  - ➢ > 6 mm, no inflammation, + wall thickening
  - ➢ Surgery
- Definitely appendicitis
  - ➢ > 6 mm, + inflammation, + wall thickening
  - ➢ Surgery

Appendicitis: CT Features

Figure 2-12-9

- Periappendiceal inflammation/soft tissue/fluid
- Appendiceal wall thickening/contrast enhancement
- Appendicolith
- Wall thickening of cecum and TI
- Focal cecal changes
  - ➢ Apical thickening
  - ➢ Cecal bar
  - ➢ "Arrowhead" sign
- Adenopathy
- Pneumoperitoneum

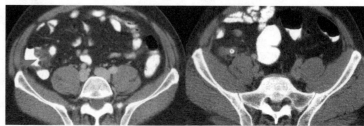

Acute appendicitis showing the "arrowhead sign"

Acute Appendicitis "Cecal Bar"
"Arrowhead Sign" [Figure 2-12-9]

Acute Appendicitis: Cecal and Terminal Ileum Mural Thickening

Acute Appendicitis: Complications
- Abscess
  - ➢ Low attenuation (10 to 30 H.U.)
  - ➢ Poorly defined or encapsulated
  - ➢ 15% contain air (gas-forming organisms or fistulization to bowel)
  - ➢ May be found at a distance from the cecum
- Perforation (20%)
  - ➢ Free air rarely seen
- Pylephlebitis (septic thrombophlebitis)
  - ➢ Rare, high morbidity/mortality
  - ➢ Air or thrombus in the mesenteric or portal vein
  - ➢ Precursor to hepatic abscess

Appendiceal Perforation
- Conservative surgical management
- CT features
  - ➢ Abscess
  - ➢ Phlegmon
  - ➢ Appendiceal wall defect
  - ➢ Extraluminal air
  - ➢ Extraluminal appendicolith

Appendiceal Neoplasms
- <0.4% of intestinal tumors
- Carcinoid tumors
- Adenomas
  - ➢ Mucinous cystadenoma
  - ➢ Adenoma
- Adenocarcinomas
  - ➢ Mucinous cystadenocarcinoma
  - ➢ Non-mucin producing adenocarcinoma
- Pseudomyxoma peritonei
- Others: adenocarcinoid, neurofibroma, mets, lymphoma

Appendiceal Carcinoid
- 50% to 85% of appendiceal tumors
- 45% of gastrointestinal carcinoids
- Affects all age groups with peak incidence at 40 years of age
- 70% to 90% discovered incidentally
- >95% of appendiceal carcinoids have benign behavior

Appendiceal Carcinoid
- Arise from neuroendocrine cells
- 71% arise in the distal tip of the appendix
- Appendectomy
  - < 1 cm diameter (95%)
- Right hemicolectomy :
  - Tumor in appendix base
  - Tumor at resection margin
  - Extension to mesoappendix
  - Tumor > 2 cm
  - Metastatic disease
  - High mitotic activity
  - Lymphatic invasion
  - Mucinous histology

Mucocele
- Descriptive term indicating dilatation of the lumen from mucus accumulation
- Does not indicate a specific underlying pathology
- Etiology
  - Retention mucoceles (hyperplastic mucosa)
  - Mucinous cystadenoma/cystadenocarcinoma
- Myxoglobulosis
  - Mucocele variant
  - Numerous mucin globules in the appendix (may calcify)

Mucinous Cystadenoma / Cystadenocarcinoma
- M = F
- 27 to 77 years of age
- Presentation
  - Right lower quadrant pain, nausea, vomiting, abdominal swelling
- Complications
  - Bowel obstruction, torsion, perforation, intussusception, appendicitis
- Gross pathology
  - Distended, mucus-filled appendix; mural fibrosis; compression of cecum
  - 20% with a synchronous colonic adenocarcinoma

Mucinous Cystadenoma / Cystadenocarcinoma
- Diagnosis of malignancy
  - Increased N:C ratio
  - Submucosal, vascular, or lymphatic invasion
  - Mets: peritoneal, nodes, distant organs
- Mucinous cystadenoma and carcinoma almost identical radiologically
- Radiologic findings suggestive of malignancy
  - Soft-tissue nodules or mass
  - Evidence of metastasis

Mucinous Cystadenoma / Cystadenocarcinoma
- Radiologic Findings
  - RLQ mass on plain film
  - Rim-like calcification
  - Mass effect medial cecal wall
  - Nonfilled appendix on BE
  - Fluid-filled, complex mass on CT or US
  - Short T1 and long T2 on MR

Mucinous Cystadenoma [Figures 2-12-10 and 2-12-11]

Pseudomyxoma Peritonei
- Presence of mucinous material on peritoneal surfaces
- Most are due to appendiceal lesions
- May occur with mucinous carcinomas from other sites: ovary, gallbladder, stomach, colorectal, pancreas, fallopian tube, urachus
- Radiologic findings
  - ➢ Ascites with high or heterogeneous attenuation
  - ➢ Loculations, septations
  - ➢ Scalloped contour of the liver and/or spleen

Mucinous Cystadenocarcinoma

Appendiceal Adenocarcinoma
[Figure 2-12-12]
- Non mucin producing
- Less common than mucinous tumors
- Histologically and radiologically resembles colonic adenocarcinoma

Appendiceal Neoplasms presenting as Appendicitis

Mucinous Cystadenoma

Appendiceal Adenocarcinoma

Non Hodgkin Lymphoma

Neoplastic vs. Nonneoplastic Appendicitis
- CT findings suggestive of neoplasm
  - ➢ Focal soft tissue mass
  - ➢ Cystic dilatation of the appendix
  - ➢ Nonspecific inflammatory changes may be seen in neoplasms of the appendix
  - ➢ 95% sensitivity for neoplasm if you combine morphologic changes with a diameter > 15 mm[1]

1. Pickhardt PJ, Levy AD, Rohrmann CA, Kende AI. *Primary Neoplasms of the Appendix Manifesting as Acute Appendicitis: CT Findings with Pathologic Correlation. Radiology 2002. 224 (3): 775-781*

Clinical Differential Diagnosis: RLQ Pain
- Appendicitis
- Inflammatory bowel disease
- Right-sided diverticulitis
  - ➢ Ileal, cecal
- Complications of GI tumors
  - ➢ Intussusception
  - ➢ Perforation
  - ➢ Obstruction
- Meckel's diverticulitis
- Small bowel obstruction
- Epiploic appendagitis
- PID

Figure 2-12-10

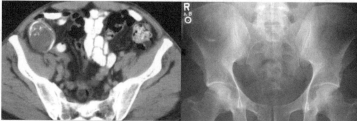

Mucinous cystadenoma

Figure 2-12-11

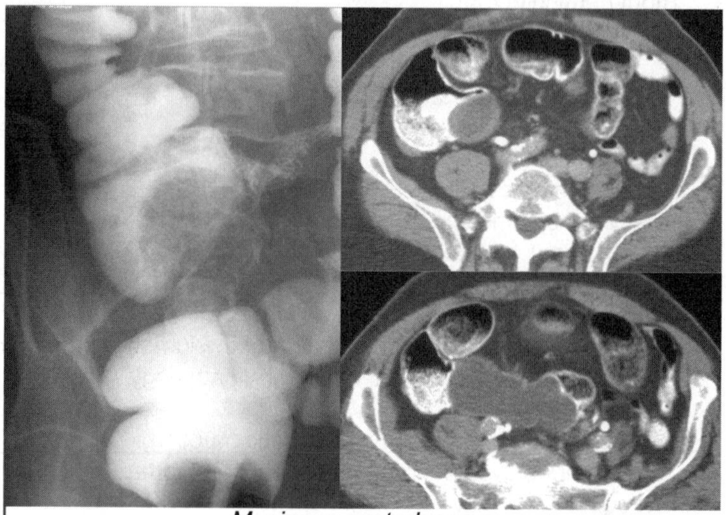

Mucinous cystadenoma

Figure 2-12-12

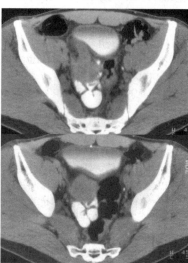

Appendiceal adenocarcinoma

- Complications of ovarian cysts
  - ➢ Hemorrhage
  - ➢ Rupture
  - ➢ Torsion
- Ectopic pregnancy
- Ureteral obstruction
  - ➢ Stones, tumors, inflammatory disease
- Mesenteric adenitis
- Omental infarction
- Peritoneal carcinomatosis
- Peritonitis/abscess

17-year-old male with RLQ pain and poor appetite
Mesenteric Adenitis *[Figure 2-12-13]*

Figure 2-12-13

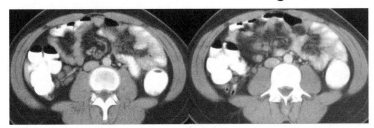

Mesenteric adenitis

50-year-old male with RLQ pain and fever
Cecal Diverticulitis *[Figure 2-12-14]*

Figure 2-12-14

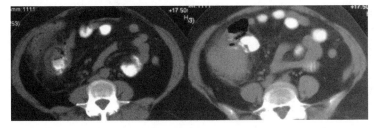

Cecal diverticulitis

64-year-old male with RLQ pain that progressed to involve the entire abdomen, fever and vomiting
Cecal Adenocarcinoma

65-year-old male with acute RLQ pain
Epiploic Appendagitis *[Figure 2-12-15]*

Figure 2-12-15

Epiploic appendagitis

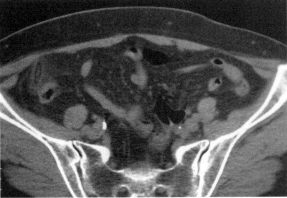

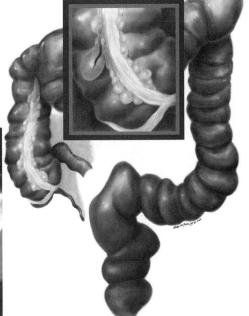

42-year-old female with RLQ pain and peritoneal signs on physical exam. Omental Infarction [Figure 2-12-16]

Figure 2-12-16

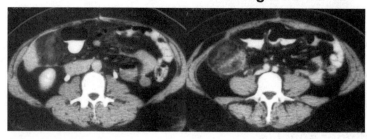

Omental infarction

35-year-old male with nausea, vomiting and RLQ pain Meckel Diverticulis [Figure 2-12-17]

Figure 2-12-17

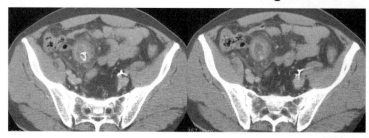

Meckel Diverticulitis

Summary

- In cases of appendicitis, carefully evaluate the surrounding bowel and mesentery for diagnostic clues in the differential diagnosis of RLQ pain
- Suspect neoplasm and use caution when interpreting scans for r/o appendicitis when
  - ➢ Atypical age
  - ➢ Atypical presentation
  - ➢ Atypical findings such as cystic dilatation (>15 mm) of the appendix or a focal soft tissue mass

Mucinous Cystadenoma

Appendiceal Adenocarcinoma

Appendicitis and Beyond References

Appendicitis

Baker SR: Unenhanced helical CT versus plain abdominal radiography: a dissenting opinion. Radiology 205:45, 1997

Balthazar EJ, Birnbaum BA, Yee J, et al: Acute appendicitis: CT and US correlation in 100 patients. Radiology 190:31, 1994

Balthazar EJ, Megibow AJ, Hulnick D, et al: CT of appendicitis. AJR Am J Roentgenol 147:705, 1986

Bendeck SE, Nino-Murcia M, Berry GJ, et al: Imaging for suspected appendicitis: negative appendectomy and perforation rates. Radiology 225:131, 2002

Birnbaum BA, Balthazar EJ: CT of appendicitis and diverticulitis. Radiol Clin North Am 32:885, 1994

Birnbaum BA, Jeffrey RB, Jr.: CT and sonographic evaluation of acute right lower quadrant abdominal pain. AJR Am J Roentgenol 170:361, 1998

Birnbaum BA, Wilson SR: Appendicitis at the millennium. Radiology 215:337, 2000

Callahan MJ, Rodriguez DP, Taylor GA: CT of appendicitis in children. Radiology 224:325, 2002

Grosskreutz S, Funaki B, Funaki C: Distal appendicitis: a possible anatomic source of error. Radiology 209:882, 1998

Jacobs JE, Birnbaum BA, Macari M, et al: Acute appendicitis: comparison of helical CT diagnosis focused technique with oral contrast material versus nonfocused technique with oral and intravenous contrast material. Radiology 220:683, 2001

Kamel IR, Goldberg SN, Keogan MT, et al: Right lower quadrant pain and suspected appendicitis: nonfocused appendiceal CT—review of 100 cases. Radiology 217:159, 2000

Lane MJ, Katz DS, Ross BA, et al: Unenhanced helical CT for suspected acute appendicitis. AJR Am J Roentgenol 168:405, 1997

Mindelzun RE, Jeffrey RB: Unenhanced helical CT for evaluating acute abdominal pain: a little more cost, a lot more information. Radiology 205:43, 1997

Pena BM, Taylor GA: Radiologists' confidence in interpretation of sonography and CT in suspected pediatric appendicitis. AJR Am J Roentgenol 175:71, 2000

Rao PM: Cecal apical changes with appendicitis: diagnosing appendicitis when the appendix is borderline abnormal or not seen. J Comput Assist Tomogr 23:55, 1999

Rao PM, Rhea JT, Novelline RA: Distal appendicitis: CT appearance and diagnosis. Radiology 204:709, 1997

Rao PM, Wittenberg J, McDowell RK, et al: Appendicitis: use of arrowhead sign for diagnosis at CT. Radiology 202:363, 1997

Raptopoulos V, Katsou G, Rosen MP, et al: Acute appendicitis: effect of increased use of CT on selecting patients earlier. Radiology 226:521, 2003

Appendiceal Neoplasms

Hinson FL, Ambrose NS: Pseudomyxoma peritonei. Br J Surg 85:1332, 1998

Horgan JG, Chow PP, Richter JO, et al: CT and sonography in the recognition of mucocele of the appendix. AJR Am J Roentgenol 143:959, 1984

Kim SH, Lim HK, Lee WJ, et al: Mucocele of the appendix: ultrasonographic and CT findings. Abdom Imaging 23:292, 1998

Lim HK, Lee WJ, Kim SH, et al: Primary mucinous cystadenocarcinoma of the appendix: CT findings. AJR Am J Roentgenol 173:1071, 1999

Madwed D, Mindelzun R, Jeffrey RB, Jr.: Mucocele of the appendix: imaging findings. AJR Am J Roentgenol 159:69, 1992

Pelage JP, Soyer P, Boudiaf M, et al: Carcinoid tumors of the abdomen: CT features. Abdom Imaging 24:240, 1999

Pickhardt PJ, Levy AD, Rohrmann CA, Jr., et al: Primary neoplasms of the appendix manifesting as acute appendicitis: CT findings with pathologic comparison. Radiology 224:775, 2002

Epiploic Appendagitis

Danielson K, Chernin MM, Amberg JR, et al: Epiploic appendicitis: CT characteristics. J Comput Assist Tomogr 10:142, 1986

Danse EM, Van Beers BE, Baudrez V, et al: Epiploic appendagitis: color Doppler sonographic findings. Eur Radiol 11:183, 2001

Ghahremani GG, White EM, Hoff FL, et al: Appendices epiploicae of the colon: radiologic and pathologic features. Radiographics 12:59, 1992

Molla E, Ripolles T, Martinez MJ, et al: Primary epiploic appendagitis: US and CT findings. Eur Radiol 8:435, 1998

Rao PM, Wittenberg J, Lawrason JN: Primary epiploic appendagitis: evolutionary changes in CT appearance. Radiology 204:713, 1997

van Breda Vriesman AC, Puylaert JB: Epiploic appendagitis and omental infarction: pitfalls and look-alikes. Abdom Imaging 27:20, 2002

Omental Infarction

Grattan-Smith JD, Blews DE, Brand T: Omental infarction in pediatric patients: sonographic and CT findings. AJR Am J Roentgenol 178:1537, 2002

van Breda Vriesman AC, Lohle PN, Coerkamp EG, et al: Infarction of omentum and epiploic appendage: diagnosis, epidemiology and natural history. Eur Radiol 9:1886, 1999

Wiesner W, Kaplan V, Bongartz G: Omental infarction associated with right-sided heart failure. Eur Radiol 10:1130, 2000

Mesenteric Masses and Cysts

Angela D. Levy, LTC, MC, USA
Department of Radiologic Pathology
Armed Forces Institute of Pathology
Washington, DC

Mesenteric Masses and Cysts
Case Based Approach
- Mesenteric and omental cysts
  - ➢ Lymphangioma
  - ➢ Enteric duplication cyst
  - ➢ Enteric cysts
  - ➢ Mesothelial cyst
  - ➢ Nonpancreatic pseudocyst
- Solid mesenteric masses
  - ➢ Mesothelioma
  - ➢ Desmoid Tumor (mesenteric fibromatosis)
  - ➢ Sclerosing mesenteritis
  - ➢ Inflammatory pseudotumor

Anatomy Definitions
- Mesentery
  - ➢ Double fold of peritoneum
  - ➢ Connects an organ to the abdominal wall
- Omentum
  - ➢ Mesentery extending from stomach to adjacent organs

Anatomy Omentum
- Greater omentum
  - ➢ Gastrocolic ligament
  - ➢ Gastrosplenic ligament
  - ➢ Gastrophrenic ligament
- Lesser omentum
  - ➢ Gastrohepatic ligament
  - ➢ Hepatoduodenal ligament

Anatomy Mesentery
- Transverse mesocolon
- Small bowel mesentery
- Sigmoid mesentery
- Mesoappendix

Mesenteric Cyst
- Descriptive term
- 5 histologic subtypes
- Different internal lining

Mesenteric Cyst
- Lymphangioma
  - ➢ Endothelial lining
- Enteric duplication cyst
  - ➢ Enteric lining with muscular wall
- Enteric cyst
  - ➢ Enteric lining with a fibrous wall
- Mesothelial cyst
  - ➢ Mesothelial lining
- Nonpancreatic pseudocyst
  - ➢ No lining

35-year-old woman with increasing abdominal girth [Figure 2-13-1]

Differential Diagnosis: Cystic Mesenteric Mass

- Mesenteric cyst
  - ➢ Lymphangioma
  - ➢ Enteric duplication cyst
  - ➢ Enteric cyst
  - ➢ Mesothelial cyst
  - ➢ Nonpancreatic pseudocyst
- Cystic neoplasm
  - ➢ Teratoma
  - ➢ Cystic malignant mesothelioma
  - ➢ Benign multicystic mesothelioma
  - ➢ Cystic soft tissue primary
  - ➢ Pseudomyxoma peritonei
- Complex ascites
- Pseudocyst

Figure 2-13-1

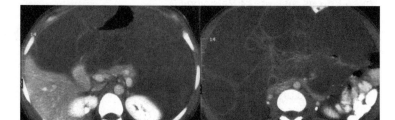

Lymphangioma

Lymphangioma

- Benign
- Vascular origin
- Affect all ages
- Many anatomic sites
  - ➢ 95% neck, axilla
  - ➢ 5% mesentery
  - ➢ Lymphangiomatosis

Lymphangioma: Mesentery

- Closely associated with small bowel
- Lack features of free fluid
  - ➢ Mass effect
  - ➢ Septations
  - ➢ No fluid in dependent spaces peritoneum

Lymphangioma: Greater Omentum

Lymphangioma: Pathology

- Interconnecting cysts
- Endothelial lining
- Dilated lymphatic spaces
  - ➢ Proteinaceous fluid
  - ➢ Chyle
  - ➢ Hemorrhage

Lymphangioma: Imaging

- Multilocular cyst
  - ➢ Fluid
  - ➢ Chyle, low attenuation
  - ➢ Enhancing septa
- Associated with small bowel
- Infiltration/insinuation
- Calcification uncommon
- Complications
  - ➢ SBO
  - ➢ Volvulus

Figure 2-13-2

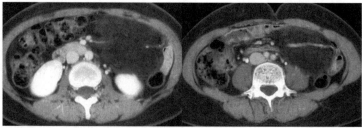

Mesenteric lymphangioma showing low attenuation and insinuating growth

Lymphangioma: Insinuating Growth and Fat Attenuation
[Figure 2-13-2]

Lymphangioma: Small Bowel Volvulus [Figure 2-13-3]

Figure 2-13-3

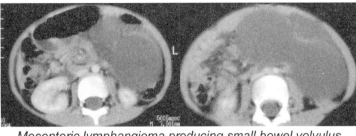

Mesenteric lymphangioma producing small bowel volvulus

71-year-old woman with abdominal pain [Figure 2-13-4]

Differential Diagnosis
- Pancreatic cystic neoplasm
  - ➢ Mucinous cystic neoplasm
  - ➢ Oligocystic adenoma
- Pancreatic pseudocyst
- Mesenteric cyst
  - ➢ Lymphangioma
  - ➢ Enteric duplication cyst
  - ➢ Enteric cyst
  - ➢ Mesothelial cyst
  - ➢ Pancreatic pseudocyst
- Cystic mesenteric neoplasm

Figure 2-13-4

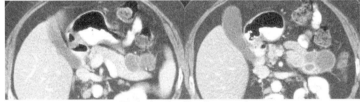

Enteric duplication cyst

Enteric Duplication Cyst

Enteric Cyst and Mesothelial Cyst
- Enteric cyst
  - ➢ Variant of enteric duplication, does not contain muscular wall
- Mesothelial cyst
  - ➢ Rare
  - ➢ Fusion failure of visceral/parietal peritoneum
- Nonspecific imaging features
- Similar appearance compared to enteric duplication cyst

Nonpancreatic Pseudocyst [Figure 2-13-5]
- Old hematoma, abscess
- No histologic lining
- Imaging
  - ➢ Thick walled
  - ➢ Internal debris

Figure 2-13-5

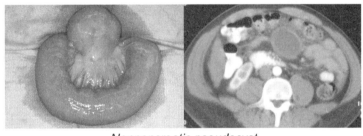

Nonpancreatic pseudocyst

55-year-old man, former shipyard worker, with worsening abdominal pain
[Figure 2-13-6]

Differential Diagnosis
- Metastatic disease
- Primary neoplasms
  - ➢ Diffuse malignant mesothelioma
  - ➢ Serous papillary carcinoma
  - ➢ Intra-abdominal desmoplastic round cell tumor
  - ➢ Leiomyomatosis peritonealis disseminata
- Diffuse Infection
  - ➢ Tuberculosis
  - ➢ Histoplasmosis

Figure 2-13-6

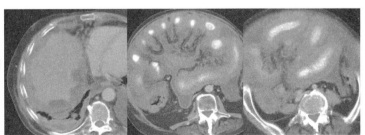

Diffuse malignant mesothelioma

Diffuse Malignant Mesothelioma
- Malignancy of mesothelial origin
- Association with asbestos
- Variants
  - ➢ Diffuse peritoneal malignant mesothelioma
  - ➢ Cystic malignant mesothelioma

Diffuse Malignant Mesothelioma

- Gross Pathology
  - ➢ Nodules, masses, caking
  - ➢ Bowel encasement
  - ➢ Thick, nodular peritoneum
  - ➢ Ascites
- Histopathologic variants
  - ➢ Desmoplastic
  - ➢ Lymphohistiocytoid
  - ➢ Small cell
  - ➢ Papillary

Diffuse Malignant Mesothelioma

- Peritoneal soft tissue nodules
- Omental and mesenteric masses, nodules
- Ascites
- Bowel wall thickening
- Fixation of small bowel

Diffuse Peritoneal Malignant Mesothelioma

Diffuse Peritoneal Malignant Mesothelioma: Peritoneal, Omental Nodules and Masses

Diffuse Malignant Mesothelioma: Small Bowel Fixation

Cystic Malignant Mesothelioma [Figure 2-13-7]

Figure 2-13-7

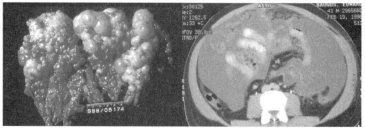

Benign Multicystic Mesothelioma

[Figure 2-13-8]
- Rare
  - ➢ Arises from pelvic peritoneum
- Unrelated to asbestos
- Unrelated to malignant mesothelioma
- Synonym
  - ➢ Multilocular peritoneal inclusion cyst
- Most common in women
  - ➢ Mean age, 37 years
- Clinical symptoms
  - ➢ Chronic pelvic pain

Cystic malignant mesothelioma

Figure 2-13-8

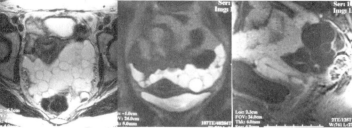

Benign Multicystic Mesothelioma

- Imaging features
  - ➢ Multicystic pelvic mass
  - ➢ Enhancing septa
  - ➢ Peritoneal surfaces of uterus, bladder
  - ➢ May extend into upper abdomen

Benign multicystic mesothelioma

Benign Multicystic Mesothelioma: Differential Diagnosis

- Metastasis
  - ➢ Mucinous adenocarcinoma
  - ➢ Serous papillary carcinoma of ovary
- Cystic malignant mesothelioma
- Primary serous papillary carcinoma of peritoneum
- Tuberculosis

11-year-old girl with cerebral palsy. She had a G-tube and Nissen repair 1-year prior and now complains of an abdominal mass [Figure 2-13-9]

Figure 2-13-9

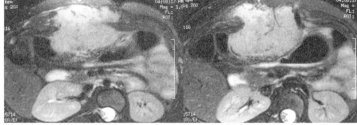

Desmoid tumor (mesenteric fibromatosis).

Differential Diagnosis: Solid Mass of Mesentery and Abdominal Wall

- Malignant
  - ➢ Soft tissue sarcoma
  - ➢ Highly aggressive lymphoma?
  - ➢ Gastrointestinal stromal tumor
  - ➢ Metastatic disease
- Benign
  - ➢ Desmoid tumor (mesenteric fibromatosis)
  - ➢ Inflammatory pseudotumor

Desmoid Tumor (Mesenteric Fibromatosis)

- Unusual
- Benign tumors
- Locally aggressive
  - ➢ Recur following resection
- Previous abdominal surgery in 2/3
- Increased incidence
  - ➢ FAP
  - ➢ *APC* germline mutations

Desmoid Tumor (Mesenteric Fibromatosis): Imaging

- Homogeneous
  - ➢ Echogenic US
  - ➢ Low attenuation CT
  - ➢ Hyperintense T2 MR
  - ➢ May enhance
- Myxoid stroma
  - ➢ Low attenuation
  - ➢ High T2 signal
- Well marginated
  - ➢ But, infiltrates bowel wall

Desmoid Tumor (Mesenteric Fibromatosis): Low attenuation, myxoid hypocellular stroma

Desmoid Tumor (Mesenteric Fibromatosis): Infiltrates small bowel wall [Figure 2-13-10]

Figure 2-13-10

- Well circumscribed
  - ➢ Locally invasive
- No capsule
- Homogenous
- No necrosis

Desmoid Tumor (Mesenteric Fibromatosis): Postoperative Recurrence

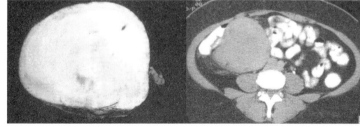

Desmoid tumor (mesenteric fibromatosis).

Desmoid Tumor (Mesenteric Fibromatosis)

Sclerosing Mesenteritis
- Rare
- Idiopathic, nonneoplastic
- Synonyms
  - Mesenteric panniculitis, fibrosing mesenteritis, mesenteric lipodystrophy
- Histologic features
  - Sclerosing fibrosis
  - Fat necrosis, lipid-laden macrophages
  - Chronic inflammation
  - Focal calcification

Sclerosing Mesenteritis *[Figure 2-13-11]*
- Variable mesenteric attenuation
  - Mixed fat/soft tissue
- Retraction of the bowel wall
  - Obstruction may occur
- May calcify

Figure 2-13-11

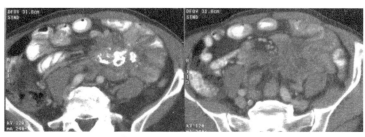

Sclerosing mesenteritis

Inflammatory Myofibroblastic Tumors (Inflammatory Pseudotumor) *[Figure 2-13-12]*
- Inflammatory infiltrates mixed with fibroblasts, collagen, and myxoid stroma
- Soft tissue mass on imaging
- Occurs in many locations
  - Liver, spleen
  - Lung
  - Lymph nodes
  - Gastrointestinal tract
  - Mesentery

Figure 2-13-12

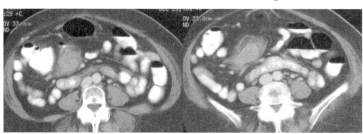

Inflammatory myofibroblastic pseudotumor

Summary: Mesenteric Cyst
- Lymphangioma
  - Endothelial lining
- Enteric duplication cyst
  - Enteric lining with muscular wall
- Enteric cyst
  - Enteric lining with a fibrous wall
- Mesothelial cyst
  - Mesothelial lining
- Nonpancreatic pseudocyst
  - No lining

Summary: Mesenteric Cyst
- <u>Lymphangioma</u>
- Most common
- Imaging
  - Multilocular
  - Enhancing septa
  - Insinuating growth

Summary: Mesenteric Cyst
- <u>Enteric duplication cyst</u>
- <u>Enteric cyst</u>
- Histologic differentiation
- Identical imaging

Summary: Mesenteric Cyst
- <u>Mesothelial cyst</u>
- Nonspecific imaging appearance

Summary: Mesenteric Cyst
- <u>Nonpancreatic pseudocyst</u>
- No histologic lining
- Old trauma/abscess
- Imaging
  - ➢ Thick wall
  - ➢ Internal debris

Summary: Mesothelioma
- Diffuse malignant mesothelioma
- Cystic malignant mesothelioma
- Benign multicystic mesothelioma

Summary: Mesothelioma
- Diffuse malignant mesothelioma
  - ➢ Asbestos
  - ➢ Nodules, masses
  - ➢ Bowel encasement
  - ➢ Bowel fixation

Summary: Mesothelioma
- Cystic malignant mesothelioma
  - ➢ Variant of DMM
  - ➢ Cystic masses
  - ➢ Ascites

Summary: Mesothelioma
- Benign multicystic mesothelioma
  - ➢ Unrelated to DMM
  - ➢ Unrelated to asbestos
  - ➢ Pelvic peritoneum
  - ➢ Multicystic mass

Summary: Fibrosing Lesions
- Desmoid tumor (mesenteric fibromatosis)
- Sclerosing mesenteritis (fibrosing mesenteritis)
- Inflammatory myofibroblastic pseudotumor

Summary: Desmoid Tumor (Mesenteric Fibromatosis)
- Benign
- Solid mass
  - ➢ Mesentery
  - ➢ Abdominal wall
- Well defined
  - ➢ Homogenous
- Infiltrates bowel wall
- Locally aggressive

Summary: Sclerosing Mesenteritis
- Rare, idiopathic
- Mixed attenuation
- Bowel retraction
- May calcify

Summary: Inflammatory Pseudotumor
- Inflammatory/fibrotic infiltrate
- Nonspecific imaging
  - ➢ Soft tissue mass

Seminar 1: Abdominal Gas

Angela D. Levy, LTC, MC, USA
Department of Radiologic Pathology
Armed Forces Institute of Pathology
Washington, DC

Case 1: 45 year old male with chronic pancreatitis and acute onset of lower abdominal pain, distension, and constipation

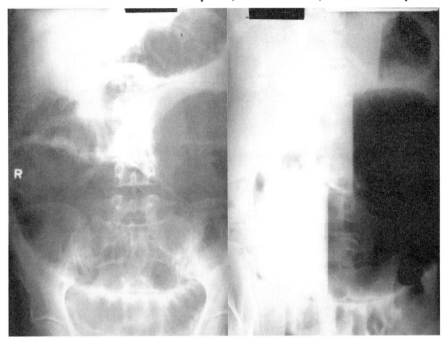

- Cecal Volvulus and Pneumatosis

Cecal Volvulus
- Acute mechanical obstruction
- Volvulus is an axial twist of at least 90 degrees
- Bascule is an anterior-cephalad fold
- Both can cause obstruction, ischemia, and necrosis
- Volvulus:Bascule = 10:1

Sigmoid Volvulus

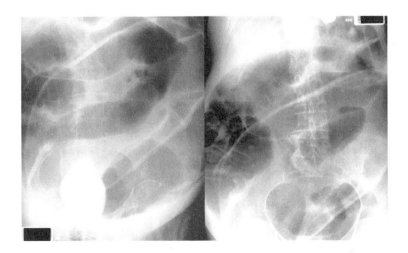

Transverse Colon Volvulus

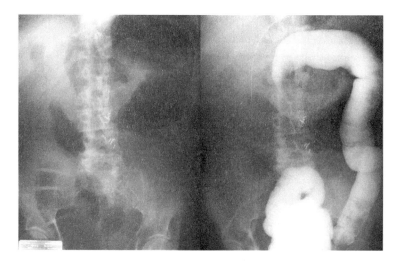

Case 2: 85 year old female with abdominal pain, fever, and shock

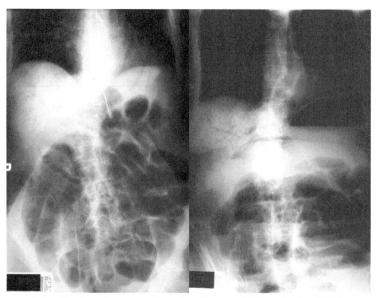

- Intestinal Ischemia with Infarction and Hepatic Portal Venous Gas

Hepatic Portal Venous Gas
- Branching radiolucencies extending to within two cm of the hepatic capsule
- Must differentiate from pneumobilia
- Differential Diagnosis:
  - ➤ Bowel Necrosis (75%)
  - ➤ IBD (10%)
  - ➤ Abscess
  - ➤ Obstruction
  - ➤ Ulcer
- Grave Prognosis

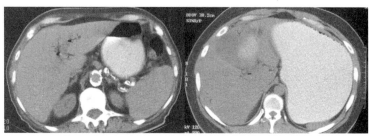

Pneumobilia   Portal venous gas

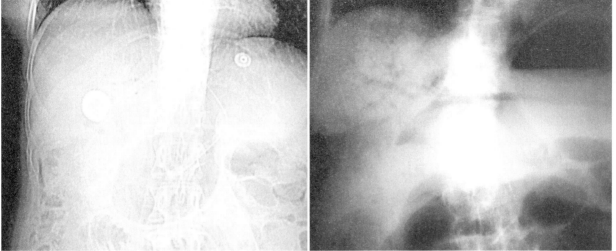

| Pneumobilia | Portal venous gas |

Pneumatosis Intestinalis
"A Sign, Not A Disease"
- Intraepithelial, submucosal or subserosal Gas
  - ➢ Aquired or generated
- Cystic
  - ➢ benign, idiopathic (pneumatosis cystoides intestinalis)
- Linear
  - ➢ benign or malignant (life threatening)
- Other terminology
  - ➢ intestinal emphysema
  - ➢ intestinal gas cysts
  - ➢ Lymphopneumatosis
  - ➢ pseudolipomatosis

Case 3: 60 year old male with progressive dyspepsia and acute, severe upper abdominal pain

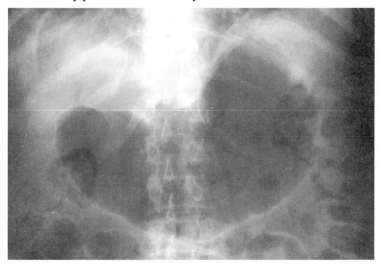

- Gastric Ulcer Perforation with Pneumoperitoneum

Pneumoperitoneum: Signs on the Supine Abdominal Film
- Central Diaphragm (Cupola)
- Diaphragmatic Slips (Leaping Dolphins)
- Morison's Pouch (Doge's Cap)
- Lesser Sac
- Falciform Ligament
- Fissure of Ligamentum Teres

Case 4: 67 year old male with severe chest pain after vomiting

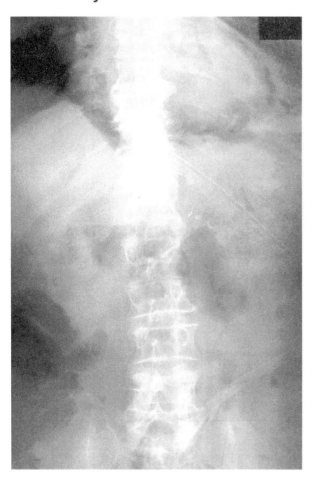

- Boerhaave's Syndrome : Described in 1724 by Dr. Hermann Boerhaave who attended to the Baron John Van Wassenaer, Grand Admiral of the Netherlands, and performed his autopsy

Boerhaave's Syndrome
- Emetogenic rupture of the distal esophagus or gastric cardia
- Left posterolateral region (1.5 - 4 cm tear)
  - ➢ reduced muscle fibers
  - ➢ entrance of nerves, vessels
  - ➢ lack of buttressing structures
- Mediastinal, pleural fluid, gas
- Left basilar pulmonary infiltrate

Causes of Esophageal Rupture
- Spontaneous
  - ➢ Boerhaave
  - ➢ Mallory-Weiss
- Iatrogenic
  - ➢ Endoscopic, Surgical Dilation
  - ➢ Tube placement
- Other
  - ➢ Caustic Ingestion
  - ➢ Trauma
  - ➢ Inflammatory
  - ➢ Neoplastic

Case 5: 50 year old male with upper abdominal pain, epigastric fullness, and constipation

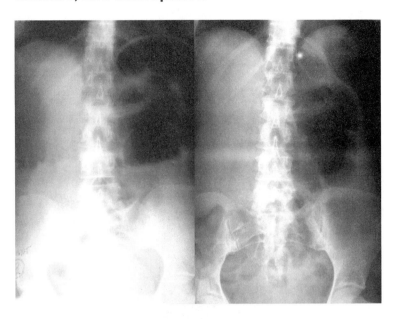

- Cecal Herniation through the Foramen of Winslow

Foramen Of Winslow Hernia
- Eight percent of internal hernias
- Large foramen
- Mobile, unfixed cecum
- Involvement:
  - ➢ Small intestine 70%
  - ➢ Cecum   25%

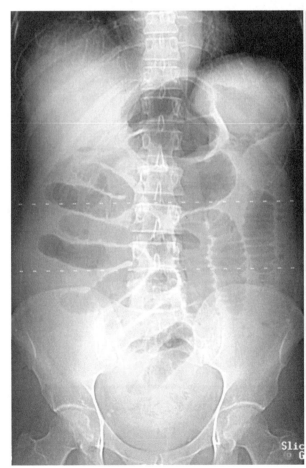

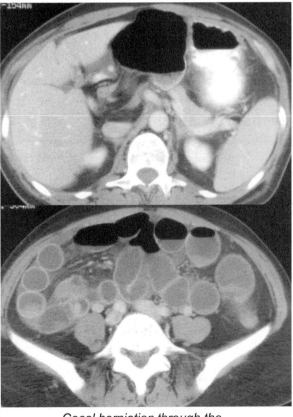

Cecal herniation through the foramen of Winslow

Seminar 2: Diffuse Diseases of the Stomach

Angela D. Levy, LTC, MC, USA
Associate Chairman
Chief, Gastrointestinal Radiology
Department of Radiologic Pathology
Armed Forces Institute of Pathology

Case 1: 65-year-old woman presents with retching and the production of little vomitus. The ER physician cannot pass a NG tube into her stomach

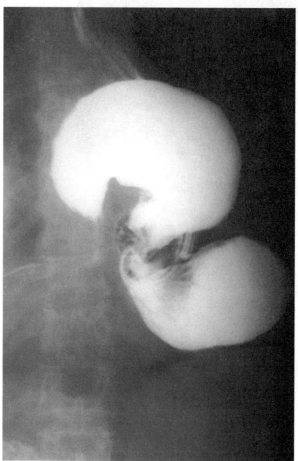

- Mesenteroaxial Volvulus

Gastric Volvulus

- Abnormal rotation of the stomach
- >180 degrees of twisting results in obstruction
- Clinical presentation
  - ➢ Severe epigastric pain
  - ➢ Violent retching with production of little vomitus
  - ➢ Inability to pass NG tube into stomach
- Organoaxial
  - ➢ Rotation about a line extending from cardia to pylorus
- Mesenteroaxial
  - ➢ Rotation about a line connecting middle of lesser curvature to middle of greater curvature
- Mixed types occur
- 30% associated with hiatal hernia

Gastric Volvulus - Radiologic Features

- Double air-fluid level on plain film
- Inversion of stomach with greater curve above lesser curve
- Positioning of cardia and pylorus at the same level
- Downward pointing pylorus and duodenum on barium studies

Mechanism for organoaxial volvulus

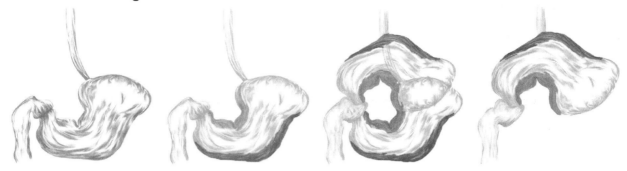

Mechanism for mesenteroaxial volvulus

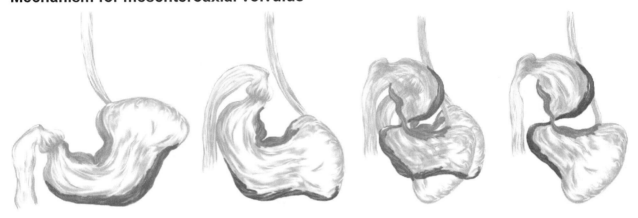

Case 2: 22-year-old woman developed epigastric pain when she was dieting in preparation for her wedding

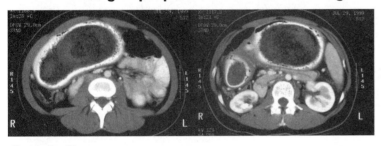

- Gastric Bezoar

Gastric Bezoar
- Accumulated ingested material
- Trichobezoar
  - ➢ Hair
- Phytobezoar
  - ➢ Vegetable material
- Pathophysiology
  - ➢ Altered gastric motility
  - ➢ Altered gastric anatomy
  - ➢ Trichotillomania

Case 3: 8-year-old girl with recurrent emesis and diarrhea

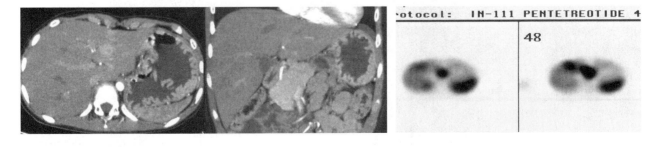

Imaging findings
- Thick gastric folds
- Thick duodenal wall
- Liver metastasis
- Large, enhancing pancreatic mass
- Positive pentetreotide scan

Zollinger-Ellison Syndrome from a Pancreatic Gastrinoma

Zollinger-Ellison Syndrome
- Affects all ages, peak 3rd to 5th decade
- Gastrin-secreting neuroendocrine tumor (gastrinoma)
  - Pancreas (75%)
  - Duodenum (15%)
  - Liver, ovary, lymph nodes
  - 60% malignant
- Clinical Features
  - One or more benign peptic ulcers
  - Diarrhea from hypergastrinemia (30%)
  - Elevated gastrin levels
- May occur in MEN I syndrome

Zollinger-Ellison Syndrome
- Radiologic features
  - Multiple ulcers
  - Increased gastric secretions
  - Thick gastric folds
- Preoperative localization of gastrinoma
  - CT
  - MR
  - Somatostatin receptor scintigraphy

Differential Diagnosis - Thick Gastric Folds
- Hypertrophic Gastropathy
  - Menetrier disease
  - Zollinger-Ellison syndrome
- Gastritis
- Neoplasm
  - Adenocarcinoma
  - Lymphoma
  - Metastasis
- Miscellaneous
  - Amyloid
  - Eosinophilic gastritis
  - Adjacent inflammation

Case 4: 70-year-old man presents epigastric pain and pedal edema

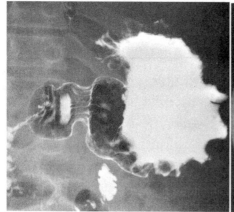 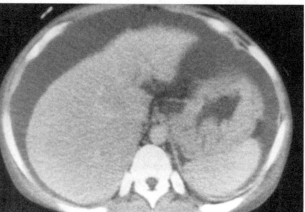

- Menetrier Disease

Menetrier Disease : Adult Form
- Most common in men, 50 to 70 years
- Symptoms
  - ➢ Epigastric pain
  - ➢ Vomiting
  - ➢ Weight loss
  - ➢ Peripheral edema
- Hypoalbuminemia and hypochlorhydria
- Diffuse enlargement of gastric folds
  - ➢ Proximal stomach
- Mucus hypersecretion
- Irreversible

Menetrier Disease : Pediatric Form
- Associated with CMV infection
- Allergic or autoimmune reaction
- Symptoms
  - ➢ Periorbital and facial edema
  - ➢ Vomiting
  - ➢ Pain
- Self-limited
- Spontaneous resolution and reversal of protein loss
- Antrum more commonly involved

Menetrier Disease : Pathology
- Pathology
  - ➢ Foveolar hyperplasia, glandular atrophy, cysts
  - ➢ Enlarged folds (1-3 cm) resembling cerebral convolutions
  - ➢ H. pylori?

Menetrier Disease : Radiology
- Thick folds
  - ➢ Non uniform
  - ➢ Tortuous
- Spiculation of greater curvature
- Antral sparing
- Flocculation of contrast

Case 5: UGI images from two different patients that complained of epigastric pain. Both patients had a history of diarrhea

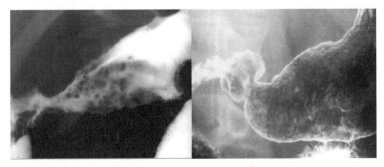

Case 5A   Case 5B

Radiologic Findings
- Narrowed antrum
- Multiple Filling defects
- Nodularity
- Ulceration?
- Effaced/nodular duodenal bulb

- Multiple ulcers
  - ➢ Aphthous ulcers
- Nodularity

Case 5 : Differential Diagnosis

- Gastritis
  - ➢ H. pylori
  - ➢ Radiation
  - ➢ Caustic ingestion
- Neoplasm
  - ➢ Lymphoma
  - ➢ Mets
  - ➢ Adenocarcinoma
- Granulomatous disease
  - ➢ Crohn
  - ➢ Sarcoid
  - ➢ Amyloid
  - ➢ TB
  - ➢ cutaneous hemangiomas, soft tissue hypertrophy of the lower extremity, congenital varicose veins

Gastric Crohn Disease

- Histologically present in up to 33% of patients with Crohn disease
- 20% of patients with ileo-colic disease have abnormal UGI [1]
- Antrum and duodenum most often affected

[1] Levine MS. Crohn's disease of the upper gastrointestinal tract. RCNA 1987

Gastric Crohn Disease

- Aphthous ulcers
- One or more large ulcers
- Nodular/cobblestone mucosa
- Abnormal gastric motility
- Tubular antrum
  - ➢ ram's horn sign
  - ➢ Shofar sign
- Obliteration of the pylorus
  - ➢ Pseudo-Billroth I sign

Seminar 3: Polyposis Syndromes

Angela D. Levy, LTC, MC, USA
Department of Radiologic Pathology
Armed Forces Institute of Pathology
Washington, DC

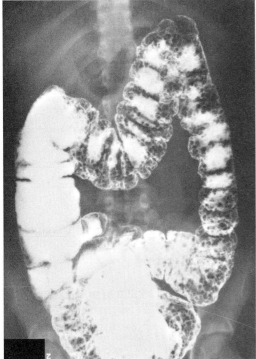

Case 1: 35-year-old woman presents with jaundice. She had a total proctocolectomy at age 20 for colonic polyps

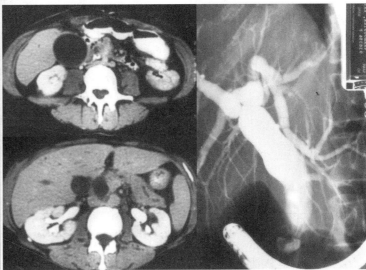

• Familial Adenomatous Polyposis Syndrome (FAP) with Ampullary Carcinoma

Familial Adenomatous Polyposis Syndrome (FAP)
• Most common polyposis syndrome
• Autosomal dominant
  ➢ Abnormal tumor suppressor gene (APC gene)
  ➢ Long arm of chromosome 5
• FAP
  ➢ Familial polyposis coli
  ➢ Gardner syndrome
  ➢ Turcot syndrome
  ➢ Attenuated adenomatous polyposis coli (AAPC)
All patients have colonic polyps
Variable extraintestinal manifestations
Incidence of 1:7000 to 1:30,000
  ➢ 20 to 30% new mutations
Diagnostic criteria
  ➢ 100 or more colorectal adenomas
  ➢ Or, mutation of APC gene
  ➢ Or, family history of FAP and an epidermoid cyst, osteoma, or desmoid tumor

FAP : Colon
• Polyps appear in adolescence
• Adenocarcinoma always occurs
  ➢ Multifocal
  ➢ Left-sided predominance
• Treatment: total proctocolectomy with ileoanal anastomosis

FAP : Duodenum and Ampulla
- Duodenal adenomas very common
- Develop in the 2nd to 5th decade of life
- Periampullary carcinoma
  - ➢ Second most frequent site of adenocarcinoma in FAP
  - ➢ Cause of death in 22% of patients following successful proctocolectomy

FAP : Stomach
- Fundic gland polyps
  - ➢ Most common gastric manifestation in western countries
  - ➢ Occur early, <20 years of age
  - ➢ Gastric fundus and body
  - ➢ Multiple and small (<8 mm)
  - ➢ Generally considered to be benign
- Adenomas
  - ➢ More common in Japan
  - ➢ Occur later than colonic adenomas, when patients are in their 30's
  - ➢ Multiple, sessile (5 to 10mm)
  - ➢ Gastric antrum
  - ➢ May develop into adenocarcinoma

FAP : Extraintestinal Manifestations
- Skin and Eye
  - ➢ Epidermoid (sebaceous) cysts, lipomas, fibromas, neurofibromas
  - ➢ Café au lait spots
  - ➢ Congenital hypertrophy of the retinal pigment epithelium (75-80%)
- Teeth and Bone
  - ➢ Supernumerary teeth, caries, dentigerous cysts, odontomas, mandibular enosteomas
  - ➢ Osteomas (mandible, skull, sinuses)
  - ➢ Cortical thickening
- Fibrous Proliferation
  - ➢ Keloids, post-op adhesions
  - ➢ Fibromatosis (desmoids)-abdominal wall, mesentery
  - ➢ Retroperitoneal fibrosis
- Thyroid Carcinoma
  - ➢ Papillary, often multifocal and affect young women
- CNS malignancies
- Other tumors
  - ➢ Hepatoblastoma, focal nodular hyperplasia, adrenal adenoma/carcinoma, carcinoid tumors

Case 2 : 22-year-old woman S/P total proctocolectomy with J-pouch. She is noted to a have an elevated fundal height during her routine OB visit

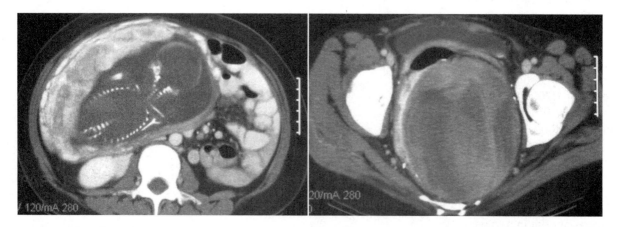

- FAP with Fibromatosis

FAP : Fibromatosis (Desmoid Tumor)
- Occurs in young patients
  - Mean age, 30 years
- 86% of patients have undergone a proctocolectomy
- Hormonal factors play a role
  - More common in women
  - May occur during with elevated estrogen (pregnancy)
- Locally aggressive
- Recurrence rate 81%

Case 3: 23-year-old man with recurrent abdominal pain

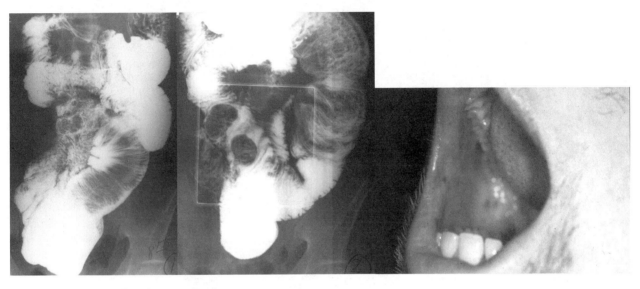

- Peutz-Jeghers Syndrome

Peutz-Jegher Syndrome (PJS)
- One-tenth as common as FAPS
- Autosomal dominant
- Two major components
  - GI hamartomatous polyps
  - Pigmented macules on skin or mucous membranes
- Presenting symptoms
  - Abdominal pain
  - GI bleeding
  - Rectal prolapse

PJS : Hamartomatous Polyp
- Smooth muscle core with overlying normal epithelium indigenous to the site of bowel in which the polyp occurs
- Carcinoma may develop
  - Adenomatous foci within the polyp

PJS : GI Manifestations
- Jejunum, ileum, colon, stomach, duodenum, and appendix affected in decreasing order of frequency
- Polyps may be sessile or pedunculated
- Few millimeter to 7 cm
- Transient intussusception common
- Treatment: polypectomy

PJS : Malignancy

- Cancer risk 50%
- GI malignancies
  - ➢ Colon, gastric, small bowel, gallbladder, biliary, pancreatic adenocarcinomas
  - ➢ Epitheliod leiomyosarcoma
- Extraintestinal malignancies
  - ➢ Breast and reproductive organs ("sex cord tumors with annular tubules" and "adenoma malignum")
  - ➢ Intraabdominal desmoplastic small cell tumors

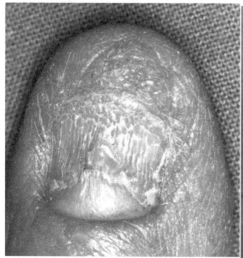

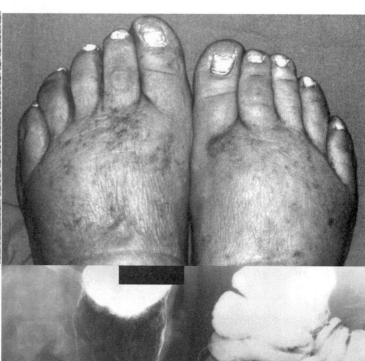

Case 4: 71-year-old woman with gradual onset of fatigue, weight loss, alopecia, loss of toe nails and finger nails, and diarrhea. Her labs show anemia and hypoproteinemia

- Cronkhite-Canada Syndrome

Cronkhite-Canada Syndrome (CCS)

- Sporadic (non-familial)
  - ➢ M=F
- Age of onset >50 years
- Syndrome components
  - ➢ GI polyps
  - ➢ Ectodermal abnormalities of skin (hyperpigmentation), hair (alopecia), and nails (onychodystrophy)
  - ➢ Malabsorption
- Presenting symptoms
  - ➢ Diarrhea, bleeding, weight loss, abdominal pain, anorexia
- Treatment: nutritional support, antibiotics, anabolic hormones
- Mortality rate 60%

CCS : GI Manifestations

- Hamartomatous polyps
- Sessile or pedunculated polyps
  - ➤ Stomach
  - ➤ Small bowel
  - ➤ Colon
- Thick gastric and duodenal folds
- Association with colon cancer

Case 5: 50-year-old man with multiple nodular growths on the face and skin

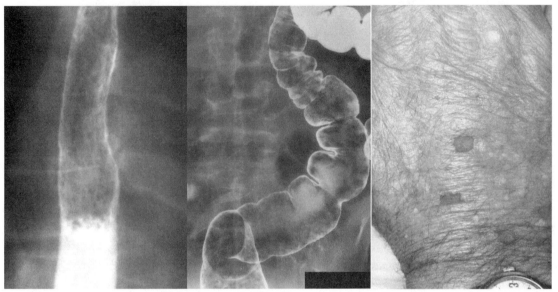

- GCowden syndrome with glycogen acanthosis

Cowden Syndrome (Multiple Hamartoma Syndrome)

- Autosomal dominant
- Usually presents by the late 20's
- Facial tricholemmomas
- Diagnostic criteria:
  - ➤ Mucocutaneous lesions
  - ➤ Breast (50%), thyroid (follicular) carcinoma
  - ➤ Lhermitte-Duclos disease
  - ➤ Macrocephaly
  - ➤ GI hamartomas
  - ➤ Mental retardation, lipomas, fibromas, GU tumors, benign thyroid and breast lesions

Cowden Syndrome: GI Manifestations

- Polyps in 70 to 85% of patients
- Multiple, small sessile polyps
- Variable histology
  - ➤ Hyperplastic, hamartoma, adenoma, juvenile, lipoma, lymphoid, ganglioneuroma, inflammatory fibroid polyp
- Any part of GI tract involved
  - ➤ Rectosigmoid most common
- Esophageal glycogen acanthosis
- Occasional, GI adenocarcinoma

Case 6: 15-year-old boy with recurrent rectal bleeding

- Juvenile Polyposis Syndromes

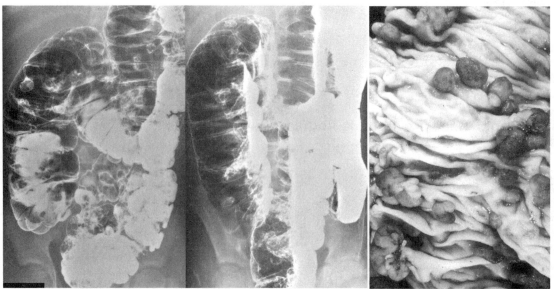

Juvenile Polyposis Syndromes
- Juvenile polyposis
  - ➢ Juvenile polyposis of the colon
  - ➢ Juvenile polyposis of the gastrointestinal tract
- Juvenile polyposis of infancy (infantile Cronkhite-Canada syndrome)

Juvenile Polyposis
- Autosomal dominant
- Two-thirds present within the first two decades of life
- Juvenile polyps
  - ➢ Hamartomatous polyps
  - ➢ Colorectum, stomach, small intestine
- Diagnostic criteria
  - ➢ >5 juvenile polyps of the colorectum
  - ➢ or, juvenile polyps throughout the GI tract
  - ➢ or, any number of juvenile polyps with a positive family history

Juvenile Polyposis of Infancy
- Autosomal recessive
- Associated congenital anomalies
  - ➢ Cardiac, CNS, GU, GI
- Diarrhea, anemia, hypoalbuminemia
- Fatal before age 2
- Generalized GI polyps

Juvenile Polyposis : Malignancy
- Increased incidence of colorectal carcinoma (30 to 40%)
  - ➢ Coexisting adenomas
  - ➢ Adenomatous change within a juvenile polyp
- Increased risk of upper GI cancers (10 to 15%)

Colon Cancer Syndromes
- Sporadic cancers, but other family members have colon cancer (30%)
- Colon cancer family syndrome (5%)
  - ➢ Hereditary nonpolyposis colon cancer (HNPCC)
- Polyposis syndromes (1%)

Hereditary Nonpolyposis Colon Cancer Syndromes (HNPCC)

Lynch I

Early onset, right-sided, frequently multiple, colon cancers

Lynch II

Lynch I + extracolonic tumors

Extracolonic tumors: small intestine, stomach, pancreas, biliary, renal, transitional cell, ovary, endometrium, laryngeal, breast, glioblastoma

Muir-Torre

Similar to Lynch II + skin lesions

Skin lesions: sebaceous adenoma, kerato-acanthoma, squamous cell, basal cell, cysts, fibromas

Summary : Polyposis Syndromes

- FAP is the most common
- Increased risk of malignancy in all polyposis syndromes
- Autosomal dominant inheritance pattern, except
  - ➢ Cronkhite-Canada (sporadic)
  - ➢ Juvenile polyposis of infancy (autosomal recessive)
- Colonic disease predominates
  - ➢ Except Peutz-Jegher, mostly small bowel
- Esophagus rarely involved
  - ➢ Except Cowden, glycogen acanthosis

Seminar 4: Pancreatic Duct

Angela D. Levy, LTC, MC, USA
Department of Radiologic Pathology
Armed Forces Institute of Pathology

Normal Pancreatic Embryology

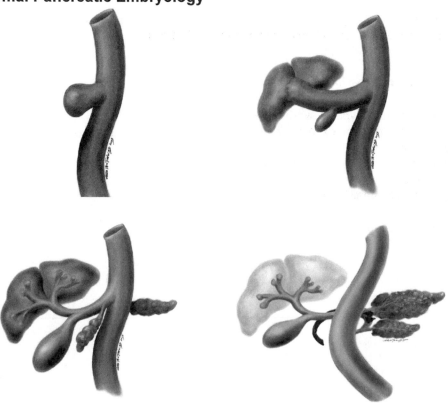

Normal pancreatic and biliary duct anatomy

- Minor Papilla
  - ➢ Accessory PD
  - ➢ Duct of Santorini
- Major Papilla
  - ➢ Main PD
  - ➢ Duct of Wirsung

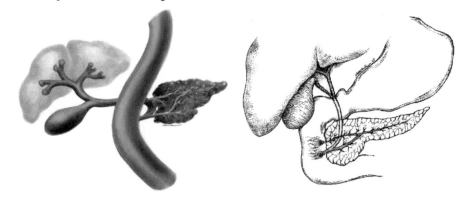

Anatomic variants of the pancreatic duct

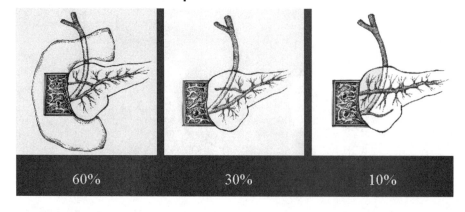

60%   30%   10%

Normal Pancreatic Duct

Case 1: 25-year-old woman with a long history of nausea, vomiting, and abdominal distension

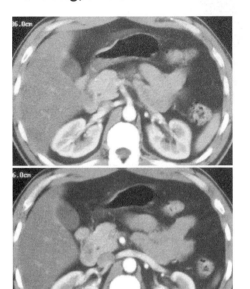

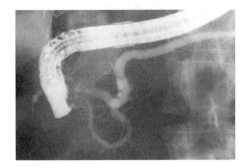

Annular Pancreas
- Bilobed ventral pancreatic bud
- Buds migrate in opposite directions
- Duodenal obstruction

Case 2: 17-year-old female with abdominal pain and elevated LFTs

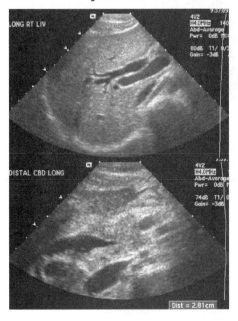

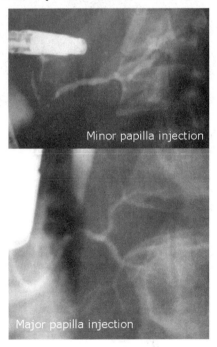

Pancreatic Divisum
- Incomplete fusion of dorsal and ventral pancreas
- Body and tail drain through the duct of Santorini, minor papilla
- Incidence
  - ➢ 4 to 11% (autopsy)
  - ➢ 3 to 4% (ERCP)
- Most asymptomatic
- 12-24% develop idiopathic recurrent pancreatitis

Case 3: Two Different Patients with the same Disease

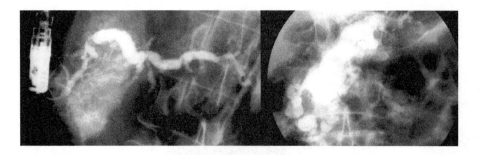

Chronic Pancreatitis : Ductal Features

- Ectasia
  - ➢ Loss of normal tapering
- Contour irregularity
- Side branches
  - ➢ Clubbing
  - ➢ Stenosis
  - ➢ Opacification of cavities
- Stenoses or occlusion
  - ➢ "Chain of lakes"
- Intraductal calculi

Case 4: 50-year-old man with abdominal pain

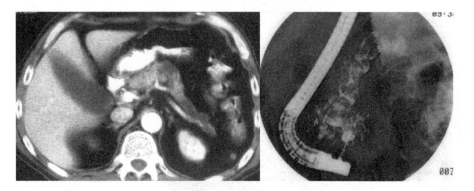

Intraductal Papillary Mucinous Neoplasm

Main Duct IMPT

Side Branch IPMT

Bulging Papilla

Case 5: 45-year-old man with chest pain and elevation of serum amylase

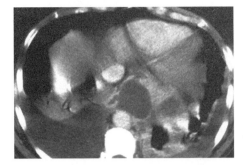 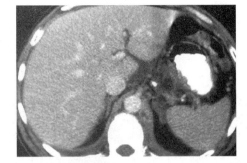

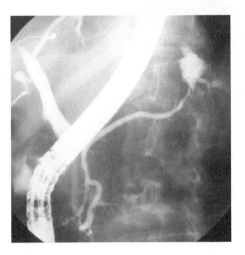

Mediastinal Pseudocyst

Fluid Collections and Pancreatitis
- 50% of patients
  - ➢ Rupture of pancreatic duct
  - ➢ Exudation of fluid from gland surface
- Most disappear
- Pseudocysts
  - ➢ Unresorbed fluid with a fibrous capsule

Seminar 5: Hepatic Imaging

Angela D. Levy, LTC, MC, USA
Department of Radiologic Pathology
Armed Forces Institute of Pathology
Washington, DC

Case 1: 50-year-old woman with vague abdominal discomfort

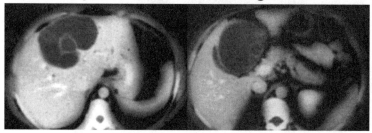

Differential Diagnosis: Complex Hepatic Cyst

- Nonneoplastic
  - ➢ Echinococcal cyst
  - ➢ Simple cyst with hemorrhage/infection
  - ➢ Post-traumatic cyst
  - ➢ Abscess
  - ➢ Ciliated hepatic foregut cyst
- Neoplastic
  - ➢ Biliary cystadenoma
  - ➢ Biliary cystadenocarcinoma
  - ➢ Cystic metastasis
  - ➢ Peliosis
  - ➢ Teratoma

Biliary Cystadenoma

- Cystic neoplasms
  - ➢ Uni- or multilocular
  - ➢ Malignant potential
  - ➢ Biliary cystadenocarcinoma
- Middle-aged women
  - ➢ Age range, 42-55 years
- Ovarian stroma histologically
- Imaging
  - ➢ Complex cyst
  - ➢ Septations
  - ➢ Mural nodules

Biliary Cystadenoma

Simple Cyst

Echinococcus granulosus

Pyogenic Hepatic Abscess

Case 2: 10-year-old girl with right upper quadrant pain

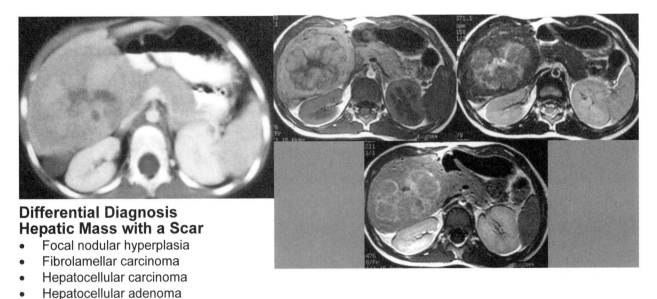

Differential Diagnosis
Hepatic Mass with a Scar
- Focal nodular hyperplasia
- Fibrolamellar carcinoma
- Hepatocellular carcinoma
- Hepatocellular adenoma
- Hemangioma

Hepatic Mass with a Scar

Focal Nodular Hyperplasia (FNH)

FNH: Sonography
- Subtle
- Similar to liver echotexture
- Doppler
  - ➢ Peripheral and central vessels
  - ➢ Radiating pattern

FNH: Computed Tomography
- Rapid arterial enhancement
- Isodense with liver in the portal venous phase
- Hypodense central scar
- Late enhancement
  - ➢ Scar
  - ➢ Peripheral vessels

FNH: Magnetic Resonance
- T1
  - ➢ Isointense
  - ➢ Low signal scar
- T2
  - ➢ Iso or slightly hyperintense
  - ➢ High signal scar
- Gd-DTPA
  - ➢ Arterial phase homogeneous enhancement
  - ➢ Delayed enhancement of the scar
- T2 with SPIO's
  - ➢ Decreased signal
  - ➢ Except scar

FNH: Sulfer Colloid
Fibrolamellar Carcinoma
Hepatocellular Carcinoma (HCC)
Hepatocellular Adenoma (HCA) with Fibrosis
Hemangioma
Hemangioma: Tagged RBC Scan

Case 3: 54-year-old man with right upper quadrant pain and jaundice

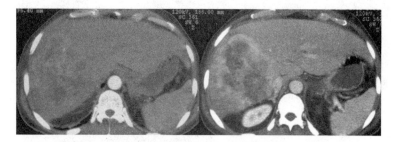

Differential Diagnosis: Rim-like Enhancement
- Hemangioma
- Metastatic disease
- Hepatocellular carcinoma
- Intrahepatic cholangiocarcinoma
- Angiosarcoma
- Epithelioid hemangioendothelioma

Intrahepatic Cholangiocarcinoma
- Delayed, rim-like enhancement
- Central hypoattenuation
- Capsular contraction
- Biliary dilatation peripheral to the mass

Intrahepatic Cholangiocarcinoma
Hemangioma
Epithelioid Hemangioendothelioma

Case 4: 50-year-old male with vague abdominal pain

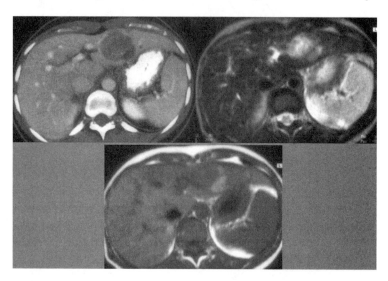

Differential Diagnosis: Liver Mass with Fat
- Hepatocellular carcinoma
- Angiomyolipoma
- Myelolipoma
- Hepatocellular adenoma
- Metastasis
  - Liposarcoma
- VERY RARE, Teratoma

Hepatocellular Carcinoma
Hepatocellular Adenoma: Focal fat and Capsule
Hepatocellular Adenoma: Diffuse Hypodensity

Angiomyolipoma
Myelolipoma
Hepatic Teratoma

Case 5: 26-year-old woman with RUQ pain and mild elevation of serum AST

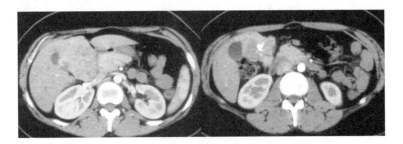

Differential Diagnosis: Calcified Liver Mass
- Nonneoplastic
  - ➢ Hematoma
  - ➢ Simple cyst
  - ➢ Parasitic infection
  - ➢ Healed infection
- Benign neoplasm
  - ➢ Hemangioma
  - ➢ Teratoma
- Malignant neoplasm
  - ➢ Fibrolamellar carcinoma
  - ➢ Epithelioid hemangioendothelioma
  - ➢ Hepatoblastoma (kids)

Fibrolamellar Carcinoma
Colon Adenocarcinoma Metastases
Echinococcus multilocularis

Seminar 6: Complications of Meckel Diverticulum

Angela D. Levy, LTC, MC, USA
Department of Radiologic Pathology
Armed Forces Institute of Pathology
Washington, DC

Cases 1-5

- All patients have the same disease
- The underlying disease is a congenital anomaly
- Each presents with a different manifestation

Case 1: 22-year-old man with fever and guaiac positive stool

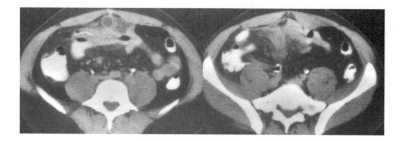

Case 2: 22-year-old man with chronic abdominal pain and anemia

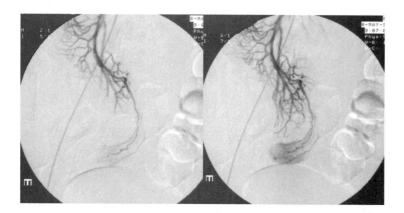

Case 3: 61-year-old woman with intermittent abdominal pain

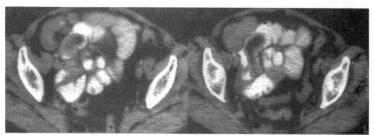

Case 4: 57-year-old man with abdominal pain and fever

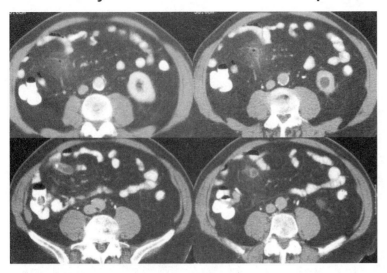

Case 5: 40-year-old man with pain and vomiting

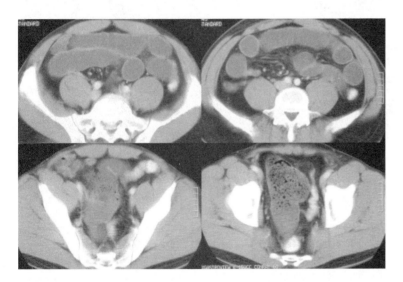

Meckel Diverticulum
- Most common anomaly of the GI tract
- 2% - 3% of the population
- M = F
- Symptoms more common in males
- 60% of patients present before age 10
- Omphalomesenteric duct anomaly
  - Improper closure and absorption

Omphalomesenteric (Vitelline) Duct
- Embryonic connection between yolk sac and midgut
- 10th week of embryogenesis
  - Midgut returns to abdomen
  - Duct is a thin fibrous band connecting midgut to umbilicus
  - Disintegrate
  - Absorption

Omphalomesenteric (Vitelline) Duct Anomalies

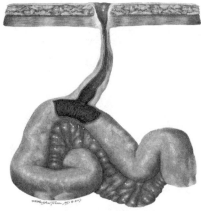

Umbilico-ileal fistula

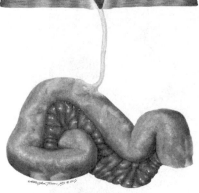

Umbilical sinus

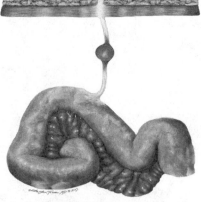

Umbilical cyst

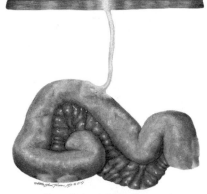

Persistent fibrous cord

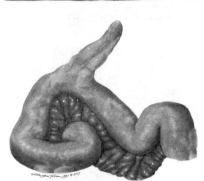

Meckel diverticulum

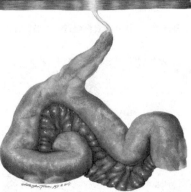

Meckel diverticulum with a fibrous attachment to the umbilicus

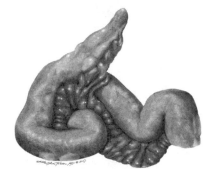

Meckel diverticulum supported by a mesentery

Omphalomesenteric (Vitelline) Duct Anomalies
- Umbilico-ileal fistula
- Umbilical sinus
- Umbilical cyst
- Persistent fibrous cord
- Meckel diverticulum
  - With a fibrous cord
  - With a portion of mesentery

Meckel Diverticulum: Pathology
- Antimesenteric side of distal ileum
  - Within 100 cm of ileocecal valve
- True diverticulum
  - Composed of all layers of the small bowel wall
- Heterotopic tissue
  - 50% of resected diverticula
  - Gastric most common (23% - 50%)
  - Pancreas (5% to 16%)
  - Rare, Brunner glands, colonic, biliary

Meckel Diverticulum: Heterotopic Gastric Mucosa

Meckel Diverticulum: Heterotopic Pancreatic Mucosa

Case 1: 22-year-old man with fever and guaiac positive stool

Differential Diagnosis
- Inflammatory bowel disease
- Urachal remnant
- Diverticulitis
- Meckel diverticulitis
- Idiopathic ileal diverticula

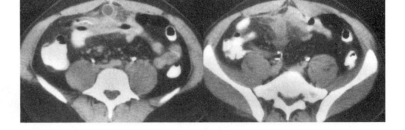

Meckel Diverticulitis

Case 2: 22-year-old man with chronic abdominal pain and anemia

Differential Diagnosis
- Neoplasm
- Ulcer
- Vascular ectasia
- Meckel diverticulum

Hemorrhagic Meckel Diverticulum

Angiographic Features of Meckel Diverticulum
- Vitellointestinal artery
  - ➤ Arises from a distal ileal branch of the SMA
- Tubular shaped angiographic blush
- Intraluminal contrast if brisk bleeding

Hemorrhage in Meckel Diverticulum
- Most frequent complication
- Tc99-pertechnetate
  - ➤ Localizes in ectopic gastric mucosa
  - ➤ Modality of choice in pediatric population
  - ➤ Sensitivity 85%, specificity 95% in kids
  - ➤ Sensitivity 63%, specificity 2% in adults

Case 3: 61-year-old woman with intermittent abdominal pain

Differential Diagnosis
- Lipoma
- Inverted Meckel diverticula

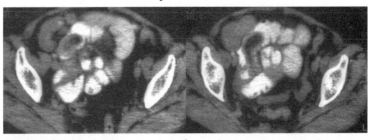

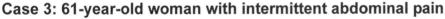

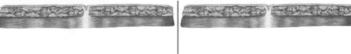

Inverted Meckel Diverticulum

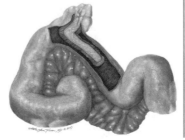

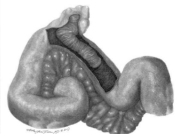

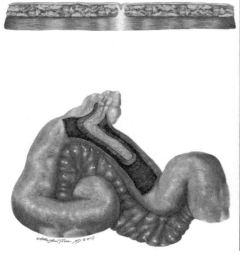 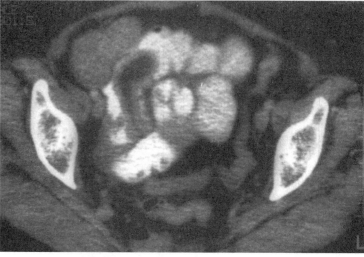

Inverted Meckel's Diverticulum with Intussusception

Case 4: 57-year-old man with abdominal pain and fever

Meckel Diverticulitis with a Stone

Meckel Diverticulitis: Etiology
- Luminal obstruction
  - ➢ Enterolith
  - ➢ Foreign body
  - ➢ Edema of orifice
- Peptic ulceration
- Torsion

Meckel Diverticulitis
- Differential diagnosis
  - ➢ Appendicitis
  - ➢ Inflammatory bowel disease
  - ➢ Idiopathic ileal diverticula
- Helpful CT features
  - ➢ Blind-ending pouch
  - ➢ Mural contrast enhancement
  - ➢ Connection to ileum
  - ➢ Midline location
  - ➢ Associated SBO

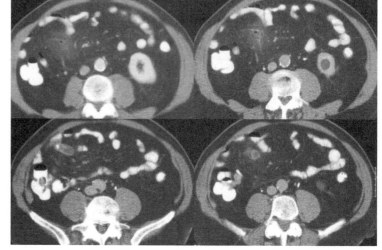

Case 5: 40-year-old man with pain and vomiting

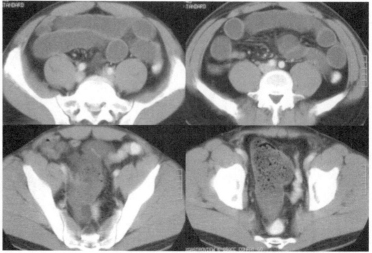

Inflamed Meckel with Small Bowel Obstruction

Obstruction in Meckel Diverticula
- Second most common complication of Meckel
- Etiology
  - ➢ Inversion with intussusception
  - ➢ Diverticulitis
  - ➢ Volvulus from attachment to umbilicus
  - ➢ Congenital mesodiverticular bands
  - ➢ Foreign body impaction
  - ➢ Inclusion of Meckel in a hernia (hernia of Littre)
  - ➢ Neoplasm
  - ➢ Inclusion of Meckel in a true knot

Summary: Complications of Meckel Diverticula
- Hemorrhage
- Obstruction
- Diverticulitis
- Inversion
  - ➢ Intussusception
- Stones
- Torsion
- Neoplasm

Cholelithiasis and Cholecystitis

Robert K. Zeman, M.D.
Professor and Chairman of Radiology
George Washington University Medical Center
Washington, D.C.

Outline/Objectives
- Detection of cholelithiasis
- Gravel versus sludge
- Acute cholecystitis
- Complications of acute cholecystitis
  - ➢ Gangrenous cholecystitis
  - ➢ Emphysematous cholecystitis
  - ➢ Empyema of the gallbladder
  - ➢ Gallbladder perforation
  - ➢ Choledocholithiasis

Premise
- The radiologist plays a central role in identifying the cause of the patient's symptoms and...
- Detecting complications of cholecystitis (inflammatory and neoplastic) that will dictate the therapeutic approach

Cholelithiasis
- 30 million American adults harbor stones
- Should "silent" stones be treated?
- 22% of patients with stones are symptomatic (Sirmione study)
- In <u>symptomatic</u> patients, 50% chance of colic in 1 year; 1–2% cumulative risk of acute cholecystitis.

Cholelithiasis
- For symptomatic stones, recommend elective laparoscopic cholecystectomy
- For acute cholecystitis:
  - ➢ Delayed surgery allows for better vizualization of surgical field
  - ➢ Early surgery means less adhesions

US of Cholelithiasis [Figure 2-20-1]
- 3 common appearances
  - ➢ Solitary stone
  - ➢ Gravel
  - ➢ Double-arc (WES)

Solitary Gallstone

Gravel

Double-Arc Sign (WES)

How Sensitive is US?
- Remember the neck of the gallbladder

Sludge vs Gravel?
- Gravel represents small, discrete calculi
- Sludge is viscous, lithogenic bile

Tumefactive Sludge
- Baseline
- After walking

Figure 2-20-1

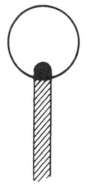 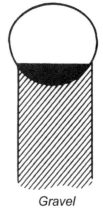 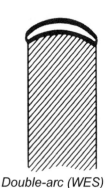

Solitary stone *Gravel* *Double-arc (WES)*

Is there any role for the OCG?
- No stones on OCG
- See 5mm stone on US

Acute Cholecystitis
- Uncomplicated vs complicated
- Cholescintigraphy vs US
- Treatment options if complications

Cholescintigraphy vs. Ultrasound
- Both equally sensitive and specific
- Emergency availability is key
- Ultrasound screens for more non-biliary diseases
- If biliary obstruction present, scintigraphy does not identify cause despite high sensitivity; US may see cause
- Scintigraphy great problem solver; can add EF when confusing symptoms

Cholescintigraphy
- The only reliable indicator of acute cholecystitis is non-visualization of the gallbladder – remember the lateral
- High sensitivity, moderate specificity

Cholescintigraphy: Positive study for acute cholecystitis

Potential Causes of False-Positive Scintigraphy For Acute Cholecystitis
- Lack of adequate fasting
- Chronic cholecystitis
- Failure to obtain delayed views
- Pancreatitis
- Hyperalimentation
- Biliary obstruction
- Prolonged fasting
- Intercurrent illness
- Alcoholism
- Overly conservative pathologic criteria of Acute Cholecystitis
- Trauma
- Gallbladder Neoplasm

Pharmacologic Enhancement of Cholescintigraphy
- Can dramatically reduce false-positives*
- Two approaches – CCK versus morphine (in setting of Suspected AC)
- Until 2002 used CCK to "pre-empt" GB
- Morphine (.04 mg/kg) given if GB fails to visualize by 30–50 minutes

*Kim et al, AJR 147:1177,1986

Use of Morphine Reduces False-Positives [Figure 2-20-2]
- 35 minutes (pre-MS)
- 55 minutes (post-MS)

Figure 2-20-2

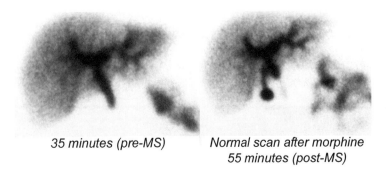

35 minutes (pre-MS)   *Normal scan after morphine 55 minutes (post-MS)*

Sonographic Findings Associated With Acute Cholecystitis

- Most useful signs
  - Cholelithiasis
  - Intramural Sonolucency
  - Sonographic Murphy Sign*
  - GB wall hyperemia**
- Secondary signs
  - Pericholecystic fluid
  - GB distention
  - Sludge
  - Gas in the Gallbladder Wall or Lumen
  - Pericholecystic Abscess

*Laing et al, Radiology 140:449, 1981
**Uggowitzer AJR 168:707, 1997

Intramural Sonolucency

- Described in 11 patients as first specific sign for acute cholecystitis*
- "Consists of a hypo-reflective or sonolucent band, continuous or interrupted, within the hyper-reflective gallbladder wall"
- Focal lucency or concentric rings (striate) most suggestive of inflammation**

*Marchal et al, Radiology 133:429, 1979
**Cohen et al, Radiology 164:31, 1987

Acute Cholecystitis-Striate GB Walls [Figure 2-20-3]

Figure 2-20-3

Acute Cholecystitis-Focal Lucency

Lucency in GB Wall is not always Edema

- Gallbladder varices in portal hypertension

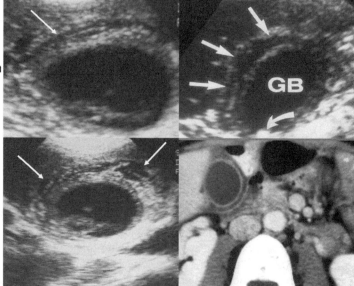

Which one has Varices?

Gallbladder Wall Thickening

- Failure to fast
- Acute cholecystitis
- Chronic cholecystitis
- Hypoalbuminemia
- Hepatitis
- Ascites
- Varices
- AIDS
- Carcinoma
- Cholesterolosis
- Mononucleosis

Multiple patients

- Beware of "sliver" of edema in some of these entities

Gallbladder Wall Thickening

- Hepatitis
- Ascites

Hyperemia of Acute Cholecystitis

Options for Treatment of Acute Cholecystitis

- PCCL
- OC
- LC
- Temporize

Role of the Radiologist in Acute Cholecystitis
- Identify findings that make temporizing ill-advised or that would potentially result in open cholecystectomy:
  - Extreme striations
  - Gangrenous cholecystitis
  - Emphysematous cholecystitis
  - Perforation
  - Biliary obstruction / Mirizzi syndrome
  - Incidental findings that preclude LC

Incidental Finding
- Hemangioma next to GB neck

Gangrenous Cholecystitis
- Not always Clostridal infection
- Implies severe inflammation
- Sonography-may see desquamated mucosa/membranes
- Scintigraphy-increased pericholecystic activity* due to:
  - delayed excretion from perihepatitis
  - hyperemia with increased tracer delivery

*Smith et al, Radiology 156:197, 1985

Gangrenous Cholecystitis-Rim Sign [Figure 2-20-4]
- Two different patients

Figure 2-20-4

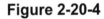
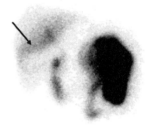
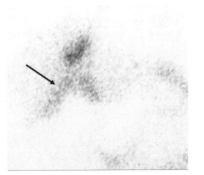

Gangrenous Cholecystitis
- Sloughed membranes

Emphysematous Cholecystitis
- Elderly patients, 20–30% are diabetic
- Male predominance
- 1/3 infected with Clostridia Welchii
- Perforation 5 times as common as for non-emphysematous cholecystitis
- "Dirty" shadowing and echogenic GB wall on sonography is suggestive
- Don't forget plain film – differential diagnosis of RUQ air

Emphysematous Cholecystitis
- US-echogenic foci=gas
- KUB

Emphysematous Cholecystitis
- US-ring-down
- KUB

Not all GB Walls with Ring-Down contain Gas
- Diagnosis?

Not all GB Walls with Ring-Down contain Gas
- Adenomyomatosis

Emphysematous Cholecystitis-CT
- Gas confined to GB wall
- Gas in lumen, hepatic ducts

Gallbladder Empyema [Figure 2-20-5]

- Infection in obstructed, inflamed gallbladder
- 25% incidence-rises to 80% if untreated after 7 days [*]
- Results in marked GB distention in 38% of patients [**]
- US, CT-Nonspecific. See distention, bile/debris level, "snow storm"

[*] Goldman et al, Gastro 11:318, 1948
[**] Fry et al, Am J Surg 141:366, 1981

Figure 2-20-5

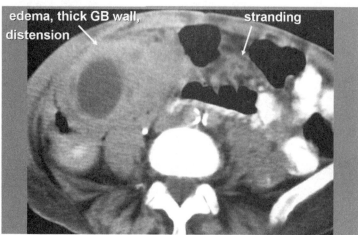

edema, thick GB wall, distension   stranding

Perforation of the Gallbladder

- Seen both in the context of chronic cholecystitis (eg., gallstone ileus) and AC
- In older literature, occurs in 3–15% of patients with acute cholecystitis
- The patient feels transiently better and then develops peritoneal signs
- Cholescintigraphy – extravasated activity – maybe
- Sonography, CT-pericholecystic collection, non-specific

Gallstone Ileus (Not AC)

- Gallstone ileus usually has chronic symptoms plus bowel obstruction

Figure 2-20-6

GB Perforation in AC [Figure 2-20-6]

GB Perforation

Choledocholithiasis

- May occur as primary duct stone (usually pigment), secondary to gallstones, or following cholecystectomy
- Most small stones will pass spontaneously. The duct caliber and dynamics may rapidly change
- CT and US are approx. 70-80% sensitive for detection of choledocholithiasis
- If you suspect CBD stones...options are MRCP, ERCP, intraop cholangiogram

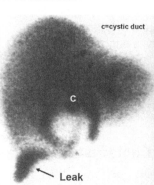
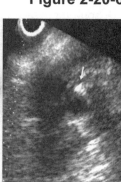

c=cystic duct

Leak

When to Perform MRCP

- Jaundice
- Dilated ducts on US
- Delayed egress on IDA
- Anatomic finding that suggests process that may result in altered duct anatomy or make laparoscopic cholecystectomy risky
- Post-cholecystectomy complications

MRCP

- T2 wt TSE or FSE, thin sections or "slab"
- Extra sections as needed

RUQ Pain (789.01) and Fever: Approach

- "R/O Acute calculous cholecystitis"...IDA, US
- "R/O Stones"...US
- "R/O Acute acalculous cholecystitis"...?
- "R/O a reason to operate"... if suspect biliary do US, if suspect acute abdomen/GI disease do CT
- Remember MRCP

Cholelithiasis and Cholecystitis References

Zeman RK, Garra BS. Gallbladder Imaging: The State-of-the-art. Gastroent Clin N. Am 2:127, 1991.

Garra BS, Davros WJ, Lack EE, Horii SC, Zeman RK: Visibility of gallstone fragments at ultrasound and fluoroscopy. Implications for monitoring of gallstone lithotripsy. Radiology 174:343, 1990.

Mathieson JR, So CB, Malone DE, Becker CD, Burhenne HJ: Accuracy of sonography for determining the number and size of gallbladder stones before and after lithotripsy. AJR 153:977, 1989.

duPlessis DJ, Jersky J. Management of acute cholecystitis. Surg Clin North Am 53:1071, 1973.

Halasz NA. Counterfeit cholecystitis: A common diagnostic dilemma. Am J Surg 130:189, 1975.

Zeman RK, Burrell MI, Cahow CE, Caride V. Diagnostic utility of cholescintigraphy and ultrasonography in acute cholecystitis. Am J Surg 141:446, 1981.

Weissmann HS, Badia J, Sugarman LA et al. Spectrum of 99m Tc-IDA cholescintigraphic patterns in acute cholecystitis. Radiology 138:167, 1981.

Eikman EA, Cameron JL, Colman M et al. A test for patency of the cystic duct in acute cholecystitis. Ann Int Med 82:318, 1975.

Fonseca C, Greenberg D, Rosenthall L et al. Assessment of the utility of gallbladder imaging with 99m Tc-IDA. Clin Nucl Med 3:437, 1978.

Freitas JE. Cholescintigraphy in acute and chronic cholecystitis. Semin Nucl Med 12:18, 1982.

Shuman WP, Gibbs P, Rudd TG et al. PIDIDA scintigraphy for cholecystitis: False positives in alcoholism and total parenteral nutrition. AJR 138:1, 1982.

Kalff V, Froelich JW, Lloyd R et al. Predictive value of an abnormal hepatobiliary scan in patients with severe intercurrent illness. Radiology 146:191, 1983.

Laing FE, Federle MP, Jeffrey RB et al. Ultrasonic evaluation of patients with acute right upper quadrant pain. Radiology 140:449, 1981.

Ralls PW, Colletti PM, Lapin SA et al. Real-time sonography in suspected acute cholecystitis: Prospective evaluation of primary and secondary signs. Radiology 155:767, 1985.

Cohan RH, Mahony BS, Bowie JD, Cooper C, Baker ME, Illescas FF: Striated intramural gallbladder lucencies on US studies. Predictors of acute cholecystitis. Radiology 164:31–35, 1987.

Teefey SA, Baron RL, Bigler SA: Sonography of the gallbladder. Significance of striated (layered) thickening of the gallbladder wall. AJR 156:945, 1991.

Shaler WJ, Leopold GR, Scheible FW: Sonography of the thickened gallbladder wall. A nonspecific finding. AJR 136:337, 1981.

West MS, Garra BS, Horii SC, Zeman RK et al. Gallbladder varices: Imaging findings in patients with portal hypertension. Radiology 179:179, 1991.

Weissmann HS, Berkowitz D, Fox MS et al. The role of technetium-99m iminodiacetic acid (IDA) cholescintigraphy in acute acalculous cholecystitis. Radiology 146:177, 1983.

Shuman WP, Rogers JV, Rudd TG et al. Low sensitivity of sonography and cholescintigraphy in acalculous cholecystitis. Radiology 142:531, 1984.

Swayne LC. Acute calculous cholecystitis: Sensitivity in detection using technetium-99m iminodiacetic acid cholescintigraphy. Radiology 160:33, 1986.

Mirvis SE, Vainright JR, Nelson AW, et al. The diagnosis of acute acalculous cholecystitis: A comparison of sonography, scintigraphy, and CT. AJR 147:171, 1986.

Jeffrey RB, Laing FC, Wong W, Callen PW. Gangrenous cholecystitis: Diagnosis by ultrasound. Radiology 156:797, 1985.

Wales LR. Desquamated gallbladder mucosa: Unusual sign of cholecystitis. AJR 139:810, 1982.

Smith R, Rosen J, Gallo LN, Alderson PO. Pericholecystic hepatic activity in cholescintigraphy. Radiology 156:797, 1985.

Siskind B, Hawkins M, Cinti D, Zeman RK, Burrell MI. Perforation of the gallbladder: Radiologic-pathologic correlation. J Clin Gastroenterol 9:670–78, 1987.

Clemett AR, Lowman RM. The roentgen features of the Mirizzi syndrome. AJR 94:480, 1965.

Weltman D, Zeman RK. Imaging of acute diseases of the gallbladder and bile ducts. Radiological Clinics of North America 32:933-950, 1994.

Fulcher AS, Turner MA, Capps GW. Technical Advances and Clinical Applications. RAdiographics 19:25-41, 1999.

Inflammatory Diseases of the Esophagus

Marc S. Levine, MD
Professor of Radiology
Hospital of the University of Pennsylvania

Figure 2-21-1

Technique
- Double-contrast:
  - ➢ Upright
  - ➢ Right lateral cardia
- Single-contrast:
  - ➢ Separate swallows
  - ➢ Prone esophagus

Reflux Esophagitis
- Most common inflam condition
- Purpose of Ba study not simply to show HH/GER but to R/O morphologic sequelae of GERD

Pathogenesis
- Frequency of GER
  - ➢ Decreased LES tone
  - ➢ Mult trans LES relaxations
- Duration of GER
  - ➢ Abnormal motility
  - ➢ (scleroderma)

Pathogenesis
- Acidity of refluxate
  - ➢ ZES (increased acid)
  - ➢ Billroth II (bile or panc)
- Resistance of mucosa
  - ➢ Age
  - ➢ Debilitation

Clinical Findings
- Heartburn and regurg
- Epigastric or RUQ pain
- Upper GI bleeding
- Dysphagia (peptic stx)

Hiatal Hernia and GER
- Occur independently
- Spont GER at fluoro:
  - ➢ 30–60% in esophagitis
  - ➢ 40–50% in volunteers

Reflux Esophagitis: Radiographic Findings
[Figures 2-21-1 and 2-21-2]
- Abnormal motility
- Granularity
- Thickened folds
- Inflammatory EG polyp
- Ulceration

Peptic Scarring: Radiographic Findings
- Radiating folds
- Deformity of wall
- Peptic stricture
- Sacculations
- Transverse folds

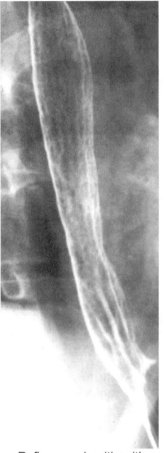

Reflux esophagitis with granular mucosa

Figure 2-21-2

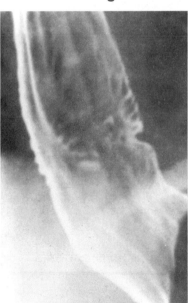

Reflux esophagitis with ulceration

Radiologic Dx of Esophagitis

	Gr 1	Gr 2	Gr 3
Koehler	13%	90%	100%
Ott	22%	83%	95%
Creteur	53%	93%	100%

Schatzki Ring
- Variant of peptic stx
- Episodic dysphagia (meat)
  - ➤ (Steakhouse syndrome)
- Symm ringlike constriction
- Vertical height 2–4 mm
- Usually sx if < 13 mm diam
- Best seen on prone views

Barrett's Esophagus
- Prog columnar metaplasia from GER and esophagitis
- Prevalence:
  - ➤ 10% with esophagitis
  - ➤ 40% with peptic stx

Clinical Findings
- Men > Women, W > B
- Reflux sx, dysphagia
- 40% asymptomatic
- Tx of GER may not cause Barrett's to regress

Histologic Findings
- Projections or islands of columnar epith separated by squam epith
- Foveolar epith > 3 cm above LES or intestinal metaplasia with goblet cells

Figure 2-21-3

Premalignant Condition
- Risk of adenocarcinoma
- Dysplasia-Ca sequence
- Endoscopic surveillance

Radiographic Findings [Figure 2-21-3]
- Classic: High stx or ulcer or reticular pattern
- Common: GER, hiatal hernia, reflux esophagitis, or peptic stricture

Dx of Barrett's by D/C Tech
- 200 pts with reflux sx
- Classified at high, mod, or low risk for Barrett's

AJR 150:97–102, 1988

Classification of Risk
- High: High stx or ulcer or reticular pattern
- Mod: Distal stx or reflux esophagitis
- Low: None of above

Radiologic vs Endoscopic Dx

Risk		Endo
High	10	9 (90%)
Moderate	73	12 (16%)
Low	117	1 (1%)

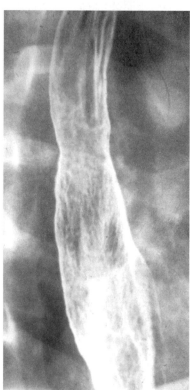

*Barrett esophagus
with mid esophageal stricture
and reticular pattern*

Radiologic Diagnosis
- Less sensitive than endoscopy
- Most false negative exams in mild disease
- Vast majority do not have Barrett's esophagus

Reflux Symptoms

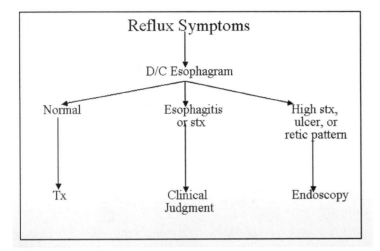

Reflux Symptoms

D/C Esophagram

Normal → Esophagitis or stx → High stx, ulcer, or retic pattern

Normal → Tx

Esophagitis or stx → Clinical Judgment

High stx, ulcer, or retic pattern → Endoscopy

Candida Esophagitis
- Most common type
- Immunocompromised (75%)
- Local esophageal stasis (25%)
  - ➤ (achalasia, scleroderma)

Clinical Findings
- Dysphagia/odynophagia
- OP Candidiasis (50%)
- Marked clinical response to antifungal agents (ketoconazole)

Radiographic Findings *[Figures 2-21-4 and 2-21-5]*
- Mucosal Plaques (90%)
  - ➤ Linear
  - ➤ Etched in white
- "Shaggy" esophagus (AIDS)
  - ➤ Plaques and membranes
  - ➤ Superimposed ulcers

Herpes Esophagitis
- 2nd most common type
- Herpes simplex virus type 1
- Immunocompromised
- Viral Cx or Bx (intranuclear inclusions in cells adjacent to ulcers)

Clinical Findings
- Dysphagia/odynophagia
- Oropharyngeal herpes
- Marked clinical response to antiviral agents (acyclovir)

Radiographic Findings *[Figure 2-21-6]*
- Discrete ulcers in upper and midesophagus
- Ulcers and plaques (mimics Candida)

Herpes Esophagitis in Healthy Pts
- Young men (15–30 y/o)
- Sexual partners with OP herpes
- Flu-like prodrome (3–10 days)
- Severe odynophagia
- Multiple tiny ulcers
- Sx resolve in 3–14 days

Figure 2-21-4

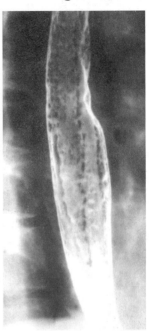

Candida esophagitis with plaques

Figure 2-21-5

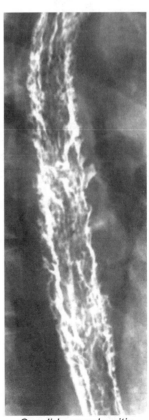

Candida esophagitis with shaggy esophagus

CMV Esophagitis
- Pts with AIDS
- Odynophagia
- Viral Cx or Bx (intranuclear inclusions in cells at ulcer base)
- Tx with ganciclovir (endo for confirmation)

Radiographic Findings [Figures 2-21-7]
- Nodular mucosa
- Small ulcers (mimics herpes)
- Giant ulcers

Figure 2-21-6

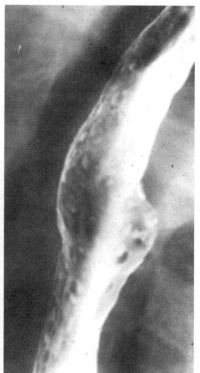

*Herpes esophagitis
with tiny ulcers*

Figure 2-21-7

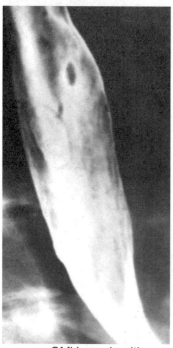

*CMV esophagitis
with giant ulcer*

Figure 2-21-8

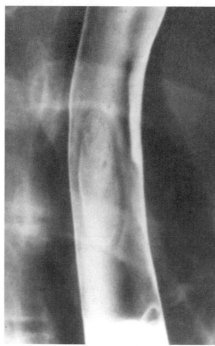

*HIV esophagitis
with giant ulcer*

HIV Esophagitis
- Odynophagia and giant ulcers
- Palatal ulcers
- Maculopapular rash
- Recent seroconversion
- Dx of exclusion (No CMV)
- Treatment with steroids

Radiographic Findings [Figure 2-21-8]
- Giant ulcers
  - ➢ (mimics CMV)
- Satellite ulcers

Giant Ulcers in 21 HIV + Pts

Cause	No Pts	%
HIV	16	76
CMV	3	14
Both	2	10

Radiology 194:447–451, 1995

Giant Ulcers in 21 HIV + Pts
- All had AIDS (CD4 ct < 200)
- Avg time from serodetect 2 yrs
- Only 1 pt had palatal ulcers or rash

Conclusions
- Most giant ulcers in HIV+ Pts caused by HIV not CMV
- Impossible to diff by clin or rad criteria
- Endoscopy for definitive Dx

Drug-Induced Esophagitis [Figure 2-21-9]
- Contact esophagitis (doxycycline, tetracycline, KCl, quinidine, NSAIDs, alendronate)
- Aortic arch or lt main bronchus
- Superficial ulcers
- Severe odynophagia but rapid clinical improvement after withdrawal of offending agent

Radiation Esophagitis
- 2–5000 rad: self-limited esophagitis (1 – 2 weeks)
- 5000 or more rad: stx, progressive dysphagia (4–8 months)
- Adriamycin potentiates XRT (only 500 rad)

Radiographic Findings
- Acute
  - Ulceration
  - Granular mucosa
  - Decreased distensibility
- Chronic
  - Abnormal motility
  - Strictures

Caustic Esophagitis
- Strong acids or alkali (liquid lye)
- Three phases of injury:
  - Acute necrosis
  - Ulceration and granulation
  - Cicatrization
- Chest pain, odynophagia, hematemesis, shock

Radiographic Findings
- Acute
  - Abnormal motility
  - Ulceration
  - Perforation
- Chronic
  - Strictures
  - (1–3 months)

Esophageal Intramural Pseudodiverticulosis
- Dilated excretory ducts
- Ductal obstruction
- Candida, diabetes, alcohol
- High strictures classic
- Peptic stx more common

Radiographic Findings
[Figures 2-21-10 and 2-21-11]
- Flask-shaped outpouchings
- "Floating" outside wall
- Associated strictures
  - (especially peptic stx)

Figure 2-21-9

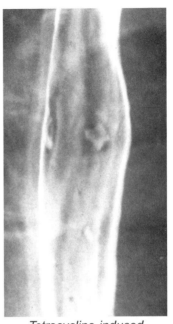

Tetracycline-induced esophagitis with three ulcers

Figure 2-21-10

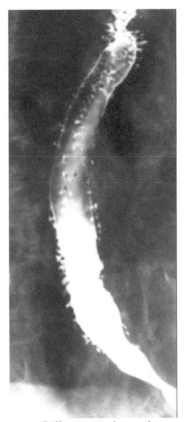

Diffuse esophageal intramural pseudodiverticulosis with high stricture

Figure 2-21-11

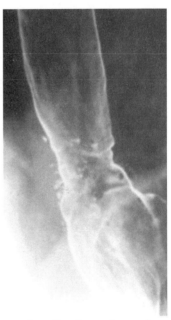

Localized esophageal intramural pseudodiverticulosis with peptic stricture

Tumors of the Esophagus

Marc S. Levine, MD
Professor of Radiology
Hospital of the University of Pennsylvania

Mucosal Lesions
- Squamous papilloma
- Adenoma
- Glycogenic acanthosis

Squamous Papilloma: Pathologic Findings
- Coral-like excrescence
- Fibrovascular core
- Hyperplastic squamous epithelium

Clinical Findings
- Usually asymptomatic
- Malignant degeneration rare
- Multiple papillomas (papillomatosis)

Radiographic Findings
- Small, sessile polyp
- Lobulated mass
- Bubbly appearance
- Diff Dx – early Ca

Glycogenic Acanthosis
- Accum of cytoplasmic glycogen
- White nodules/plaques
- Rarely causes esophageal sx
- No risk of malignant degeneration

Radiographic Findings [Figure 2-22-1]
- Round nodules/plaques
- 1–5 mm in diameter
- Predominantly midesophagus
- DDx – Candidiasis

Intramural Lesions
- Fibrovascular polyp
- Leiomyoma
- Granular cell tumor
- Duplication cyst
- Idiopathic varix

Leiomyoma: Pathologic Findings
- Most common benign tumor
- Bands of smooth muscle
- 60% DT, 30% MT, 10% PT
- Up to 20 cm in diameter
- Patterns – submucosal, exophytic, intraluminal, circumferential

Clinical Findings
- Most pts asx
- Dysphagia
- GI bleed rare
- Enucleation

Figure 2-22-1

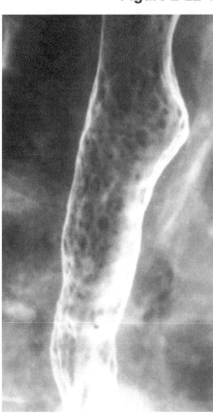

Glycogen acanthosis with nodules

Radiographic Findings [Figure 2-22-2]
- CXR – soft tissue mass, Ca++ rare
- Ba – submucosal mass
- CT – soft tissue mass
- DDx – fibroma, hemangioma, granular cell tumor, duplication cyst

Unusual Findings
- Annular lesion
- Giant intraluminal mass
- Gastric involvement
- Multiple lesions
- Leiomyomatosis

Leiomyomatosis
- Proliferation of smooth m.
- Children/adolescents
- Long-standing dysphagia
- Familial – autosomal dominant
- Alport's syndrome (nephritis, deafness, ocular lesions)

Radiographic Findings
- Ba – tapered narrowing of distal esophagus (1° achalasia?)
- Length > achalasia
- Symmetric fundal defects
- CT – thickened wall (2° achalasia?)

Fibrovascular Polyp: Pathologic Findings
- Benign intraluminal tumor
- Fibrous/adipose/vascular tissue with nl squam epith
- Hamartoma/fibroma/lipoma/fibrolipoma/angiolipoma
- All classified as FVPs
- Malig degen rare

Pathologic Findings
- Arises in cervical esophagus
- Loose submucosal conn tiss
- Dragged inf by peristalsis
- Occas prolapses into fundus
- Pedicle in cervical esophagus

Clinical Findings
- Dysphagia
- Resp sx – inspiratory stridor, choking, wheezing
- Regurgitation of fleshy mass
- Asphyxia/sudden death

Radiographic Findings [Figures 2-22-3 to 2-22-5]
- CXR
  - ➢ Rt sup med mass
  - ➢ Retrotracheal bowing
- Ba
  - ➢ Smooth, expansile intraluminal mass
  - ➢ Var size & location
  - ➢ Lobulation common
  - ➢ Prox pedicle rare
- DDx
  Air bubble, achalasia, malignant tumor

Figure 2-22-2

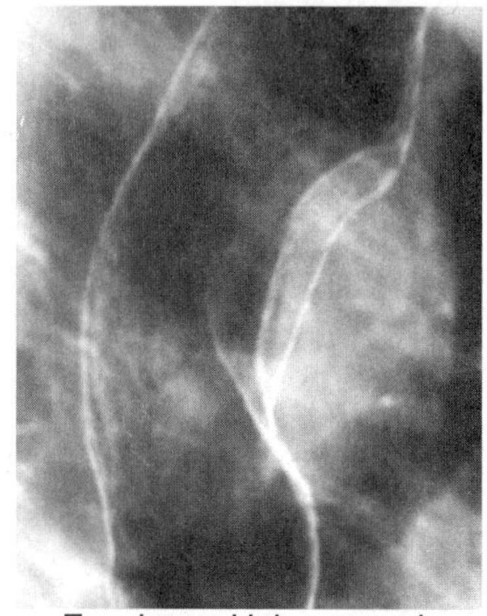

Esophageal leiomyoma in profile

Figure 2-22-3

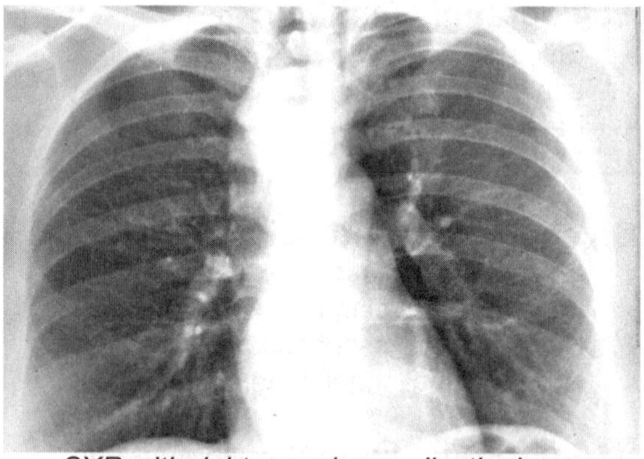

CXR with right superior mediastinal mass caused by fibrovascular polyp

Figure 2-22-4

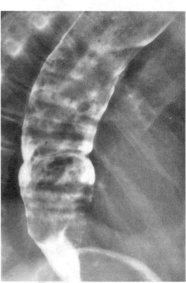

Esophagram shows fibromuscular polyp as smooth expansile mass is esophagus

Figure 2-22-5

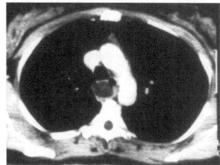

Fibrovascular polyp with fat attenuation on CT

Radiographic Findings [Figures 2-22-5 and 2-22-6]

Path	CT
• Adipose	Lipid density [1]
• Mixed	Heterogeneous
• Fibrous	Soft tissue density

[1] High-signal intensity on T1MR / High echo on endoscopic U/S

Duplication Cyst
- Abnl embryo development
- Sequest from prim foregut
- Ciliated columnar epith
- Most pts asymptomatic
- Occas bleeding/infection

Radiographic Findings
- CXR: Mediastinal mass
- Ba: Submucosal mass
- CT: Homogen low atten
- MR: High-signal on T2

Malignant Tumors
- Squamous cell carcinoma
- Adenocarcinoma
- Spindle cell carcinoma
- Small cell carcinoma
- Leiomyosarcoma
- Kaposi's sarcoma
- Malignant melanoma
- Lymphoma
- Metastases

Squamous Cell Carcinoma:
- Epidemiological Factors
- Tobacco and alcohol
- Geographic variations (China, Iran, S Africa)
- Low molybdenum in soil (accum of nitrosamines)

Predisposing Factors
- Achalasia
- Lye strictures
- Head and neck tumors
- Celiac disease
- Plummer-Vinson
- Tylosis

Definitions
- Early: mucosa or submucosa without lymph node mets
- Superficial: mucosa or submucosa with or without lymph node mets
- Small: < 3.5 cm regardless of depth of invasion or lymph node mets

Routes of Spread
- Direct extension – trachea, bronchi, lungs, pericard, aorta, diaphragms
- Lymphatic spread – nodes in med, neck, upper abdomen (paracardiac, lesser curv, celiac)
- Hematogenous – lungs, adrenals, liver

Clinical Findings
- Dysphagia and wt loss
- Odynophagia (if ulcerated)
- Chest pain (poor sign)
- Paroxysmal coughing (if TEF)
- 5-year survival < 10%

Figure 2-22-6

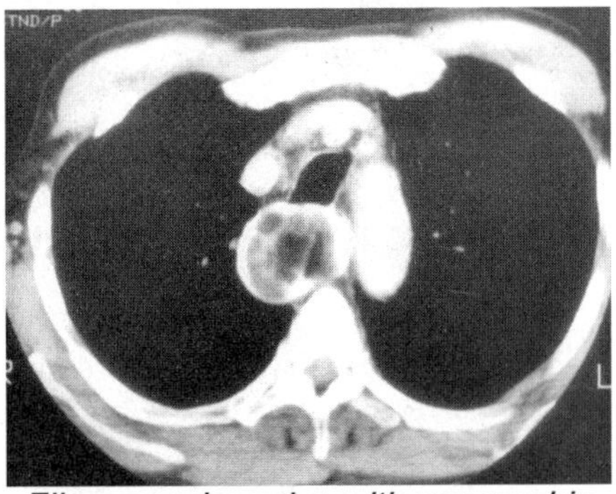

Fibrovascular polyp with geographic areas of fat and soft tissue attenuation on CT

Early Squamous Cell Carcinoma: Radiographic Findings
[Figure 2-22-7]
- Small, sessile polyp
- Plaquelike (central ulcer)
- Focal irregularity in wall
- Superficial spreading

Adv Squamous Cell Carcinoma [Figures 2-22-8 and 2-22-9]
- Plain Film
  - ➢ Widened med
  - ➢ Ant tracheal bowing
  - ➢ Thick RT stripe
  - ➢ A/F level in esoph
- Barium
  - ➢ Infiltrating
  - ➢ Polypoid
  - ➢ Ulcerative
  - ➢ Varicoid

Squamous Cell Carcinoma: Staging
- CT: Sens limited by adenopathy (mets in nl-sized nodes)
- MRI: Comparable to CT
- US: Depth of invasion & lymph node mets

Adenocarcinoma
- Arises in Barrett's mucosa
- Dysplasia-Ca sequence (low-grade, high-grade, ca-in-situ, invasive)
- Comprises 20–50% of esoph Ca's
- Predominantly in distal esophagus
- Often invades proximal stomach
- Prevalence 10% in Barrett's esoph
- 30–40X greater risk than gen pop
- Dysphagia and weight loss
- Same prognosis as squamous Ca
- Endoscopic surveillance

Figure 2-22-7

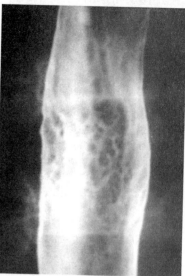

Superficial spreading carcinoma with focal nodularity

Figure 2-28-9

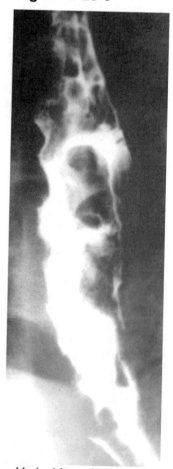

Varicoid carcinoma with large submucosal defects in lower esophagus

Figure 2-28-8

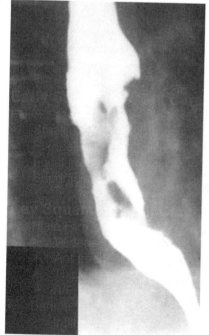

Primary ulcerative carcinoma with giant meniscoid ulcer surrounded by rind of tumor

Radiographic Findings [Figures 2-22-10 and 2-22-11]
- Early: sessile polyp, plaque, sup spreading, stricture
- Adv: infiltrating, polypoid, ulcerative, varicoid (often invades cardia)

Figure 2-22-10

Figure 2-22-11

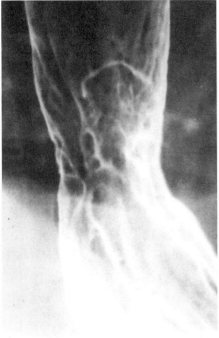

Early adenocarcinoma in Barrett's esophagus with plaque-like lesions

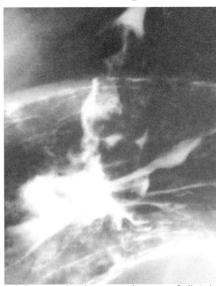

Advanced adenocarcinoma of distal esophagus invading stomach with nodularity and ulceration at cardia

Spindle Cell Carcinoma
- Carcinomatous and sarcomatous elements
- Spindle cell metaplasia
- Dysphagia and weight loss
- Same prognosis as squamous Ca

Radiographic Findings [Figure 2-22-12]
- Ba-polypoid intraluminal mass expanding lumen without obstruction
- CT-expansile esophageal mass
- DDx-malignant melanoma

Figure 2-22-12

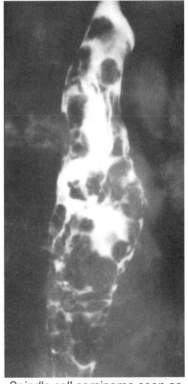

Spindle cell carcinoma seen as polypoid mass expanding esophagus without causing obstruction

Radiology of Peptic Ulcer Disease

Marc S. Levine, MD
Professor of Radiology
University Hospital of Pennsylvania

Hypertrophic Gastritis [Figures 2-23-1 and 2-23-2]

- Glandular hyperplasia
- Increased acid secretion
- Thickened folds
- Diff Dx:
  - ➢ Menetrier's
  - ➢ Lymphoma

Figure 2-23-1

Figure 2-23-2

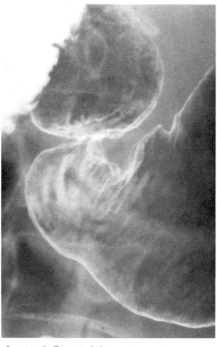

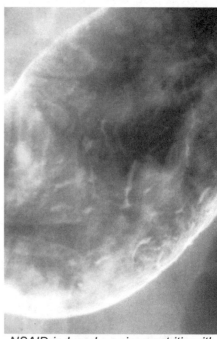

Erosive gastritis with varioloform erosions in antrum

Antral gastritis with hypertrophied antral-pyloric fold on lesser curvature of distal antrum

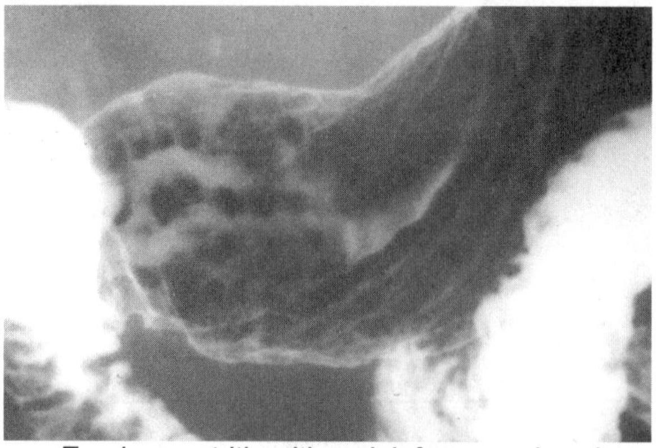

Figure 2-23-3

Antral Gastritis [Figure 2-23-1]

- Thickened antral folds
- Longitudinal or Transverse
- Crenulation of lessercurvature
- Hypertrophic antral-pyloric fold

Causes of Erosive Gastritis [Figure 2-23-3]

- PUD
- NSAIDs
- Alcohol
- Stress
- Trauma
- Crohn's

Acute Aspirin Ingestion (2–8 tabs/day in nl pts)

Finding	Time Span
• Erosions	8–24 hrs
• Max damage	1–3 days
• Healing	3–7 days

Duodenitis

- Spastic bulb
- Thickened folds
- Nodules
- Erosions

NSAID-induced erosive gastritis with linear erosions clustered in gastric body near greater curvature

Gastric Ulcers

- Shape
- Size
- Location
- Morphology

Figure 2-23-4

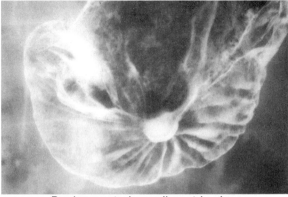

Benign posterior wall gastric ulcer

Figure 2-23-5

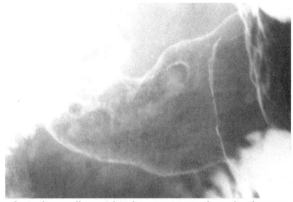

Anterior wall gastric ulcer seen as ring shadow on double contrast view

Figure 2-23-6

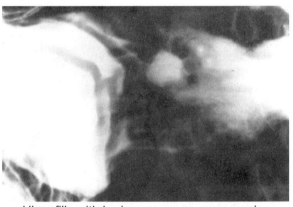

Ulcer fills with barium on prone compression

Figure 2-23-7

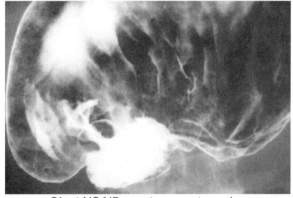

Giant NSAID greater curvature ulcer

Multiple Gastric Ulcers

- 2–30% of pts with GUs
- Association with aspirin in 80%
- Each ulcer evaluated separately

Upper GI vs Endoscopy

- More than 95% GUs Dx in North America are benign
- 6–16% of benign-app GUs on S/C studies are malignant
- Is endo always necessary?

Benign Gastric Ulcers [Figures 2-23-4 to 2-23-8-]

- En Face
  - ➢ Round or ovoid crater
  - ➢ Smooth mound of edema
  - ➢ Symmetric radiating folds
- In Profile
  - ➢ Projection outside lumen
  - ➢ Hampton's line or ulcer mound or collar

Figure 2-23-8

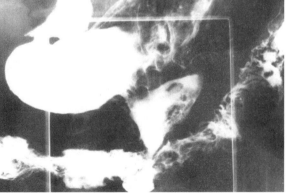

NSAID-induced greater curvature ulcer with gastrocolic fistula

Malignant Gastric Ulcers [Figure 2-23-9]

- En Face
  - Irregular crater in mass
  - Loss of areae gastricae
  - Nodularity, clubbing, or fusion of radiating folds
- In Profile
  - Projection of crater inside lumen within mass
  - Acute angles of mass

Equivocal Ulcers

- Irregularity of ulcer shape
- Asymmetry of mass effect
- Nodularity, irregularity, or clubbing of radiating folds
- Enlarged areae gastricae
- Location on greater curve

Figure 2-23-9

Malignant lesser curvature ulcer with clubbed folds abutting ulcer on prone compression

Radiologic Dx of Gastric Ulcers

Rad Dx	No Pts	Endo	Final Dx
• Benign	191	164	All ben
• Equiv	69	63	56 ben / 7 malig
• Malig	72	68	2 ben / 66 malig

AJR 141:331–333, 1983

Radiologic Dx of Gastric Ulcers

Rad Dx	No Pts	Endo	Final Dx
• Benign	68	24	All ben
• Equiv	37	33	All ben
• Malig	3	3	All malig

AJR 164:9–13, 1987

Gastric Ulcer Investigation

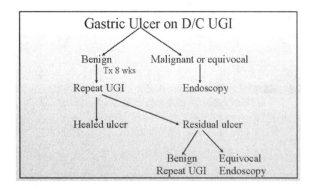

Advantages of Upper GI over Endoscopy

- Shorter procedure time
- Negligible risk
- Lower cost

Upper GI vs Endoscopy

	Cost
• D/C upper GI	$218
• Endoscopy procedure	$540
• Pathology	$180
• Hospital	$102
• **Total**	$822

Cost of Evaluating 1 Million GUs in United States

• UGI + endo	$1 billion
• UGI + sel endo	$490 million
• Diff in Cost	$510 million

Ulcer Healing
- Change in size and shape
- Avg pd for healing 8 wks
- Ulcer scar in 90%

Ulcer Scar
- Central pit or depression
- Radiating folds
- Retraction of adjacent wall

Duodenal Ulcers *[Figure 2-23-10]*
- 90% < 1 cm in size
- 50% on anterior wall
- 85% with deformed bulb
- 5% linear
- 15% multiple

Giant Duodenal Ulcers
- Greater than 2 cm in size
- Higher frequency of complix (bleeding, obst, perforation)
- Fixed configuration at fluoro

Postbulbar Duodenal Ulcers *[Figure 2-23-11]*
- 5% of all duodenal ulcers
- Medial wall of prox descending duodenum above papilla
- Indentation of lateral wall
- Notoriously difficult to Dx
- Can result in development of ring stricture

Investigation of Duodenal Ulcers

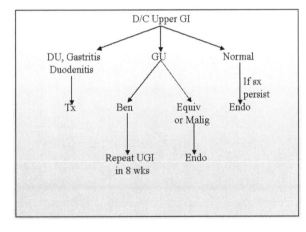

H. Pylori
- Gram-negative bacillus
- Increases with age (50% of pop > age 60)
- Eradicated by antibiotics and antisecretory agents

Radiographic Findings *[Figure 2-23-12]*
- Thickened gastric folds (predom antrum and body)
- Polypoid gastritis with thickened, lobulated folds
- Enlarged areae gastricae

Association with Gastric Carcinoma
- Increased risk of gastric Ca
- Less than 1% develop Ca
- Not enough evidence to treat all pts with *H.pylori*

Figure 2-23-10

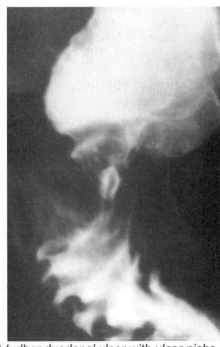

Duodenal bulbar ulcer

Figure 2-23-11

Post-bulbar duodenal ulcer with ulcer niche in proximal descending duodenum

Figure 2-23-12

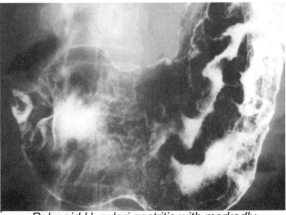

Polypoid H. pylori gastritis with markedly thickened, lobulated folds in gastric body

H. Pylori & Gastric Lymphoma
- Stomach devoid of lymphoid tissue
- Development of lymph follicles with *H. pylori* (MALT)
- Low-grade MALT lymphoma (MALTOMA)
- Characteristic pathologic features

Gastric MALT Lymphoma
- Regress with antibiotics in 70-80%
- Precursor of high-grade lymphoma
- 50-72% of all gastric lymphomas
- More common than prev recognized

Radiographic Findings [Figure 2-23-13]
- Nodularity of mucosa (rounded 2-7 mm nodules)
- Diff Dx:
  - ➢ Focal gastritis
  - ➢ Intest metaplasia
  - ➢ Enlarged areae gastricae

Risk of Ulcers
	Prevalence
Gastric ulcer	60-80%
Duodenal ulcer	95-100%

Detection of H.Pylori
- Endoscopic bx
- Urea breath test
- Serum Ab test

Figure 2-23-13

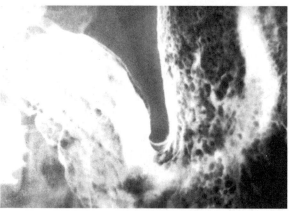

Gastric MALT lymphoma with confluent nodules in gastric body

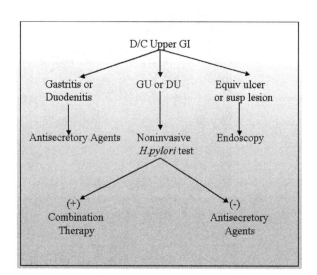

Pancreatitis: Imaging Has Made a Difference

Bruce P. Brown, MD
University of Iowa Hospitals and Clinics

Acute Pancreatitis
- (Marseilles 1985)
- Sudden onset abdominal pain
- Increased pancreatic enzymes, blood, urine
- Pancreatic edema, fat and gland necrosis, hemorrhage
- Variable involvement of regional or remote tissues (Atlanta 1992)

"Is this heaven?" "No. It's the anterior pararenal space."

Normal Pancreas

Chronic Pancreatitis
- (Marseilles 1985)
- Recurrent or persistent abdominal pain
- +/- increased enzymes
- Irreversible morphologic change in pancreas
  - ➢ Fibrosis
  - ➢ Acinar destruction
  - ➢ Calcification
- Diffuse, Focal
- Loss of function

Acute Pancreatitis: Who Gets It?
- Biliary stones (45%)
- Alcohol (35%)
- Idiopathic (10–15%)
- Hypercalcemia
- Hypertriglyceridemia
- Drugs
- Post ERCP
- Hereditary
- Trauma
- Infection
- Vasculitis
- Pancreas cancer
- Pancreas divisum
- Sludge?

Acute Pancreatitis: Pathophysiology
- Alcohol
  - ➢ Alters duct permeability -> protein precipitation in ductules
- Gallstones
  - ➢ Common channel of bile and pancreatic ducts -> bile reflux into pancreatic duct

Acute Pancreatitis: A Cascade of Events

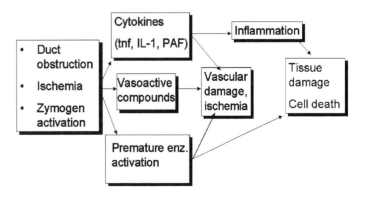

Acute Pancreatitis: Good and Bad
- Interstitial
  - Edema
  - Architecture preserved
  - No hemorrhage
- Hemorrhagic
  - Tissue necrosis, pancreas, fat
  - Hemorrhage
  - Vascular thrombosis & inflammation

Acute Pancreatitis: Clinical Dx
- Abdominal pain->back
- Nausea, vomiting
- DDx
  - Perforated ulcer, bowel ischemia, cholecystitis
- Labs
  - Hyperamylasemia
  - Elevated lipase, more specific for pancreatitis
  - Degree of enzyme elevation: no correlation w. severity

Acute Pancreatitis: Complications
- Early (2-3 days) multi-organ failure
  - Cardiovascular, pulmonary, renal
  - Phospholipase A2, elastase, tumor necrosis factor, cytokines, IL-1,2,6, trypsinogen activated peptide (TAP)
- Intermediate (2-5 weeks)
  - Infection, pseudocyst, GI, biliary
- Late (months – years)
  - Vascular, pseudoaneurysm

Balthzar 2002 Radiol Clin

Acute Pancreatitis: Plain Films
- Chest film
  - Pleural effusion 43% w. severe pancreatitis
  - ARDS
  - Pulmonary infarction
- Duodenum or colon distention
  - Sentinal loop = focal dilation
  - Colon cutoff = gas-filled colon -> abrupt cutoff at splenic flexure

Acute Pancreatitis: GI Contrast
- No primary role; may screw up CT
- Perigastritis, duodenitis, colitis -> Thick folds
- Mucosa intact
- Mass effect from pancreatic fluid
- Fundal varices from splenic vein thrombosis

Acute Pancreatitis: Ultrasound
- Of limited use in Dx
- Is pancreatitis associated w gallstones?
- Are there pancreatic fluid collections?
- Vascular complications?
- Intervention

Acute Pancreatitis: MRI
- Advantages
  - Gadolinium easy on kidneys
  - Able to view biliary tract
- Sick Patients
  - Motion artifacts
  - Difficult to monitor
  - Specialized equipment
  - Intervention difficult

Acute Pancreatitis: CT
- Best overall modality
- Global view
- Prognosis & followup
- Understand widespread nature of pancreatitis
- Routes for intervention

Acute Pancreatitis: Terminology
Atlanta Symposium 1992
- Confusion of terms
- Acute pancreatitis
  - Mild = minimal organ involvement, uncomplicated recovery w. supportive Rx
  - Severe = organ failure or complications eg. pseudocyst, necrosis, infected necrosis, abscess

Acute Pancreatitis: Acute Fluid Collections
- Extravasated pancreatic fluid
- Anterior pararenal space, lesser sac
- Not loculated
- No capsule
- 40% patients w. acute pancreatitis
- 50% resolve spontaneously
- May develop into pseudocyst

Acute Pancreatitis: Pseudocyst [Figure 2-24-1]
- Loculated collect. of panc. Enzymes
- Non-epithelialized wall of fibrous or granulation tissue
- 4-6 wks to develop
- Arise from acute fluid collect. (30-50%)
- 50% resolve spontaneously
- > 5 cm less likely to resolve

Pseudocyst: Complications [Figure 2-24-2]
- Infection
- Bile duct or GI obstruction
- Perforation -> adjacent organs
- Vascular
  - Venous stenosis,occlusion
  - Gastric varices
  - Pseudoaneurysm
  - Hemorrhage

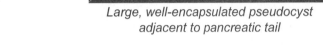

Figure 2-24-1

Large, well-encapsulated pseudocyst adjacent to pancreatic tail

Figure 2-24-2

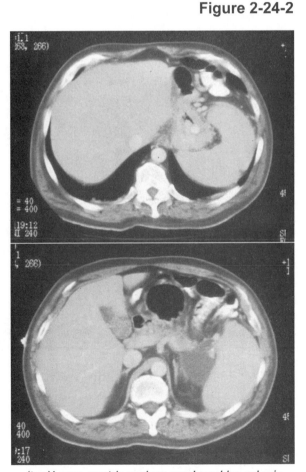

(top)Large gastric varices produced by splenic vein thrombosis from pancreatic pseudocyst adjacent to splenic hilum.
(bottom) Pseudocyst projecting from the pancreatic tail to the splenic hilum with no visualization of hilar splenic vein

Acute Pancreatitis : Necrosis
- Non-enhancing pancreas or peripancreatic tiss. – old "phlegmon"
- Non-viable tissue
- Poor prognosis
- Type determines Rx
  - Sterile-trial of med Rx
  - Infected-Debridemant – 1st two weeks, abscess takes sev wks.
  - Mortality15-50%
- Needle aspiration to Dx

Acute Pancreatitis: Abscess
- Circumscribed collection of pus
- Develops after several weeks
- Needle aspiration
- Percutaneous drainage
-

Acute Pancreatitis: Location
- Central location affords several routes for spreading disease
- Anterior pararenal space
  - Pancreas
  - Colon
  - Duodenum
- Bare area = reflection of post parietal peritoneum to form the transverse mesocolon
- Root of the small bowel mesentery contiguous w. transverse mesocolon
- Tail = intraperitoneal -> splenorenal ligament
- Posterior to the lesser sac

Barium Left Anterior Pararenal Space-o-Gram *[Figure 2-24-3]*

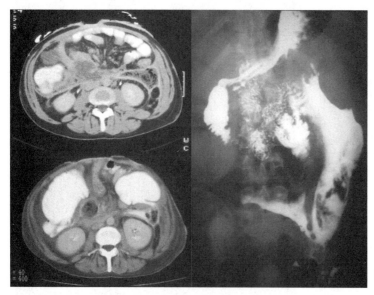

Figure 2-24-3

*(top left) Extensive necrosis in the anterior pararenal space on both sides with air anterior to the left kidney mistaken for air in the colon.
(bottom left). Delayed views showing contrast anterior to the left kidney.
Thought to be in the colon.
(right) Barium upper gi contrast study showing erosion of the pancreatic inflammation into the small bowel with barium contrast leaking throughout the entire left anterior pararenal space*

Acute Pancreatitis: Good and Bad
- Interstitial (Good) 80-90%
  - < 10% organ failure
  - 1-3% mortality
- Hemorrhagic (Bad) 10-20%
  - Necrosis
  - 50-60% organ failure
  - 15-20% mortality

Banks. Gastro Endoscopy 2002

Acute Pancreatitis: Can we predict trouble?

- 75% acute pancreatitis resolve w/o complications
- 5–20% mortality
- Can't biopsy
- Who is really sick?
- Clinical Predictors
  - Ranson Criteria Sens = 57–85%; Spec = 68–85%
  - APACHE II = 77% pos. pred. Val on admit; 88% after 48 hrs

Clinical Assessment of Pancreatitis Severity

- RANSON
- Non-Gallstone pancreatitis
  - Admission (any 3)
    - ❖ > 55yrs old; WBC > 16K,
    - ❖ Blood sugar >200
    - ❖ LDH >350 ; AST > 250
  - At 48 hrs (any 3),
    - ❖ Hct decr >10
    - ❖ Rise in BUN > 5
    - ❖ Calcium < 8
    - ❖ PO2 < 60
    - ❖ Fluid deficit > 6L
    - ❖ Base deficit > 4

- APACHE II
  - Vitals signs
  - PO2
  - pH
  - Electrolytes
  - Creatinine
  - HCT; WBC
  - Glasgow coma score

Can Imaging Alone Predict Trouble? Yes

- CT grading (Balthazar 1985;1990)
  - A = Normal
  - B = Focal or diffuse enlargement
  - C = Peripancreatic inflammation
  - D = Single fluid collection outside gland
  - E = 2 or more fluid collections or gas in or near panc.
  - 83 PTS
    - ❖ All A's discharged w/o complications within 2 wks
    - ❖ A or B -> no abscess
    - ❖ D or E -> 5 of 6 deaths; 89% of abscesses

Imaging Predicts Trouble. Can we refine this further?

- Problem: After classifying patients as high-risk, fluid collections resolved in 54%
- Pancreatic necrosis
  - Poor gland enhancement correlates w. degree of necrosis at surgery (Kivisaari GI Radiol 1984)
  - Gland necrosis correlates with development of complications (Balthazar Radiol 1990)
    - ❖ No necrosis = no mortality; 6% morbidity
    - ❖ Necrosis = 23% mortality; 82% morbidity

Acute Pancreatitis: Can we predict trouble? [Figure 2-24-4]
- CT Severity Index (Balthazar Radiol: 1990)
- CT anatomic changes
  - ➤ A = 0, B = 1, C =2, D = 3, E = 4
- Gland necrosis
- < 30% = 2, 30-50% = 4, > 50 = 6
  - ➤ 0-1 = no mortality or complications
  - ➤ 2 = no mortality; 4% complications
  - ➤ 7-10 = 17% mortality; 92% complications

Acute Pancreatitis: The Power of CT
- Suspected pancreatitis – Dx in doubt
- Severe pancreatitis suspected of complications
- Pancreatitis w/o improvement in 72 hrs of med. Rx
- Improving pancreatitis that deteriorates
- Severe pancreatitis w. initial scan (D-E; CTSI 3–10) – follow-up may detect asymptomatic complications

Chronic Pancreatitis
- Definition (Marseilles 1985)
  - ➤ Recurrent or persistent abdominal pain
  - ➤ May or may not see increase enzymes
  - ➤ Irreversible morphological change in pancreas
    - ❖ Fibrosis
    - ❖ Acinar destruction
    - ❖ Calcification, duct /parenchyma
  - ➤ Focal, segmental, diffuse
  - ➤ Progressive loss of exocrine/endocrine function

Chronic Pancreatitis
- Who Gets It?
  - ➤ Chronic alcohol abuse (60–70%)
  - ➤ Idiopathic (30%)
  - ➤ Biliary tract disease
  - ➤ Hereditary
  - ➤ Hyperlipidemia
  - ➤ Hyperparathyroid
  - ➤ Pancreas divisum
- Clinical
  - ➤ Recurrent abdominal pain (95%),
  - ➤ Pancreatic insufficiency ,
    - ❖ Malabsorption,
    - ❖ Diabetes,
  - ➤ Amylase/Lipase levels +/– abnormal

Chronic Pancreatitis: Pathophysiology
- Poorly understood
  - ➤ Etoh increases ductal secretion ->
  - ➤ Precipitation of protein plugs ->
  - ➤ Calcification
    - ❖ chain of lakes / dilated duct
  - ➤ Inflammatory infiltrate + fibrosis

Chronic Pancreatitis: Plain Films
- Pancreas Ca++ (75-90%)
  - ➤ Most common in Etoh pancreatitis,
  - ➤ Ductal or parenchymal
  - ➤ May be focal
  - ➤ Increase w. progression pancreatic dysfunction
  - ➤ Also w. hereditary pancreatitis, cystic fibrosis

Figure 2-24-4

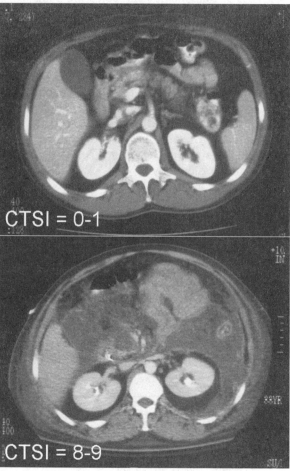

CTSI = 0-1

CTSI = 8-9

Balthazar Classification of severity of acute pancreatitis

(top). Mild Pancreatitis: CTSI = 0-1. Small amount of peripancreatic stranding. No fluid collections. Entire gland enhances.

(bottom). Severe Pancreatitis: CTSI = 8-9. Pancreas outlines are obliterated with necrosis. No enhancement with contrast

Chronic Pancreatitis: Barium [Figure 2-24-5]
- Inflammation/scar -> perigastritis
- Not primary disease of bowel

Figure 2-24-5

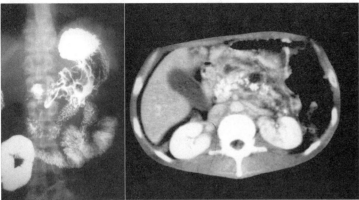

(left) Severe distortion of the gastric contours on double-contrast barium study from chronic pancreatitis with inflammatory changes and scar in the perigastric tissues, so-called "perigastritis." There is no primary gastric disease.

(right) CT appearance of the same patient showing changes of chronic pancreatitis with parenchymal calcifications and gland atrophy

Chronic Pancreatitis: Ultrasound
Heterogenous echotexture
- Hyperechoic foci = Ca++/ fibrosis,
- Bile &/or pancreatic duct dilation
- 40% focal mass DDx = cancer
- Complications
  - Pseudocyst portal / splenic vein thrombosis
- Endoscopic ultrasound?
  - 98% sensitivity / 90% specificity?

Chronic Pancreatitis: Endoscopic Ultrasound
- Difficult to establish a gold standard esp. for mild to moderate disease
- EUS high negative predictive value for moderate to severe chronic pancreatitis, but low positive predictive value for mild to moderate disease.
- Few studies with histology
  - Sens = 87%; Spec = 64%

Chronic Pancreatitis: CT
- Gland enlargement (30%)
- Mass (30%) ? Cancer
- Atrophy (15%)
- Sens. 50-90%: Spec. 55-85%
- Acute + chronic w. exacerbation of disease

Chronic Pancreatitis: MRI
- Parenchyma
  - T1 fat-supressed, pre & post Gd dynamic
  - Decreased signal/Delay in peak vs. controls
  - Sens = 79%; Spec = 75%
  - Better than morphologic changes alone
- MRCP
  - 5% post ercp pancreatitis; 10-15% failure to cannulate
  - Highly T2 weighted, single breath-hold sequences
  - 85-90% agreement w. ERP for duct caliber
  - Limited ability to dx early chronic pancreatitis -> functional exam, secretin, studies not conclusive.

Remer EM Radiol. Clin. of N. Am. 40(2002) 1229-1242, 2002

Chronic Pancreatitis: ERCP
- Cambridge Classification of chronic pancreatitis
  - ➢ Mild = 3 side branches dilated; main duct 2–4 mm
  - ➢ Moderate = small cysts, irregular duct
  - ➢ Severe = any of above +
    - ❖ Cyst >10mm, intraductal filling defect, calculi, main duct obstruction, severe irregularity

Pancreatitis Requests We Have Known and Loved

Acute Pancreatitis: "I see something there. Why don't you stick a drain in it?
- What do you see?
  - ➢ No go if no flow
    - ❖ Liquid or solid?
    - ❖ Necrosis won't flow
    - ❖ Hemorrhage? May not flow; may release tamponade
  - ➢ Vascular?
    - ❖ The big red surprise

Pancreatitis: "Febrile. Please aspirate fluid." What then?
- You are in charge of thinking ahead.
- Modality?
- Route?
  - ➢ Transgastric? Not for diagnosis only
- What is the plan?
  - ➢ Pus -> tube
  - ➢ Indeterminate -> Gram stain +/- tube
  - ➢ Clear fluid -> Gram stain, culture
  - ➢ Solid stuff -> no flow -> saline -> culture. BX?

Pancreatic Pseudocyst

Pancreatic Fluid Collection: "I am happy to help, but what is the indication for drainage? My staff wants it"
- Indication for access to evolving fluid collection or necrosis decided on full evaluation of clinical, lab, and imaging
- Percutaneous drain useless if won't flow through tube
  - ➢ No tube for necrosis or hematoma
  - ➢ Aspiration to dx infected necrosis
- Uninfected collections and small pseudocysts may resolve on their own

Pancreatitis References

Topazian M, Gorelick GS. Acute Pancreatitis. In: Yamada T, Textbook of Gastroenterology, Third Edition, Volume 2. Lippincott Williams and Wilkins, 1999, 2121-2150.

Owyang C. Chronic Pancreatitis. In: Yamada T, Textbook of Gastroenterology, Third Edition, Volume 2, Lippincott Williams and Wilkins, 1999, 2151-2177.

Banks PA. Epidemiology, natural history, and predictors of disease outcome in acute and chronic pancreatitis. Gastrointestinal Endoscopy 2002; 56 (6) S226-S230

Meyers MA. Dynamic Radiology of the Abdomen Normal and Pathologic Anatomy, Fifth Edition.Springer, New York 2000.

Balthazar EJ. Staging of Acute Pancreatitis. Radiol. Clin. of N. Am. 2002;40:6, 1199-1209.

Balthazar EJ. Complications of Acute Pancreatitis. Radiol. Clin. of N. Am 2002; 40:6, 1211-1227.

Remer EM, Baker ME. Imaging of Chronic Pancreatitis. Radiol. Clin of N. Am 2002; 40:6, 1229-1242.

Fulcher AS, Turner MA. MR Cholangiopancreatography. Radiol. Clin of N. Am 2002: 40:6, 1363-1376.

Strate T, Knoefel WT, Yekebas E, Isbicki JR. Chronic Pancreatitis: etiology, pathogenesis, diagnosis, and treatment. Int. J Colorectal Dis. 2003; 18: 97-106,.

Chatizicostas C, Roussomoustakaki M, et al. Balthazar Computed Tomography Severity Index Is Superior to Ranson Criteria and APACHE II and III Scoring Systems in Predicting Acute Pancreatitis Outcome. J. Clin. Gastroenterol. 2003; 36: 3, 253-260.

Wiersema MJ, Hawes RH, et al. Prospective evaluation of endoscopic ultrasonography and endoscopic retrograde cholangiopancreatography in patients with chronic abdominal pain of suspected pancreatic origin. Endoscopy 1993;25:555-564.

Gastrointestinal Bleeding In The Age of the Endoscope. What Does a Radiologist Have To Contribute?

Bruce P. Brown, MD
University of Iowa Hospitals and Clinics

GI Bleeding: Demographics
- Older
- Male
- Use alcohol, tobacco
- Aspirin, non-steroidal anti-inflammatory
- Anticoagulants

Peura et al, Am.J.Gastro. 1997

Gastrointestinal Bleeding: Presentation
- Hematemesis – Bloody vomitus, red, coffee grounds; indicates upper GI bleeding
- Melena – Black, tarry stools; usually indicates upper GI bleeding
- Hematochezia – Red blood per rectum; lower GI bleed, large-volume upper GI bleed (> 1000 cc)

Acute GI Bleeding: Demographics
- Upper GI 76%
  - ➤ Duodenal & gastric ulcers >50%,
- Lower GI 24%
  - ➤ Diverticular 30-50%
- 79% Anemia
- 31% Hypovolemia
- 59% Transfused
- 45% Endoscopic Rx
- 7% Surgery
- 2% Death

Peura et al, Am.J.Gastro. 1997

Gastrointestinal Bleeding: How Bad Is It?
- Hypovolemia - 30% of GI bleeders
  - ➤ 5 L (10 Units) = normal volume
  - ➤ Hct poor measure of acute bleeding
  - ➤ 20% blood loss -> 10 mmHg drop BP w. standing
  - ➤ 40% blood loss = Shock = resting supine tachycardia, hypotension, pallor, agitation
  - ➤ Massive GI bleed = > 6 units transfusion needed in 24 hours

Acute Gastrointestinal Bleeding: Diagnosis is NOT the first priority
- Resuscitation
  - ➤ Two BIG lines 18 gauge
  - ➤ Fluids immediately
  - ➤ Blood when available; 6 u typed & crossed
  - ➤ ICU

Gastrointestinal Bleeding: Where Is It?

- Upper GI
  - Proximal to ligament of Treitz,
  - Usually melena
  - NG tube – 16% negative even w. UGI bleed
- Lower GI
  - Distal to the ligament of Treitz
  - Usually hematochezia

Lower GI Bleeding: Causes

- Diagnosis   % of total
  - Duodenal Ulcer   24
  - Gastric Erosions   23
  - Gastric Ulcer   21
  - Varices   10
  - Mallory-Weiss tear   7
  - Esophagitis   6
  - Neoplasm   3
  - Other   11

Silverstein et al, Gastro.Endosc. 1981

Lower GI Bleeding: Causes

- Diagnosis   % of total
  - Diverticulosis   43
  - Vascular Ectasia   20
  - Idiopathic   12
  - Neoplasia   9
  - Colitis
    - ❖ Radiation   6
    - ❖ Ischemia   2
    - ❖ Ulcerative colitis   1
  - Other   7

Reinus et al GI Clin NA 1990

GI Bleeding: Endoscopy

- First line procedure in UGI bleed
  - 90–95% accurate Dx
  - Useful for prognosis, treatment
- Performed immediately
  - Alcoholics,
  - Large volume loss
  - Aorto-enteric fistula
- Performed more "electively"
  - Young, no evidence of hypovolemia

Nuclear Scintigraphy

- Most sensitive non-invasive test
- Detects bleeding rates 0.1ml/min
- Two techniques
  - Tc 99m sulfur colloid
  - Tc 99m labeled red blood cells
- Used to
  - Delineate obscure sources – small bowel, intermittent bleeding
  - Enhance the efficacy of angiography

Angiography
- Usually preceded by RBC study
- Detects 0.5 ml/min
- Upper GI bleeding
  - When endoscopy inconclusive
  - Anticipation of transcatheter intervention
- Lower GI bleeding
  - Procedure of choice?

Upper GI Bleeding: Peptic Ulcer Disease
- Gastric, duodenal, stomal ulcers = 50% UGI bleeding
- Etiology: Non-steroidals, H. Pylori
- Anatomic risk factors
  - High lesser curve
  - Posterior-inferior duodenal bulb
  - Giant gastric (>3 cm) & duodenal (>2 cm)
- Endoscopic risk factors

Risk of Rebleeding: Endoscopy
- Peptic ulcer disease rebleeding
  - Clean fibrin base   5%
  - Flat spot   10%
  - Adherent clot   22%
  - Visible vessel   43%
  - Spurting vessel   90%

Lainm NE JM; 717; 1994. UCLA-CURE studies.

Gastritis
- Hemorrhage, erythema, erosions
- Erosion = superficial break in mucosa w. punctate bleeding, fibrin base
- Causes
  - Non-steroidals -> antral erosions, ulcer
    - ❖ bleeding usually not severe, resolve w. D/C
  - Alcohol ingestion
    - ❖ Direct toxin? ->erythema

Gastritis
- Portal hypertension
  - Diffuse or patchy erythema, punctate bleeding, vascular ectasia
- Requires reduction of portal hypertension
- Stress Erosions
  - ICU patients
  - One or more bleeding erosions
    - ❖ Bleeding may be severe

Acute Hemorrhagic Gastritis

Esophageal Varices
- 50% cirrhotics develop esoph. varices.
- 1/3 of these bleed
- Portal v. pressure >12 mmHg. Hep.v
- At risk to bleed
  - Large size
  - Located near GE Junct.
  - Vascular ectasia on the varices
- Rapid bleeding
- Emergent endoscopy
- 50% of cirrhotics w. bleed = non-variceal
- Poor prognosis
  - 30–50% mortality for first bleed
  - 2/3 die within one year

Esophageal Varices: Rx

- Vasopressin (somatostatin/octreotide)
  - 50% effective
- Sclerotherapy – 85–95% effective
  - Probably improves survival; complications
- Band ligation
  - As effective as sclero Rx; few complications
- Balloon tamponade
  - 70–90% effective
  - 30–50% rebleed after balloon down,
  - 10–30% severe complications
- TIPS (Transjugular Intrahepatic Portosystemic Shunt)
  - Expandable stent – hepatic to portal v.
  - 95% technically successful
  - As effective as sclero Rx
  - 10–15% complications
  - 10–25% encephalopathy
  - 30–50% stenosis at 1 year
- Surgical porta-caval shunts
  - 50–80% mortality for emergency shunt
  - Elective shunts for endoscopic Rx failures

Gastric Varices Without Esophageal Varices

Mallory-Weiss Tear

- 5–10% GI bleeds
- Hx of retching; 40% no retching
- Non-penetrating linear tear(s) near GEJ
  - 25% multiple lesions; 75% have o. pathol.
- 90% resolve spontaneously
- Rx ->endo.oversewing

Gut Hemangioma

- Rare
- Described in young and old
- Esophagus, stomach, sm. bowel, colon
- Classification
  - Capillary – collection of thin-walled vess.
  - Cavernous – large, dilated channels w. thrombosis -> Ca++
    - ❖ Tendency to bleed
  - Angiomatosis – large area of hemangioma

Gut hemangioma

- Cavernous hemangioma
  - Phleboliths on plain film
  - UGI = Submucosal mass
- CT
  - Thick wall
  - Early enhancement – network of vessels & sinuses thickening the wall
  - Late enhancement – confluent sinus fill-in
- Endoscopy
  - Soft, submucosal mass or thickened folds, blue-red discoloration

Small Bowel Bleeding: Tough to Dx

- 3–5% GI bleeds occur in small bowel (2nd portion duod. to ileocec. valve)
- Bleeding is intermittent
- Most common causes are vascular
- Inaccessible
- Anatomy variable

Small Bowel Bleeding: Causes
- Vascular lesions most common
  - Angiodysplasia, hemangioma, AVM, vasculitis
- Small bowel tumors
  - Leiomyoma/sarcoma, adenoma/carcinoma, lymphoma, mets
- Ulcers
  - Crohn's, Meckel's diverticulum, ZE syndrome
- Diverticula
- Aortoenteric fistula

Small Bowel Bleeding: How Well Does Imaging Do?
- Small bowel series vs enteroclysis
  - 71% lesions missed on small bowel series [1]
- Small bowel series for occult bleeding
  - 5% yield for bleeding site [2]
- Enteroclysis
  - 10 % yield for bleeding site [3]
- Enteroscopy
  - Cumbersome, not generally available

[1] Maglinte, Radiol 144:737; 1982
[2] Rabe, Radiol. 140:47; 1981
[3] Rex, Gastro 58;89; 1997

Small Bowel Bleeding

Nuclear Scintigraphy
- Most sensitive non-invasive test
- Detects bleeding rates of 0.1 ml/min
- Two techniques
  - Tc 99m sulfur colloid
  - Tc 99m labeled RBC's
- Used to
  - Delineate obscure sources – small bowel, intermittent bleeding
  - Enhance the efficacy of angiography

Technetium 99m Labeled RBC's
- New in vitro process (Ultratag) >95% eff.
- Continuous dynamic imaging
  - Large FOV camera over abdomen
  - 60 images q 15 min
  - Stored for dynamic playback to detect labeled RBC's outside normal blood pool

Technetium 99m Labeled Red Blood Cells
- Disadvantages
  - Origin of bleed unclear on delayed scans
  - Vascular organs may interfere w. detection
  - Loss of tag can produce false +/-
- Advantages
  - Detects intermittent bleeding
- Labeled RBC's
  - Sensitivity = 85–95%; Specificity = 70–85%,
  - Method of choice

Meckel's Diverticulum
- Most common congenital GI tract anom.
- Vitelline duct fails to resorb
- True diverticulum –
  - 2% of population
  - 2 x more common in males
  - 2 cm long (1–10 cm),
  - 2 feet from ileocecal valve
- 50% ectopic gastric or pancreatic mucosa
- 25–40% symptomatic
- Complications
  - Bleeding – usually in kids <5 yr,
  - Intussusception – kids & adults
  - Volvulus, diverticulitis, perforation
- Bleeding – ulceration of gastric mucosa

Aortoenteric Fistula
- Erosion of aorta into 3rd portion of duod,
- Dacron graft, atheroma, mycotic aneurysm
- "Herald bleed" stops spontaneously followed by exsanguinating bleed
- High index of suspicion
- Preemptive surgery

Pill Endoscopy
- Ingestible capsule
- 7 hour recording
- 2 images per second
- Localizing surface antennae
- View in "real-time"
- Contraindicated w. obstruction

Lower GI Bleeding: Causes
- Diagnosis   % of total

Diagnosis	% of total
Diverticulosis	43
Vascular Ectasia	20
Idiopathic	12
Neoplasia	9
Colitis	
❖ Radiation	6
❖ Ischemia	2
❖ Ulcerative colitis	1
Other	7

Reinus et al GI Clin NA 1990

Colonic Diverticulosis
- Colon Diverticula = herniations of mucosa and submucosa through muscular layers at site of penetration of vasa recta through bowel wall.

Colonic Diverticular Bleeding
- 35–50% prevalence of diverticula
- 15% pts. tics bleed
- 5% massively
- The major cause of lower GI bleed
- 75% of tics in left colon
- 70% of bleeding tics in right colon [1]
- 80% resolve spontaneously
- Not asst's w. diverticulitis

[1] Cassarella, NEJM 286:450;1972

Colonic Diverticular Bleeding: RX
- Colonoscopic vasoconstrictor injection, heater probe, laser – select patients
- Angiography
  - ➢ Selective catheterization
    - ❖ Vasopressin 50-90% success
    - ❖ Embolo Rx – Gelfoam, coils
- Surgery

Angiodysplasia
- 20–40% acute LGI bleeding
- Vascular ectasia
  - ➢ 2/3 in pts >70 yrs old
  - ➢ Aortic valve disease
    - ❖ Von Willebrand factor depletion?
- < 5mm vascular tufts
- Cecum & right colon
- Bleeding
  - ➢ Not massive, intermittent
  - ➢ Stop spontaneously, 85% bleed again
- Pathogenesis
  - ➢ Increased tension in cecal wall
  - ➢ Repeated, intermittent obstruction of submucosal veins -> dilation & tortuosity
  - ➢ Develop small A-V malformation
- Colonoscopy 80–90% sensitive
- Angiography
  - ➢ early tangle of vessels
  - ➢ early filling & slow emptying dilated veins
- Treatment
  - ➢ Abnormal vessels – poor response to vasoconstrictors; may temporize
  - ➢ Endoscopic electrocoagulation
  - ➢ Embolo Rx
  - ➢ Diffuse disease – estrogen-progesterone
  - ➢ Surgery

Gastrointestinal Bleeding References

Peura DA, Lanza FL. Gostout CJ, Foutch PG. The American College of Gastroenterology Bleeding Registry: preliminary findings. Am J Gastroenterol. 1997 Jun;92(6):924-8.

Reinus JF, Brandt LJ. Upper and lower gastrointestinal bleeding in the elderly. Gastroenterol Clin North Am. 1990 Jun;19(2):293-318.

Mitros, FA, Atlas of Gastrointestinal Pathology. Gower Medical Publishing.

Elta, GH Approach to the Patient With Gross Gastrointestinal Bleeding. In Textbook of Gastroenterology, Lippincott Williams and Wilkins, Philadelphia, 1999, Yamada, T et al Eds.

Fritscher-Ravens A, Swain CP. The wireless capsule: new light in the darkness. Dig Dis. 2002;20(2):127-33.

Small Bowel Obstruction

Francis J. Scholz, M.D.
Radiologist, Lahey Clinic
Clinical Professor of Radiology,
Tufts University School of Medicine

Small Bowel Obstruction
- "Impaired passage of contents thru SB."
- Partial vs Complete ("High Grade")
- Intermittent vs Continuous
- Mechanical vs Paralytic ("Ileus")

SBO
- Review
  - Mechanical
  - Classic Acute "Complete" SBO
  - Classic Appearances
    - ❖ Intermittent SBO
    - ❖ Partial SBO

SBO
- Motility
  - Paralytic Ileus
  - Intestinal Pseudo-obstruction
  - Scleroderma Collagen Vasc
  - Radiation enteritis, earliest stage
  - Sprue, MAB diseases
  - DYSMOTILITY is a FUNCTIONAL SBO !
  - Slow passage acts / looks obstructive

Chronic vs Acute SBO: Concept to help analyze SB in CT, KUB, SB Series
- Distention vs Dilatation: 2 variables
  - Dilatation: bowel diameter is larger than expected
    - ❖ It may be a few loops or entire small bowel
    - ❖ It may or may not be Distended
  - Distention: bowel has uniform appearance of maximum possible diameter
    - ❖ Like a small, medium, or large sausage shaped balloon inflated to its capacity
    - ❖ Appears tensely filled, to capacity

Chronic vs Acute SBO [Figures 2-26-1 to 2-26-3]
- Distention vs Dilatation
- Distended, not Dilated:
  - Acute, initial
- Dilated, not Distended:
  - Chronic, intermittent
  - DYSMOTILITIES !
- Dilated <u>and</u> Distended:
  - Acute, recurrent

Figure 2-26-1

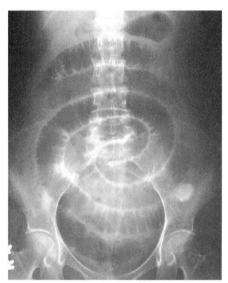

Acute mechanical SBO showing uniformly distended bowel

Figure 2-26-2

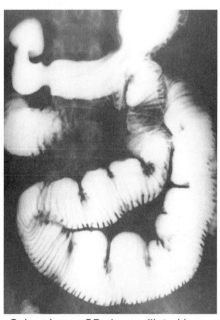

Scleroderma SB shows dilated loops with segments whose diameter are greater than preceding case of acute SBO. Loops are not uniformly distended with segments that are partly collapsed

Bloating, Obstruction [Figure 2-26-4]
- Prior Colectomy for constipation with
- Ileo-rectal anastomosis

SBO-CT
- SBO suspected
- SB distended on KUB
  - No need oral contrast.
  - IV useful to maximize Dx
- See extra-luminal cause
- Diff Paralytic vs Mech.
- See Complications: Ischemia

CT: Acute SBO [Figure 2-26-5]
- Holy Grail = Transition Point
  - Define Lesion
  - Absent a "Lesion" = Adhesion
  - Study
    - ❖ Colon ? Collapsed
    - ❖ Ileocecal Valve
    - ❖ Duodenal Crossing
    - ❖ Mesenteric Vessels

CT: Acute SBO
- Points to Remember:
  - Critical to find & Dx SBO
  - Ischemia may result (or cause of SBO)
  - May resolve before surgery, (NG suction, bezoar passage)
  - Surgeon may
    - ❖ Miss at surgery
    - ❖ Cure unknowingly by dissection
    - ❖ Underestimate degree of disease you Dx

Figure 2-26-3

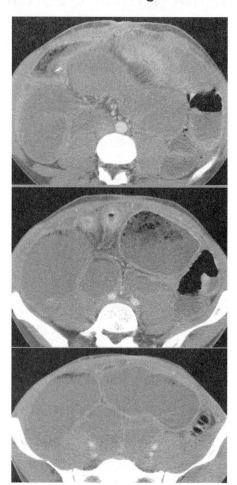

Crohn Disease: Acute obstruction in pt with chronic obstructive episodes. SB appears both dramatically dilated and uniformly distended. This suggests acute obstruction in a patient with chronic recurring obstruction

Figure 2-26-4

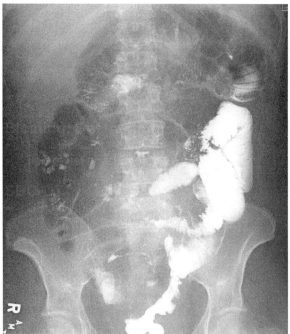

48 Hr films shows barium in proximal SB. Chronic dysmotility diseases may produce massive dilatation. Segments that do not propel act like mechanical obstruction

Figure 2-26-5

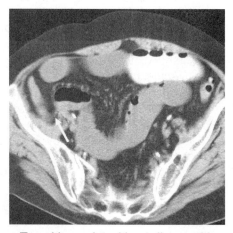

Transition point without discernable mass or hernia indicates adhesion

SBO - Enema [Figure 2-26-6]
- 1. Ileus vs SBO
- 2. Partial, intermittent
- 3. If ? Is SBO vs LBO
- (Possibly define very distal SBO cause)

SBO - SB Study [Figure 2-26-7]
- Partial, intermittent
- Enteroclysis

SBO - SB Study
- Dedicated SB Series
  - "Serious" SB Series
    - Freq films & fluoroscopy
    - Spot: Compress & Palpate
    - Oblique & Tangent
    - Valsalva

SBO
- Motility
  - Paralytic Ileus
  - Intestinal Pseudo-obstruction
  - Sprue, MAB diseases
- Mechanical
  - Adhesions ~ 50%
  - Tumor
    - Intussuscept, encase
  - Inflammation (SB, Colon Ticitis, Crohns)
  - Volvulus
  - Hernia
  - Bezoar
  - Ischemia

Adhesion Causes
- Benign Adhesions
  - Surgical
  - Inflammatory
  - Radiation
  - Ischemia
- Neoplastic Adhesions
  - (Carcinoid)

Adhesion Types
- Inter-loop
- Intra-loop
- Loop to Solid Organ
- Loop to Omentum
- Mesenteric Adhesion
  - (retractile mesenteritis)
- Combinations of all

Figure 2-26-6

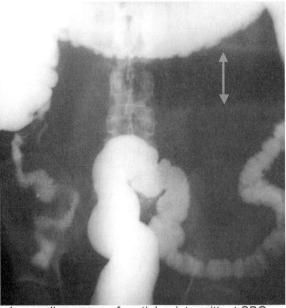

In puzzling cases of partial or intermittent SBO, barium enema will prove that the colon is not involved and reflux into the terminal ileum will confirm SB diameter differences diagnostic of mechanical SBO and may define cause

Figure 2-26-7

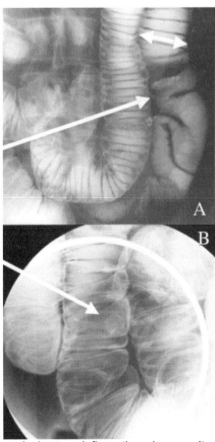

Enteroclysis may define otherwise occult cause of SBO. Abrupt diameter change in A indicates point of partial adhesion. Image B shows a small polyp, a lead point for intussusception

Adhesion Rad [Figure 2-26-8]
- Crossing Band
- Zig-Zag
- Acute angulation
- Spiculation
- Abrupt diameter transition
- Bunch / Twist of Mesentery
- Fixed Loops over time

Crossing Band

Tethering Tenting Adhesion [Figure 2-26-9]

Figure 2-26-9

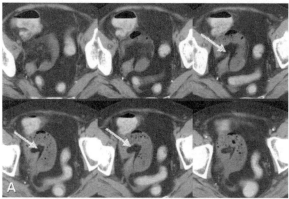

Focal adhesion (image A) causes tenting, (arrow) with bezoar or "SB feces" above tented transition point

Multiple Zig-Zag Adhesions

Focal Adhesion, Mass Like (Mesentery)

Tumor - SBO
- Applecore
- Matted Mess
- Extrinsic Compress
- Intussusception
- Adhesion
- Any / all of above

Lead Point
- None : normal physio
- Tumor
- Lymphoid hyperplasia
- Inverted Meckels
- Sprue

Inverted Meckel's Diverticulum [Figure 2-26-10]
- Pain
- Bleeding
- SBO
- Intussusception

Figure 2-26-8

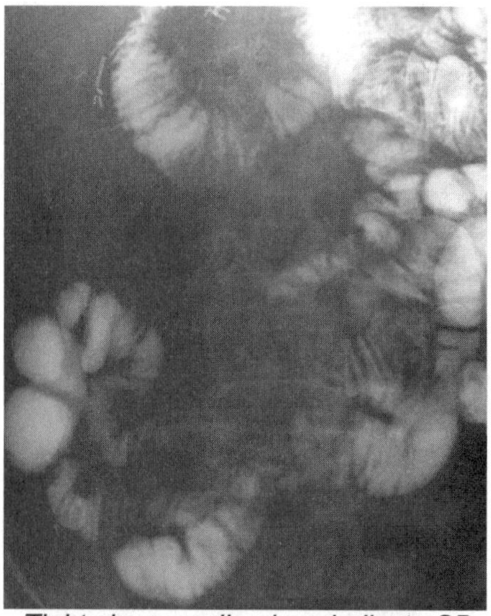

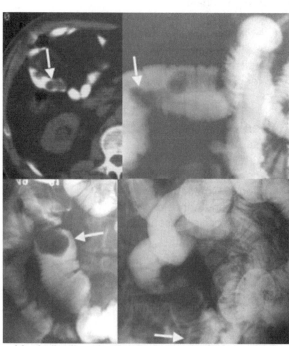

Tight zig zag adhesions indicate SB loops are bound by adhesion usually due to simple scar but such binding may be caused by tumor or inflammation

Figure 2-26-10

Meckel's diverticula may invert and cause SBO. Elongated polyps should raise suspicion

Intussusception of Inverted Meckels [Figure 2-26-11]
Figure 2-26-11

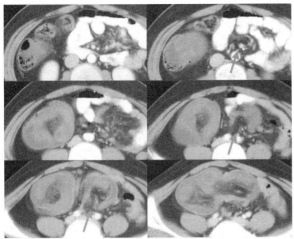

Intussusception may progress deeply into colon creating large confusing pseudotumor. "Intratumoral" fat and vessels are a clue to an intussusception

Carcinoid SBO [Figure 2-26-12]
- 1° Tumor obscured
- 2° Tumor:
  - ➢ Adhesions
  - ➢ Extrinsic Mesenteric Mes Mass(es)
  - ➢ Calcify
  - ➢ Vascular Compromise
  - ➢ Intussusception
  - ➢ Any or all above

Closed Loop Obstruction [Figure 2-26-13]
- Lumen occluded at 2 adj. sites
  - ➢ Adhesion
  - ➢ Hernia - Internal, External
  - ➢ Tumor
  - ➢ Volvulus
- Obstructed loop fills w fluid
- Distends, elongates
- Base narrows, loop twists
- Venous & Art Occlusion results

Bezoar
- Rarely sole cause SBO:
  - ➢ THINK: motility dis.
  - ➢ Radiation, scleroderma
  - ➢ NI person: Fiber binge
- More often part of SBO:
  - ➢ Fibrous Food impaction above "lesion" (adhesion)
  - ➢ "SB Feces sign"

Adhesion Traps Bezoar. SBO results

SBO in Colonic Diverticulitis
- SB can be sicker than Colon
- ~5-15% present w SBO
  - ➢ Adhesions
  - ➢ SB abscess
  - ➢ Fistula

Figure 2-26-12

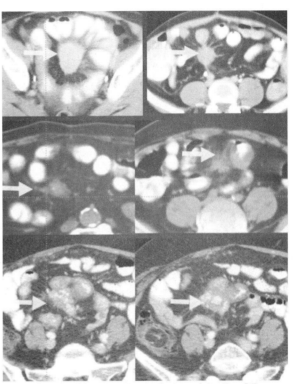

Carcinoid metastases (arrows) to the SB mesentery may cause fibrous retraction and obstruction of bowel, veins, and arteries

Figure 2-26-13

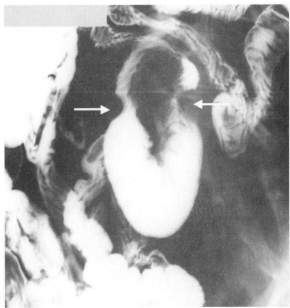

Closed loop obstruction with compression of two limb produce distention between two points of obstruction. These have high risk of torsion and vascular compromise

SBO, Abscess in Colonic Diverticulitis [Figure 2-26-14]

- SBO also in any inflamm condition
  - Appendicitis
  - PID

SBO, Chronic partial. Endometriosis with Adhesion [Figure 2-26-15]

Figure 2-26-15

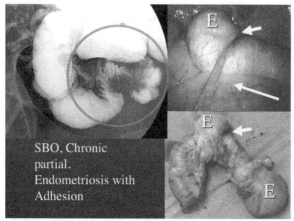

Endometrial Deposits: Chronic recurring pain, bloating in 47 year old woman. Other exams negative. Enteroclysis shows non distensible SB with angulation. At surgery, adhesions (long arrow) from endometrial deposit (labeled E) on SB distorts a pelvic SB loop (short arrows). The resected specimen shows a second endometrial deposit (2nd E).

Mesenteric Volvulus [Figure 2-26-16]

- Assoc w
  - Malrotation
    - Left Colon
    - Right SB
    - "Weak" Treitz
  - Internal Hernia
  - External Hernia
  - Post operative
- Short / bunched mesentery

Ligament of Treitz

"Corkscrew", "Helix", "Barberpole", "Whirl" [Figure 2-26-17]

Abdominal Hernias

- 1.5 % of population
- 500,000 ops yearly
- External (most) or Internal
- Hiatal, Inguinal, Femoral, Ant Abd Wall
- Majority include peritoneal sac & fat
- Contents:
  - Greater Omentum
  - SB or Colon
  - Other organs possible

Figure 2-26-14

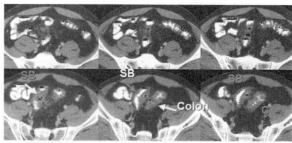

Diverticulitis causing SBO. Any inflammatory process may involve SB and present with SBO

Figure 2-26-16

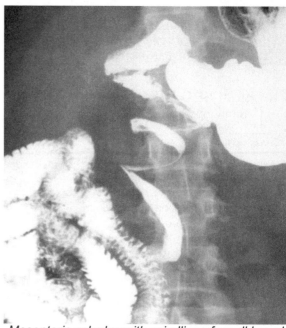

Mesenteric volvulus with spiralling of small bowel

Figure 2-26-17

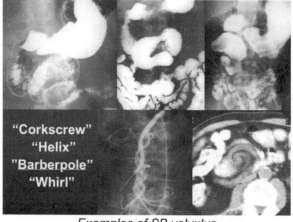

Examples of SB volvulus

External Abdominal Hernias
Diaphragmatic, Pelvic, Abd Wall

- Diaphragmatic
  - ➢ Esophageal Hiatus
  - ➢ Foramen of Bochdalek
  - ➢ Foramen of Morgagni
  - ➢ Acquired diaphragmatic defects
  - ➢ Congenital diaphragmatic defects

Morgagni Hernia

- Embryo defect in fusion of sternal & costal diaphragm
- Majority on R
- = 10% congenital diaphragm defects
- True membranous sac
- Majority asymptomatic
- Complications 10%

Morgagni Hernia with SB

External Abdominal Hernias
Diaphragmatic, Pelvic, Abd Wall

- Hernias of Pelvis
  - ➢ Inguinal
  - ➢ Femoral
  - ➢ Obturator
  - ➢ Sciatic
  - ➢ Vaginal Enterocele
  - ➢ Rectal Enterocele
  - ➢ Levator Hernia

Obturator Hernia *[Figure 2-26-18]*

- Rare
- 3 Types
  - ➢ 1. Into Pectineus muscle
  - ➢ 2. Between Superior & Middle fasciculi Obturator Externus
  - ➢ 3. Between Internal & External Obturator membranes (rare)

Enterocele *[Figure 2-26-19]*

- Common
- SB descent into
  - ➢ Pouch of Douglas
  - ➢ Into - out Vagina
  - ➢ Into - out Rectum

Richter's Hernia *[Figure 2-26-20]*

- Contains part of antimesenteric wall
- 90% inguinal - femoral
- Prone to strangulation
- Patent lumen despite strangulation

Littre's Hernia

- Pre-existing diverticulum herniates.
  - ➢ Colonic
  - ➢ Meckel's
- 50% Inguinal
- 30% Umbilical
- (Amyand Hernia
  = inguinal hernia with appendix in it.)

Figure 2-26-18

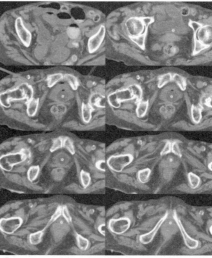

Obturator Hernia of SB (Short Arrow) . This patient also had an asymptomatic right SB inguinal hernia downstream

Figure 2-26-19

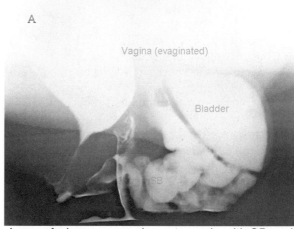

Image A shows a massive enterocele with SB and bladder everting or evaginating out of the vagina. Enteroceles cause defecation difficulties, pelvic pain, but rarely cause SBO

Figure 2-26-20

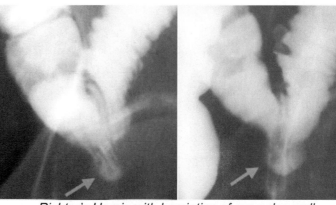

Richter's Hernia with herniation of one colon wall without lumen obstruction

External Abdominal Hernias
Diaphragmatic, Pelvic, Abd Wall

- Abdominal Wall
  - Umbilical
  - Ventral
    - ❖ Epigastric
    - ❖ Spigelian
    - ❖ Parastomal
  - Lumbar
  - Incisional (Anywhere)

Small Pediatric Umbilical Hernia

- Congenital "outies":
  - Protrusion of fat (viscera) thru patent umbilical ring
  - Rarely symptomatic
  - (Omphalocele: not hernia but failure of abd wall closure: viscera never in abdomen)

Umbilical Hernia

- Adult:
  - 4% of all hernias
  - May incarcerate / strangulate
  - Middle age F, usually obese
  - Spont rupture in pregnancy or ascites

Epigastric Hernia

- Hernia of linea alba
- Most small, asymptomatic
- Usually above umbilicus
- Symptoms incr reclining 2° pull on incarcerated tissue
- 5% @ autopsy
- Contents usually omentum & properitoneal fat

Spigelian Hernia [Figure 2-26-21]

- Hernia thru Spigelian line
  - Lateral to Rectus
- Usually Omentum, Colon, SB
  - Occasionally:
    - ❖ Stomach, Ovary, Meckel's

Incisional Hernias [Figure 2-26-22]

- True iatrogenic hernia
- Common association: wound infection
- Lower incidence w transverse incisions
- Incarceration common (33%)
- Strangulation rare (5%)
- Recurrence, esp w obesity

Parastomal Hernias

- Assoc w any stoma
- Common
- Majority Asymptomatic
- Symptoms:
  - Stoma dysfunction
  - Incarceration common
  - Strangulation rare
  - Recurrence, esp w obesity

Figure 2-26-21

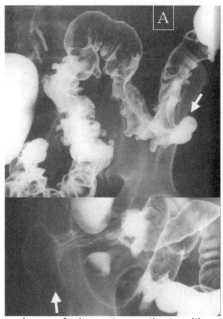

Image A shows two patients with Spigelian Hernias. Upper image shows a loop of Sigmoid entering a left Spigelian Hernia. The lower image shows a Richter type hernia of the lateral cecal wall(arrow) into a Spigelian Hernia

Figure 2-26-22

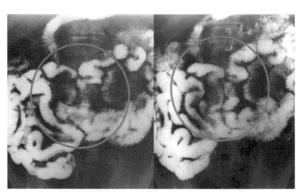

Fixed loops of SB on films taken 30 minutes apart are abnormal

Incarcerated Hernia [Figure 2-26-23]
- SB Distension
- Neck
- Efferent limb collapsed
- Sac Fluid
- Compressed Abd Wall

Strangulated and incarcerated

Internal Hernias
• Paraduodenal	A	53%
• Pericecal	B	13%
• Foramen of Winslow	C	8%
• Transmesenteric	D	8%
• Pelvis	E	7%
• Transmesosigmoid	F	6%

Gahremani & Whalen Curr Prob Radiol 5:1-30,1975

Internal Abdominal Hernias
- Also:
  - ➢ Trans-omental
  - ➢ Retro-anastomotic
    - ❖ Antecolic
    - ❖ Retrocolic
    - ❖ Roux -en Y

Internal Hernias except paraduodenal
- Associated w prior bowel surgery (Clips)
- Look for
  - ➢ Mesenteric:
    - ❖ Bunching
    - ❖ Vein Engorgement
    - ❖ Misty Mesentery
  - ➢ Criss-crossed vessels
  - ➢ Hairpin Veins and arteries
  - ➢ Ascitic fluid, local or diffuse

Paraduodenal Hernia
- All Internal Hernias: < 1% SBO, (LBO)
- 50% IH = Paraduodenal
- Mortality high in pre-CT era (20%)
- Clinically: asymptomatic, pain, SBO,
- Left   3X > R;   M > F
- Congen failure of fusion mesentery w parietal peritoneum

J Comp. Assist. Tomo. 10:542, 1986

Left Paraduodenal Hernia [Figure 2-26-24]
- Extends into desc & transv mesocolon
- Stomach displaced to right
- Colon ant. or inf. to hernia
- Neck contains IMVein & Left Colic Art.
- IM Vein displaced ant. by hernia
- Treitz OK

Figure 2-26-23

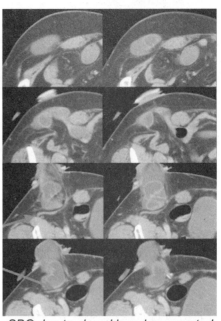

SBO due to closed loop Incarcerated parastomal hernia. Even though the bowel wall is white indicating perfusion, signs accompanying signs are worrisome for strangulation

Figure 2-26-24

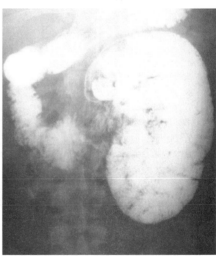

Left Paraduodenal Hernia. SB appears wrapped. Left PD hernia displaces the stomach to the right

Right PD Hernia [Figure 2-26-25 and 2-26-26]

- Assoc w absent Ligament of Treitz
- Displaces stomach to left
- SB behind duodenum
- RPDH into ascending mesocolon
- Behind Right & Transverse Colon

Figure 2-26-25

Figure 2-26-26

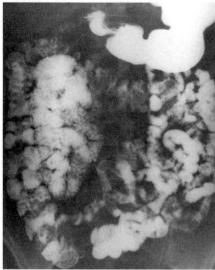

Right Paraduodenal Hernia: Image A shows a right PDH with clustered loops behind the proximal transverse colon

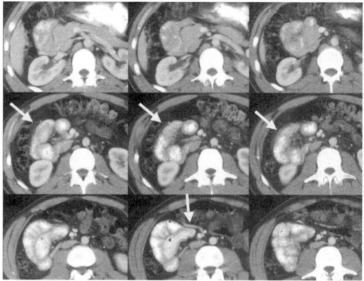

Right Paraduodenal Hernia: Note duodenum does not cross between SMA and Aorta. Note duodenum merges into SB in right gutter. Ileocolic vessels cross in front of SB to pass to right colon. The vessels that usually are posterior to SB in front of right kidney and confuse when we search for appendix in RLQ now arc in front of SB indicating a right PDH

Figure 2-26-27

Foramen of Winslow [Figure 2-26-27]

- "Epiploic Foramen"
- Ant:R free margin of Lesser Omentum - Porta Hepatis to Lesser curve of stomach
  - ➢ PortalVein
  - ➢ Hepatic Art
  - ➢ CBD

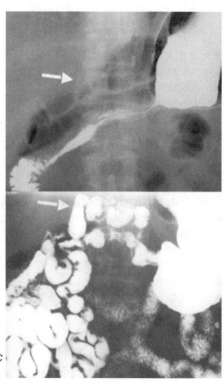

Hernia into Foramen of Winslow: Upper image shows air filled small bowel loops (arrow) above stomach displacing and compressing distal stomach and duodenum. Lower image shows same findings in a patient with barium filled loops within lesser sac

Cecal Volvulus into lesser sac [Figure 2-26-28 and 2-26-29]
* SBO
    * Potential in Cecal Volvulus
    * SB follows IC Valve

Figure 2-26-28

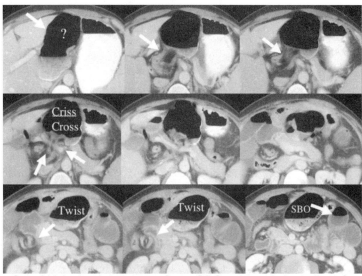

Cecal Volvulus into Lesser Sac. SBO evident in last slice. Gas filled structure (labeled" ?") in first slice is posterior to stomach. See criss-cross sign of internal hernia first slice second row. See vovlulus of compressed bowel and vessels leading away from gas and fluid filled structure posterior to stomach

Trans-mesocolic hernia [Figure 2-26-30]

Pre op DX: Infarcting Internal Hernia [Figure 2-26-31]
* Complex Subject
    * Many Causes
* Vital to diagnose and "stage"
    * Common problem
    * Delay in DX disastrous
    * Incomplete DX fatal

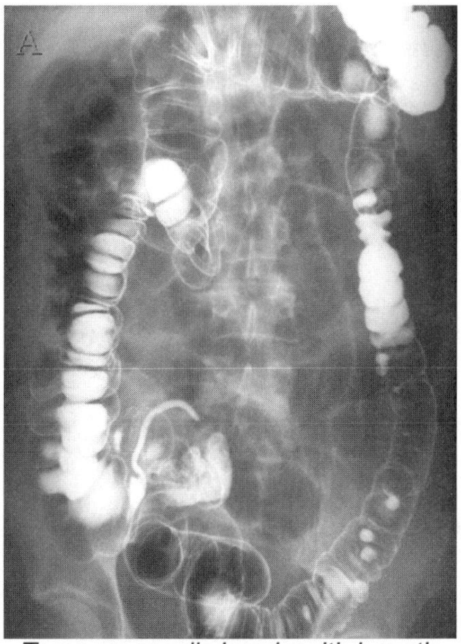

Figure 2-26-31

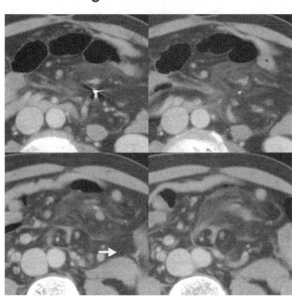

Figure 2-26-29

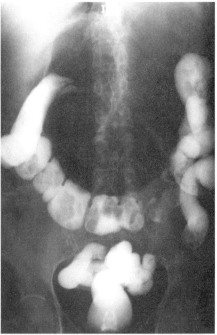

Cecal Volvulus herniating into lesser sac: Barium Enema shows beak like colon termination with a kidney bean gas collection

Figure 2-26-30

Trans-mesocolic hernia with hepatic flexure displaced inferiorly by bunched air distended loops of SB. A similar appearance could be seen in pt with a right paraduodenal hernia

Ischemic internal hernia. Note surgical clip in image one. Engorged mesentery in all images. Bottom left image shows Criss Cross mesentery (arrow) indicating internal hernia

Trans-mesenteric hernia [Figure 2-26-32]

Internal Hernia [Figure 2-26-33]
- Bezoar above IH
- Engorged distal SMV branch
- Hairpin Vein
- Misty Mesentery

Figure 2-26-32

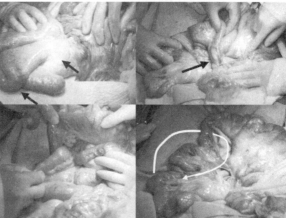

Transmesenteric Hernia: top image shows distended SB loops with white lymphatic engorged mesentery (arrows). The mesentery could be traced back in top right image to a hole in the mesentery seen in bottom left image. With reduction of this hernia (curved arrow bottom right), bowel deflated and the ischemic blue bowel the arrow points to in bottom right turned to normal pink within minutes of reduction

Figure 2-26-33

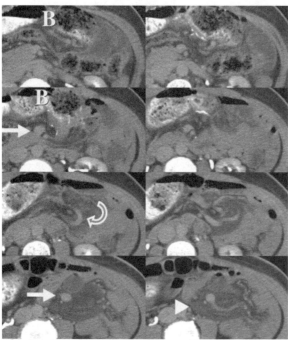

Obstructing Closed Loop Internal Hernia year plus after Laparascopic Bypass for morbid obesity. Bezoar (B) is seen in SB proximal to the internal hernia. Note engorged distal SMV (lowest arrow) is equal in diameter to proximal SMV (upper arrow). Curved arrow is a hairpin or sharply turning vein. Arrowhead shows misty mesentery from lymphatic engorgement

Internal Hernia
- Engorged Vessels
- Engorged Mesentery
  - Swollen veins
  - Yellow swollen fat
  - Pale exuded lymph fluid
- Lymph fluid coagulum (bottom

Gallstone Ileus [Figure 2-26-34]

SBO
- Complex Subject
  - Many Causes
- Vital
  - Common
  - Delay in DX disastrous
  - Incomplete DX fatal

Figure 2-26-34

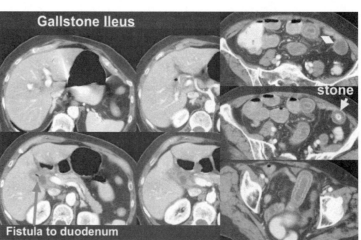

Gallstone Ileus with compromised bowel. Note fistula to duodenum, air in hepatic bile duct, and stone in distal SB. Top right image shows a target sign loop (left of diamond) with white internal mucosa and (right of diamond) adjacent loop which has less mucosal enhancement

Mesenteric Ischemia

Francis J. Scholz, M.D.
Radiologist, Lahey Clinic
Clinical Professor of Radiology,
Tufts University School of Medicine

Bowel Ischemia
- Small Bowel or "Mesenteric" ischemia
  SMA distribution: SB, Right Colon
- "Colonic Ischemia" - a different disease
  Watershed: Sigmoid, Splenic
- ESD: never: unless surgery - radiation

The Radiology of Mesenteric Ischemia
- 1. Review classifications & pathophysiology
- 2. Rad Findings: Ischemia & Infarction
- 3. Clues to Etiology, emphasis on CT

Mesenteric Ischemia
Acute, Sub Acute, Chronic
- 3 categories
  - ➢ Arterial Occlusive
  - ➢ Venous Occlusive
  - ➢ Non-Occlusive Arterial - Low Flow

Pathophysiology of Ischemia
- Mucosa & submucosa
  - ➢ Most sensitive, high metabolism
  - ➢ Edema, hemorrhage, & slough
- Muscularis propia
  - ➢ Initial spasm
  - ➢ Then atonia
  - ➢ Then perforation or:
    - ❖ healing with stricture
    - ❖ healing with no sequelae
- Serosa
  - ➢ With healing may see adhesions

Ischemia
- Rad Findings, Symptoms & Prognosis depend on:
  - ➢ Duration
    - ❖ Momentary to Permanent
  - ➢ Degree
    - ❖ 1-100%
  - ➢ Extent
    - ❖ % of SB

Fast Ischemia
- Cell, Tissue, Organ & Organism death -24-48 H
  - ➢ Eg. Embolus to SMA
  - ➢ Eg. Hypotension: Profound & prolonged

Slow or Minimal Ischemia
- Cellular & localized tissue death →
- Organ dysfunction
  - ➢ Eg Radiation Enteritis
  - ➢ Eg Scleroderma
  - ➢ Eg Arteriosclerotic Abdominal Angina

Ischemia
- Chronic - recurrent - slow
- Acute - sudden - fast
- Often both
  - ➢ Chronic for months then Acute

Wet vs Dry Ischemia
- Wet: Ischemia w arterial inflow p insult ("reperfusion")
  - ➢ SEE: Thickest wall, bleeding into wall, ascites.
  - ➢ Eg: Venous occlusion, Transient hypotension, fleeting, partial embolism
- Dry: Ischemia w no arterial inflow.
  - ➢ SEE: "Thinner" or normal wall, no ascites.
  - ➢ Eg. Complete proximal SMA embolus, sudden thrombosis.

Chou C, CT Manifestations of Bowel Ischemia. AJR2002;178-87

Wet vs Dry Ischemia : Personal experience
- Two extremes: Prune vs Plum
- Wet: Classic
  - ➢ Radiologists overcall on CT
  - ➢ Surgeons undercall at Surgery
- Dry: Puzzling SBO
  - ➢ Radiologists undercall - miss completely
  - ➢ Surgeons baffled by our stupidity
  - (SECRET: Study Mesenteric Vessels I+)

Most Specific Single Finding of Ischemia
- Absent perfusion of bowel wall on CT
- 100% specific, 30-50% sensitive
- Diagnosis therefore depends on
  - ➢ History
  - ➢ Summation of findings
    - ❖ Wall thickening
    - ❖ Mesenteric Edema
    - ❖ Ascites

Acute Mesenteric Ischemia
- WBC
- Elevated Lactic Acid
- History
  - ➢ Suggestive History:
    - ❖ Pain in excess of Physical Exam
  - ➢ Risk Factors

High Risk Patients (Boley, Clark)
- Pt > 50 yrs with:
- Valvular or Atherosclerotic Ht Dis
- Longstanding CHF
- Arrythymia
- Hypovolemia or hypotension
- Dig or diuretic Rx
- Recent MI
  - ➢ Boley
- Also: AAA w or wo repair, Any Abd, Cardiac, Thoracic Surg

Dry Infarct [Figure 2-27-1]

- Tendency to:
  - ➤ Thinner Wall
  - ➤ Absent "Target"
  - ➤ No intramural blood
  - ➤ Ascites min /absent
- Beware: "Ileus or SBO" in Sick Pt at high risk

Spectrum: Ischemia to Infarction [Figure 2-27-2]

- Gasless abdomen
- Ileus
- Thick Folds
  - ➤ Target - CT, US
  - ➤ Stack of Coins - Films
- Loss of Folds in Unchanging Thick-walled Loop
- Focal ulcer
- Shaggy gas pattern
- Collar button ulcers
- Intramural fistulas
- Intraluminal mucosal cast
- Mesenteric or portal vein gas
- Intraperitoneal air
- Stricture
- Pseudodiverticulum
- Many findings possible in same pt

Figure 2-27-1

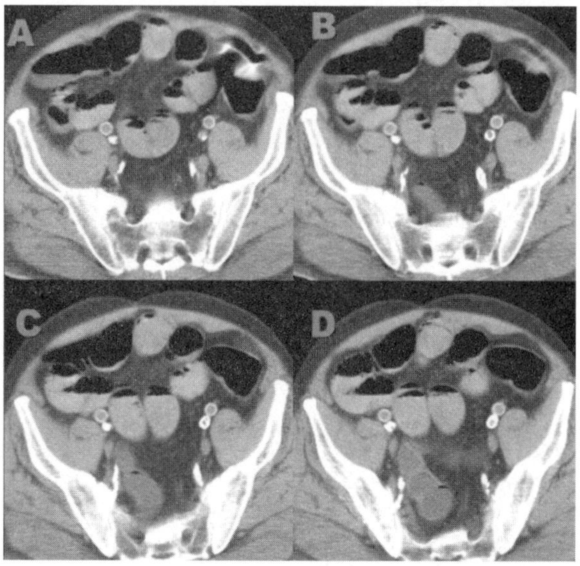

Four sequential images (A-D) of a patient with infarction without reperfusion. Thin walls without target sign or intramural blood. No ascitic fluid. Good example of a dry infarct with minimal or absent inflow of arterial blood. Dry infarcts may be due to a large central SMA embolus or lack of collaterals to allow inflow from smaller emboli or thrombi

Figure 2-27-2

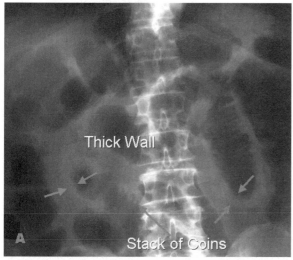

Thick Wall

Stack of Coins

With reperfusion ischemia the wall thickens with fluid and blood from leaking capillaries. Stack of coin appearance is due to fluid and blood in the valvulae conniventes

Figure 2-27-3

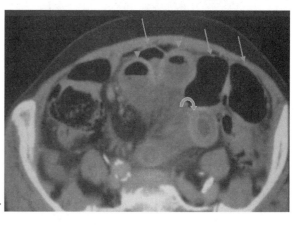

Remember the low of Burps & Farts
[Figure 2-27-3]

- Air rises & thins normal walls
  Note engorged mesentery

Image shows normal thin wall effaced by air (arrows) while arrowheads show thick wall not effaced by air. A loop with a target sign is also noted (curved arrow).The slightest amount of SB (or colon) air will rise and thin the wall of normal bowel. Walls that are thickened by blood or tumor will not thin out. Understanding this concept allows for easy detection of abnormal bowel

Regular Stack [Figure 2-27-4]
- Blood / Edema in Wall
- Suggests:
  - ➢ Acute
  - ➢ Recent
  - ➢ Severe

Hemorrhage vs Ischemia?

Hemorrhage vs Ischemia [Figure 2-27-4]
- Some CT features overlap: target, hemoperitoneum
- Short segment < 15 cm with wall thickening of 1 cm or greater typical intramural hemorrhage
- Long segment > 30 cm with wall thickening of less than 1 cm is typical ischemia
- 15 -30 cm overlap

Macari M, et al Intestinal ischemia versus intramural hemorrhage: CT evaluation. AJR. 2003 Jan;180(1):177-84.

Irregular Stack
- Blood / Edema in wall
- Suggests:
  - ➢ Chronicity
  - ➢ Recurrence
  - ➢ Fibrosis

Loss of Folds in Unchanging Loop

Thick Wall
- May be oral contrast between "valvulae conniventes" or "valves of kerckring", "plicae", "folds"

Thick Wall & Ulcers

Ischemic Pneumatosis [Figure 2-27-5]

Intramural and Intravenous Air [Figure 2-27-6]

Figure 2-27-4

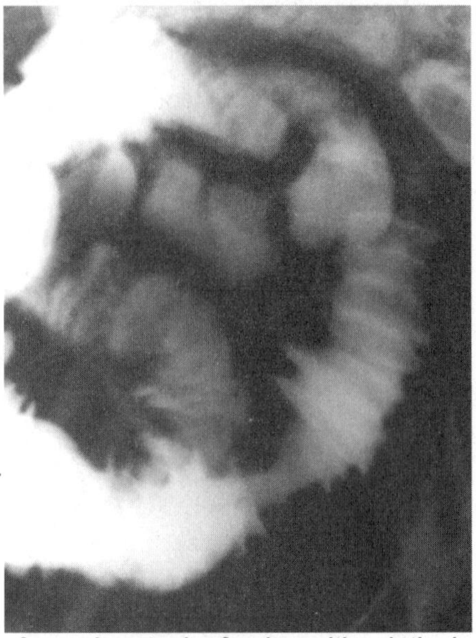

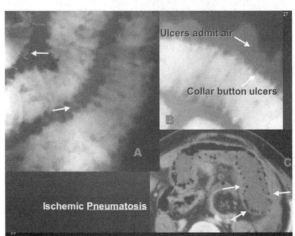

A regular stack of coins with relatively uniform appearance of folds is suggestive of recent bleeding into the wall. A stack of coins appearance can be due to blood or fluid. Patients with coagulopathies or with leaking capillaries due to vasculitis will have a similar appearance

Figure 2-27-5

Two spot films(images A & B) from a water soluble contrast ileostomy enema shows multiple ulcerations filling with contrast or with air. The CT scan slice (image C) shows pneumatosis

Figure 2-27-6

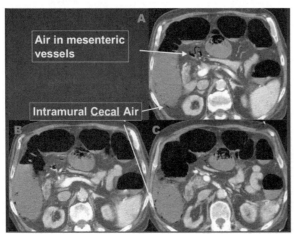

Intramural and intravenous air is seen (arrows). This is evidence of a degree of bowel infarction. The degree of infarction is difficult to determine and may not correlate with amount of air. A small focus of wall infarction may allow large amounts of air to enter veins. Once air enters a vein it may travel long distances. When SBO is present air may be under pressure and large amounts may enter veins through even tiny foci of loss of mucosal integrity

Intrahepatic Portal Venous Air [Figure 2-27-7]

Splanchnic air will go everywhere splanchnic. It doesn't stay near its origin

Sloughed Mucosa / Serosa

Mucosal Cast [Figure 2-27-8] Two CT images, A & B, show shaggy irregular intramural air, suggesting a mucosal cast, or sloughing of the mucosa
Inside Serosa

Figure 2-27-8

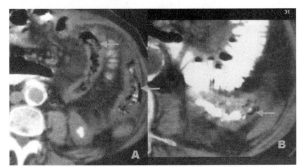

Two CT images, A & B, show shaggy irregular intramural air, suggesting a mucosal cast, or sloughing of the mucosa

SBO Pearl [Figure 2-27-9]

- SBO makes isch / Infarxn look worse
- Rads overestimate Infarxn
- Edema greater
- Air dissects great distances under pressure:
  - ➢ Example: neck crepitus
- Pneumatosis not = Infarxn

Mucosal Cast Inside Serosa

Figure 2-27-7

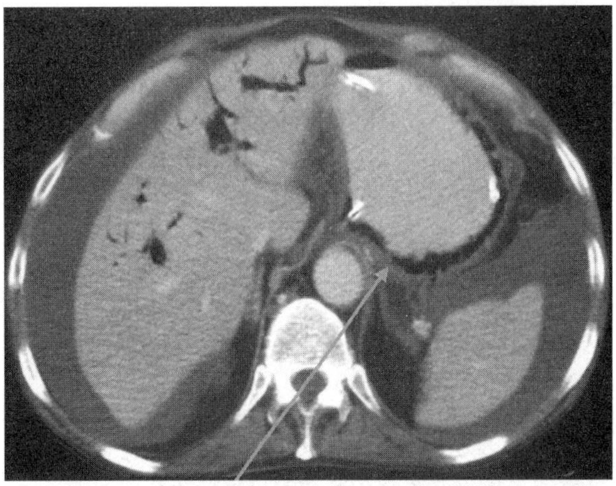

Air is seen in portal branches and within veins in the otherwise normal stomach. (Arrow) Air in the portal system may distribute anywhere within the portal circulation by gravity. In the prone position, air in the intrasplenic veins would likely be seen

Figure 2-27-9

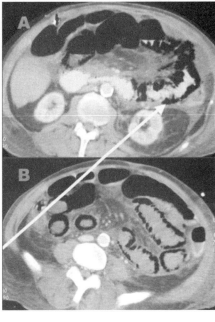

Two slices from a patient show a shaggy irregular mucosal cast (image A) indicating a mucosal slough (long arrow). There are other loops of bowel with extensive pneumatosis (image B). The length of bowel involved with pneumatosis may greatly exceed the amount of bowel that is infarcted because air travels long distance in veins and in areolar submucosal tissue

Reperfusion [Figure 2-27-10]
- Blood Vessels damaged
  - ➢ Tiniest in mucosa
    - ❖ Dead, clotted,
    - ❖ Mucosa non-perfused
  - ➢ Bigger vessels
    - ❖ Loss of vessel muscular tone
    - ❖ Hyperemic bowel musculature,
    - ❖ Shunt to veins

Ischemia may cause strictures [Figure 2-27-11]

Figure 2-27-11

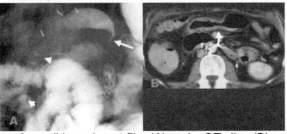

A small bowel spot film (A) and a CT slice (B) show a tapered stricture (arrows) and a long tubular stricture (arrowheads).
With recovery from a severe ischemic insult, healing with stricturing can occur

Etiologies of Ischemia
- Arterial Occlusive
  - ➢ Atherosclerosis - Thrombosis
  - ➢ Emboli
  - ➢ Mechanical -
    - ❖ Volvulus,
    - ❖ Incarceration
    - ❖ Avulsion
  - ➢ Radiation Endarteritis Obliterans
- Venous Occlusive
- Arterial Non-Occlusive

Embolus
- Atrial Fibrillation
- Valvular heart disease
- Sharp cut off
- Filling defect

Embolism [Figure 2-27-12]

Figure 2-27-10

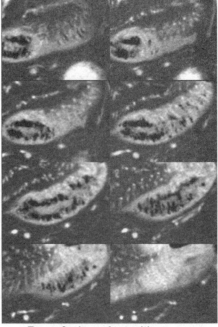

Reperfusion: A pt with severe unexplained pain. CT scan within hours before surgery shows pneumatosis with early shaggy mucosal cast formation. The central mucosal cast is gray, non perfusing. The thickened wall shows prominence of blood vessels on its surface and throughout the wall. The patient had viable bowel at surgery and recovered without requiring resection. The mucosal vessels are hypoperfused and the muscularis has the bowel equivalent of "luxury perfusion"

Figure 2-27-12

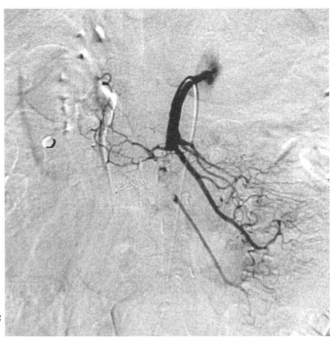

Embolism: Abrupt cut off due to embolus

Orifice Clot [Figure 2-27-13]

Venous Air & Lack of Wall Perfusion [Figure 2-27-14]

Figure 2-27-14

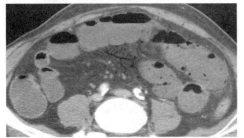

Venous air and lack of perfusion of SB wall

Thrombosis [Figures 2-27-15 and 2-27-16]
- Absent segment
- Slow filling distal vessel
- Large collaterals
- Reconstitution
- Vascular calcification
- Irregular lumen

Figure 2-27-13

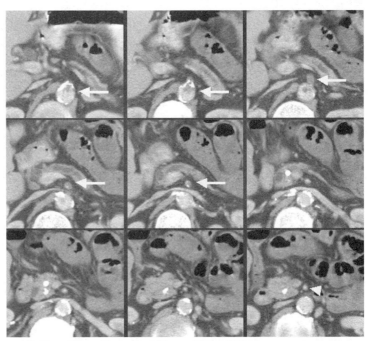

Orifice Clot: Clot straddling orifice of SMA, some in aorta, some in SMA. In lower sections there is some collateral inflow with more opacification. It may be difficult to determine if native aortic mural clot extension in orifice has occurred or, more likely, embolism from heart has wedged here

Figure 2-27-15

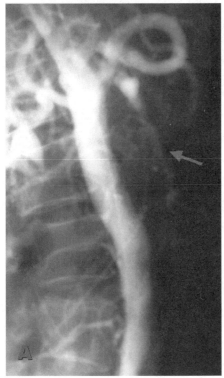

Figure 2-27-16

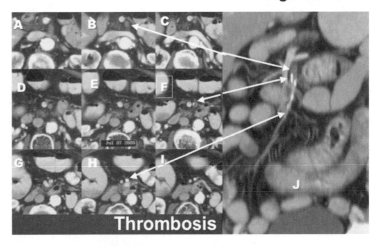

2-27-15: Slow filling of an irregular faint SMA (arrow). This is usually indicative of atherosclerotic thrombotic disease

2-7-16: Nine axial images(A-I) show non-opacification of the SMA proximally (Images A-G) with contast in the SMA distally(Image H t& I) indicating distal perfusion by collaterals, confirmed with a coronal reconstruction (image J).

Peripheral focal lesion
Ulcerating Plaque [Figure 2-27-17]

Dysplasia

Chronic Radiation Enteritis
- Recurrent attacks:
  - ➢ Abd pain
  - ➢ SBO
  - ➢ Diarrhea
- 6 wks to decades after radiation.
- Increasing frequency & severity
  - ➢ Symptoms progress for 1 - 3 years until S / D
- Initially dysmotility.
- Later morphologic changes.

Radiation Enterocolitis
- Endarteritis obliterans
- "Onion - skinning"
- Fibrosis
- "Slow motion ischemia"
- "Regional Premature Arteriosclerosis"

Radiation Enteritis [Figure 2-27-18]
- Regional abnormality with:
  - ➢ SBO, dilated proximal to dis.
  - ➢ Hypermotility, (non-propulsive)
  - ➢ Thickened folds
  - ➢ Fixed loops & Stiff walls
  - ➢ Narrowed loops - Strictures
  - ➢ Adhesions
  - ➢ Fistulas

Scleroderma
- Patchy Smooth Muscle disease 2° to Vascultitis
- Dilated, <u>dry</u>, delayed
- Thin crowded folds, "Hidebound" walls
- Pseudosacculations, SB, Colon
- Accordion or Pipestem Contractions
- (Wet if bacterial overgrowth)
- Also: Esoph dysmotility / Stricture, Balanced pneumoperitoneum, soft tissue calcinosis, interstitial fibrosis at bases.

Pseudosacculations [Figure 2-27-19]

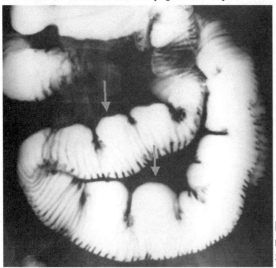

Figure 2-27-17

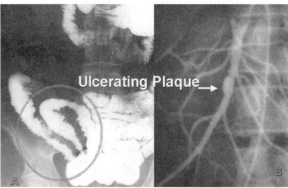

A SB series (Image A) shows a stack of coins appearance (within circle).
An angiogram (Image B) shows a bulging segment of the SMA (arrow), consistent with an ulcerating plaque showering cholesterol emboli.
(This could also be a mycotic aneurysm if the patient were septic.)

Figure 2-27-18

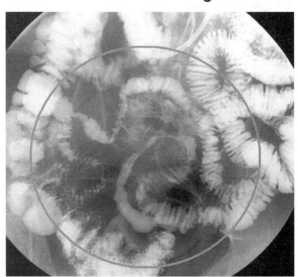

Enteroclysis shows abnormal SB. Small bowel within circle shows distinct regional differences from more proximal bowel. There is fold thickening producing stack of coins appearance, a tubular segment indicating strictures (arrows).

Figure 2-27-19

Eccentric wide mouthed "diverticula" (arrows) on the mesenteric wall are characteristic psuedosacculations of Scleroderma

Hidebound [Figure 2-27-20]

Figure 2-27-20

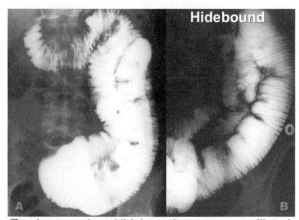

Two images show Hidebound appearance, dilated loops, and crowding together of folds. A "Hidebound" appearance makes the SB look as if the bowel is wrapped in plastic food wrap and then distended with the edges flattened against the wrap. The loops are dilated but the thin folds remain crowded together, with up to 10 folds per inch. Were normal SB to be distended to the same degree, the folds would be spaced far apart.

Accordion - Pipecleaner Contractions [Figure 2-27-21]

Figure 2-27-21

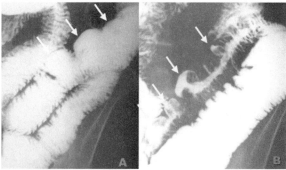

Detail from two sequential SB films, A & B, demonstrate several features of Scleroderma. Psuedosacculations (arrows) are seen in one segment in the image A. That segment contracts in image B with linear shortening but without circumferential contraction, like an accordion and the pseudosaccules (arrows) do not contract because of loss of muscle. This produces an a pipecleaner pattern. This transient appearance should not be mistaken for the fixed stack of coins appearance of hemorrhage

Colonic Pseudosacculations

Etiologies of Ischemia
- Arterial Occlusive
  - ➢ Atherosclerosis
  - ➢ Embolus
- Venous Occlusive
  - ➢ Proximal Obstruction
  - ➢ Distal Disease
- Arterial Non-Occlusive

SMV Thrombosis Etiology
- Idiopathic
- Recent Surgery
- Hypercoagulable States
  Protein S, C defic, P Vera
- Cirrhosis
- Portal Vein Thrombosis
- Pancreatic Inflamm / Neoplasm
- Mesenteric disease
- Pelvic Infectious Processes

Figure 2-27-22

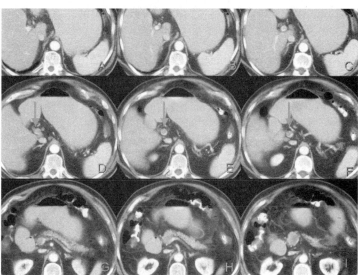

Images A-I: Sequential CT images show thrombus (arrows) in Portal Vein

Symptoms SMV Thrombosis [Figure 2-27-22]
- Mean duration of symptoms
  - ➢ 9.1 days, range 1-42 d
- Pain 84%, N & V 56%, Fever & Chills 56%
- Diarrhea 23%, Blood in Stools 23%
- Ischemia in 21%
  - ➢ Bowel Wall Thickening
  - ➢ Mesenteric Congestion
- Mortality in 7%

Warshauer DM, Lee JKT, Mauro MA, White GC; Superior Mesenteric Vein Thrombosis w Radiologically Occult Cause: Retrospective Study of 43 Cases; AJR2001;177:837-841

Splanchnic Vein Thrombus
- May begin in peripheral IM or SMV & spread toward liver
  - ➤ Eg diverticulitis, SMV occlusion, ischemia
- May begin in liver and propagate distally
  - ➤ Eg Cirrhosis, Budd Chiari,

Cirrhosis
- P Hyper
- Slow flow
- PV Thrombosis
- P Vein Calcification

Mesenteric Disease *[Figure 2-27-23]*
- Lymphoma of SB Mesentery
- Nodes Compress Veins
- Engorged Mesentery
- Infarction / Slough

Etiologies of Ischemia
- Arterial Occlusive
  - ➤ Atherosclerosis
  - ➤ Embolus
- Venous Occlusive
- Arterial Non-Occlusive
  - ➤ Low Flow States
    - ❖ Shock
    - ❖ Steals
    - ❖ Arterial Vasospasm
    - ❖ SBO

Abdominal Angina, a <u>clinical</u> syndrome
- 1. Pain following eating
- 2. Weight loss
- 3. Diarrhea, rapid transit
- "Classic"
  - ➤ Occlusion of 2 of 3: Celiac, SMA, IMA
  - ➤ May be 1 vessel occlusion, part others
  - ➤ May be absent with full 3 vessel occlusion
- Vasculitis, Radiation, Median Arcuate Ligament Syndrome, Steal Syndromes, CA Pancreas

Figure 2-27-23

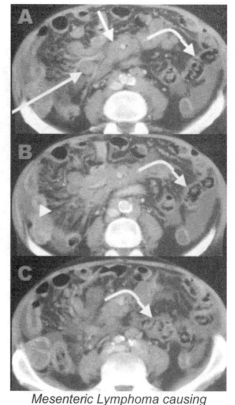

Mesenteric Lymphoma causing Ischemia: Images A-C show bulky nodes in the SB mesentery (straight arrow). The mesentery is engorged (arrowhead) indicating compression of mesenteric vessels. Shaggy irregular intramural air (curved arrows) indicates infarction with mucosal slough. Compression of SB veins may lead to venous engorgement and bowel infarction

Abdominal Angina: Median Arcuate Ligament

[Figure 2-27-24]
- Median Arcuate Ligament of diaphragm
- Compression / fibrosis of Celiac Artery (occ SMA too)
- Collateral Steal from SMA

Figure 2-27-24

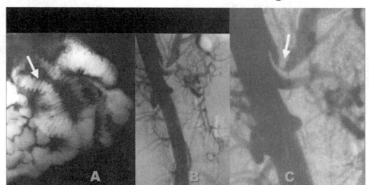

Image A in a patient with chronic intermittent abdominal pain shows a stack of coins appearance to the jejunum. Image B and a detail from it, image C, show that there is a short segment narrowing of the Celiac Axis with a normal SMA just caudal to it. The appearance allows the diagnosis of median arcuate ligament syndrome. The median arcuate ligament of the diaphragm may compress the Celiac Axis. This forces a physiologic steal from the SMA which may be asymptomatic when the bowel is at rest. Following eating, classic abdominal angina may occur because the steal creates a functional mesenteric ischemia

Expiration / Inspiration

Median Arcuate Ligament
Collateral Steal from SMA [Figure 2-27-25]

Vasculopath
- Lush vasculature in upper abdomen
- Abrupt SMA end.
- Paucity lower abdomen

Vasculopath
Collateral Steal from SMA [Figure 2-27-26]
- See steal from SMA to SMA, IMA and beyond
Reflex Arterial Vasospasm in SMA

CT Hypotension: "Shock Bowel" [Figure 2-27-27]
- Systolic BP < 100 mm
  - < 80 in children
- Small aorta < 6mm
- Flat vena cava & renal vein
- Small spleen
- Prolonged "White"
  - Mesentery
  - Mucosa
  - Kidneys

Figure 2-27-26

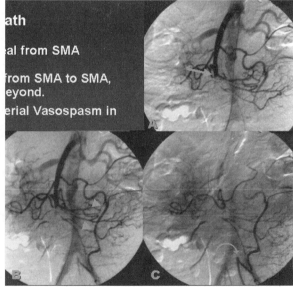

Three images from SMA injection (A-C) show abrupt termination (arrow) and collateral flow filling an enlarged marginal arcade vessel (arrowheads) and filling of IMA branches (curved arrow). Chronic steal syndromes in vasculopaths have variations in amount stolen depending on varying demand. Walking may deplete visceral flow and produce Reflex Arterial Vasopasm and abdominal angina

Figure 2-27-25

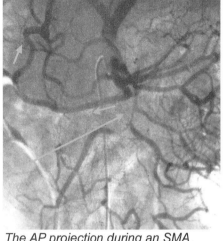

The AP projection during an SMA injection, image A, shows collateral filling of the Celiac vessels and reflex mesenteric vasoconstriction of the mid and distal branches of the SMA, placing them at risk of thrombosis. Celiac artery disease may be the cause of mesenteric angina, ischemia, or infarction due to collateral steal

Figure 2-27-27

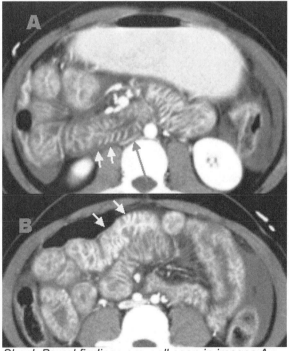

Shock Bowel findings are well seen in images A, B. The mucosa has bright white enhancement defining the mucosal valvulae conniventes (small arrows). There is submucosal edema, flat Inferior Vena Cava (long arrow), bright arterial contrast and bright kidneys. The images have the appearance of arterial phase even though they are well beyond the normal venous phase time period. "Delayed Nephrogram" and "Delayed Mucosagram" should alert the radiologist to a patient in shock on the CT table

Target sign

- Blood, Serum, Plasma, Interstitial Fluid, Fat, Air
- Ischemia
- Vasculitis
- Intramural Hemorrhage
- Crohns: edema (or fat)
- Angioedema
- Portal Hypertension
- NSAIDs Enteritis

Angioedema: Leaking Capillaries

[Figures 2-27-28 to 2-27-30]

- Enhancement of mucosa
- Edema of submucosa
- Fluid in lumen
- Ascites
- Etio
  - ➢ Allergic reaction,
  - ➢ Hereditary,
  - ➢ ACE inhibitors.

DeBacker AI, et al; CT of Angioedema of the Small Bowel, AJR 2001; 176: 649-52

Figure 2-27-28

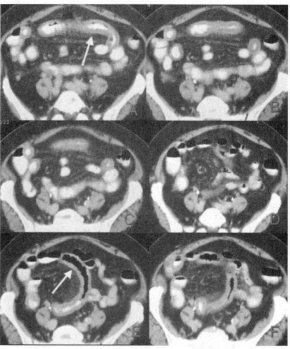

Six sequential axial CT images (A-F) show wall thickening with fluid density (The law of burps and farts is apparent and helpful here in judging extent of disease) in a patient with angioedema. This is a process where the capillaries leak. It may be due to allergies to food, drugs, or other exogenous allergens. There is an hereditary form where it occurs without specific causation. Angiotensin Converting Enzyme inhibitor drugs may produce this finding alone or in association with glottic or generalized edema. It may be dose related or seen with only certain ACE inhibitors. Those with bowel angioedema from ACE inhibitors may present with a radiographic and clinical picture suggesting mesenteric ischemia. Patients on hypertensive or cardiac medications should be questioned about recent change in antihypertensive medication or dosage to exclude this as an etiology. Cessation of the offending ACE inhibitor may provide relief and radiographic return to normal within 24 to 48 hours

Figure 2-27-29

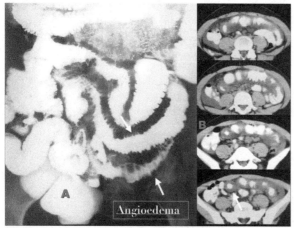

Image A is a small bowel series film in an hypertensive patient who recently was changed to an ACE inhibitor and complained of pain and cramps. A stack of coins appearance is seen in several loops of small bowel (Arrows). Sequential CT images (Images B) show diffuse wall thickening with water density as well as ascites

Figure 2-27-30

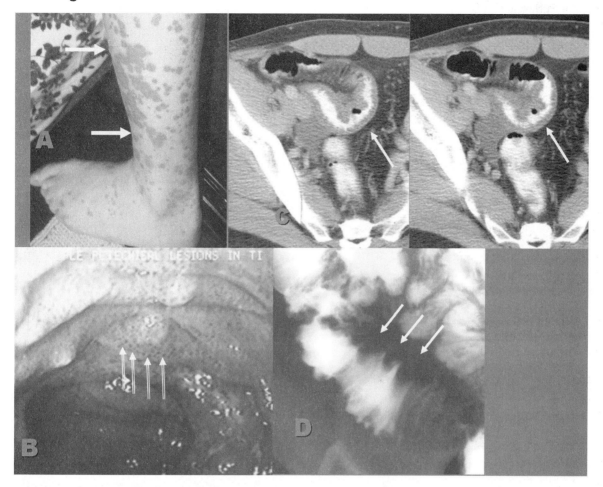

Henoch Schonlein is a transient but often recurring immune mediated vasculitis, usually affecting children. It can be seen in adults. Usually the characteristic palpably raised itchy red lesions (Arrows Image A) are present and allow a diagnosis. Petechiae (arrows in image B of ileal endoscopy) and purpuric lesions also occur in the bowel. Abdominal involvement is seen in 50-75% of patients who present with dramatic colicky abdominal pain and bleeding, which may be massive in 1-2% of patients. Bleeding into the wall of the bowel thickens it (Image C arrows) and gives a stack of coins appearance (Image D arrows). This intramural bleeding may cause obstruction, GI bleeding, infarction, perforation, or intussusception in the distal small bowel. While there is no effective treatment, the patients must be monitored for the complications until the attack subsides

Bowel Damage Pathways [Figure 2-27-31]

- Loss of Barrier Integrity
  - ➤ Vascular Barrier
    - ❖ Leak of serum, plasma, cells
    - ❖ Edema
    - ❖ Ischemia
    - ❖ Loss of mucosal barrier
  - ➤ Mucosal Barrier
    - ❖ Inflow of excluded molecules
    - ❖ Edema
    - ❖ Loss of vascular barrier
    - ❖ Vascular compromise
    - ❖ Ischemia

Ischemia CT Mimics

- Vascular or Mucosal Barrier Interruption
  - ➤ Ischemia
  - ➤ Vasculitides HSP, SLE,
  - ➤ Coagulopathies
  - ➤ Regional Inflammation - tic app it is
  - ➤ Crohns
  - ➤ Infectious Enteritis
  - ➤ Neutropenic Enterocolitis
- Many diseases may have phases of overlap

Mesenteric Ischemia

- Diagnosis
  - ➤ Imperative in Acute & Chronic Ischemias
  - ➤ Now earlier Dx by MDCT - IV contrast
  - ➤ Think of it in every abd pain CT.
- Physiological understanding is critical
- Remember Steal
- Surgeons undercall some, be brave, stay bold
- We undercall some, explain plums & prunes

Figure 2-27-31

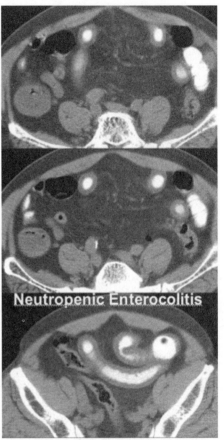

Neutropenic Enterocolitis, or "typhlitis" is an example of loss of mucosal barrier allowing transmural injury to mimic ischemic disease. Differing diseases may have convergent paths or common pathways at times in the course of those diseases

Malabsorption

Francis J. Scholz, M.D.
Radiologist, Lahey Clinic
Clinical Professor of Radiology,
Tufts University School of Medicine

The Radiology of Malabsorption (MAB)
- Review
  - ➤ The physiology of MAB
  - ➤ The "MAB Pattern"
  - ➤ Sprue - "Celiac Disease"- in detail
  - ➤ Other Diseases of MAB

Myths About MAB & CD
- "New" barium prevents Dx.
- Enteroclysis is necessary.
- A clinical or lab diagnosis.
- Diarrhea is always present.

Sprue Presentations
- Diarrhea   85%
- Weight loss   57%
- Abd distress   29%
- Edema   29%
- Bone pain   19%
- Tetany   10%
- Failure to grow, hematuria, foot drop, hypovolemic shock, each 2%

Trier J, Celiac Sprue NEJM 1991

Sprue Presentations
- 50% of adult pts present w Fe Defic Anemia

Farrell RJ, Kelly CP. Celiac Sprue.N Engl J Med. 2002 Jan 17;346(3):180-8

Back and Leg Pain
- Primary Care
- Neurologist - back pelvis films
- Radiologist - GI series
- Gastroenterologist

Absorption: A Synchronized Symphony
- Endocrine hormones
- Exocrine secretions
- Enzymes
- Muscular mixing + propulsion
- pH variations
- Arterial + venous flow variations

The Clinician's MAB
- "Significant decreased uptake of nutrients into the vascular pool"
- End result of many diseases
- Inability to absorb isolated nutrients or any nutrient

The Physiologist's MAB
- Maldigestion (no enzymes, no mixing)
  - ➤ biliary - panc insuff, ZE, bacterial overgrowth, SB diverticulosis "Lumenal"
- Cellular MAB (Columnar Cell uptake failure)
  - ➤ sprue, ischemia, villous tip infiltration
- Malassimilation (Columnar Cell exit failure)
  - ➤ lymphangiectasia, abetalipoproteinemia, mesenteric diseases
    "Mesenteric"

The Radiologist's MAB: "Malabsorption Pattern"

- Dilution
- Dilatation
- Delay
- "MP" → to chronic enteric fluid overload

Figure 2-28-1

"Malabsorption Pattern"

- Historically, radiologic MAB Pattern = Sprue
- Sprue is king of MAB pattern BUT
- Other disease can cause MAB pattern
- Not all Sprue pts have "MAB pattern"

Sprue: Gold Standard Dx

- SB Biopsy
- Antiendomysial antibody ("EMA")
  - ➤ IgA Ab to extracellular reticular fibers
  - ➤ 90% sensitive, 98% specific
- Tissue Transglutaminase antibody (tTGab)
  - ➤ 86% sens; 84% spec
- AntiGliadin IGA antibody
  - ➤ 76% sens, 79% spec

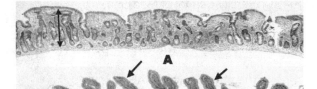

Image shows a biopsy of Sprue at the top contrasted with a normal biopsy at the bottom. With Sprue there is loss of the normal fingerlike villi (arrows) seen below and Crypt Hyperplasia (compare thickness of double arrowheads)

Johnston SD, et al A comparison of antibodies to tissue transglutaminase with conventional serological tests in the diagnosis of coeliac disease. Eur J Gastroenterol Hepatol. 2003 Sep;15(9):1001-4.

Villous Atrophy and Crypt Hyperplasia - Normal Villi and Crypts [Figure 2-28-1]

Entero-enteric Circulation

- Crypts <u>secrete</u> fluid into lumen
- Villi <u>absorb</u> fluid + nutrients from lumen
- Nutrients into portal veins, lymphatics
- Crypts recycle fluid back into lumen

Sprue – Pathophysiologic Sequence

- Mucosal Villous Atrophy + Crypt hypertrophy →
- Chronic Fluid Overload →
- Dilatation (SB Muscle pooped- "CGF") →
- Delay in Transit –> Incr Malabsorption

Figure 2-28-2

Sprue 1° Rad findings I [Figure 2-28-2]

- Dilution   WET !!
- Dilatation   WIDE !!
- Delay in transit   WAY LATE !!
- Segmentation
- Folds: normal –> nodular –> flat
- MALABSORPTION PATTERN

Jejunal Peristalsis "Feathery Fishtails" - Ileal Peristalsis "Esophageal"

Look at the difference in "tone": diameter and peristalsis

Sprue 1° Rad Findings II

- Proximal SB <u>mucosal villous atrophy</u>
  - ➤ reversal of jejuno-ileal fold pattern
  - ➤ toothpaste jejunum (moulage, < 4 folds/inch)
  - ➤ "jejunization" of ileum (increased ileal folds)
  - ➤ flattened duodenal mucosa
  - ➤ foamy mucosal pattern "mosaic"
- Intussusceptions, momentary + non-obstructing

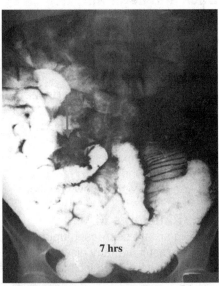

The "Malabsorption Pattern" is characterized by Dilution evident with watery low density of barium (arrow) caused by fluid mixing with it, Dilatation evident by wide diameter (double arrow head) and Delay evident by a 7 hour marker without any barium reaching the colon

Toothpaste – Reversal [Figures 2-28-3]

Foamy, Thick, Bald [Figure 2-28-4]

Foamy, Thick, Bald
- The Jejunum looks like the Ileum, the Ileum looks like the Jejunum, and the Duodenum looks like hell.

Figure 2-28-4

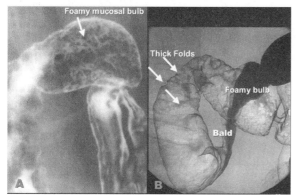

Image A shows a nodular lacy mucosal pattern (arrow) in the duodenal bulb. This is due to atrophy of the mucosa allowing the normal submucosal glands to become apparent.
Image B shows fold thickening of duodenitis

Mosaic Pattern [Figure 2-28-5]

Mucosal Atrophy
- Fissures
- Pits
- Acid burns thinned mucosa

Ulcer
- "Occult GI Bleeding (FOBT+)…detected in half of pts with Sprue"

Fine KD, Prevalence of occult GI bleeding in celiac sprue, NEJM 1996 334:1163-7

Figure 2-28-3

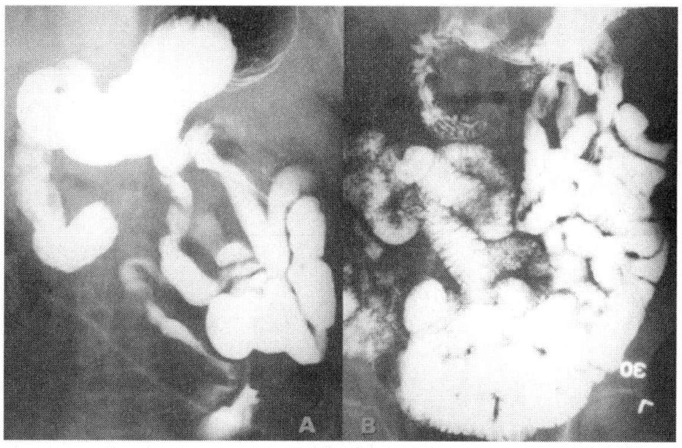

Image A shows a smooth fold-free segment of the jejunum, called "toothpaste" or "moulage" caused by atrophy of mucosal villi and thickening of the wall by crypt hyperplasia

Image B shows a bald jejunum in the LUQ and a feathery abundant fold pattern in the ileum RLQ. Chronic increase in the nutrient mix presented to the ileum because of lack of jejunal absorption cause compensatory hypertrophy of ileal mucosa, hence "Reversal of Fold Pattern".

Figure 2-28-5

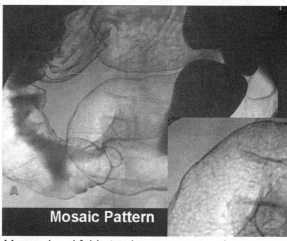

Mucosal and fold atrophy may create a lacy granular or "mosaic" pattern in the jejunum with double contrast or mucosal detail compression images

Jejunal Webs [Figures 2-28-6 to 2-28-8]

Figure 2-28-6

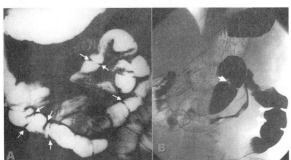

Recurrent ulceration and healing may lead to multiple short segment web-like strictures (arrows).

Figure 2-28-8

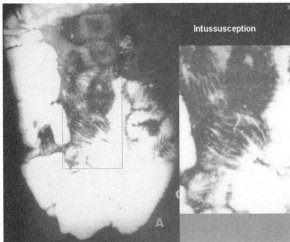

An intussusception is apparent in image A. These are usually transient with dilated flaccid thin walled loops of bowel sliding easily into each other

Figure 2-28-7

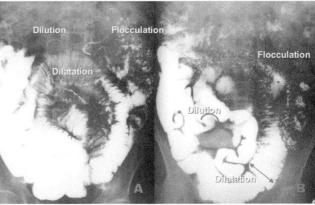

Image A and B are small bowel films having classic MAB pattern. Dilution is evident with watery appearing barium (curved arrows). Dilatation is seen (double arrowheads). Puddles of isolated barium are evident (red dots) which if large can be called "segmentation", if small, "flocculation". Fluid and poor peristaltic activity in MAB causes segmentation and flocculation. An arrowhead in image A shows a worm or threadlike collection of barium caused by a small amount of barium settling out in a fluid filled length of bowel that has not had enough peristalsis to keep the barium and water mixed.

CT in Sprue [Figure 2-28-9]
- Fluid-filled, dilated, non-distended SB
- Fragmentation of contrast
- Intussusceptions - transient
- Mesenteric nodes 1-2 cm
- Large colon w foamy feces "Stool Whip"
- Loss of body fat
- Small Spleen
- Fatty Liver

Figure 2-28-9

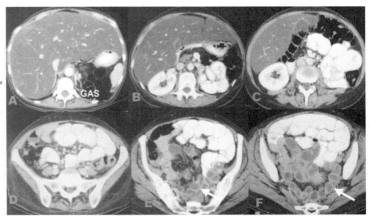

Sprue and its metabolic consequences. There is minimal subcutaneous and intra-abdominal fat from the chronic malnutrition from malaborption. Fatty change is apparent in the liver. The Spleen is small. There is a large amount of gas in the colon from fermentation of unabsorbed nutrients not absorbed in the SB. The small bowel is dilated and the distal loops are fluid filled. (The left kidney was remotely resected for unrelated ? ! neoplasm)

Dilated non-distented SB, Fluid filled distal SB loops, Slow transit of contrast *[Figure 2-28-10]*

Figure 2-28-10

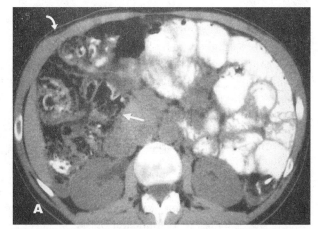

Large amount of stool (arrow), lack of body fat in subcutaneous tissues (curved arrow) and in peritoneal cavity, and dilated flaccid appearing SB loops are consistent with MAB. Sprue should be suggested if the history is appropriate

Reactive Lymphadenopathy *[Figure 2-28-11]*

Figure 2-28-11

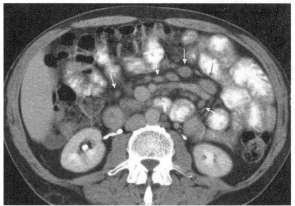

Multiple small and moderate sized lymph nodes are seen in the SB mesentery (arrows) surrounding mesenteric vessels

Figure 2-28-12

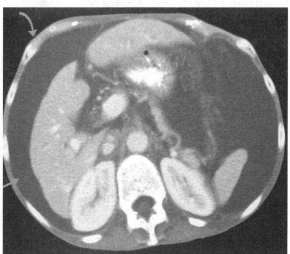

Nutritional Collapse: With severe untreated Sprue, patients may suffer widespread nutritional collapse. This patient presented with cachexia. Ascites (arrow) and absent subcutaneous fat (curved arrow) is apparent

Nutritional Collapse in Sprue *[Figure 2-28-12]*
- Hypoproteinemia
  - ➢ Hypoalbulminemia
  - ➢ Ascites
- Vitamin deficiencies
  - ➢ K Coagulation defects
- Iron Deficiency Anemia
  - ➢ Jejunum absorbs Fe
  - ➢ Slowwww bleeding
- Electrolyte Disturbances
  - ➢ Tetany
  - ➢ Seizures

Sprue = "Immune Disease"
- Lymphadenopathy on CT (reactive hyperplasia)
  - ➢ Mesenteric & para-aortic LNs
  - ➢ Large cavitating nodes = poor prognosis
- Peripheral lymphadenopathy
- Splenic atrophy & clinical hyposplenism

"Genetic Disease"
- HLA B8 , DR3 histocompatility gene in 80% of sprue
- (vs 20% of "normal" population)
- Increased prevalence of Sprue in families
- 10% latent Sprue in 1st order relatives

"Allergic Disease"
- Wheat, rye, barley
- Alpha-gliadin component of Gluten
- "Grass Allergy"

Sprue: Immune Sequence
- Genetic susceptibility
- ?Viral exposure → immune memory
- Gluten + endothelium → antigen
- Lymphocytes flood villous tips
- Antibodies destroy villi

Marsh biopsy categories
- 1 normal
- 2 infiltration with lymphocytes
- 3 early villous atropy
- 4 severe villous atrophy and crypt hyperplasia

Marsh M N, Gluten, major histocompatibility complex, and SB. A molecular and immunobiologic approach to spectrum of gluten sensitivity ('celiac sprue') Gastroenterology 1992 Jan;102(1):330-54)

Sprue Associated Autoimmunities
- Dermatitis Herptetiformis
- Macroamylasemia
- IGA mesangial glomuleronephritis
- Bilateral Occipital Calcif, Epilepsy
- Insulin dependant diabetes
  - ➢ 300% increase incidence of Sprue
- Alopecia areata

Dermatitis Herpetiformis
- Pruritic papulovesicular lesions
- IG A deposits - dermal-epidermal junction
- Goes away with gluten restriction

Nodules !! In Celiac Sprue ??

Healing Sprue
- Folds slowly return, first
- Diameter slowly shrinks
- May take 3-4 years

Sprue
- Occult
  - ➢ Nl SB exam, Asympt,
  - ➢ bx +, labs +
  - ➢ Intraepithelial lymphocytes
  - ➢ 1° relatives of sympt pts: 5-15 %
- Classic MAB pattern
  - ➢ Wet, wide, way late
- Nodular
  - ➢ Sandy Nodules, irritable
- Non-responsive
  - ➢ Diet errors, misdiagnosis
  - ➢ True recalcitrant 5-20%
  - ➢ Lymphoma

Recalcitrant Sprue
- Non responsive to initial Rx 8+yrs
- Loss of responsiveness
- Smoldering symptoms
- Thick folds
- "Ulcerative Jejunitis"
- High incidence of Lymphoma

"Recalcitrant" "Relapsing" Sprue
- Misty Mesentery
- Perivascular Cloaking

Lymphoma in Sprue
- Loss of response to gluten restriction.
- Rising Ig A, Sepsis.
- Increasing lymphadenopathy.
- Thickened bowel loops.
- Mesenteric Perivascular Cloaking ???
- 1 yr lymphoma survival - 31 %, 5 yr - 11%
- 3.4% malignancy in CD (Lymphoma, CA Esophagus, other)

MAB Differential
- Viral, bacterial, parasitic gastroenteritis
- Sprue
- Chronic ischemia
- Advanced scleroderma
- Multiple adhesions
- Multiple mets
- SB diverticulosis
- Retroperitoneal + mesenteric tumors
- Diabetes
- Gastric surgery, esp vagotomy
- Surgical blind loop
- Pancreatic insufficiency
- Mediterranean lymphoma ("IPSID")
- VIPoma & gastrinoma (ZE)

Think Physiologically
- Maldigestion (no enzymes, no mixing)
  - biliary - panc insuff, ZE, bacterial overgrowth, SB diverticulosis "Lumenal"
- Cellular MAB   (columnar C uptake failure)
  - sprue, ischemia, villous tip infiltration
- Malassimilation   (columnar cell exit failure)
  - lymphangiectasia, abetalipoproteinemia, mesenteric diseases "Mesenteric"

Lumenal [Figures 2-28-13 and 2-28-14]

Lumenal MAB: Shwachman - Diamond Syndrome [Figure 2-28-15]
- Exocrine Pancreatic Insufficiency
  - 50% outgrow in adolescence
- Neutropenia
- Chronic Infections
- Myeloid Leukemia
- Metaphyseal Chondrodysplasia
  - Dwarfism

Figure 2-28-13

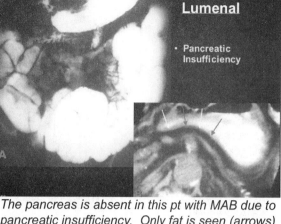

The pancreas is absent in this pt with MAB due to pancreatic insufficiency. Only fat is seen (arrows) where pancreas should be

Figure 2-28-14

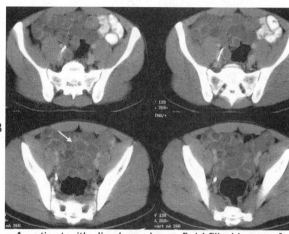

A patient with diarrhea shows fluid filled loops of SB (arrow) in the pelvis indicating MAB and slow transit

Figure 2-28-15

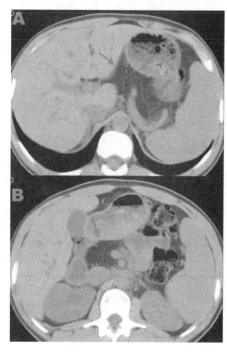

CT of upper abdoment shows fat in the pancreatic bed (arrows) with no glandular tissue. Patient had been diagnosed with Shwachman Diamond previously and had stopped therapy at the start of college

Lumenal MAB: ZE Syndrome [Figure 2-28-16]

- MAB X-Ray pattern 2° to
  - ➤ increased volume of gastric fluid
  - ➤ decreased pH
  - ➤ > enzyme non-activation
  - ➤ > poor digestion
  - ➤ > hypermotility
  - ➤ > edema/hyperemic folds
- Clinical MAB variable

ZE

- Excess fluid
- Thick folds
- Hyperemic mucosa

Lumenal MAB: Gastric Surgery [Figure 2-28-17]

- MAB pattern 2° to
  - ➤ Vagotomy
  - ➤ Loss of pylorus –> bolus into SB
  - ➤ > Poorly mixed food
  - ➤ > Lack of acid digestion
  - ➤ > Poor enzyme synchronization
- Clinical MAB not common 1yr p Surg
  - ➤ Absorption occurs distally

Villous Dysfunction

- Sprue
- Cong / Acq Enzyme Deficiencies
  - ➤ Sugar splitting enzymes (Lactase)
- Bacterial Toxins
  - ➤ Crypts Hypersecrete
  - ➤ Capillaries Leak
  - ➤ Enterocytes Malfunction
  - ➤ Lymphatic Congestion

Malabsorption from Bacterial Overgrowth [Figure 2-28-18]

- Motility Diseases, eg Scleroderma
- SB Diverticulosis

Figure 2-28-16

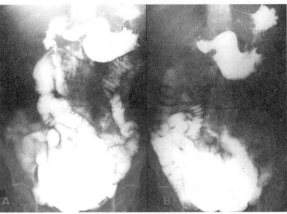

See dilution, dilatation from ZE syndrome

Figure 2-28-17

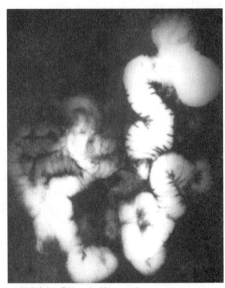

With a Bilroth II or other surgery to increase gastric emptying, the proximal SB will become dilated due to surges of fluid and poor synchronization of the digestive process. Absorption equilibrates and occurs in the distal SB and patients usually become asymptomatic as they accommodate their dietary habits

Figure 2-28-18

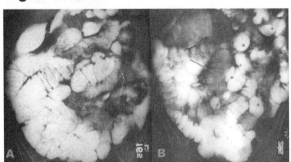

Bacterial infections affect absorption in a number of ways. Invasive bacteria may stun or destroy the absorptive endothelial cells, may impair small capillary or lymphatic vessel drainage, compete for nutrients, or degrade critical enzymes. A MAB pattern is apparent with dilated loops (double arrow in A) and diluted barium (arrows A & B). Delay in transit is evident in image B at 285 minutes. In this patient numerous diverticula (red dots) shelterr bacteria from peristaltic cleansing, allowing them to multiply to such a degree that they degrade or utilize nutrients and enzymes. Note how more diverticula are apparent in image B, diverticula may be difficult to assess, hiding amid dilated loops. Megaloblastic anemia from B12 deficiency may result in patients with numerous large SB diverticula.

Tropical Sprue

- Villous and Crypt Atrophy
- Malabsorption
- Glossitis, wt loss, diarrhea, skin changes
- Folate & B12 deficiency prominent
  - Rx folate, B12 improves partly
- Antibiotic Rx cures
- Relapses common in tropics

Westergaard H.Tropical Sprue Curr Treat Options Gastroenterol. 2004 Feb;7(1):7-11.

Haghighi P, Wolf PL. Tropical Sprue and subclinical enteropathy.. Crit Rev Clin Lab Sci. 1997 Aug; 34(4): 313-41.

Scleroderma [Figure 2-28-19]

Giardiasis - Campylobacter [Figure 2-28-20]

Figure 2-28-20

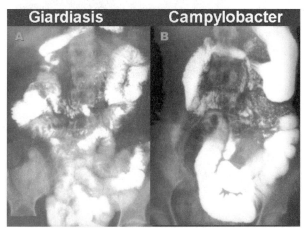

Image A shows MAB associated with Giardiasis. Image B is a patient with MAB from Campylobacter

Figure 2-28-19

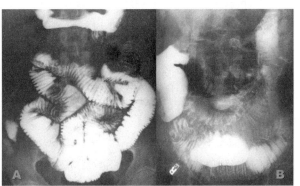

In image A, typical changes of Scleroderma involving SB are apparent with dilated loops, hidebound appearance and pseudo-sacculations. Scleroderma creates a motility disturbance without affecting absorption, creating a dry pattern without dilution. However, with severe Scleroderma and dysmotility, patients may have episodes of bacterial overgrowth which then produce MAB as seen in the patient in image B with dilution apparent

Cryptosporidium [Figure 2-28-21]

Figure 2-28-21

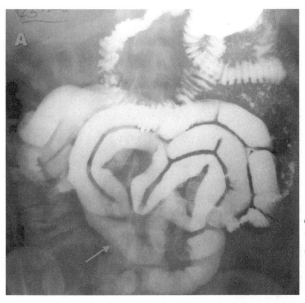

Cryptosporium is an invasive organism that with produce edema, effacing folds, and will cause MAB evident by dilute barium (arrow). Cryptosporidiosis is one of the causes of toothpaste pattern in addition to Sprue in proximal SB, Lymphoma in segments, Crohns, Graft versus Host, and Mastocystosis

Mastocytosis [Figure 2-28-23]
- Lymph cells: Lymphoma, Nodular Lymphoid Hyperplasia, Lymph Cell Granulomas of Crohns or TBC, Immunoproliferative Small Intestinal Disease (IPSID)
- Eosinophils: Eosinophilic Gastroenteritis
- Mast Cells: Mastocystosis
- Macrophages: Chronic infections: IPSID, Tropical Sprue, Amyloid, Whipples
- Pearl:
  - Small nodules diff
- Think:
  - White Blood
- Cell Differential:
  - PMN
  - Lymph
  - Eo
  - Mast
  - Macroph

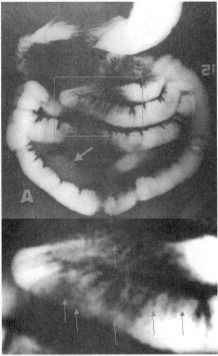

Image A. Mastocystosis is a disease that may infiltrate the SB with mast cells. The infiltration may cause loss of folds or toothpaste appearance and nodularity. MAB in varying degrees may be seen (dilute barium arrow in A)

Figure 2-28-23

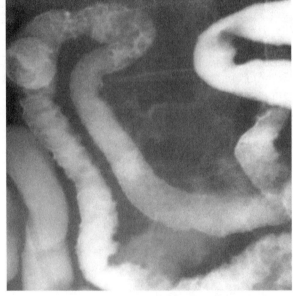

Nodules in the SB are usually caused by cellular infiltrates. To ease your differential brain pain, think of a WBC smear and all the types of WBCs seen. So nodularity in the SB from ordinary PMNs caused by infections, acute or chronic - eg Whipples

MAB: 2° Villus Blockage by
- Lymph cells (immune disease, lymphoma, Crohn Disease)
- PMNs (infections)
- Eosinophils (eosinophilic gastroenteritis)
- Mast cells (mastocytosis)
- Macrophages (Whipples)
- Amyloid (amyloidosis)

Villus Dysfunction
- Engorged Veins & Lymphatics
- Blocked Arteries (ischemia)

Villus Dysfunction
- Paraplegic with diarrhea
- MAB pattern
- Villous atrophy on Bx
- No response to gluten restricted diet
- Physical Exam ->

Arterial Insufficiency *[Figure 2-28-24]*

Figure 2-28-24

Venous Insuffic - Cavernous Transformation and Portal Hypertension

Lymphangiectasia *[Figure 2-28-25]*

Uremia: Multi-faceted MAB
[Figure 2-28-26]

Malabsorption
- Radiologists may still be first on scene in pts with Sprue & MAB diseases
- MAB major radiographic pattern
- Fluid is the hallmark of MAB pattern

Sprue is King of Rad MAB
- Nodular Phase
  - ➤ Rarely seen, ? short phase
- MAB Phase
  - ➤ Commonest
- Recalcitrant
  - ➤ Dietary indiscretions, edema, nodes, MALIG
- Lymphoma
  - ➤ Nodes, weight loss, loss of gluten response

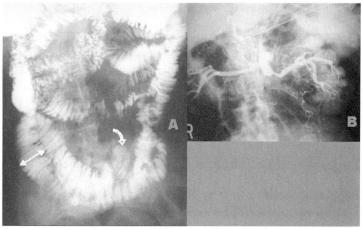

Arterial insufficiency may cause dysfunction of all cells of SB creating dysmotility and malabsorption. Note dilatation (double arrow) and dilution (curved arrow). Usually these bowel symptoms are accompanied by abdominal pain leading to a correct diagnosis. This paraplegic patient had an element of sensory denervation which caused the diagnosis of aortic thrombosis (image B arrow) to be missed initially

Figure 2-28-25

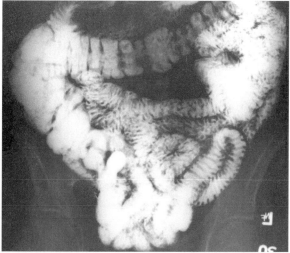

Lymphangiectasia (Image B) may cause degrees of clinical and radiographic MAB due to engorged lymphatics and mucosal edema which will impede absorption. Usually folds remain prominent

Figure 2-28-26

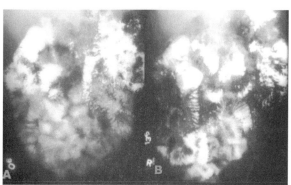

Severe metabolic disturbances may cause MAB, both clinical and radiographic. Here dilution, dilatation, fragmentation are apparent. Usually end stage metabolic diseases with major failure, eg hepatic or renal, or cardiac insufficiency, will have severe MAB. The diagnosis is usually well known and the clinical features of MAB are intermixed or lost among the other severe disturbances present

Malabsorption References

Trier J, Celiac Sprue NEJM 1991

Farrell RJ, Kelly CP. Celiac Sprue.N Engl J Med. 2002 Jan 17;346(3):180-8

Marsh M N,   Gluten, major histocompatibility complex, and the small intestine. A molecular and immunobiologic approach to the spectrum of gluten sensitivity ('celiac sprue') Gastroenterology 1992 Jan;102(1):330-54)

Fine KD, Prevalence of occult GI bleeding in Celiac Sprue, NEJM 1996 334:1163-7

Westergaard H.Tropical Sprue Curr Treat Options Gastroenterol. 2004 Feb;7(1):7-11.

Haghighi P, Wolf PL. Tropical Sprue and subclinical enteropathy.. Crit Rev Clin Lab Sci. 1997 Aug; 34(4): 313-41.

Johnston SD, et al A comparison of antibodies to tissue transglutaminase with conventional serological tests in the diagnosis of coeliac disease. Eur J Gastroenterol Hepatol. 2003 Sep;15(9):1001-4.

Lomoschitz F, et al Enteroclysis in adult celiac disease: diagnostic value of specific radiographic features. Eur Radiol. 2003 Apr;13(4):890-6.

Schweiger GD, Murray JA Postbulbar duodenal ulceration and stenosis associated with celiac disease.Abdom Imaging. 1998 Jul-Aug;23(4):347-9.

The Spleen

Robert M. Abbott, M.D.
University of Maryland Medical Center
Baltimore, MD

Introduction
- Embryology
- Anatomy
- Function
- Imaging Appearance
- Differential Diagnosis

Embryology
- Spleen is derived from a mass of mesenchymal cells between the layers of the dorsal mesogastrium during the 6th wk of gestation
- Mesenchymal cells form capsule and all parenchymal and supporting tissues
- Spleen achieves its characteristic shape and position by the 3rd month of fetal life
- Hematopoietic cells produce red and white cells until late in fetal life

Embryology
- Pancreas, spleen and celiac artery are b/w the layers of the dorsal mesogastrium
- Stomach rotates and the left side of the mesogastrium fuses with the peritoneum over the left kidney.
- Fusion explains the dorsal attachment of the lienorenal (splenorenal) ligament and why adult splenic artery passes to the left behind the peritoneum to enter ligament.

Anatomy
- Spleen is a soft, reddish purple highly vascular organ
- Usually a completely intraperitoneal
- Underlies the posterior 9-11 ribs
- Oblique orientation with long axis along course of posterior 10th rib

Anatomy
- Separated from 9-11 ribs, left lung and pleura by diaphragm
- Lateral to the greater curvature of the stomach
- Contacts posterior aspect of tail on pancreas
- Related to upper anterior surface of left kidney
- Superior to splenic flexure

Ligaments
- Splenorenal – reflection of peritoneum running from the diaphragm and anterior aspect of left kidney to hilum of spleen
  - ➢ Pancreatic tail enters the splenorenal ligament as it exits the retroperitoneum
  - ➢ Contains splenic vessels
- Gastrosplenic - dorsal mesentery b/w spleen and stomach
  - ➢ Contains short gastric and left gastroepiploic vessels
- Phrenicocolic – beneath the caudal end of spleen

Bare Area
- Occurs when fusion of the dorsal mesogastrium with the parietal peritoneum of the posterior abdominal wall proceeds too far
- Splenorenal ligament is oliterated - creating a "bare area"
- Result: surface of the spleen is not intraperitoneal in location
- Spleen in direct contact with the kidney

Anatomy
- 2 poles- anterior and posterior
- 3 major surfaces that are molded by the surrounding organs
- Diaphragmatic surface - convex
- Gastric surface - concave
- Renal surface – concave
- Splenic flexure - may leave an impression on the inferior pole

Anatomy
- Hilum
  - Major vessels enter and exit
  - Most often on the gastric surface
- Capsule – 1mm thick
  Covers entire spleen except at hilum
- Splenic artery
  - Branch of celiac artery
  - Tortuous
- Splenic vein
  - Runs in groove on back of pancreas below artery
  - Joins SMV to form portal vein

Histology
- Spleen is comprised of a dense connective tissue stroma and functional parenchymal cells
- The functional parenchyma is comprised of red and white pulp

Histology
- The splenic sinuses are composed of long anastomosing dilated capillary like channels
- These channels join together by longitudinal slit like spaces - all types of blood cells can pass through these spaces into the splenic cords
- Splenic sinuses coalesce to form pulp veins which drain into trabecular and then splenic veins
- The splenic cords occupy all of the red pulp b/w the pulp arteries, sinuses and veins

White Pulp
- The white pulp is composed of round or ellipitcal areas of dense aggregated lymphocytes, plasma cells, macrophages and other free cells.
- Cells are arranged as periarterial lymphatic sheaths or nodules which are known as Malpighian or splenic corpuscles.
- Gross color of the white pulp results from the closely packed lymphocytes

Red Pulp
- Surrounds white pulp
- Comprised of terminal branches of the central arteries, splenic sinuses and cords which are filled with systemic blood
- High content of RBCs produces the gross color of the red pulp

Open vs. Closed Circulation (Blood traveling through the red pulp)
- Open
  - Portion of blood is transferred from the splenic sinuses and perfuses slowly through the splenic cords before entering the venous sinuses
- Closed
  - Blood bypasses splenic cords and travels from the splenic sinuses directly into the endothelial lined venous sinuses

Function
- Largest component of the reticuloendothelial system
- Important in the initiation of humoral and cellular immune response
- Responds to blood borne antigens, removes aged RBCs, abnormal cells and foreign particles
- Stores RBCs and sequesters 30% of all platelets
- Lymphocyte and monocyte production after birth

Location and Size
- Typically in left upper quadrant
- Considerable variation in size and shape
- Average size 12 L x 7 W x 4 AP cm
- Normal < 13 cm
- Weight approx 150g (nl range of 100-250g)
- Receives 4% of cardiac output with 350L of blood perfusing each day - transit time is 25 secs

Symptoms of an Abnormal Spleen
- LUQ Pain
- Splenomegaly
- Mass
- Fever
- Anemia
- Thrombocytopenia

Imaging Modalities
- Plain films
- Radionuclide scan
- Ultrasound
- CT
- MR
- Angiography

Evaluation of the Spleen
- Present or Absent
- Size
- Location (ectopic?)
- Margins
- Homogeneity
- Mass lesions
- Accessory Spleen

Ultrasound Appearance
- Homogeneous pattern of echoes
- Scattered echogenic foci representing blood vessels
- Overall echogenicity slightly greater than liver
- Need to evaluate size, shape, relationship to other organs and position of hilum

CT Technique
- Helical scanning
- Single breath hold
  - Eliminates artifacts, respiratory motion and misregistration
- Arterial and redistribution phase imaging
- Noncontrast for Ca++ and for evaluating change in enhancement
  - Spleen homogeneous and slightly less dense than liver (40-60HU)

CT Technique: CECT
- To evaluate lesions and differentiate from pancreatic adrenal abnormalities
- Contrast: Oral and intravenous contrast
- Injection rate: 3-5 ml/sec for 125 ml (Optiray 320)
- Scan Delay: "Smart Prep" - ROI over liver (40 HU above baseline)
- Slice thickness 5mm pitch 1:1

CT Appearance: Pitfalls
- Initial heterogeneous enhancement becomes homogeneous with time (enhanced parenchyma should be 5-10 HU less dense than liver)
- Arterial phase appearance should not be mistaken for disease
- More rapid the injection the more pronounced the pattern

Heterogeneous Enhancement
- Serpentine, cord like, mottled or striped aka "zebra spleen".
- By 2 min post injection homogeneous enhancement
- DDx
  - Decreased cardiac output
  - SV thrombosis
  - Portal HTN

MR Technique
- Single breath hold techniques
- IV Gd
- T1 and T2 relaxation times of spleen similar to kidney but longer than liver
- PD of spleen similar to liver

MR Technique
- T1 (SE or SPGR)
- T2 (SE, FSE or STIR)
- Gd use is routine usually SPGR with FS 30 sec after bolus
- MR appearance similar to CT

Variants
- Accessory Spleen
- Splenic Clefts
- Lobulation
- Splenorenal fusion
- Splenosis
- Wandering spleen

Accessory Spleen
- Mesenchymal cells that form the spleen fail to coalesce completely
- Seen in 10-30% of autopsies
- Usually no significance except when confused with a mass

Accessory Spleen
- Can in increase in size over time in patient s/p splenectomy
- Can extend into the adrenal fossa and mimic an adrenal nodule
- Spect or MPR may be useful

Accessory Spleen
- Splenic hilum 75%
- Embebbed in pancreatic tail 20%
- Gastrohepatic ligament
- Along splenic artery in retroperitoneum

Accessory Spleen
- Should demonstrate a synchronous pattern of enhancement with the spleen during all phases of scanning
- May resemble a mass or adenopathy

Variations in Splenic Contour
- Mesenchymal masses may only partially fuse which can create lobuations, notches and clefts - may be supplied by a separate splenic artery
- Lobulation more sublte variation of a cleft
- Cleft 2-3 cm deep and well defined - Do not confuse with a laceration
- Splenic tongue remnant of nl tissue in the splenic hilum - ddx from pancreatic tail or with mass effect on stomach

Splenosis
- Autotransplantation of splenic tissue after trauma or rarely splenectomy
- Location
  - Mesentery, peritoneum, omentum
  - Pleura
  - Diaphragm

Splenosis: Features and DDX
- Small enhancing implants
- RBC or Tc sulfur colloid scan
- Accumulation in most dependent locations: Morrison's pouch, perihepatic space and paracolic gutter
- DDX
  - Accessory spleen
  - Endometriosis
  - Hemangioma
  - Peritoneal mesothelioma

Figure 2-29-1

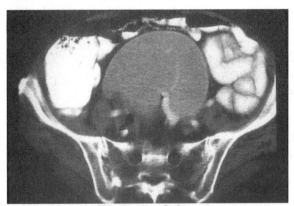
Wandering Spleen

Variations in Position
- Position related to the length of splenorenal ligament (usually several cm)
- SR ligament is formed by the fusion of the dorsal mesogastrium and the parietal peritoneum of the posterior parietal wall
- If incomplete fusion occurs the SR ligament can be elongated and create wandering spleen - position can vary over time

Wandering Spleen [Figure 2-29-1]
- May be symptomatic as a result of torsion
- Can be intermittant or result in infarction
- May remain asymptomatic

Figure 2-29-2

Splenic Torsion [Figure 2-29-2]

Asplenia vs. Polysplenia

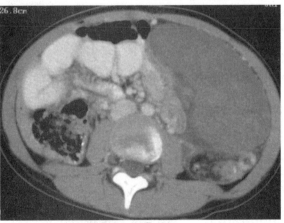
Splenic Torsion

	Asplenia	Polysplenia
Cardiac Anomalies	Yes	Yes
Lungs	Trilobed	Bilateral Bilobed
Pulmonary Vascularity	Decreased	Increased
Stomach	Midline	Malpositioned
Gallbladder	Midline	Absent

Polysplenia [Figure 2-29-3]
- Bilateral left sidedness
- Presentation: infancy or adulthood; M<F
- A/W cardiac, GI, and GU anomalies
- Bilateral morphologic left lungs (2/3rds)
- Bilateral SVC (50%)
- IVC interruption of hepatic segment with azygous/hemiazygous continuation
- Large azygous vein may mimic aortic arch
- Normal to increased PBF
- Polysplenia
- Hepatic symmetry
- Absent GB
- Malrotation of bowel
- Stomach right/left
- Poor prognosis – 90% mortality by midadolescence

Figure 2-29-3

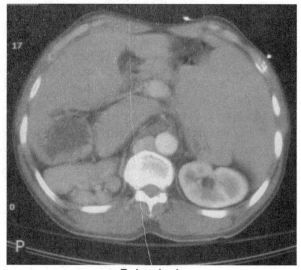
Polysplenia

Asplenia (Ivemark Syndrome)
- Bilateral right sidedness
- 1:1,750 to 1:40,000 births; M.F
- A/W CHD (50%) – TAPVR most common
- GI/GU anomalies
- Situs anomalies
- Absent spleen (see Howell -Jolly bodies = RBC inclusions)
- Bilateral trilobed lungs = bilateral minor fissures
- Decreased PBF
- Bilateral SVC
- Hepatic symmetry
- Stomach: R/L/midline
- Abdominal aorta and IVC same side
- 80% mortality 1st year

Splenomegaly
- Length >13 cm
- Splenic Index: L x W x AP > 480 cm3
- Spleen tip extending below the right lobe of the liver
- AP diameter > 2/3 of AP diameter of the abdomen

Splenomegaly: Huge
- CML
- Myelofibrosis
- Malaria
- Visceral leishmaniasis (aka Kala-azar = Hindi term – "black fever" or dumdum fever)
- Gaucher's disease
- Lymphoma

Splenomegaly: Moderately Large
- As above
- Storage diseases
- Hemolytic anemia
- Portal hypertension
- Leukemia

Splenomegaly: Mildly Large
- As above
- Infection
  - ➢ Hepatitis, mononucleosis, brucellosis, typhoid and TB
- Infiltrative
  - ➢ Sarcoid and amyloid
- Collegen Vascular
  - ➢ RA, SLE and polycythemia vera

Lymphoma

- Hodgkin's or NHL
- Spleen involved in 70%
- Splenomegaly due to diffuse infiltration
- Miliary nodules but may be larger (2-10 cm in up to 25%)
- Adenopathy in hilum (NHL), uncommon in Hodgkin's

Lymphoma: CT Appearance

- Homogeneous enlargement
- Solitary Mass
- Multifocal
- Diffuse infiltration

Lymphoma: Solitary mass [Figure 2-29-4]

Lymphoma: Diffuse Infiltration [Figure 2-29-5]

Gaucher's Disease

- Radiographic Findings
  - ➢ Liver
    - ❖ Hepatomegaly
  - ➢ Spleen
    - ❖ Splenomegaly (marked)
    - ❖ Focal lesions (usually infarcts)
  - ➢ MSK
    - ❖ Erlenmeyer flask deformity of distal femur
    - ❖ Generalized osteopenia
    - ❖ Multiple lytic bone lesions
    - ❖ AVN of femoral head

Small Spleen

- Hereditary Hypoplasia
- Irradiation
- Infarction
- Polysplenia
- Atropy

Calcifications

- Disseminated
  - ➢ Phleboliths
  - ➢ Granulomas (histoplasmosis, TB brucellosis)
- Capsular and parenchymal
  - ➢ Pyogenic/TB abscess
  - ➢ Infarction
  - ➢ Hematoma
- Vascular
  - ➢ Splenic artery calcification
  - ➢ Splenic artery aneurysm
  - ➢ Splenic infarcts
- Calcified cyst wall
  - ➢ Congenital cyst
  - ➢ Posttraumatic cyst
  - ➢ Echinococcal cyst
  - ➢ Cystic dermoid
  - ➢ Epidermoid
  - ➢ Pseudocyst

Figure 2-29-4

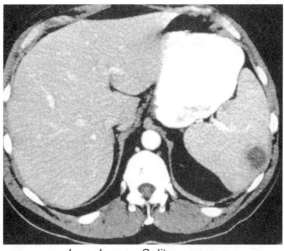

Lymphoma - Solitary mass

Figure 2-29-5

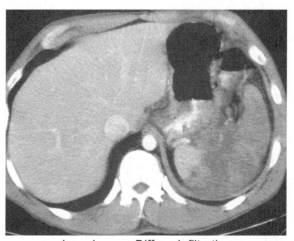

Lymphoma - Diffuse Infiltration

Splenic Masses
- Solitary vs multiple
  - Cystic
    - Cysts
    - Infection
    - Metastases
    - Tumor
  - Solid
    - Congenital
    - Infarct
    - Primary Tumors
    - Metastases

Cystic Lesions
- Solitary
  - Congenital cyst
  - bscess
  - Parasitic cyst
  - Pseudocyst
  - Cavernous hemangioma
  - Lymphangioma
  - Metastasis
- Muliple
  - Cysts - rare
  - Lymphangioma
  - Hemangioma
  - Metastases
  - Infection

Figure 2-29-6

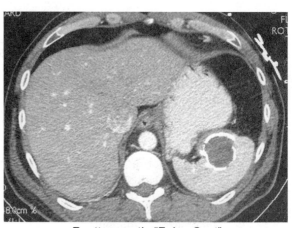

Posttraumatic "False Cyst"

Posttraumatic Cyst
- Most common cyst – 80% of all splenic cysts
- No epithelial lining
- Calcification in up to 25%
- Thought to reflect end stage of intrasplenic hematoma

Posttraumatic "False Cyst" *[Figure 2-29-6]*

Echinococcus *[Figure 2-29-7]*
- Caused by Echinococcus granulosus
- Usually liver or lung but can involve spleen
- Endemic areas include Argentina, Greece and Spain
- Uni or multilocular
- Hydatid sand, daughter cysts and Ca++

Figure 2-29-7

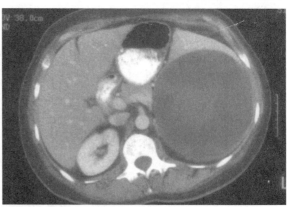

Echinococcus

Solid Splenic Lesions
- Solitary
  - Congenital bulge
  - Infarct
  - Primary tumors
  - Metastasis
- Multiple
  - Granulomas
  - Infection
  - Lymphoma
  - Primary tumors
  - Sarcoid
  - Metastases

Solitary Solid Lesion: Primary Tumors

- Benign
  - Hemangioma
  - Lymphangioma
  - Hamartoma
  - Lipoma
  - Pseudotumor

Cavernous Hemangioma [Figure 2-29-8]

- Most common benign tumor
- Usually asymptomatic
- Cystic or solid
  - Vascular channels lined with a single layer of endothelium and filled with RBCs
- Varaible appearance
  - Ca++ peripheral or central
  - Delayed enhancement

Solitary Solid Lesion: Lymphangioma

- Resemble hemangiomas but filled with lymph
- Single or multiple
- 3 types of vascular channels
  - Capillary
  - Cavernous
  - Cystic

Lymphangioma: Imaging [Figure 2-29-9]

- US - well defined, hypoechoic with sepatations and debris
- CT- Sharp margins, thin walled, low attenuation – no enhancment
- Similar to cyst - low T1 and high T2 signal

Solitary Solid Lesion: Hamartoma

[Figure 2-29-10]
- Rare
- Mixture of normal splenic elements – more red pulp
- Usually asymptomatic
- Imaging
  - US - hyperechoic
  - CT - Isodense NCCT
  - CECT or MR – immediate and intense diffuse enhancement
  - Note: difference from hemangioma with delayed fill in

Solitary Solid Lesion: Pseudotumor

- Rare – Unknown etiology
- Composed of localized area of inflammatory change
- Fibroblastic and granulomatous changes
- Looks malignant but benign

Pseudotumor: Imaging

- US – hypoechoic
- CT
  - Discrete hypodense mass
  - Ca++
  - Delayed contrast enhancment
  - Central Stellate area
- MR
  - T1 hypo, T2 hetero
  - Low SI central Ca++ does not enhance

Figure 2-29-8

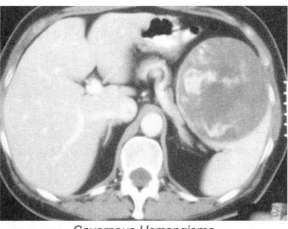

Cavernous Hemangioma

Figure 2-29-9

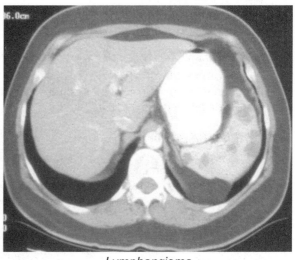

Lymphangioma

Figure 2-29-10

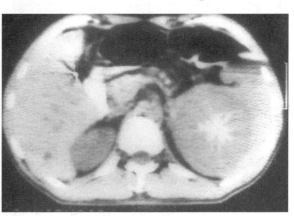

Hamartoma

Primary Tumors
- ? Benign
  - Hemangiopericytoma
  - Epithelioid Vascular Tumor
  - Littoral Cell Angioma
- Malignant
  - Angiosarcoma
  - Lymphoma

Hemangiopericytoma
- Found frequently in the muscles of the lower extremities and SC tissues
- Variable biologic behavior
- High rate of local recurrence and malignant potential
- Biologically aggressive esp abdominal locations
- Several forms ranging from true benign form to malignant form
- Reported CT findings - large mass with polylobular contours with smaller lesions throughout spleen
- Speckled Ca++ maybe present
- Often bleed due to hypervascular nature and expansile growth
- With contrast see discete hyperdensity of solid portions and septations

Epithelial Hemangioendothelioma
- Vascular neoplasm of intermediate malignancy
- Imaging nonspecific
- CT - changes suggestive of malignancy
  - Necrosis
  - Bleeding
  - Ill defined borders
  - Infiltrative growth
- Features may not be present making dx difficult
- Almost never displays a capsule

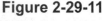

Figure 2-29-11

Littoral Cell Angioma [Figure 2-29-11]
- Very Rare
- Arise from cells lining splenic sinus
- US - isoechoic with anechoic blood filled spaces
- CT - splenomegaly with multiple low attenuation nodular masses
- MR - hypointense T1 and T2 due to the presence of hemosiderin in the neoplastic cells
- Don't confuse with Gamma -Gandy Bodies

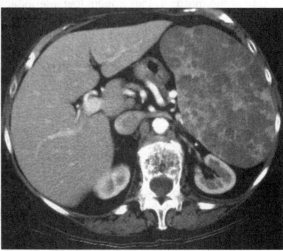

Littoral Cell Angioma

Gamma-Gandy Bodies
- Foci of iron deposition
- Seen in patients with cirrhosis and portal HTN
- Due to microhemorrhage in the splenic parenchyma

Gamma-Gandy Bodies
- Lesion usually < 1cm
- Signal void on all pulse sequences
- Susceptibility artifact on GE images seen as blooming artifact

Splenic Angiosarcoma
- Exceedingly rare
- Most common nonlymphoid primary malignant tumor of the spleen
- More common in patients with thorotrast exposure
- Splenomegaly with well defined nodules or diffuse involvement

Angiosarcoma [Figure 2-29-12]

- Frequent spontaneous rupture (30%)
- CT/MR - very vascular and enhance intensely
- May see evidence of hemorrage precontrast and findings of hemosiderin on MR
- Very poor prognosis

Solid Splenic Lesions

- Multiple
  - ➢ Granulomas
  - ➢ Infection
  - ➢ Lymphoma
  - ➢ Primary tumors
  - ➢ Sarcoid
  - ➢ Metastases

Multiple Solid Lesions: Infection

- Majority of cases a/w generalized sepsis
- Maybe only site in immunocompromised
- Appearance
  - ➢ Single wedge lesion
  - ➢ Larger multiple lesions
  - ➢ Subphrenic
  - ➢ Miliary appearance (e.g. Candida)

PCP [Figure 2-29-13]

Lymphangiomatosis

- Dilated endothelial lined channels
- Supported by fibrous tissue
- Filled with proteinaceous material

Multiple Solid Lesions: Peliosis

- Rare - unknown etiology
- Usually found incidentally and pts asymptomatic
- Maybe a/w malignant hematologic disease, metastatic cancer, TB, steroids, thorotrast and viral infection
- Characterized by widespread blood filled cystic spaces
- +/- endothelial lining or thrombosis

Peliosis: Imaging

- US
  - ➢ Hypo or hyperechoic lesions
  - ➢ May occupy entire spleen
- CT
  - ➢ Low attenuation foci
  - ➢ Post contrast pattern similar to hemangiomas

Sarcoid [Figure 2-29-14]

- Splenic involvement
- ➢ Isolated
- ➢ With liver involvment (20-30%)
- ➢ Both can occur w/o chest disease
- ➢ Does not correlate with CXR stage
- ➢ 60% symtomatic
- ➢ 90% elevated ACE

Figure 2-29-12

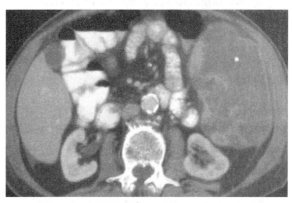

Angiosarcoma

Figure 2-29-13

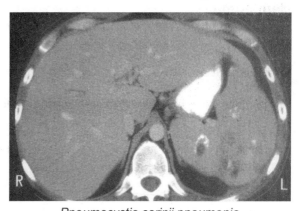

Pneumocystis carinii pneumonia

Figure 2-29-14

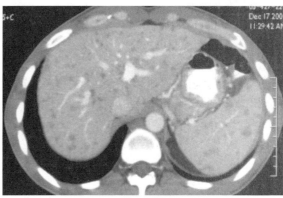

Sarcoid

Splenic Trauma
- Spleen prone to injury and very vascular
- CT procedure of choice
- US used to detect peritoneal fluid
- Plain films can see rib fxs
- Blunt or penetrating trauma
- Splenectomy not done in stable patients

Figure 2-29-15

Splenic Trauma
- Hematoma
  - Sucapsular
  - Intrasplenic
  - Perisplenic
- Look for sharp margin b/w spleen and peritoneal fluid
- Fluid will accumulate in dependent areas

Laceration [Figure 2-29-15]

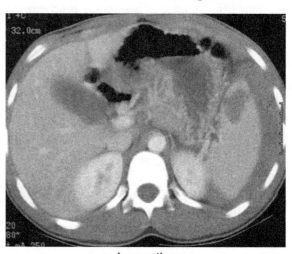

Laceration

Hematoma
- Fresh blood has same density as adjacent organ
- Unclotted blood - decreased density
- Clotted blood - increased density
- Clot retraction - increased density
- Clot lysis – fluid density
- Sentinel clot – high density, nonenhancing = site of injury
- Delayed complications
  - Rebleed, infection and rupture
- Rebleed – 2 wks in 75% and 4 wks in 90% of those who bleed

Intervention
- Percutaneous aspiration
- Drainage
- Biopsy
- Embolization
- Splenectomy

Post Splenectomy
- Patients more susceptible to infection
- Higher risk <2 yrs or severe hematological disorders
- Immune changes more significant in infants than adults

Summary
- Embryology
- Anatomy
- Function
- Imaging Appearance
- Differential Diagnosis

Summary
- Variants
- Splenomegaly
- Small spleen
- Calcifications

Summary: Splenic Masses

- Solid vs multiple
  - Cystic
    - Cysts
    - Infection
    - Metastases
    - Tumor
  - Solid
    - Congenital
    - Infarct
    - Primary Tumors
    - Metastases

Summary: Cystic Lesions

- Solitary
  - Congenital cyst
  - Posttraumatic cyst
  - Abscess
  - Parasitic cyst
  - Pseudocyst
  - Cavernous Hemangioma
  - Lymphangioma
  - Metastasis
- Muliple
  - Cysts - rare
  - Lymphangioma
  - Hemangioma
  - Metastases
  - Infection

Summary: Solid Splenic Lesions

- Solitary
  - Congenital Bulge
  - Infarct
  - Primary Tumors
  - Metastasis
- Multiple
  - Granulomas
  - Infection
  - Lymphoma
  - Primary tumors
  - Sarcoid
  - Metastases

Summary: Primary Tumors

- Benign
  - Hemangioma
  - Lymphangioma
  - Hamartoma
  - Lipoma
  - Pseudotumor

Summary: Primary Tumors

- ? Benign
  - Hemangiopericytoma
  - Epithelioid Vascular Tumor
  - Littoral Cell Angioma
- Malignant
  - Angiosarcoma
  - Lymphoma

Summary

- Trauma
  - ➢ US/CT
  - ➢ Hematoma
- Intervention
- Post splenectomy

Spleen References

Dobritz M, Nomayr A, Bautz W, Fellner FA. Gamna-Gandy bodies of the spleen detected with MR imaging: a case report. Magn Reson Imaging 2001; 19:1249-1251.

Faer M, Lynch R, Lichtenstein J, Madewell J, Feigin D. Traumatic splenic cyst: radiologic-pathologic correlation from the Armed Forces Institute of Pathology. Radiology 1980; 134:371-376.

Ferrozzi F, Bova D, Draghi F, Garlaschi G. CT findings in primary vascular tumors of the spleen. AJR Am J Roentgenol 1996; 166:1097-1101.

Freeman J, Jafri S, Roberts J, Mezwa D, Shirkhoda A. CT of congenital and acquired abnormalities of the spleen. Radiographics 1993; 13:597-610.

Fulcher AS, Turner MA. Abdominal Manifestations of Situs Anomalies in Adults. Radiographics 2002; 22:1439-.

Levy AD, Abbott RM, Abbondanzo SL. Littoral cell angioma of the spleen: CT features with clinicopathologic comparison. Radiology 2004; 230:485-490.

Maves CK, Caron KH, Bisset GS, 3rd, Agarwal R. Splenic and hepatic peliosis: MR findings. AJR Am J Roentgenol 1992; 158:75-76.

Ramani M, Reinhold C, Semelka R, et al. Splenic hemangiomas and hamartomas: MR imaging characteristics of 28 lesions. Radiology 1997; 202:166-172.

Ros P, Moser R, Jr, Dachman A, Murari P, Olmsted W. Hemangioma of the spleen: radiologic-pathologic correlation in ten cases. Radiology 1987; 162:73-77.

Shimono T, Yamaoka T, Nishimura K, et al. Peliosis of the spleen: splenic rupture with intraperitoneal hemorrhage. Abdom Imaging 1998; 23:201-202.

Tang S, Shimizu T, Kikuchi Y, et al. Color Doppler sonographic findings in splenic hamartoma. J Clin Ultrasound 2000; 28:249-253.

Torres GM, Terry NL, Mergo PJ, Ros PR. MR imaging of the spleen. Magn Reson Imaging Clin N Am 1995; 3:39-50.

Urrutia M, Mergo PJ, Ros LH, Torres GM, Ros PR. Cystic masses of the spleen: radiologic-pathologic correlation. Radiographics 1996; 16:107-129.

Warnke R, Weiss, LM., Chan, JK., Clearly, ML., Dorfman, RF. Tumors of the Lymph Nodes and Spleen. Washington, DC: Armed Forces Institute of Pathology, 1995.

Inflammatory Bowel Disease

Robert M. Abbott, M.D.
University of Maryland Medical Center
Baltimore, MD

Inflammatory Bowel Disease Classification
- Idiopathic
- Ischemic
- Infectious
- Drug Induced
- Graft vs. Host
- Diverticular

Inflammatory Bowel Disease: Introduction
- Idiopathic
  - Ulcerative colitis
  - Crohn's disease
- Specific
  - Behcet's
  - Pseudomembranous colitis
  - Typhlitis
  - Graft vs. host disease
  - Diverticulitis

Inflammatory Bowel Disease: Introduction
- Pathogenesis
  - Genetic
  - Immunologic
  - Infectious
  - Environmental, dietary
  - Intrinsic GI tract: enteric plexus, hormones, mucin
  - Psychological

Inflammatory Bowel Disease: Introduction
- Genetic
  - 30-100x risk in first degree relatives
  - 15% of patients have first degree relative with IBD
  - Higher rates in monozygotic twins

Inflammatory Bowel Disease: Role of Imaging Studies
- Determine initial site
- Evaluate extent of disease
- Therapeutic response
- Detection of complications
- Differential diagnosis

Ulcerative Colitis: Epidemiology
- Incidence:2-10 per 100,000
- Geography:Developed countries: Northern Europe, United States, Israel
- Ethnic/Racial: White, Jewish (2-5x risk)
- Age:15-25; smaller peak @ 50-70
- Sex:Slight female preponderance

Ulcerative Colitis
- Unknown origin
- Colorectal mucosa
- Other layers of the bowel wall
- Begins in the rectum and extends proximally

Layers of the Bowel Wall
- Mucosa
- Muscularis Mucosa (MM)
- Submucosa (SM)
- Muscularis propria (MP)
- Serosa

Ulcerative Colitis: Plain Film Features [Figure 2-30-1]
- Widening of the haustral markings
  - \> 5-6 mm - early bowel wall edema
  - More obvious than mucosal granularity or ulceration
  - Only assess if colon adequately distended
  - Distal half of colon often decreased haustration in the elderly

Ulcerative Colitis: Plain Film Features
- Caliber of the air filled colon
  - Normal diameter of the transverse colon < 5.5 cm
  - Chronic "burned out" UC colon narrow and tubular
  - Diameter of > 6-7 cm suggests toxic megacolon

Ulcerative Colitis: Plain Film Features
- Mural Thickness
  - Normally 3-5 mm
  - =/> 10 mm chronic UC or granulomatous colitis

Toxic Megacolon
- Up to 5% of patients with UC
- Mortality 20%
- Pathology
  - Transmural inflammation
    - ❖ Muscularis propria
    - ❖ Serosa
  - May lead to peritonitis w/o perforation

Toxic Megacolon
- Pathology
  - Vasculitis of small arterioles
  - Inflammation and destruction of the myenteric and submucosal plexus
  - Myocytolosis in the muscularis propria

Toxic Megacolon [Figure 2-30-2]
- Colonic dilatation
- Mean diameters between 8.2-9.2 cm
- Lumen diameter > 5cm indicates ulceration to the muscle layer
- Early - may be limited to a short segment
- Transverse colon least dependent on supine film

Toxic Megacolon
- Residual mucosal islands
  - Severe mucosal disruption
- Subserosal or omental edema
  - Accounts for thickened colonic wall
- Normal haustral pattern
  - Always lost
  - Profound inflammation and ulceration

Ulcerative Colitis: Barium Enema Indications
- Confirm the clinical diagnosis
- Assess the extent and severity of disease
- Differentiate UC from Crohn disease and other colitides
- Follow course of disease
- Detect complication

Figure 2-30-1

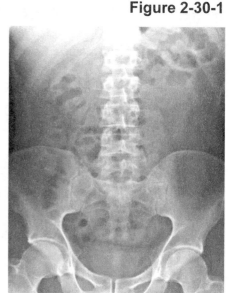

KUB demonstrating widening of haustra due to bowel wall edema

Figure 2-30-2

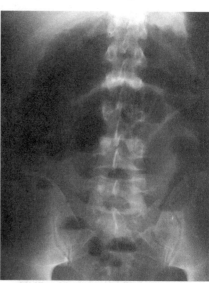

KUB with colonic dilatation in a patient with toxic megacolon. The transverse colon is the least dependent portion of the colon a supine film.

Ulcerative Colitis: Granular Pattern
- Progressive edema and hyperemia of the mucosa
- Smooth colonic margin is replaced by a thickened indistinct mucosal line
- Chronic UC - mucosal pattern is coarser with colonic contour changes

Ulcerative Colitis: Granular Pattern
- Acute disease
  - ➢ Abnormality of the mucus produced by the involved mucosa
  - ➢ Histology - reduction in the number of goblet cells
- Chronic, burned-out disease
  - ➢ Granulation tissue that re-epithelializes the mucosa

Ulcerative Colitis: Mucosal Stippling
- Acute granular phase
  - ➢ Inflammatory cells
  - ➢ Cellular debris
  - ➢ Crypt abscesses
  - ➢ Microabscesses erode into the lumen
  - ➢ Barium flecks adhere producing stippling

Figure 2-30-3

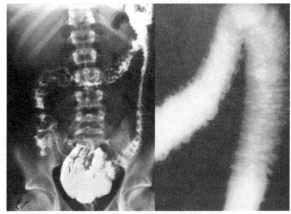

Ulcerative Colitis: Collar-Button Ulcers
[Figure 2-30-3]
- Ulcers breach the lamina propria, muscularis mucosae and submucosa
- Submucosal ulcers extend laterally
- Ulcers are contained by the muscularis propria and muscularis mucosae
- Mucosal defect small in relation to undermining

Collar-button ulcers in ulcerative colitis

Ulcerative Colitis: Collar-Button Ulcers
- Frequently related to taeniae
- Ulcers enlarge and interconnect
  - ➢ Collar-button configuration is lost
  - ➢ Residual islands of mucosa and inflammatory pseudopolyps results

Ulcerative Colitis: Inflammatory Pseudopolyps
- Severe UC - extensive mucosal and submucosal ulceration
- Small islands of mucosa and submucosa survive
- Inflamed edematous mucosa produces pseudopolyp

Ulcerative Colitis: Inflammatory Pseudopolyps
- Progression of collar-button ulcers
- Typically UC but can occur in Crohn disease
  - ➢ Cobblestoning in Crohn disease is a type of pseudopolyp
  - ➢ Preserved mucosa are surrounded by linear and transverse ulcerations

Figure 2-30-4

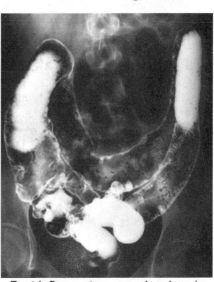

Ulcerative Colitis: Postinflammatory Pseudopolyps
[Figure 2-30-4]
- During mucosal healing
- Regenerated mucosa
- Polypoid lesions
  - ➢ Small and round
  - ➢ Long and filiform
  - ➢ Bushlike simulating a villous adenoma
- Not a neoplasm
- Follows severe attack of colitis

Post Inflammatory pseudopolyps in ulcerative colitis

Ulcerative Colitis: Postinflammatory Pseudopolyps
- Mucosal bridges
  - Islands of mucosa surrounded by ulceration
  - Ulcer re-epithelialize
- PI polyps can also be seen in
  - Crohn colitis
  - Ischemic colitis
  - Infectious colitis

Ulcerative Colitis: Backwash Ileitis
- 10-40% of patients with chronic ulcerative pancolitis
- Distal 5-25cm of ileum is inflamed
- Occurs only in pancolitis
- Resolves 1-2 weeks after colectomy

Ulcerative Colitis: Backwash Ileitis [Figure 2-30-5]
- ? reflux of colonic contents into the small bowel
- Patulous and fixed ileocecal valve
- Persistent dilatation of the TI
- NL fold pattern is absent
- Mucosa granular

Ulcerative Colitis: Blunting or Loss of Haustral Clefts
- Loss of haustra in the proximal colon is always abnormal
- Acute disease
  - Taenaie become relaxed
- Chronic disease
  - Fixed contraction and massive hypertrophy
  - Contraction causes shortening of the colon

Ulcerative Colitis: CT Features [Figure 2-30-6]
- Early mucosal changes are not seen on CT
- Large pseudopolyps may be seen
- Perforation
- Pneumotosis in toxic megacolon
- Mural thickening

Ulcerative Colitis: CT Features - Mucosal Thickening
- Subacute and chronic UC
- Due to hypertrophy of muscularis mucosa
- Lamina propria thickening
- Submucosa thickened due to deposition of fat or edema

CT Features: Mural Stratification [Figure 2-30-7]
- Axial CT - target or halo appearance
- Lumen is surrounded by a ring of soft tissue attenuation
  - Mucosa, lamina propria, and hypertrophied muscularis mucosa
- Middle low attenuation ring
  - Edema or fatty infiltration of submucosa
- Outer ring of soft tissue attenuation
  - Muscularis mucosa

Figure 2-30-5

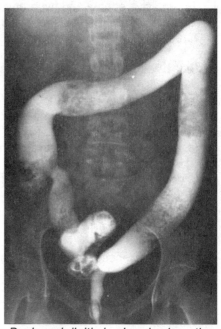

Backwash ileitis in chronic ulcerative pancolitis. Patulous and fixed ileocecal valve.

Figure 2-30-6

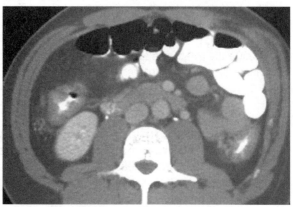

Mural thickening in ulcerative colitis

Figure 2-30-7

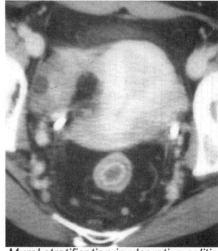

Mural stratification in ulcerative colitis

CT Features: Mural Stratification
- Not specific
- Crohn's disease
- Infectious entercolitis
- Pseudomembranous colitis
- Ischemic and radiation entercolitis
- Mesenteric venous thrombosis
- Bowel edema
- Graft vs. host disease

Chronic Ulcerative Colitis: Rectal findings
- Subacute and chronic UC
- Due to hypertrophy of muscularis mucosa
- Lamina propria thickening
- Submucosa thickened due to deposition of fat or edema

Ulcerative Colitis: Extraintestinal Manifestations [Figure 2-30-8]
- Musculoskelatal
  - ➢ Sacroiliitis
  - ➢ Enteropathic arthropathy
  - ➢ Peripheral arthritis

Ulcerative Colitis: Extraintestinal Manifestations
- Ocular
  - ➢ Uveitis
- Dermatologic
  - ➢ Erythema nodosum
  - ➢ Pyoderma gangrenosum

Inflammatory Bowel Disease: Hepatobiliary Manifestations
- Fatty infiltration   50%
- Chronic active hepatitis   1%
- Cirrhosis   1.5%
- Pericholangitis   50%
- Sclerosing cholangitis   1-4%
- Cholangiocarcinoma   1%
- Cholesterol gallstones (Crohn's)   40%

Inflammatory Bowel Disease: Genitourinary Manifestations
- Crohn's > U.C.
- Urolithiasis : 2-10%
- Amyloidosis
- Ureteral obstruction
- Fistulas

Ulcerative Colitis: Carcinoma [Figure 2-30-9]
- Risk related to extent, duration
- 10% per decade after 10 years
- Synchronous: 25%
- Difficult to detect:
  - ➢ Flat, plaque
  - ➢ Infiltrating, stricture

Crohn's Disease: Epidemiology
- Incidence:1-6 per 100,000
- Geography: Developed countries:
  - ➢ Northern Europe, United States, Israel
- Ethnic/Racial:White, Jewish(2-8x risk)
- Age:15-25, smaller peak @ 50-70
- Sex:Slight female preponderance

Figure 2-30-8

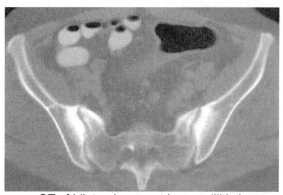

CT of bilateral symmetric sacroiliitis in inflammatory bowel disease

Figure 2-30-9

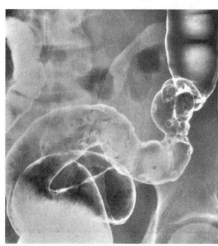

Colon Carcinoma in longstanding ulcerative colitis

Crohn's Disease
- Chronic granulomatous process
- Transmural inflammation
- Extends to serosa and mesenteric lymph nodes
- Any portion of GI tract
- TI and proximal colon most common

Crohn's Disease: Distribution
Colon only	20%
Small intestine only	20%
Colon and small intestine	60%
Rectum	50%
Perianal disease	40%
UGI tract	5-10%

Crohn's Disease: Plain Film Features
- Small bowel obstruction can occur
- Stenotic segments and dilated loops
- Confined to colon similar to UC
- Gas filled stricture in colon is not specific
- Toxic megacolon

Crohn's Disease: Barium Enema Features
- Small bowel mucosal granularity - earliest finding
  - ➢ Due to alteration in villous morphology
    - ❖ Edema
    - ❖ Hyperplasia
    - ❖ Clubbing
    - ❖ Fusion
    - ❖ Inflammatory cell infiltrate

Crohn's Disease: Lymphoid Hyperplasia
- Lymphoid follicles on BE
  - ➢ 50% of children and 13% of adult DCBE
  - ➢ Appear as 1-3mm elevations in the mucosa without a ring shadow
  - ➢ May enlarge in a variety of infectious, neoplastic, immunologic and inflammatory diseases of the gut including Crohn's disease

Figure 2-30-10

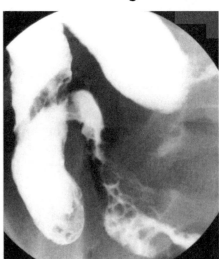

Crohn's Disease: Aphthous Lesions
- Lymphoid follicles enlarge and overlying mucosa ulcerate
- Small superficial ulcers with erythematous margins
- Punctate central collections of barium surrounded by a radiolucent halo - target or bull's-eye appearance

Crohn's Disease: Aphthous Lesions
- 44-72% Crohn's disease
- Nonspecific
  - ➢ Amebiasis
  - ➢ Salmonella
  - ➢ Shigellosis
  - ➢ Herpes
  - ➢ CMV
  - ➢ Behcet disease
  - ➢ Ischemic colitis
  - ➢ Yersinia entercolitis

Crohn disease with cobblestoning. Terminal ileum demonstrates nodular mucosa caused by islands of preserved epithelium surrounded by a network of ulcerations.

Crohn's Disease: Cobblestoning [Figure 2-30-10]
- Adjacent aphthous ulcers coalesce
- Longitudinal linear ulceration and transverse fissuring
- Edematous intervening mucosa
- Form of inflammatory pseudopolyposis

Crohn's Disease: Deep Ulceration [Figure 2-30-11]
- Fissuring ulcers
- Penetrate beyond submucosa
- Result in knife-shaped or "rose-thorn" fistula
- Do not result in pneumoperitoneum due to inflamed adherent loops

Crohn's Disease: Complications
Perianal disease:	40%
Fistula:	20-40%
Stricture, obstruction:	20%
Abscess:	15-20%
Toxic colon:	3%
Carcinoma:	<1%

Crohn's Disease: Pericolic Sinus Tracts
- Long interconnecting fistula
- Occur in muscularis mucosa or subserosa
- Parallel the bowel lumen
- Highly suggestive of Crohn's disease

Crohn's Disease: Fistula and Sinus Tracts [Figure 2-30-12]
- 20-40% of patients
- Enteroenteric
- Enterocolic
- Colocolic
- Enterovesical
- Enterovaginal
- Enterocutaneous
- Anorectal
- Duodenopancreatic
- Gastrocolic
- Colobronchial
- Enterospinal

Crohn's Disease: String Sign [Figure 2-30-13]
- TI becomes markedly narrowed
- Originally reported in acute prestenotic disease
- Now commonly used to describe fixed chronic narrowing
- Fibrosis and thickening of the bowel wall
- Cicatrizing phase of Crohn's

Figure 2-30-11

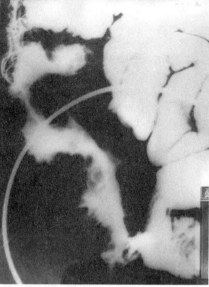

Rose-thorn fistulae in Crohn disease.
Represent deep fissuring ulcers.

Figure 2-30-12

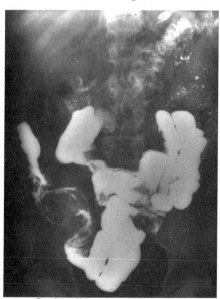

Crohn disease with multiple
enteroenteric fistulae.

Figure 2-30-13

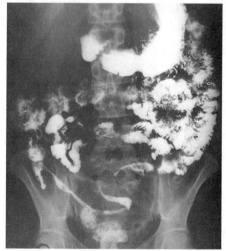

Crohn disease "string sign"

Crohn's Disease: Lumen Narrowing
- Transmural inflammation
- Bowel wall thickening and fibrosis
- Shortening of the gut

Crohn's Disease: Strictures
- Aysmmetric
- Less smooth and circumferential than UC
- 21% of patients with small bowel disease
- 8% with Crohn's colitis

Crohn's Disease: Sacculations [Figure 2-30-14]
- Transmural fibrosis is asymmetric
  - Mesenteric side of bowel
- Unaffected antimesenteric side tends to bulge
- Outpouchings may develop

Crohn's Disease: CT Features
- Bowel wall thickening 1-2 cm
- 83% of patients
- Most often TI
- Acute noncicatrizing phase
- Mural stratification maintained
- Target or double-halo appearance

Crohn's Disease: CT Features
- Inflamed mucosa and serosa may enhance
- Degree of enhancement correlates with disease activity
- Mural stratification
  - Present - no transmural fibrosis
  - Absent - transmural fibrosis
    - Long-standing disease
    - Homogeneous attenuation
    - Irreversible fibrosi

Crohn's Disease: Separation of Bowel Loops [Figure 2-30-15]
- Abscess
- Phlegmon
- Creeping fat or fibrofatty proliferation
- Bowel wall thickening
- Mesenteric lymphadenopathy

Crohn's Disease: Mesenteric Fibrofatty Proliferation
- AKA creeping fat
- CT- sharp interface b/w bowel and mesentery lost
- Small mesenteric lymph nodes may be present
- Lymph nodes > 1cm
  - Exclude lymphoma and carcinoma
    - Occur with > frequency in Crohn patients

Crohn's Disease: Comb Sign
- Hypervascularity of the mesentery
  - Vascular dilatation
  - Tortuosity
  - Wide spacing of the vasa recta
- "Vascular jejunization of the ileum"
- Hypervascularity suggests active disease

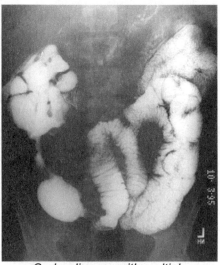

Figure 2-30-14

Crohn disease with multiple strictures, asymmetric fibrosis and sacculations on antimesenteric border.

Figure 2-30-15

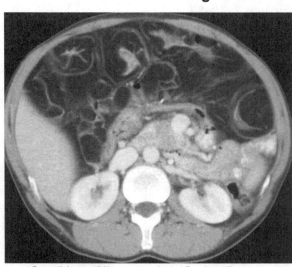

Small bowel lipomatosis in Crohn disease.

Crohn's Disease: Abscess
- 15-20% of patients
- Most frequent with small bowel disease or ileocolitis
- Etiology
  - Sinus tracts
  - Fistulas
  - Perforations
  - Post-surgical

Crohn's Disease: Phlegmon
- Ill-defined inflammatory mass in mesentery or omentum
- Common cause of mesenteric mass effect in patients with Crohn disease
- CT- "smudgy" or "streaky" appearance of mesenteric or omental fat

Ulcerative Colitis: Summary
- Contiguous disease
- Confluent
- Circumferential
- Symmetric
- Begins in rectum and extends proximally
- Granular mucosa
- Colectomy curative

Crohn's Disease: Summary
- Patchy
- Discontinuous
- Asymmetric
- Pseudodiverticula
- Anal and perianal disease
- Fistula and sinus tracts
- Ulcers
  - Aphthoid
  - Discrete, deep (greater than 3mm)
  - Fissuring
  - Rose thorn
- Recurrent Disease

UC vs. Crohn's Disease

Feature	UC	Crohn's
Skip Lesions	5% - during healing	Common - 80%
Terminal Ileum	BW ileitis 10-40%	>80%
Rectum	95%	25-50%
Lymphoid Follicles	Rare	Common
Granularity	Common	Less Common
Aphthous	Rare	70%
Inflamm PP	Common	Less Common
Linear Ulcers	Rare	Common
Cobblestone	Rare	Typical
Fistula and Sinus	Rare	Typical
Toxic Colon	10%	3%
Carcinoma	10%/decade after 10 yrs	Rare 3%

UC vs. Crohn's Disease

CT Finding	Chronic UC	Crohn's
Mural Stratification	60%	10%
Mean Wall Thickness	<10mm	>10mm
Outer Bowel Wall Contour	Smooth and regular 95%	Serosal Irregularity 80%

IBD: Radiologic-Pathologic Correlation

Radiology	Pathology
Granular Mucosa	Hyperemia, abn mucin, Inflamm cells, edema
Mucosal Stippling	Crypt abscess, edema
Aphthous Lesion	Erosion over lymph follicle Mucosal edema
Collar Button	Undermining of crypt Abscesses into submucosa
Intramural Tracts	Communicating crypt Abscesses or deep ulcers
Linear Ulcers	Long. and Trans. Ulceration Isolated NL mucosa
Cobble-stoning	Intersecting linaear and Trans. Ulcers around IPs
Fistula	Deep transmural ulcers Epithelial communication
Thumb printing	Fold thickening, submucosal Edema and inflammation
String Sign	Luminal narrowing-inflamm Edema and/or fibrosis/scar
Mural Stratification	Hypertrophy of MM Fat infiltration of SM
Tubular Shortened	Hypertrophy/contraction MM. SM thick. Relax taenia
IP	Residual inflamed mucosal islands surrounded by ulcer
Post IP	Regenerated epithelium on Mucosal islands
Sacculation	Eccentric transmural dz antimesenteric sparing

Behcet's Syndrome
- Vasculitis, multisystemic
- Orogenital ulceration, skin and ocular inflammation
- GI tract: 20%
- Male > female, 10-30 years

Behcet's Syndrome
- Ileocolitis:
  - ➢ Similar to Crohn's or U.C.
  - ➢ Perforation, hemorrhage frequent
- Esophagitis
  - ➢ Discrete, shallow ulcers
  - ➢ Mid ? distal

Pseudomembranous Colitis
- Immunosuppressed patients or
- Prolonged antibiotic therapy
- Complicated by Clostridium difficile enterotoxin overgrowth
- Usually pancolonic but may be isolated
- CT appearance of PMC is nonspecific and may be NL

Pseudomembranous Colitis: CT Findings
[Figure 2-30-16]
- Typically pancolitis
- Mural thickening - often marked
- Mural stratification
- Ascites
- Mucosal enhancement
- Accordion sign

Pseudomembranous Colitis : Accordion sign
- Barium trapped b/w thickened mucosal folds
- DDx
  - ➢ PMC
  - ➢ Other onfections
  - ➢ Ischemic colitis
  - ➢ Cirrhosis/ascites
  - ➢ Lupus vasculitis

Pseudomembranous Colitis: Differential Diagnosis
- UC
- Crohn disease
- Ischemia
- Infection
- Typhlitis
- Lymphangiec-tasia
- Leukemia
- Lymphoma
- Hemorrhage
- Diverticulitis

Typhlitis [Figure 2-30-17]
- Inflammation of the cecum
- Unknown etiology - likely infection
- Neutropenia, fever, RLQ pain and diarrhea
- Neutropenic colitis/enterocolitis
  - ➢ Extension to entire colon and small bowel

Typhlitis: CT Findings [Figure 2-30-18]
- Segmental bowel wall thickening
- Intramural edema/necrosis
- Pneumatosis coli
- Pericolic fluid
- Stranding in the adjacent fat

Figure 2-30-16

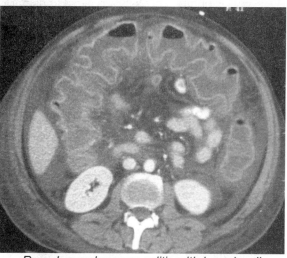

Pseudomembranous colitis with bowel wall thickening, mucosal enhancement and ascites.

Figure 2-30-17

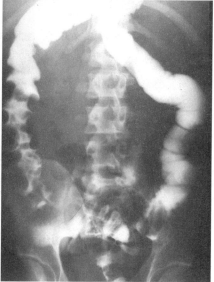

Typhlitis with marked bowel wall thickening of the right colon.

Figure 2-30-18

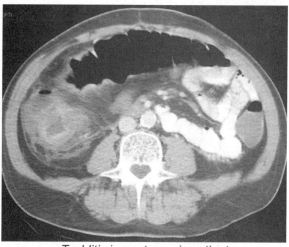

Typhlitis in neutropenic patient

Typhlitis
- Early Dx and Rx necessary to avoid transmural necrosis and perforation
- DDX
  - PMC
  - Graft vs. host
  - CMV Colitis

Graft vs. Host Disease
- Bone marrow transplant patients - most common
- Allogenic Tx of immunocompetent lymphocytes
- Donor cytotoxic T lymphocytes attack
  - Skin
  - Gut
  - Liver
  - Mucous membranes

Graft vs. Host Disease
- Small most common
- Thickened mucosal folds
- Increased secretions
- Rapid transit
- Prolonged coating
- "Toothpaste" appearance

Graft vs. Host Disease: Toothpaste Bowel
- Globally featureless
- Tubular
- Mucosal folds effaced
- Separated
- Edematous

Diverticulitis
- Diverticula most common in sigmoid
  - Smallest diameter-highest intraluminal pressure
  - Occur where the vasa recta perforate the bowel wall
- Inspissated fecal matter leads to intramural abscess and perforation

Figure 2-30-19

Diverticulitis: CT Findings *[Figure 2-30-19]*
- Pericolonic edema and inflammation
- Diverticula
- Bowel wall thickening
- Abscess
- Obstruction

Diverticulitis: Complications
- Sinus tract/fistula
- Bowel obstruction
- Peritonitis
- Hemorrhage
- Remote Abscess
- Osteomyelitis

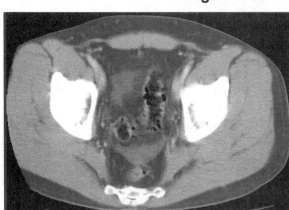

Sigmoid Diverticulitis

Diverticulitis vs. Colon Cancer
- Findings atypical for diverticulitis
  - Asymmetric or eccentric wall thickening
  - Short segment of colonic involvement
  - Pericolic lymph nodes
- Findings atypical for colon cancer
  - Pericolic inflammation
  - Extraluminal air/fluid
  - Long segment involvement
  - Fluid at the root of the sigmoid mesentery

Inflammatory Bowel Disease: Summary
- Idiopathic
  - Ulcerative colitis
  - Crohn's disease
- Specific
  - Behcet's
  - Pseudomembranous colitis
  - Typhlitis
  - Graft vs. host disease
  - Diverticulitis

Inflammatory Bowel Disease Selected References

Bayraktar Y, Ozaslan E, Van Thiel DH. Gastrointestinal manifestations of Behcet's disease. J Clin Gastroenterol 2000; 30:144-154.

Carucci LR, Levine MS. Radiographic imaging of inflammatory bowel disease. Gastroenterol Clin North Am 2002; 31:93-117, ix.

Chintapalli KN, Chopra S, Ghiatas AA, Esola CC, Fields SF, Dodd GD, 3rd. Diverticulitis versus colon cancer: differentiation with helical CT findings. Radiology 1999; 210:429-435.

Fenoglio-Preiser C. Gastrointestinal Pathology: Atlas and Text. New York: Lippincott-Raven, 1999.

Giardiello FM, Bayless TM. Colorectal cancer and ulcerative colitis. Radiology 1996; 199:28-30.

Gore RM. CT of inflammatory bowel disease. Radiol Clin North Am 1989; 27:717-729.

Gore RM, Balthazar EJ, Ghahremani GG, Miller FH. CT features of ulcerative colitis and Crohn's disease. AJR Am J Roentgenol 1996; 167:3-15.

Gore RM, Ghahremani, G.G., Miller, F.H. Inflammatory Bowel Disease: Radiologic Diagnosis: RSNA Categorical Course in Diagnostic Radiology, 1997; 95-109.

Horton KM, Corl FM, Fishman EK. CT evaluation of the colon: inflammatory disease. Radiographics 2000; 20:399-418.

Jacobs JE, Birnbaum BA. CT of inflammatory disease of the colon. Semin Ultrasound CT MR 1995; 16:91-101.

Lichtenstein JE. Radiologic-pathologic correlation of inflammatory bowel disease. Radiol Clin North Am 1987; 25:3-24.

O'Sullivan SG. The accordion sign. Radiology 1998; 206:177-178.

Wills JS, Lobis IF, Denstman FJ. Crohn disease: state of the art. Radiology 1997; 202:597-610.

Notes

Notes

Genitourinary Radiology

Imaging of Uterine Disorders

Paula J. Woodward, MD
Chief, Genitourinary Radiology
Department of Radiologic Pathology
Armed Forces Institute of Pathology

Overview
- Normal Anatomy
- Imaging Techniques
- Congenital Anomalies
- Benign Lesions
- Malignancies

Uterus
- Fundus
- Corpus
- Cervix

Uterine Corpus
- Serosa
  - peritoneal reflection
- Myometrium
  - involuntary smooth muscle
- Endometrium
  - stratum basalis
  - stratum functionalis

Cervix
- Internal os
- Endocervical canal
  - columnar epithelium
  - plicae palmatae
  - surrounded by fibrous stroma and muscular layer
- External os
  - squamocolumnar junction

Uterine Ligaments
- Broad ligaments
  - double sheet of peritoneum
- Cardinal ligaments
- Uterosacral ligaments
- Uterovesical ligaments
- Round ligaments

Blood Supply
- Uterine artery
  - branch of internal iliac
  - passes superficial to the ureter
  - enters myometrium at internal os
- Ovarian artery
  - branch of the aorta
  - anastomosis with uterine artery

Imaging Techniques
- Ultrasound
- Hysterosalpingography
- Sonohysterography
- MRI

Ultrasound
- Transabdominal
  - full baldder
  - 2.5–5.0 MHz transducer
- Transvaginal
  - empty bladder
  - 5.0–7.5 MHz transducer

Myometrium
- Homogeneous intermediate echogenicity
- Can sometimes see hypoechoic inner and outer layers
- Blood supply
  - uterine
  - arcuate
  - radial
  - spiral (endometrium)

Endometrium [Figure 3-1-1]
- Early proliferative phase
  - thin echogenic line
- Late proliferative phase
  - hypoechoic thickening, 4–8mm
- Secretory phase
  - hyperechoic thickening, 7–14mm
- Menstrual phase
  - thin broken echogenic line

Hysterosalpingography: HSG
- First ten days of menstrual cycle
- Active PID contraindication
- Radiation dose 75–750 mrad
- Only visualizes internal contour
- Primary use tubal patency

Pelvic MRI
- Phased Array Coils
- Fast T2WI images

Pelvic Protocol
- Pelvic Coil
- 1 mg IM glucagon
- Coronal localizer – FMPSPGR
- FSE T2 – sagittal, axial, coronal, oblique
  - TR 4,000–5,000
  - TE 90–130
  - ETL 16
  - FOV 20–24 cm
  - Thickness 4–5 mm, 1 mm gap
  - Matrix 256x256
  - 2–4 NEX
- T1 SE
  - Axial
  - TR 300–500
  - TE min
- T1 Fat Sat with Gd

Uterus
- T1 – uniform intermediate signal
- T2 – zonal anatomy
  - Endometrium – high signal
  - Junctional zone – low signal
  - Myometrium – intermediate signal

Figure 3-1-1a

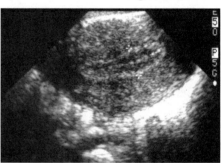

Endometrium, proliferative phase

Figure 3-1-1b

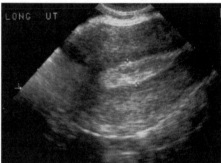

Endometrium, secretory phase

Normal Uterus

[Figure 3-1-2]

Normal Cervix

[Figure 3-1-3]

Embryology

[Figures 3-1-4 and 3-1-5]

Figure 3-1-2

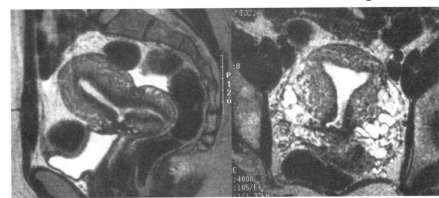

Normal Uterus: Sagittal T2WI and HSG view

Figure 3-1-3

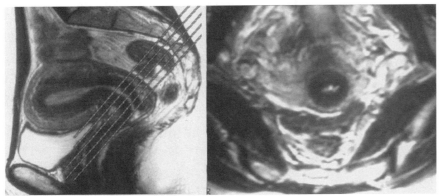

Normal Cervix: sagittal and donut view

Figure 3-1-4

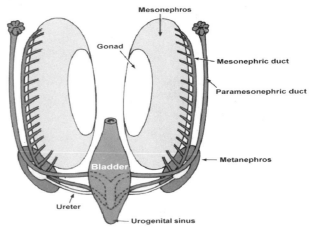

Embryologic paramesonephric ducts

Figure 3-1-5

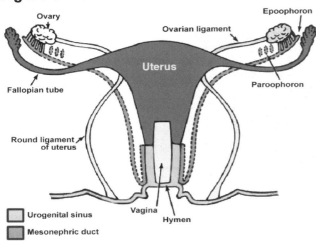

Uterus forms from fused paramesonephric ducts.

Mullerian Duct Anomalies

[Figure 3-1-6]

•	Class	Description
•	I	Agenesis or hypoplasia
•	II	Unicornuate
•	III	Didelphys
•	IV	Bicornuate
•	V	Septate
•	VI	VIDES-related

Unicornuate / Didelphys

[Figure 3-1-7]

- Low rate of pregnancy loss
- Limited surgical options
- Unicornuate – highest rate of renal agenesis
- Didelphys – 75% have vaginal septum

Bicornuate

[Figures 3-1-8 and 3-1-9]

- Partial fusion of ducts
- Concave external contour
- Bicollis or unicollis

Figure 3-1-7

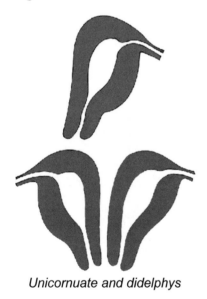

Unicornuate and didelphys

Figure 3-1-6

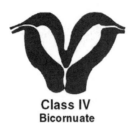
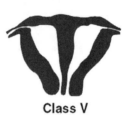
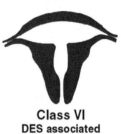

Classification of Mullerian duct anomalies

Figure 3-1-8

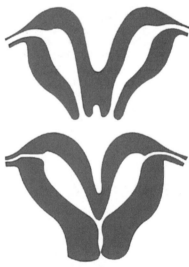

Bicornuate bicollis (2 cervices) and bicornuate unicollis (1 cervix)

Figure 3-1-9

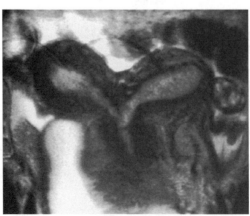

Bicornuate, unicollis

Septate

Figure 3-1-10

[Figures 3-1-10 and 3-1-11]
- Most common uterine malformation
- Highest spontaneous abortion rate
- Septum may be complete or partial
- Septum may be fibrous or composed of myometrium

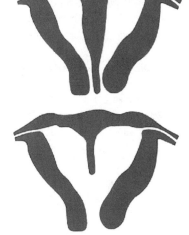

Complete and partial septum

Figure 3-1-11

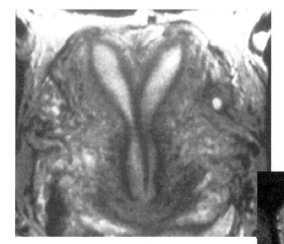

Septate uterus with a complete fibrous septum through the cervix

Bicornuate vs. Septate

[Figure 3-1-12]

	Bicornuate	Septate
Angle between horns	>90%	<90º
External morphology	concave	normal
Complications	abnormall lie premature labor	increased spontaneous abortion rate
Treatment	metroplasty	hysteroscopic resection

Arcuate Uterus

[Figure 3-1-13]

Figure 3-1-12

Figure 3-1-13

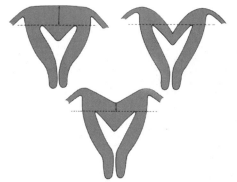

At least 1 cm of myometrium should be present for hysteroscopic resection

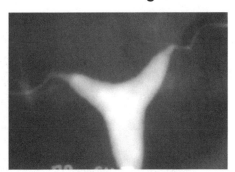

Arcuate uterus

Diethylstilbestrol: DES – Related

[Figure 3-1-14]

Figure 3-1-14

- 1–1.5 million female progeny exposed
- 50% have a uterine anomaly
- Associated with clear cell carcinoma of the vagina
- No associated urinary tract abnormality

Mullerian Duct Anomalies

- Form a continuum
- Renal anomalies in 25%
- Obstructions are common – risk for endometriosis and adenomyosis
- Septate has highest spontaneous abortion rate
- DES exposure risk factor for clear cell carcinoma of the vagina

Benign Uterine Masses

- Leiomyomas
- Adenomyosis

Leiomyoma

- Benign smooth muscle tumor
- Dysmenorrhea, hypermenorrhea, fertility problems
- 25% of premenopausal women

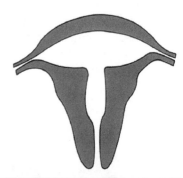
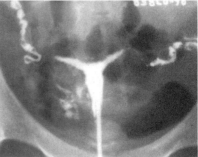

DES exposure

Leiomyoma

[Figure 3-1-15]

- Submucosal, intramural, subserosal
- Well circumscribed
- US – generally hypoechoic
- MRI – low signal on T1 and T2 unless they have undergone degeneration

Figure 3-1-15

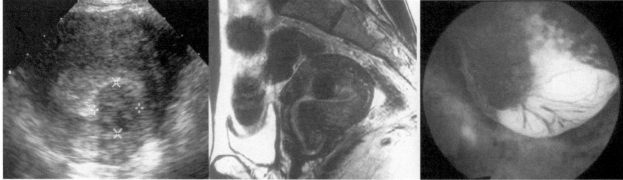

US, MRI, and hysteroscopic image of a submucosal fibroid

Leiomyoma Degeneration *[Figure 3-16]*

- Hyaline
- Myxomatous
- Cystic
- Hemorrhagic (carneous)
- Sarcomatous

Figure 3-1-16

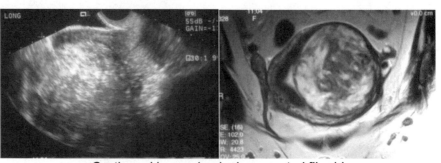

Cystic and hemorrhagic degenerated fibroid

Indications for MRI
- Pre-myomectomy
- Rapidly growing fibroid
- When US is confusing

Adenomyosis [Figure 3-1-17]
- Heterotopic implants of endometrium within the myometrium
- Dysmenorrhea, hypermenorrhea
- 25% of hysterectomy specimens

Adenomyosis
- Diffuse or focal (adenomyoma)
- Irregular borders
- US
  - ➢ enlarged heterogeneous uterus
- MRI
  - ➢ junctional zone > 1 cm
  - ➢ low signal on T1 and T2
  - ➢ punctate areas of high signal

Endometrial Thickness
- < 15 mm in premenopausal patient (secretory phase)
- ≤ 8mm in asymptomatic post-menopausal patient (if on hormones scan after withdrawl bleeding)
- ≤ 4mm postmenopausal and bleeding

Abnormal Uterine Bleeding
- Polyps
- Submucosal fibroids
- Hyperplasia
- Carcinoma
- Atrophy
  - ➢ most common cause of post-menopausal bleeding

Sonohysterography
[Figure 3-1-18]

Endometrial Polyps
[Figure 3-1-19]
- Focal overgrowth of endometrial tissue
- Pedunculated or sessile
- 20% are multiple
- May be cystic

x

Figure 3-1-17

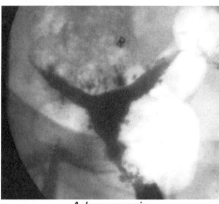

Adenomyosis

Figure 3-1-18

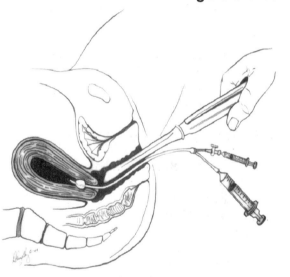

Figure 3-1-19

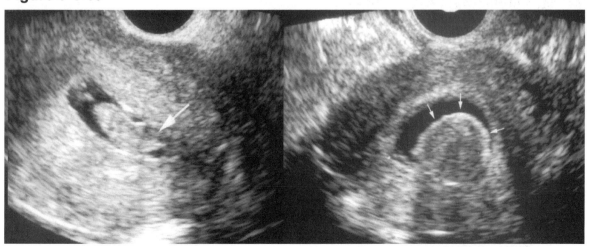

Endometrial polyp   *Submucosal fibroid*

Endometrial Hyperplasia [Figure 3-1-20]

- Increased estrogen stimulation
  - ➢ hormone replacement (unopposed estrogen)
  - ➢ tamoxifen
  - ➢ anovulatory cycles, polycystic ovarian disease
  - ➢ obesity
  - ➢ estrogen producing tumors (granulosa cell, thecoma)
- Risk factor for carcinoma

Tamoxifen [Figure 3-1-21]

- Has an antiestrogen effect on the breast but weak estrogen effect on the uterus
- Increased risk of endometrial carcinoma, hyperplasia, and polyps
- Cystic changes often present

Postmenopausal Bleeding

- ≤ 4mm – atrophy
- \> 4mm – sonohysterogram
  - ➢ diffuse thickening – random bx or D&C
  - ➢ focal thickening – hysteroscopy

Endometrial Carcinoma

- Most common GYN malignancy- 33,000 cases/year
- Risk factors:
  - ➢ unopposed estrogens, tamoxifen
  - ➢ nulliparous
  - ➢ diabetes
  - ➢ obesity

Endometrial Carcinoma

- Histology
  - ➢ adenocarcinoma (80–90%)
  - ➢ adenosquamous
  - ➢ papillary serous **
  - ➢ clear cell carcinoma **
- Grade
  - ➢ I – well differentiated
  - ➢ II – moderately well differentiated
  - ➢ III – poorly differentiated

Endometrial Carcinoma: FIGO – Staging

Stage	Description
0	Carcinoma in situ
Ia	Limited to endometrium
Ib	Less than 1/2 myometrium
Ic	Greater than 1/2 myometrium
II	Invades cervix but not beyond uterus
III	Beyond uterus but not outside pelvis
IVa	Outside true pelvis / bladder / bowel
IVb	Distant metastases

Figure 3-1-20

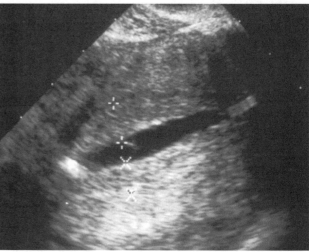

Endometrial hyperplasia

Figure 3-1-21

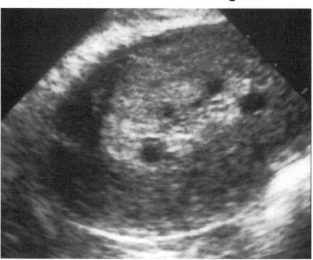

Cystic endometrium from tamoxifen

MRI Findings [Figure 3-1-22]

- Intermediate signal mass
- Expands endometrial cavity
- Enhances less than myometrium
- Not for screening

MRI Staging

- Disruption of junctional zone
- Depth of myometrial invasion
- Extension into cervix
- Extension beyond uterus
- Adenopathy

Prognostic Factors

- Histology
- Tumor grade
- Depth of myometrial invasion
- Lymph node involvement

Figure 3-1-22

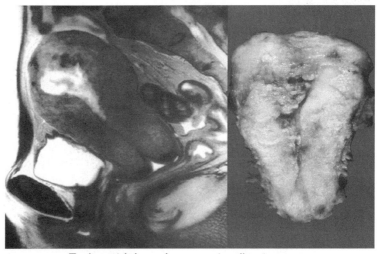

Endometrial carcinoma extending to serosa

Cervical Carcinoma

- 14,000 cases/year, 4,900 deaths/year
- Begins at squamocolumnar junction
- 90% are squamous cell
- Association with papilloma virus, herpes, and HIV

Cervical Carcinoma

Stage	Description
0	Carcinoma in situ
I	Confined to cervix
II	Invades beyond cervix but not to pelvic sidewall or lower third of vagina
IIa	No parametrial invasion
IIb	Parametrial invasion
III	Extension to pelvic sidewall / lower third of vagina / causes hydronephrosis
IVa	Invasion into bladder / rectum
IVb	Distant metastases

Staging

- Clinical
  - errors in 32% for stage IB (greater than 5mm deep and 7mm wide)
  - 62% for II-IV
- MRI
  - 93% accuracy for tumor size within 5mm
  - Staging accuracy 87%- 92%

Prognosis

- Tumor size
- Depth of invasion
- Parametrial extension
- Lymph node involvement

MRI

- Intermediate signal T2WI
- Check list
  - tumor size
  - depth of stromal invasion
  - parametrial invasion
  - hydronephrosis
  - lymphadenopathy

Cervical Carcinoma Stage I

[Figure 3-1-23]

Cervical Carcinoma Stage II

[Figure 3-1-24]

Figure 3-1-23

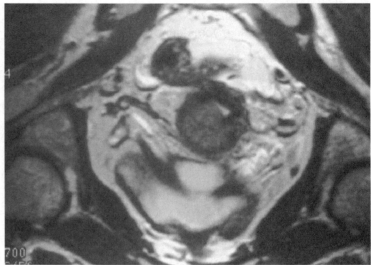

Stage I cervical carcinoma

Figure 3-24

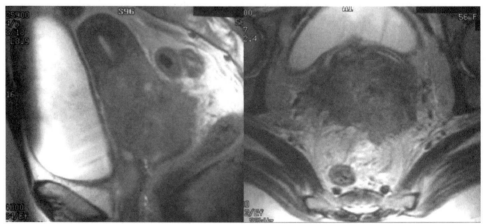

Stage IIB cervical carcinoma with obvious parametrial invasion

Renal Neoplasms
Approach to Renal Masses

Paula J. Woodward, MD
Chief, Genitourinary Radiology
Department of Radiologic Pathology
Armed Forces Institute of Pathology

Approach to Renal Masses: 4 Questions
- Cyst vs Solid
- Infiltrative vs Expansile
- Fatty vs Soft Tissue
- Solitary vs Multiple

Tumor Growth: Ball vs. Bean
- Expansile – "Ball"
- Infiltrative – "Bean"

Expansile Renal Mass
- Spherical, exophytic, frequently encapsulated
- DDx
  - Malignant – adenocarcinoma, metastases, lymphoma
  - Benign – cyst, angiomyolipoma, oncocytoma, etc.

Infiltrative Renal Masses
- Invades parenchyma, preserves renal contour, poorly marginated
- DDx
  - Malignant – transitional cell, squamous cell, lymphoma, atypical adenocarcinoma
  - Benign – pyelonephritis, XGP, TB

Intravenous Urography
- Only good for expansile masses
- Misses 1/3 of masses <3cm
- All lesions require further work up
  - US, CT, MRI

Ultrasound
- Cyst
  - anechoic
  - acoustic enhancement
  - sharp posterior wall
- RCCA
  - can be hypo, iso, or hyperechoic

Computed Tomography
- 94% sensitive for lesions 3 cm or less
- 90- 95% accuracy in staging
- Pre and post contrast of lesion
- Scan in both corticomedullary and nephrographic phase

Volume Averaging – All Tissues in the Slice Volume are Averaged

[Figures 3-2-1 to 3-2-3]

Phases of Excretion
- Corticomedullary phase 25 –80 sec
- Nephrographic phase 90–120 sec
- Excretory phase 3 –5 min
  - Varies with injection rate, cardiac output, and renal function

Corticomedullary Phase (CMP)
- Cortex and medulla > 100 HU difference
- Best for metastases and vascular invasion
- Pitfalls: Can miss hyperdense cortical masses and hypodense medullary masses, pseudotumor in the IVC

Nephrographic Phase
- Renal lesions are best seen in the nephrographic phase
- 1.1 ——> 2.4 more masses detected

Venous extension
[Figure 3-2-4]

Excretory Phase
- Decreasing density of nephrograms
- Worsening streak artifact especially with non-ionic contrast

Excretory Phase
- New role in CT-urography

Figure 3-2-1

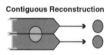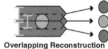

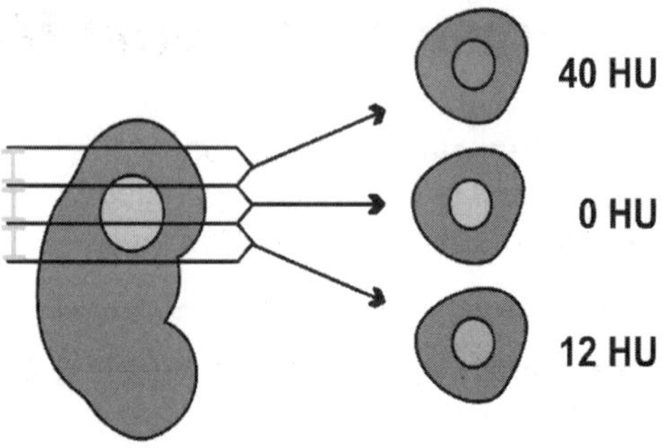

Volume averaging

Figure 3-2-2

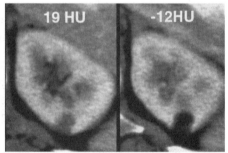

Figure 3-2-3

Affect of volume averaging on an AML

Figure 3-2-4

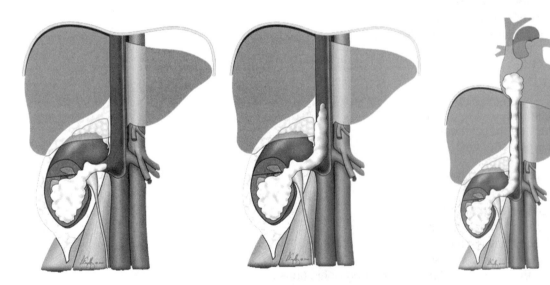

Surgical approach is based on extent of venous invasion

Enhancement
- < 10 HU no enhancement
- > 15 HU enhancement
- 10–15 HU gray zone

De-enhancement
- Decrease 15 HU at 15 minutes

CT Technique for Renal Mass Characterization
- Scan kidneys both pre and post contrast
- Slice thickness of 5–7mm
- Scan during corticomedullary and nephrograhic phase
- Perform overlapping reconstruction if the lesion is small
- Delayed scans

Magnetic Resonance Imaging
- Equivalent to CT in accuracy with Gd
- Calcification difficult to detect
- Excellent for vascular invasion

Magnetic Resonance Imaging
- Cysts
  - low-signal T1WI
  - high-signal T2WI
  - no enhancement
- Solid
  - 15% enhancement with Gd

Calculating % Enhancement
- (Post SI – Pre SI) / Pre SI x 100 = % enhancement

Malignant Neoplasms
- Adenocarcinoma
- Uroepithelial tumors
  - Transitional cell
  - Squamous cell
- Lymphoma
- Metastases

Renal Cell Carcinoma
- 25,000 –30,000 new cases and 12,000 deaths per year
- 12,000 deaths per year
- Peak incidence – sixth and seventh decade
- M:F (2–3:1)
- Bilateral 2%, multicentric 15%

Renal Cell Carcinoma
- expansile cortical mass
  - 90% originate from the proximal convoluted tubule

Renal Cell Carcinoma
- Slow growing low grade malignancies may be encapsulated
- Can have areas of necrosis, cyst formation, hemorrhage, or calcification

Histology
- Clear cell – 70–80%
  - Deletion on chromosome 3p
  - Lipid rich
- Papillary – 10–15%
  - Slower growing, less vascular, calcification more common, often encapsulated, better prognosis
- Other – chromophobe, sarcomatoid, medullary, etc.

Renal Cell Carcinoma - Risk factors

- Dialysis *[Figure 3-2-5]*
- von Hipple Lindau *[Figure 3-2-6]*
  - often multiple RCCAs
  - multiple renal cysts
  - affects other abdominal organs
- Tuberous sclerosis (much less common)

Renal Cell Carcinoma: Presentation

- "Classic triad" – hematuria, flank pain, mass < 50%
- Paraneoplastic – hypertension, erythrocytosis, hypercalcemia
- Other – fever, weight loss, anemia, varicocele
- 30% present with metastases

Calcification

- 20–30% of RCCA
- 1–2% of benign cysts
- Rim calcification – 80% benign
- Central calcification – 87% malignant

"Cystic" Changes

- 15–25% of RCCA
  - Necrosis 75%
  - Cystic 25% – often papillary histology
    - ❖ Mural nodule or septations *[Figure 3-2-7]*
    - ❖ Malignant cell lining (VHL)

Benign Lesions

- Simple Cyst
  - Water density
  - Thin (1-2 mm) wall
  - No enhancement
- Minimally Complicated Cyst
  - High density cysts (protein or blood)
  - Thin septations
  - Thin curvilinear calcifications

Surgical Lesions

- Enhancing lesions
- Nodularity
- Thick wall (>2mm)
- Thick septations
- Irregular or central calcifications
  - Less important

Spontaneous Renal Hemorrhage

- RCAA (men)
- AML (women)
- Infarction
- Infection
- AV malformation
- Vasculitis
- Glomerulonephritis

Infiltrating Renal Cell

- 7% of adenocarcinomas
- Arise from the renal medulla – difficult to differentiate from invasive uroepithelial tumor
- Medullary carcinoma, collecting duct carcinoma, sarcomatoid neoplasms
- Poor prognosis

Figure 3-2-5

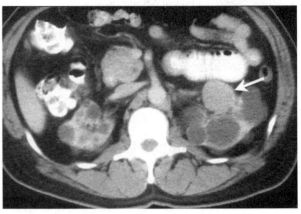

Cystic disease of dialysis with RCCA

Figure 3-2-6

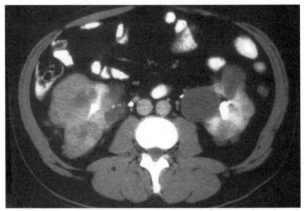

VHL with multiple RCCA

Figure 3-2-7

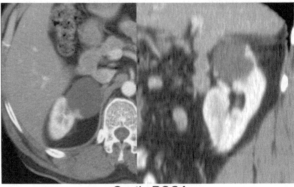

Cystic RCCA

Medullary Carcinoma [Figure 3-2-8]
- Young black male with sickle cell trait
- From epithelium of papilla or distal collecting duct
- Survival < 4 mos.

Robson Staging [Figure 3-2-9]
- I – Confined to kidney
- II – Within Gerota's fascia
- III A – renal vein or IVC invasion
- III B – lymph nodes
- III C – vascular invasion plus nodes
- IV A – direct organ invasion
- IV B – distant metastases

Figure 3-2-8

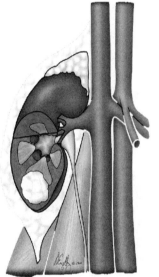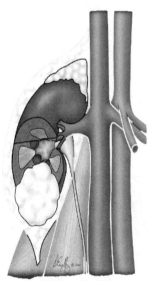

Medullary carcinoma with infiltrative pattern

TNM Staging
- T1 – < 7cm
- T2 – > 7 cm
- T3a – local invasion not beyond Gerota's fascia
- T3b – venous invasion below diaphragm
- T3c – venous invasion above diaphragm
- T4 – extension beyond Gerota's fascia
- N0 – no regional lymph nodes
- N1 – metastasis in a single regional lymph node
- N2 – metastasis in more than one regional lymph node
- M0 – no distant metastasis
- M1 – distant metastasis
- Stage I
  - ➢ T1,N0,M0
- Stage II
  - ➢ T2,N0,M0
- Stage III
  - ➢ T1,N1,M0
  - ➢ T2,N1,M0
  - ➢ T3a,N1,M0
  - ➢ T3b,N0,M0
  - ➢ T3b,N1,M0
  - ➢ T3c,N0,M0
  - ➢ T3c,N1,M0
- Stage IV
  - ➢ T4,N0,M0
  - ➢ T4,N1,M0
  - ➢ Any T,N2,M0
  - ➢ Any T,any N,M1

Figure 3-2-9

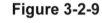

Stage 1　　*Stage II with invasion into Gerota's fascia*

Nephron-sparing Surgery
- Margins of at least 5 mm normal tissue
- < 4cm, away from renal hilum (polar, cortical)
- Survival rates comparable to radical nephrectomy

Stage II vs. Stage I
[Figure 3-2-10]
- Nodule in perinephric space most specific but present < 50%
- Perinephric stranding unreliable

Figure 3-2-10

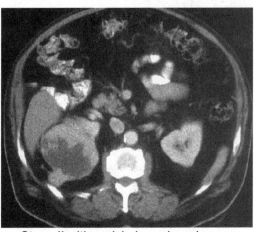

Stage II with nodule in perirenal space

Stage III a,b,c
[Figure 3-2-11]

Figure 3-2-11

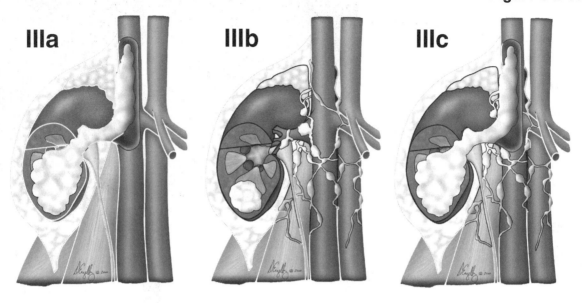

Stage III renal carcinoma: Imaging
[Figure 3-2-12]

Figure 3-2-12

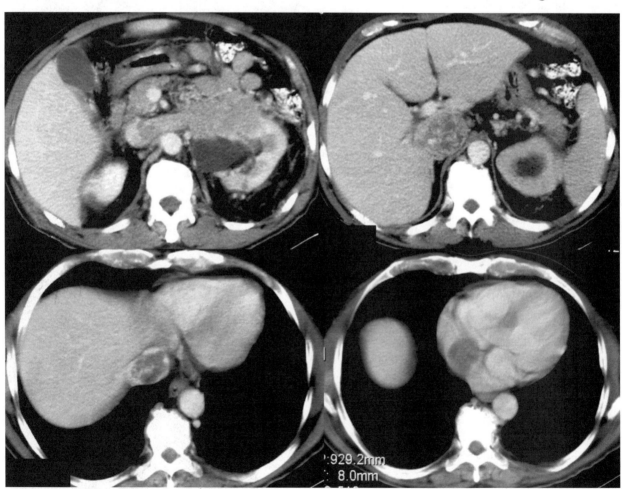

Vascular invasion extending to the right atrium

Stage IV
[Figure 3-2-13]

Figure 3-2-13

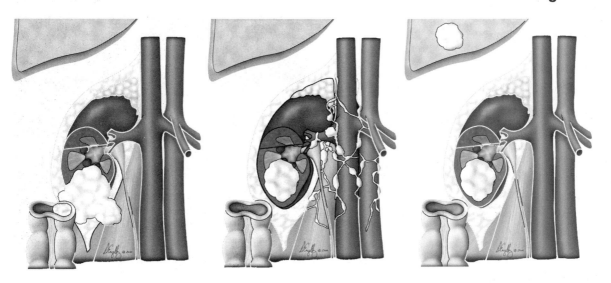

Stage IV renal carcinoma: Imaging
[Figure 3-2-14]

Figure 3-2-14

Renal Cell Carcinoma: Metastases
- Lung   69%
- Bone   43%
- Liver   34%
- Nodes   22%
- Brain   5%
- Adrenal   4%

Abdominal CT Checklist
- Renal vein, IVC
- Regional lymph nodes
- Adrenal glands
- Contralateral kidney
- Review lung and bone windows

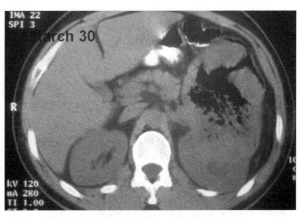

Stage IV with invasion into the descending colon

Uroepithelial Neoplasms
- 5–10% of all urinary tract malignancies
- Transitional cell 85– 95%
- Squamous cell carcinoma 5–10%
- Rare – adenocarcinoma, sarcoma, metastases

Transitional Cell Carcinoma
- 50–70 yo
- Males > females (3:1)
- Risk factors
  - Smoking
  - Aniline dyes
  - Benzene
  - Analgesic nephropathy (phenacetin)
  - Balkan nephropathy

Transitonal Cell Carcinoma
- Hematuria 75%
- Multicentric 30 – 50%
- Bilateral 10%
- Incidence by location:
  - Bladder 92%
  - Pelvis 6%
  - Ureter 2%

Transitional Cell Carcinoma
[Figure 3-2-15]
- Small, hypovascular masses
- Majority papillary with endophytic growth
- Renal invasion in 25%
- Imaging
  - Retrogrades, IVP with compression
  - CT urography
  - US and conventional poor

Figure 3-2-15

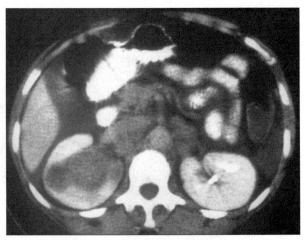

Invasive transitional cell carcinoma presenting as a renal mass

Squamous Cell Carcinoma
[Figure 3-2-16]
- Squamous metaplasia from chronic irritation
- Associated with stones (>50%)
- Aggressive behavior, commonly infiltrative
- Survival < 1 yr

Figure 3-2-16

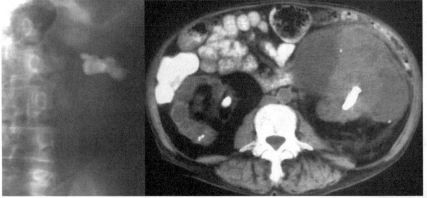

Sqaumous cell carcinoma with a staghorn calculus and large soft tissue mass

Renal Lymphoma
[Figures 3-2-17 and 3-2-18]
- Common in widespread disease
- Primary lymphoma very rare
- Hematogenous spread or direct invasion
- 50-70% bilateral
- Homogeneous
- Multiple masses   50%
- Infiltrating hilar mass   25%
- Perirenal   10%
- Renal enlargement   10%
- Solitary mass   5%

Figure 3-2-17

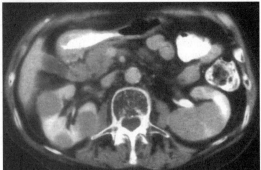

Renal lymphoma with homogeneous expansile and infiltrative masses

Figure 3-2-18

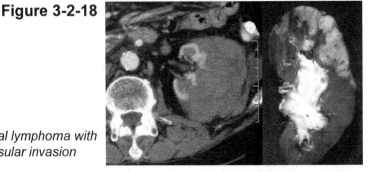

Perirenal lymphoma with capsular invasion

Metastases

- 7 – 20% of autopsy cases
- Generally asymptomatic
- Primaries
  - ➢ Lung
  - ➢ Breast
  - ➢ GI (esp colon)
  - ➢ Melanoma

Metastates

- Spread
  - ➢ Hematogenous – usually cortical
  - ➢ Lymphatic – perirenal
  - ➢ Direct invasion
- Expansile or infiltrative pattern
- Solitary or multiple masses

Benign Renal Neoplasms

- Cystic
  - ➢ Multilocular cystic nephroma
- Solid
  - ➢ Parenchymal
    - ❖ Adenoma
    - ❖ Oncocytoma
    - ❖ Juxtaglomerular tumor
  - ➢ Mesenchymal
    - ❖ Angiomyolipoma
    - ❖ Lipoma
    - ❖ Leiomyoma
    - ❖ Angioma
    - ❖ Fibroma

Figure 3-2-19

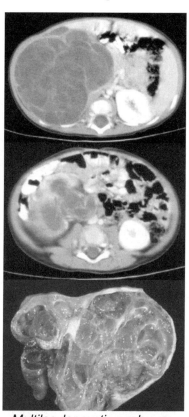

Multilocular cystic nephroma with herniation into the renal pelvis

Multilocular Cystic Nephroma

[Figure 3-2-19]

- Bimodal age distribution
  - ➢ < 2 yo (M:F, 3:1)
  - ➢ >40 yo (F:M, 9:1)
- Multiple well-defined cysts with enhancing septa, no hemorrhage
- Can herniate into renal pelvis
- DDx: cystic renal cell carcinoma, MCDK complicated benign cyst, abscess

Adenoma

- Benign (?) cortical neoplasm
- Small (<1cm)
- Often found at autopsy
- Robbins Pathologic Basis of Disease: "these tumors do not differ from low-grade papillary renal cell adenocarcinoma"

Figure 3-2-20

Oncocytoma

[Figure 3-2-20]

- Oncocyte – Greek "swollen cell"
- Large epithelial cells with granular eosinophilic cytoplasm (abundant mitochondria)
- Found in kidney, salivary glands, thyroid, parathyroid, and pancreas

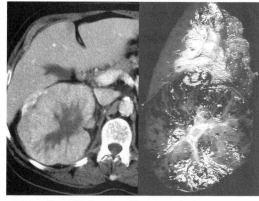

Oncocytoma with a central scar

Oncocytoma
- Usually asymptomatic
- Large – 7 cm avg. at detection
- Older males
- Solid exophytic enhancing mass
- Can not distinguish from RCCA

Oncocytoma
- Helpful features – all non-specific
  - Central scar
  - "Spoke wheel" angio appearance
  - Necrosis, hemorrhage, calcification rare
  - No adenopathy or metastases
- Gross – tan/brown tumor with pale central scar

Juxtaglomerular Cell Tumor
- Renin producing tumor
- Rare cause of hypertension, may also have headache and muscle weakness
- Young adults (F:M, 2:1)
- Hypovascular mass – imaging non-specific

Angiomyolipoma: AML
- Renal hamartoma with blood vessels, smooth muscle, and fat
- Prevalence 0.3–3%
- 80% sporadic
  - Females 30–50 yo
  - Usually solitary
- 20% tuberous sclerosis

Figure 3-2-21

Angiomyolipoma: Imaging
- Ultrasound non-specific *[Figure 3-2-21]*
- AML
  - Shadowing
  - Markedly hyperechoic
- RCCA
  - Hypoechoic rim
  - Cystic spaces
- Must prove with CT or MRI

Angiomyolipoma: Imaging
- CT
  - HU < –10 will detect 85% of AMLs
  - no calcifications
  - Vascular phase imaging can detect aneurysms

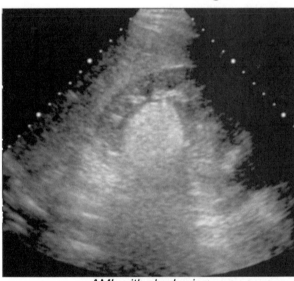

AML with shadowing

- MRI
  - fat bright on T1 and T2
  - fat saturation sequence
- Angiography
  - Tortuous, abnormal vessels with small aneurysms
  - Embolization

Figure 3-2-22

Tuberous Sclerosis *[Figure 3-2-22]*
- Autosomal dominant
- Clinical triad – seizures, adenoma sebaceum, mental retardation
- Multiple hamartomatous lesions including: retinal hamartoma, cortical tubers, subependymal nodules, ungual fibroma, angiofibroma, pulmonary lymphangiomyomatosis, cardiac rhabdomyoma

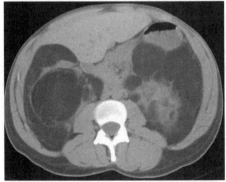

Tuberous sclerosis with large bilateral AMLs

Tuberous Sclerosis

[Figure 3-2-22]

- Renal involvement
  - ➢ Approx 3/4 will have AML
    - ❖ 75% multiple
    - ❖ 50% bilateral
  - ➢ Cysts can also be seen especially in children
  - ➢ 1–2% develop RCCA

Angiomyolipoma: Presentation

[Figure 3-2-23]

- Incidental finding
  - ➢ Usually < 4 cm
- Hemorrhage
  - ➢ Usually > 4cm
  - ➢ May be spontaneous or minor trauma
- Bleeding may be life-threatening in up to 25% of cases
- Vessels thick walled with decreased elastin
- Predisposition for aneurysm formation

RCCA with Fat

[Figure 3-2-24]

- Osseous metaplasia – calcification
- Lipid necrosis – large necrotic masses
- Engulfed perirenal or sinus fat – irregular invasive appearance

Helpful Tips

- No enhancement (etc.)
  - ➢ Benign cyst
- Fat
  - ➢ AML
- Multiple AMLs
  - ➢ Tuberous sclerosis
- Infiltrative + expansile
  - ➢ Lymphoma
- Herniation into renal pelvis + female
  - ➢ Multilocular cystic nephroma
- Cysts + solid masses
  - ➢ VHL or dialysis
- Central scar + no adenopathy or vein invasion
  - ➢ Oncocytoma

Figure 3-2-23

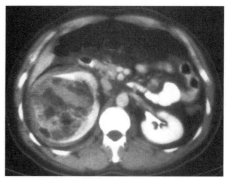

Angiomyolipoma with bleed

Figure 3-2-24

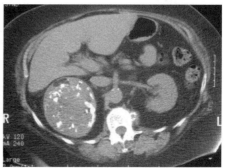

RCCA with osseous metaplasis

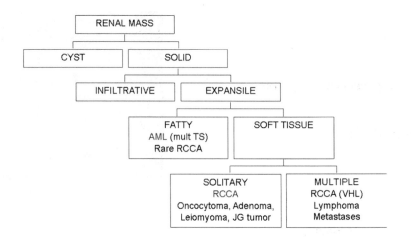

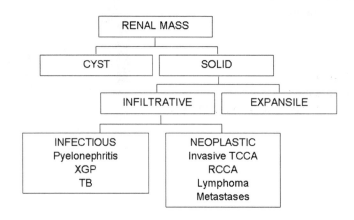

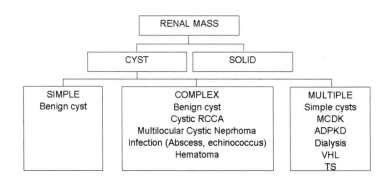

Urinary Tract Trauma

Paula J. Woodward, MD
Chief, Genitourinary Radiology
Department of Radiologic Pathology
Armed Forces Institute of Pathology

Hematuria
- Penetrating
  - ➢ all require evaluation
- Blunt
  - ➢ gross hematuria of >30rbc/hpf
  - ➢ microhematuria with shock
  - ➢ microhematuria >24hrs
  - ➢ high energy impact, multiple organ injury
  - ➢ may have significant injury without hematuria

GU Trauma
- Evaluate lower tract before upper tract if both may be injured
- Males always perform retrograde urethrogram before foley is inserted if there is blood at the meatus or pubic rami fx/diastasis

Male Urethra [Figure 3-3-1]
- Posterior
  - ➢ Membranous
  - ➢ Prostatic
- Anterior
  - ➢ Penile
  - ➢ Bulbous

Retrograde Urethrogram: RUG
[Figure 3-3-2]
- Inflate pediatric foley (3–5cc) in fossa navicularis
- 50 cc of 30–60% contrast
- Inject 20–30 cc and take film while continuing to inject
- Oblique if possible or gently move penis laterally
- May perform pericatheter RUG if foley is in place

Figure 3-3-1

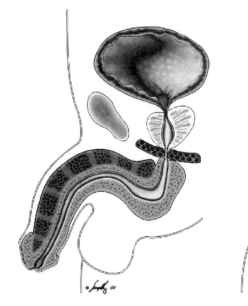

Normal urethra

Figure 3-3-2

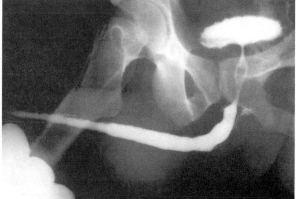

Intact urethra

Urethral Trauma

[Figures 3-3-3 to 3-3-10]

- Posterior – pelvic fractures
  I – stretch
  II – rupture above UGD
  ➢ retropubic extravasation
  III – rupture above and below UGD
  ➢ perineal/scrotal extravasation
  IV – bladder neck and urethra
  V Anterior urethral trauma– straddle
  ➢ bony injury uncommon
  ➢ partial/complete
    ❖ corpora/venous extravasation
  ➢ associated scrotal trauma

Complications

- Strictures
- Fistulas

Figure 3-3-3

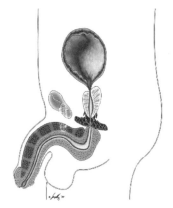

Type 1 - Stretch injury

Figure 3-3-4

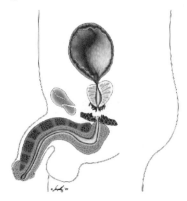

Figure 3-3-5

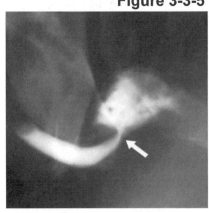

Type II – rupture above UGD

Figure 3-3-6

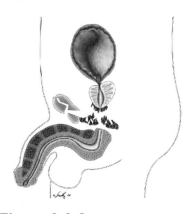

Figure 3-3-7

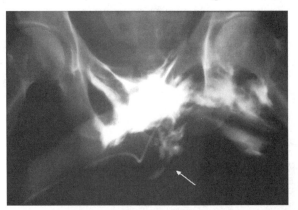

Type III – rupture above and below UGD

Figure 3-3-8

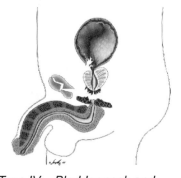

Type IV – Bladder neck and urethra

Figure 3-3-9

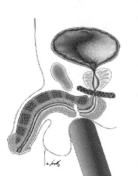

Figure 3-3-10

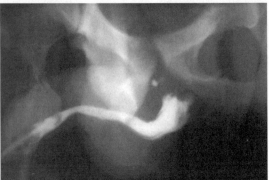

Type V – Anterior urethral trauma (straddle injury)

Bladder Trauma

- Blunt or penetrating
- 5–10% of pubic rami fx
- Pelvic fractures in 80% of ruptures
  - 83% of extraperitoneal
  - 62% of intraperitoneal

Bladder Trauma Evaluation

- Standard cystogram
  - 300–500cc
    incomplete filling may miss leak
  - 15–30% I concentration
  - AP, obliques
  - post drainage important for small leaks
- CT
  - clamp foley
  - delayed images, post drain

Extraperitoneal Bladder Rupture

[Figures 3-3-11 and 3-3-12]

- 60%
- focal extravasation, "flame-shaped"
- conservative therapy

Intraperitoneal Bladder Rupture

[Figures 3-3-13 and 3-3-14]

- 40%
- free flowing extravasation, outlines intraperitoneal organs
- surgical therapy

Bladder Trauma Evaluation

[Figure 3-3-15 and 3-3-16]

- CT cystogram
  - perform routine CT
  - drain bladder
  - refill with 2–3% I solution (300 cc)
  - scan full and post drain

Ureteral Injury

- Least common site of injury (<3%)
- Penetrating trauma – anywhere
- UPJ disruption

Figure 3-3-11

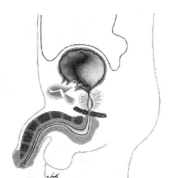

Extaperitoneal bladder rupture

Figure 3-3-12

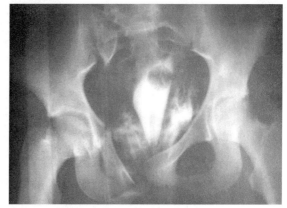

Extaperitoneal bladder rupture

Figure 3-3-13

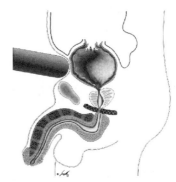

Intraperitoneal bladder rupture

Figure 3-3-14

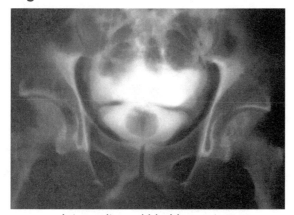

Intraperitoneal bladder rupture

Figure 3-3-15

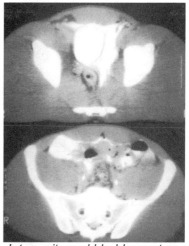

Intraperitoneal bladder rupture on CT cystogram

Figure 3-3-16

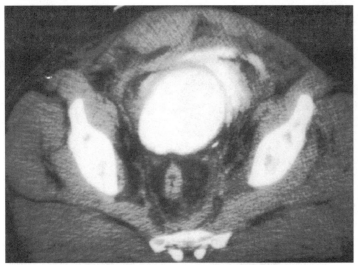

Extraperitoneal bladder rupture on CT cystogram

Renal Injuries

[Figures 3-3-17 to 3-3-33]

- Category I
  - ➢ Minor (85%)
    - ❖ contusion
    - ❖ intrarenal hematoma
    - ❖ small subcapsular/perirenal hematoma
    - ❖ segmental infarction
    - ❖ superficial laceration
  - ➢ Conservative management
- Category II
  - ➢ Serious (10%)
    - ❖ deep lacerations
    - ❖ laceration through the collecting system
    - ❖ large perinephric/subcapsular hematoma
  - ➢ Conservative management vs. surgery
- Category III
  - ➢ Catastrophic
    - ❖ fractured/shattered kidney
    - ❖ renal artery occlusion/avulsion
    - ❖ rim sign
    - ❖ renal vein occlusion/avulsion
    - ❖ UPJ avulsion, discruption
  - ➢ Usually surgical treatment

**Figure 3-3-17:
Contusion**

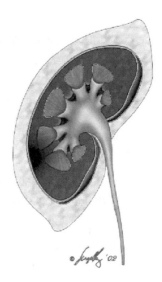

**Figure 3-3-18:
Hematoma**

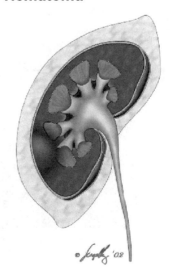

**Figure 3-3-19:
Subcapsular Hematoma**

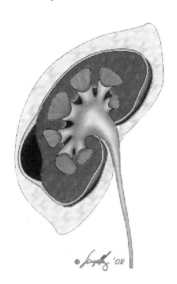

Figure 3-3-20

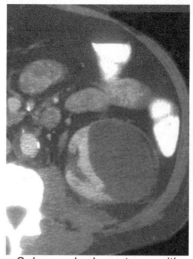

*Subcapsular hematoma with
delayed nephrogram*

**Figure 3-3-21:
Laceration**

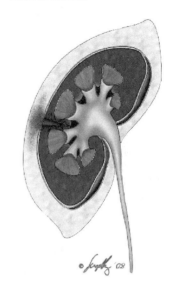

**Figure 3-3-22:
Segmental infarction**

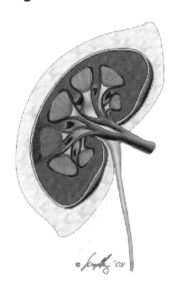

**Figure 3-3-23:
Laceration with urine
leak**

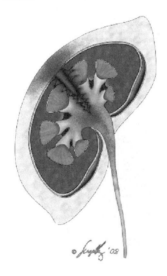

Figure 3-3-24

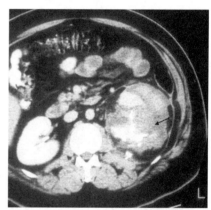

*Laceration into the collecting
system with urine leak*

**Figure 3-3-25:
Shattered kidney**

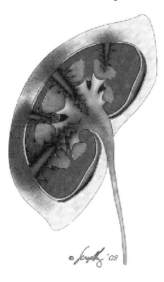

**Figure 3-3-26:
Vascular Avulsion**

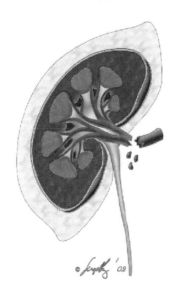

Figure 3-3-27

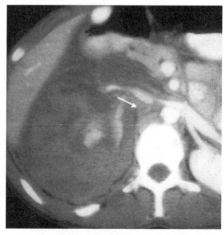

*Vascular avulsion with contrast
extravasation*

Figure 3-3-28:
Renal artery thrombosis

Figure 3-3-29:
Rim sign

Figure 3-3-30

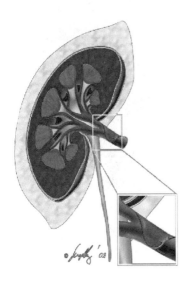

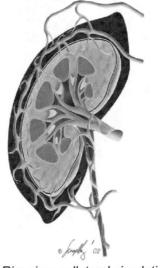

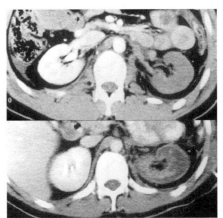

*Acute arterial thrombosis with
subsequent development
of a rim sign*

*Rim sign: collateral circulation
forming after thrombosis*

Figure 3-3-31:
Renal Vein Thrombosis

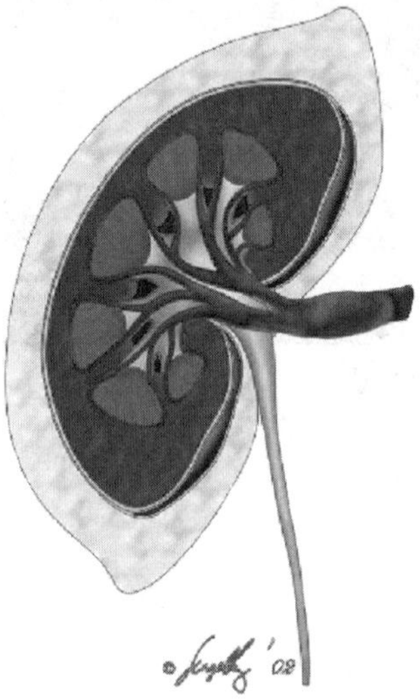

Figure 3-3-32:
UPJ disruption

Figure 3-3-33

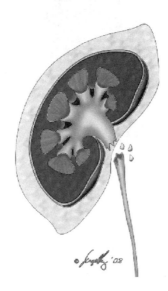

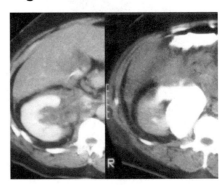

*UPJ disruption. Leak obvious on
delayed films*

UPJ disruption

- Deceleration injury
- 3:1, children:adults
- 3:1, R:L
- Stent, nephrostomy, surgery

Conclusion

- If there is blood at the meatus, perform urethrogram first
- A normal bladder on CT does not rule out a leak
- Post-drainage films are key for small leaks
- Don't forget delayed images

Selected References

1.   Ali M, Safriel Y, Sclafani SJ, Schulze R. CT signs of urethral injury. Radiographics 2003; 23:951-963; discussion 963-956.
2.   Blankenship B, Earls JP, Talner LB. Renal vein thrombosis after vascular pedicle injury[clin conference]. AJR Am J Roentgenol 1997; 168:1574.
3.   Fishman EK, Horton KM. CT evaluation of bladder trauma: a critical look. Acad Radiol 2000; 7:309-310.
4.   Goldman SM, Sandler CM, Corriere JN, Jr., McGuire EJ. Blunt urethral trauma: a unified, anatomical mechanical classification. J Urol 1997; 157:85-89.
5.   Herschorn S, Radomski SB, Shoskes DA, Mahoney J, Hirshberg E, Klotz L. Evaluation and treatment of blunt renal trauma. J Urol 1991; 146:274-276; discussion 276-277.
6.   Kamel IR, Berkowitz JF. Assessment of the cortical rim sign in posttraumatic renal infarction. J Comput Assist Tomogr 1996; 20:803-806.
7.   Kawashima A, Sandler CM, Corriere JN, Jr., Rodgers BM, Goldman SM. Ureteropelvic junction injuries secondary to blunt abdominal trauma. Radiology 1997; 205:487-492.
8.   Kawashima A, Sandler CM, Corl FM, et al. Imaging of renal trauma: a comprehensive review. Radiographics 2001; 21:557-574.
9.   McAndrew JD, Corriere JN, Jr. Radiographic evaluation of renal trauma: evaluation of 1103 consecutive patients. Br J Urol 1994; 73:352-354.
10.   Nunez D, Jr., Becerra JL, Fuentes D, Pagson S. Traumatic occlusion of the renal artery: helical CT diagnosis. AJR Am J Roentgenol 1996; 167:777-780.
11.   Roberts JL. CT of abdominal and pelvic trauma. Semin Ultrasound CT MR 1996; 17:142-169.

Retroperitoneum

Paula J. Woodward, MD
Chief, Genitourinary Radiology
Department of Radiologic Pathology
Armed Forces Institute of Pathology

Retroperitoneum

- Non-neoplastic
  - ➤ Fluid collections
    - ❖ Pancreatic
    - ❖ Urinoma
    - ❖ Hematoma
    - ❖ Abscess
  - ➤ Retroperitoneal fibrosis
  - ➤ Extramedullary hematopoiesis
- Lymphadenopathy
  - ➤ Inflammatory/infectious
  - ➤ Castleman disease
  - ➤ Lymphoma
  - ➤ Metastatic adenopathy
- Organs
  - ➤ Pancreas, colon, duodenum
  - ➤ Kidneys, adrenal, ureters
- Primary (> 100 benign and malignant tumors)
  - ➤ Neurogenic
    - ❖ Nerve sheath, ganglioneuroma, ganglioneuroblastoma, neuroblastoma
    - ❖ Paraganglioma
  - ➤ Mesenchymal
    - ❖ Lipoma/sarcoma, leiomyoma/sarcoma, malignant fibrous histiocytoma (MFH), lymphangioma, hemangioma, hemangiopericytoma, angiosarcoma
  - ➤ Germ cell
    - ❖ Teratoma (benign and malignant)

Anatomy: 3 spaces [Figure 3-4-1]

- Anterior pararenal [APRS]
- Perirenal [PRS]
- Posterior pararenal [PPRS]

Figure 3-4-1

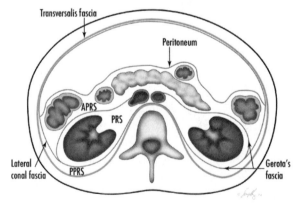

Retroperitoneal spaces

Anterior pararenal space (the GI space)

- Colon (ascending and descending)
- Pancreas
- Duodenum (2nd and 3rd portions)

Perirenal space contains (the GU space)

[Figure 3-4-2]

- Kidneys
- Adrenal glands
- Upper portion of ureters

Figure 3-4-2

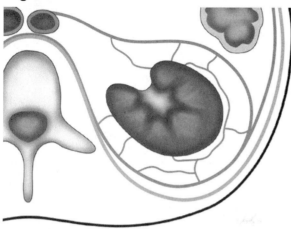

Updated view of the perirenal space with complex fascial boundaries

Figure 3-4-3

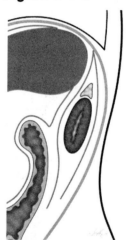

Sagittal view of the retroperitoneum

Posterior pararenal space (the nothing space): *[Figure 3-4-3]*

- no solid organs
- Fat, connective tissue, nerves

Borders:

- Parietal peritoneum separates peritoneal space from APRS
- Anterior renal fascia separates APRS from perirenal space (Gerota's fascia)
- Posterior renal fascia separates PPRS from perirenal space (Zuckerkandl's fascia)
- Lateral conal fascia demarcates the lateral extent of the APRS
- Lateral conal fascia separates the APRS from the PPRS
- All spaces communicate inferiorly

Retroperitoneal fibrosis

- Microscopically: collagen, fibroblasts, and inflammatory cells
- Typical distribution: below kidneys to bifurcation
- 40% may have atypical distribution
- 8 – 10 % malignant
  - ➢ Desmoplastic reaction to infiltrating metastases
  - ➢ Breast, lung, colon, prostate, cervix
  - ➢ Prognosis poor (3-6 months)
- Fibrotic tissue often involves IVC and aorta
- Medial deviation of ureters
- Hydronephrosis

Retroperitoneal fibrosis - Etiology

- 2/3 idiopathic (Ormand's Disease)
- Methysergide toxicity
- Aortic aneurysm
- Surgery
- Hemorrhage
- Inflammatory bowel disease
- Collagen vascular disease
- Radiation/surgery
- Fibrosing conditions elsewhere

Retroperitoneal fibrosis [Figure 3-4-4]
- IVP, retrogrades
  - Medial deviation of ureters
  - Hydronephrosis

Retroperitoneal fibrosis [Figure 3-4-5]
- CT
  - Wispy plaque-like deposits to confluent masses
  - Enhancement variable
  - Aorta is encased but not deviated
- MR
  - Fibrotic phase
    - Low on T1 and T2
    - No enhancement
  - Active phase
    - High on T2
    - Enhancement
    - Can not rule out malignancy
    - Must biopsy

Treatment
- Stents
- Steroids
- Immunosuppression
- Surgery

Neurogenic Tumors
- Nerve sheath
  - Schwannoma (neurilemmoma), neurofibroma, malignant nerve sheath tumor
- Ganglionic
  - Ganglioneuroma, ganglioneuroblastoma, neuroblastoma
- Paraganglionic
  - Paraganglioma (pheochromocytoma)

Neurogenic Tumors
- Paraspinal masses
- Mass often elongated and well-defined
- Smooth or mildly lobular
- Generally benign
- Rapid growth, increased vascularity, poorly circumscribed suggest malignancy

Neurogenic Tumors
- Low density on CT
- Low signal on T1WI
- May be hyperintense on T2WI (myxoid matrix)
- May have calcifications

Figure 3-4-4

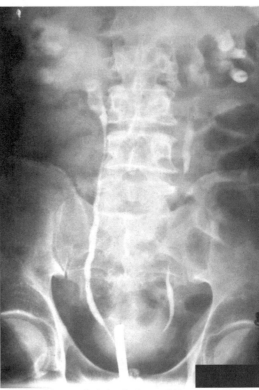

RPF with medial deviation of the ureters and hydronephrosis

Figure 3-4-5

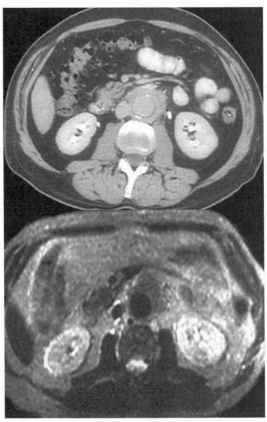

RPF with low signal on T2WI

Nerve sheath tumors [Figure 3-4-6]
- Often appears as psoas mass
- Look at neuroforamen
- May have intraspinal (extradural) extension
- Multiple consider neurofibromatosis

Ganglion Cell Tumors [Figure 3-4-7]
- Form from primitive neural crest cells
- Sympathoblast
  - Neuroblastoma
  - Ganglioneuroblastoma
  - Ganglioneuroma
- Pheochromoblast
  - Paraganglioma

Ganglioneuromas
- Benign
- More common in mediastinum
- Generally asymptomatic
- Elongated low-density masses
- Maybe be hyperintense on T2WI
- Delayed enhancement

Paraganglioma (Extra-adrenal pheochromocytoma)
- About 10% of pheochromocytomas
- Most (60–80%) have known catecholamine excess
  - Hypertension, palpitations, sweating, tremor, diarrhea, nausea
- More commonly malignant than adrenal pheochromocytomas

Paraganglioma [Figure 3-4-8]
- Organs of Zuckerkandl
- CT non-specific
  - Enhance avidly
  - Contrast contraindicated
- High signal on T2 is suggestive but is not universally seen
- Uptake on MIBG scan

Figure 3-4-6

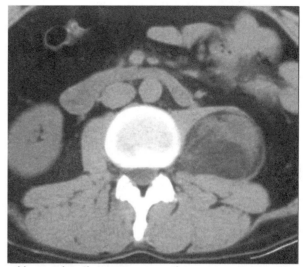

Nerve sheath tumor presenting as a psoas mass

Figure 3-4-7

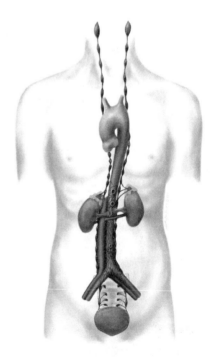

Sympathetic chain

Figure 3-4-8

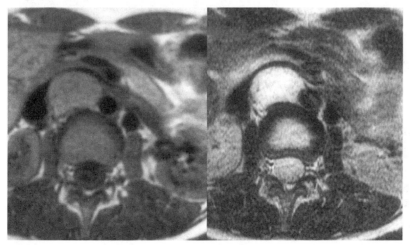

Paraganglioma

Leiomyosarcoma *[Figure 3-4-9]*
- More commonly necrotic than other tumors
- May have intravascular invasion
- May arise in the wall of the IVC

Figure 3-4-9

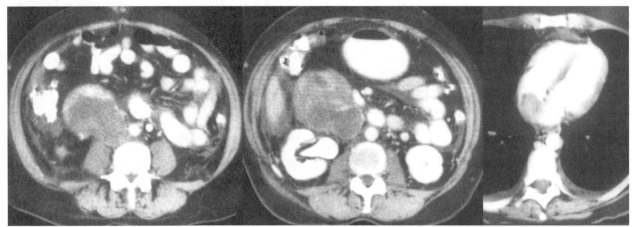

Leiomyosarcoma with IVC invasion

MFH / Malignant fibrous histiocytoma *[Figure 3-4-10]*
- Generally large masses
- Necrosis less common
- T2WI helpful – "Bowl of fruit sign"
  - ➢ Mosaic of low and high signal
    - ❖ Fibrous tissue – low
    - ❖ Myxoid stroma – hyperintense
    - ❖ Soft tissue - intermediate

Lymphangioma *[Figure 3-4-11]*
- Benign
- Fluid-filled
- Uni-multiloculated
- Insinuates itself around organs
- Can be huge

Figure 3-4-10

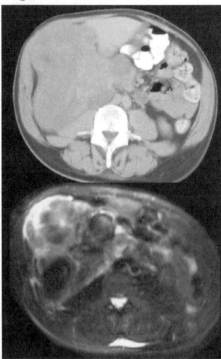

MFH with "bowl of fruit" on T2WI

Figure 3-4-11

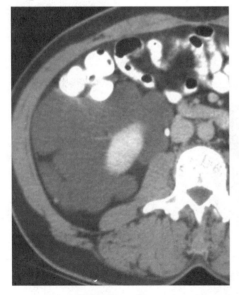

Lymphangioma

Teratoma

- Most are mature (benign) and are cured by surgery
- Children (less than 6 months) and young adults (15–25 years)
- Female:male = 3:1

Teratoma [Figures 3-4-12 and 3-4-13]

- Fat (sebum or adipose tissue)
- Calcification in 90% (may be clump-like)
- Cystic portion in 75%

Figure 3-4-12

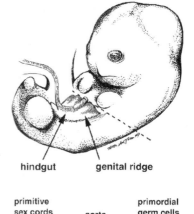

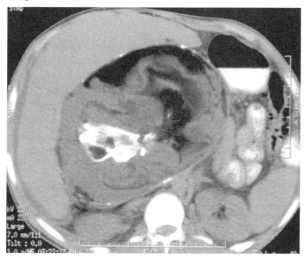

Embryo with germ cells in the retroperitoneum

Figure 3-4-13

Retroperitoneal teratoma

Malignant germ cell tumors are more common in males and are much more likely to be secondary to a testicular tumor (rather than primary retroperitoneal)

Figure 3-4-14

Liposarcoma [Figure 3-4-14 and 3-4-15]

- The most common primary retroperitoneal tumor
- 85% have fat detected by CT or MR
- Well-differentiated, pleomorphic, myxoid, de-differentiated
- Poorly differentiated tumors have no detectable fat by imaging studies

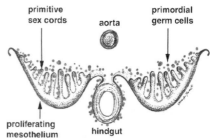

Liposarcoma

Figure 3-4-15   Myxoid liposarcoma with high signal on T2WI

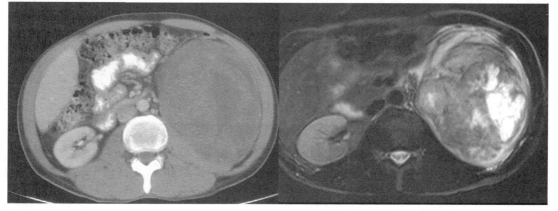

Liposarcoma
- Clinical presentation
  - Often present late
  - Weight gain
- Infiltrative margins
- Complete surgical excision may be difficult
- Local recurrence common

Hyperintense T2WI-Things with a myxoid matrix
- Neurogenic tumors
- Malignant fibrous histiocytoma
- Myxoid liposarcoma

Fat containing retroperitoneal masses
- Liposarcoma: large, heterogeneous
- Teratoma: young patients, calcification, cystic area
- Myelolipoma: usually arising from adrenal
- Angiomyolipoma: arises from kidney, but attachment may be hard to find

Selected references

1.   Engelken JD, Ros PR. Retroperitoneal MR imaging. Magn Reson Imaging Clin N Am 1997; 5:165-178.
2.   Granstrom P, Unger E. MR imaging of the retroperitoneum. Magn Reson Imaging Clin N Am 1995; 3:121-142.
3.   Kim T, Murakami T, Oi H, et al. CT and MR imaging of abdominal liposarcoma. AJR Am J Roentgenol 1996; 166:829-833.
4.   Nishimura H, Zhang Y, Ohkuma K, Uchida M, Hayabuchi N, Sun S. MR imaging of soft-tissue masses of the extraperitoneal spaces. Radiographics 2001; 21:1141-1154.
5.   Nishino M, Hayakawa K, Minami M, Yamamoto A, Ueda H, Takasu K. Primary retroperitoneal neoplasms: CT and MR imaging findings with anatomic and pathologic diagnostic clues. Radiographics 2003; 23:45-57.
6.   Morton A. Meyers. Dynamic Radiology of the Abdomen. Springer-Verlag. A must read book in your residency

Radiologic Evaluation of the Scrotum

Paula J. Woodward, MD
Chief, Genitourinary Radiology
Department of Radiologic Pathology
Armed Forces Institute of Pathology

Embryology
- Sex is chromosomally determined at fertilization
- No morphologic differentiation until week 7 ("indifferent stage")
- Testis determining factor on short arm of Y chromosome
  - ➤ induces formation of seminiferous tubules

3 Components of Gonad *[Figure 3-5-1 to 3-5-4]*
- Germ cells
  - ➤ arise from yolk sac
  - ➤ migrate to genital ridges
- Mesothelium
  - ➤ primitive sex cord
  - ➤ Sertoli cells
- Mesenchyme
  - ➤ Interstium
  - ➤ Leydig cells

Figure 3-5-1

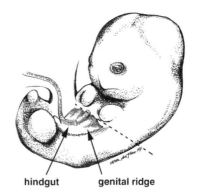

hindgut   genital ridge

*Migration of germ cells along the
hindgut to the genital ridges*

Figure 3-5-2

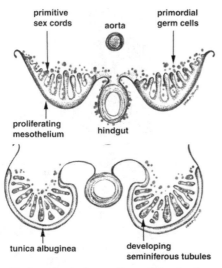

Embryologic formation of the testes

Figure 3-5-3

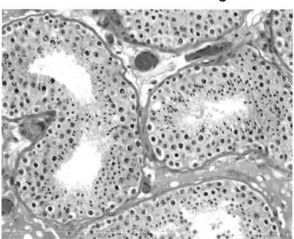

Normal seminiferous tubules

- Leydig cells secrete testosterone
  - ➤ stimulate mesonephric ducts
- Sertoli cells secrete mullerian-inhibiting factor

Figure 3-5-4

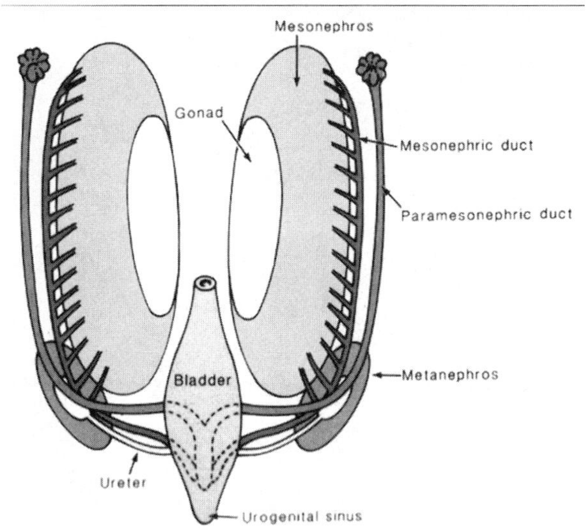

Sex organs at indeterminate stage

Mesonephric (Wolffian) Ducts
- Epididymis
- Vas deferens
- Ejaculatory ducts
- Seminal vesicles

Embryologic Remnants
- Mullerian
  - ➢ appendix testis
- Wolffian
  - ➢ appendix epididymis

Testis [Figure 3-5-5]
- 200-300 lobules
- Seminiferous tubules (300-980 meters)
- Efferent ductules (15-20) converge at mediastinum

Epididymis
- Form single convoluted tubule in head (600 cm)
- Tail loosely attached inferiorly
- Exits as single tube

Spermatic cord [Figure 3-5-6]
- Vas deferns
- Testicular, deferential, cremasteric arteries
- Pampiniform plexus
- Nerves, lymphatics

Ultrasound
- Testes
  - ➢ homogeneous low level echoes
  - ➢ linear echogenic mediastinum testis
- Epididymis
  - ➢ globus major (head), body, tail
  - ➢ iso- to slightly hyperechoic

MRI
- T1WI - homogeneous intermediate signal
- T2WI - high signal with low signal mediastinum testis and linear septations

MRI [Figure 3-5-7]
- Tumors will be low signal masses

Goals of Ultrasound
- Intra-testicular vs. extra-testicular
- Cyst vs. solid

Testicular Neoplasms
- Germ Cell Neoplasms (95%)
- Sex cord, Stromal Tumors
  - ➢ Sertoli cell
  - ➢ Leydig cell
- Lymphoma
- Metastases
- Epidermoid Cysts

Figure 3-5-5

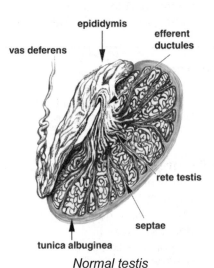

Normal testis

Figure 3-5-6

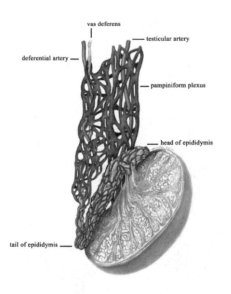

Spermatic cord

Figure 3-5-7

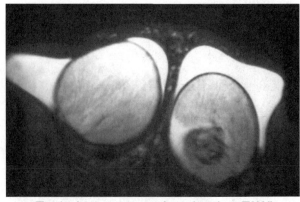

Testicular tumors are low signal on T2WI

Germm Cell Neoplasms
- Seminoma (most common "pure" tumor)
- Embryonal Cell Carcinoma
- Yolk Sac Tumor (Endodermal Sinus Tumor)
- Teratoma
- Choriocarcinoma
- MGCT - Mixed Germ Cell Tumor (most common overall)

Seminoma [Figure 3-5-8]
- Homogeneous, well-defined
- May be lobular and multifocal
- Bilateral 2%
- Peak age 30-40 years
- Radiosensitive
- Good prognosis

Non Seminomatous Germ Cell Tumor [Figure 3-5-9]
- Embryonal
  - ➢ Rare in pure form
  - ➢ 87% of MGCT
- Yolk Sac (endodermal sinus tumor)
  - ➢ Most common childhood tumor
  - ➢ 44% of MGCT
- Teratoma
  - ➢ Mature and immature (always malignant in adults)
  - ➢ Cysts/calcifications common features
- Choriocarcinoma
  - ➢ Very rare
  - ➢ Dismal prognosis

Figure 3-5-8

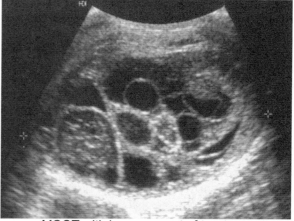

Seminoma

Figure 3-5-9

MGCT with large amount of teratoma

Non Seminomatous Germ Cell Tumor
- Mixed germ cell tumors much more common than any pure tumor
- Heterogeneous, ill-defined
- Peak age 20's
- Not radiosensitive
- Often higher stage and less favorable prognosis than seminoma

Germ Cell Tumors: Modes of Spread
- Lymphatic
  - ➢ ipsilateral renal hilum
- Hematogeous
  - ➢ common with choriocarcinoma
  - ➢ lung, liver, brain

Tumor Markers
- Alpha-fetoprotein (AFP)
  - ➢ from fetal liver, GI tract, and yolk sac
  - ➢ elevated in tumors with yolk sac elements
- Human chorionic gonadotropin (HCG)
  - ➢ produced by syncytiotrophoblasts from developing placenta
  - ➢ elevated in tumors with choriocarcinoma (occasional seminoma)
- LDH
  - ➢ Non-specific, correlates with bulk of disease
- Elevated in 80% of non-seminomatous tumors

Burned-Out Germ Cell Tumor
- Presents with metastases (often extensive)
- The primary may not contain any active tumor and may be difficult to identify
- Orchiectomy performed if any suspicious area seen

Testicular Microlithiasis
- 0.6% in general population
- Present in 40% of germ cell tumors
- Usually bilateral
- Consider annual screening

Risk Factors for Testicular Carcinoma
- Prior testicular tumor
- Cryptorchidism
- Infertility
- Family history
- Intersex syndormes (hermaphrodite)
- ??? microcalcifications

Cryptorchidism [Figure 3-5-10]
- 5% testicular agenesis
- 65% migratory testis
- 30% undescended
- Increased incidence of malignancy
- Risk is also increased in the contralateral testis

Sex Cord, Stromal Tumors [Figure 3-5-11]
- Sertoli (sex cord) and Leydig (stromal)
- 90% benign
- More common in pediatric age group
- May be be hormonally active
  - ➢ precocious puberty, gynecomastia
  - ➢ more common with Leydig
- Sertoli cell tumors may be bilateral and calcified

Testicular Lymphoma – Presentation
- Most common testis tumor > 60 yo
- 5% of testicular neoplasms
- < 1% of patients with lymphoma
- Often presents as the site of recurrent disease because of "blood-testis barrier" (Sertoli cells)

Testicular Lymphoma – Imaging [Figure 3-5-12]
- Most common bilateral tumor
- Homogeneous
- Epididymis and spermatic cord often involved

Epidermoid Cyst [Figure 3-5-13]
- Benign
- ? germ cell tumor
- Filled with keratin
- Well-defined, ringed-appearance
- Can not differentiate from a malignant neoplasm

Figure 3-5-10

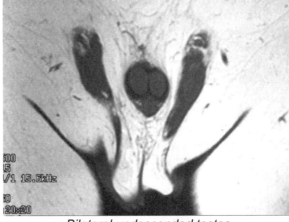

Bilateral undescended testes

Figure 3-5-11

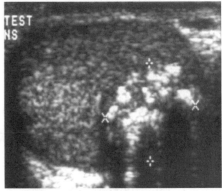

Sertoli cell tumor with calcification

Figure 3-5-12

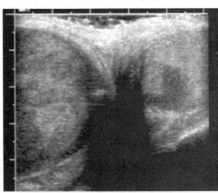

Lymphoma with bilateral testicular masses

Figure 3-5-13

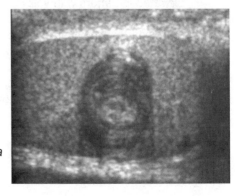

Concentric rings in a epidermoid cyst

Tumors Summary
- Children
  - ➤ Yolk sac tumor
  - ➤ Sertoli, Leydig cell
- Mixed germ cell tumor
  - ➤ Younger men (20s)
  - ➤ Heterogeneous, poorly defined
- Seminoma
  - ➤ Somewhat older (30s)
  - ➤ Homogeneous
- Lymphoma
  - ➤ Older males
  - ➤ Bilateral
  - ➤ May involve paratesticular tissues

Non-neoplastic Testicular Masses
- Tubular ectasia
- Cysts
- Sarcoidosis
- Adrenal rests
- Acute scrotum
  - ➤ infection
  - ➤ infarction
  - ➤ trauma

Tubular Ectasia
- Dilatation of the rete testis
- Often bilateral
- Associated with a spermatocele
- Tubular US appearance
- Iso- to hyperintense on T2WI

Testicular Cysts [Figure 3-5-14]
- Peripheral
  - ➤ Tunica albuginea cyst
- Central
  - ➤ Must be careful to differentiate from cystic neoplasm
  - ➤ Can not have any solid component
  - ➤ Often associated with dilated rete testis

Sarcoidosis [Figure 3-5-15]
- Multisystem chronic granulomatous disorder
- 5% will have genital involvement
- Epididymis more commonly involved
- More common in Blacks (testicular tumors are rare)

Adrenal rest hypertrophy secondary to congenital adrenal hyperplasia [Figure 3-5-16]
- Adrenal rests in 7.5-15% of newborns, 1.6% adults
- Hypertrophy when exposed to elevated ACTH
- Bilateral, multiple, eccentric
- Tx – glucocorticoids not orchiectomy

Bilateral Testicular Masses
- Lymphoma
- Seminoma (rarely)
- Metastases
- Sarcoidosis
- Adrenal rests

Figure 3-5-14

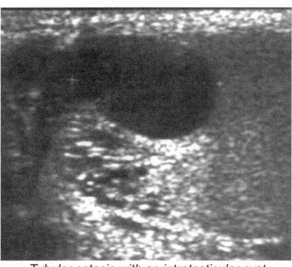

Tubular ectasia with an intratesticular cyst

Figure 3-5-15

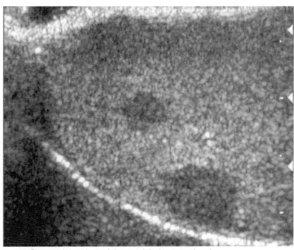

Sarcoidosis with multiple testicular masses

Figure 3-5-16

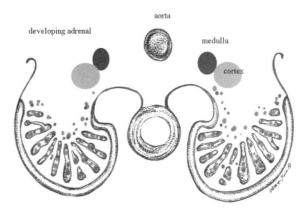

Developing adrenals

Extratesticular Scrotal Masses

Figure 3-5-17

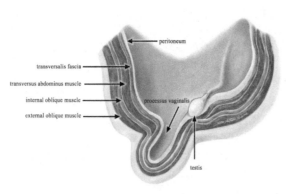

Developing scrotum

Figure 3-5-18

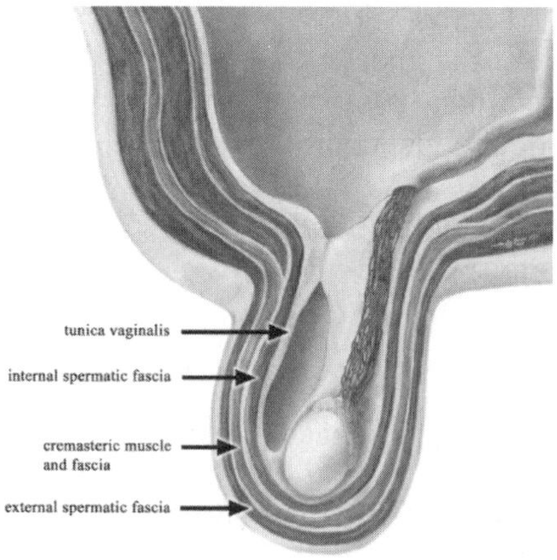

Adult scrotum

Hydrocele
- Fluid between the parietal and visceral layers of the tunica vaginalis
- Small amount is normal

Hydrocele
- Congenital
  - Patent processus vaginalis, may have an inguinal hernia
- Acquired
  - Infection, infarction, trauma, tumor

Figure 3-5-19

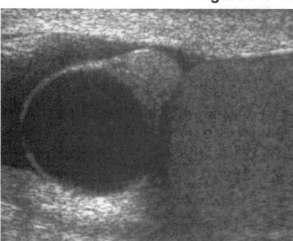

Epididymal cyst

Scrotal Calculi
- Torsion of appendix or inflammatory deposits
- Repeated microtrauma
  - bikers
- Variable size and calcification
- Mobile

Epididymal Masses
- Cyst, Spermatocele *[Figure 3-5-19*
- Infection
  - Bacterial (acute)
  - TB (chronic)
- Tumors
  - Adenomatoid tumor
  - Papillary cystadenoma (von Hippel-Lindau)
  - Lymphoma
- Sarcoidosis

Figure 3-5-20

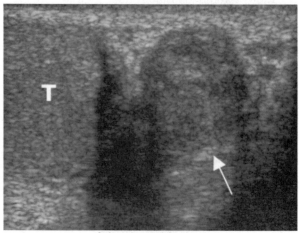

Adenomatoid tumor

Adenomatoid Tumor *[Figure 3-5-20]*
- Benign
- Most common epididymal tumor
- Solid, small, well-circumscribed

Papillary Cystadenoma
- Associated with VHL (70%)
- 40% bilateral
- Benign

Epididymal and Testicular Mass

- Lymphoma
  - Testicular involvement greater than epididymis
- Sarcoidosis [Figure 3-5-21]
  - Epididymal involvement greater than testis
  - More common in Blacks
- Infection
  - Bacterial (acute)
  - TB (chronic)

Tuberculosis

- Epididymis primary site with testis secondarily involved
- 30% bilateral
- 50% will have abscess or fistulas

Figure 3-5-21

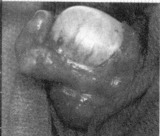

Sarcoidosis with marked epididymal enlargement

Acute Scrotum

- Trauma
- Epididymitis/orchitis
- Torsion

Acute Epididymitis

- Bacterial infection from lower urinary tract - chlamydia, gonococcus, E coli
- US findings - enlarged, hypoechoic, hyperemia, hydrocele, skin thickening
- 20% have associated orchitis

Orchitis

- Usually secondary to epididymitis
- May rarely be focal
- US findings - enlarged, heterogeneous echogenicity, hyperemia
- May lead to focal ischemia/infarction

Fournier Gangrene

- Diabetics or other immunosuppression
- Scrotal abscess with necrotizing infection of the perineum
- Surgical emergency

Torsion

- Gray scale US may be normal early
- Decreased or absent flow with Doppler
  - Compare with normal side
  - Venous compromise occurs first
- Look for mass in inguinal canal
- Testis becomes enlarged and hypoechoic with time

Torsion

- < 6 hrs at diagnosis salvage rate 80-100%
- 12 hr salvage rate 20%

Paratesticular masses

- Varicocele
- Fibrous pseudotumors
- Polyorchidism
- Neoplasms
  - Lipomas
    - Half of all spermatic cord tumors
  - Liposarcoma
  - Rhabdosarcoma, leiomyosarcoma, MFH
  - Mesothelioma

Varicocele [Figure 3-5-22]

- \> 3mm
- Idiopathic
  - ➢ incompetent valves
  - ➢ more common on left (bilateral 10%)
    - longer course
    - more perpendicular insertion
    - "nutcracker" effect of left renal vein under SMA
- Secondary to abdominal mass

Varicocele

- 15% of general population
- 40% of men with infertility
- ? increased temperature
- improved pregnancy rates (35-50%) with repair even if subclinical

Fibrous Pseudotumor [Figure 3-5-23]

- Hylanized collagen and granulation tissue
- Attached to tunica albuginea
- US non-specific
- MRI low signal intensity

Polyorchidism

- abnormal division of genital ridge
- often abnormal spermatogenesis
- increased risk of torsion

Paratesticular Neoplasms

- lipomas [Figure 3-5-24]
- liposarcoma [Figure 3-5-25]
- rhabdosarcoma
- leiomyosarcoma
- MFH
- mesothelioma

Lipoma [Figure 3-5-24]

- Most common extratesticular neoplasm
- Half of all cord tumors
- Variable by ultrasound
  - ➢ may be homogenously hypoechoic
- MR with fat suppression helpful

Figure 3-5-22

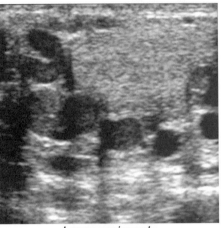

Large varicocele

Figure 3-5-23

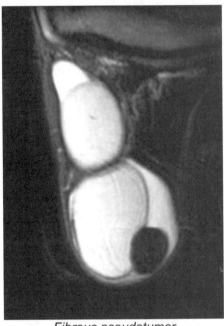

Fibrous pseudotumor

Figure 3-5-24

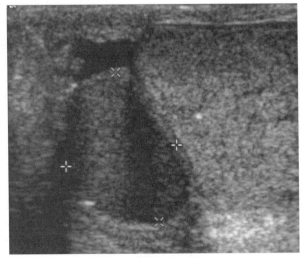

Lipoma

Figure 3-5-25

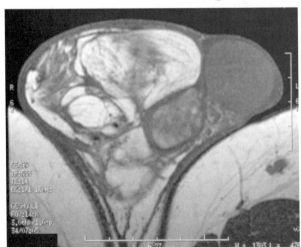

Liposarcoma

Mesiothelioma [Figure 3-5-26]

- Tunica vaginalis lined with mesothelial cells
- Much less common then pleural or peritoneal
- Benign and malignant
- Often present with hydrocele

Selected References

1. Black JA, Patel A. Sonography of the abnormal extratesticular space. AJR Am J Roentgenol 1996; 167:507-511.
2. Black JA, Patel A. Sonography of the normal extratesticular space. AJR Am J Roentgenol 1996; 167:503-506.
3. Bostwick DG. Spermatic cord and testicular adnexa. In: Bostwick DG, Eble JN, eds. Urologic surgcial pathology. St. Louis: Mosby, 1997; 647-674.
4. Chung JJ, Kim MJ, Lee T, Yoo HS, Lee JT. Sonographic findings in tuberculous epididymitis and epididymo-orchitis. J Clin Ultrasound 1997; 25:390-394.
5. Cramer BM, Schlegel EA, Thueroff JW. MR imaging in the differential diagnosis of scrotal and testicular disease. Radiographics 1991; 11:9-21.
6. Doherty FJ. Ultrasound of the nonacute scrotum. Semin Ultrasound CT MR 1991; 12:131-156.
7. Feuer A, Dewire DM, Foley WD. Ultrasonographic characteristics of testicular adenomatoid tumors. J Urol 1996; 155:174-175.
8. Frates MC, Benson CB, DiSalvo DN, Brown DL, Laing FC, Doubilet PM. Solid extratesticular masses evaluated with sonography: pathologic correlation. Radiology 1997; 204:43-46.
9. Geraghty MJ, Lee FT, Jr., Bernsten SA, Gilchrist K, Pozniak MA, Yandow DJ. Sonography of testicular tumors and tumor-like conditions: a radiologic-pathologic correlation. Crit Rev Diagn Imaging 1998; 39:1-63.
10. Grebenc ML, Gorman JD, Sumida FK. Fibrous pseudotumor of the tunica vaginalis testis: imaging appearance. Abdom Imaging 1995; 20:379-380.
11. Heaton ND, Hogan B, Michell M, Thompson P, Yates-Bell AJ. Tuberculous epididymo-orchitis: clinical and ultrasound observations. Br J Urol 1989; 64:305-309.
12. Horstman WG, Middleton WD, Melson GL. Scrotal inflammatory disease: color Doppler US findings. Radiology 1991; 179:55-59.
13. Kassis A. Testicular adenomatoid tumours: clinical and ultrasonographic characteristics. BJU Int 2000; 85:302-304.
14. Kim ED, Lipshultz LI. Role of ultrasound in the assessment of male infertility. J Clin Ultrasound 1996; 24:437-453.
15. Kutchera WA, Bluth EI, Guice SL. Sonographic findings of a spermatic cord lipoma. Case report and review of the literature. J Ultrasound Med 1987; 6:457-460.
16. Mattrey RF. Magnetic resonance imaging of the scrotum. Semin Ultrasound CT MR 1991; 12:95-108.
17. Ragheb D, Higgins JL, Jr. Ultrasonography of the scrotum: technique, anatomy, and pathologic entities. J Ultrasound Med 2002; 21:171-185.
18. Sudakoff GS, Quiroz F, Karcaaltincaba M, Foley WD. Scrotal ultrasonography with emphasis on the extratesticular space: anatomy, embryology, and pathology. Ultrasound Q 2002; 18:255-273.
19. Tessler FN, Tublin ME, Rifkin MD. Ultrasound assessment of testicular and paratesticular masses. J Clin Ultrasound 1996; 24:423-436.
20. Woodward PJ, Schwab CM, Sesterhenn IA. From the archives of the AFIP: extratesticular scrotal masses: radiologic-pathologic correlation. Radiographics 2003; 23:215-240.
21. Woodward PJ, Sohaey R, O'Donoghue MJ, Green DE. From the Archives of the AFIP: Tumors and Tumorlike Lesions of the Testis: Radiologic-Pathologic Correlation. Radiographics 2002; 22:189-216.

Figure 3-5-26

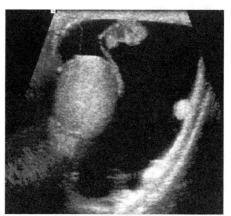

Mesothelioma with nodules and hydrocele

First Trimester Ultrasound

Paula J. Woodward, MD
Chief, Genitourinary Radiology
Department of Radiologic Pathology
Armed Forces Institute of Pathology

Figure 3-6-1

Ovarian Period: (Weeks 1–2)
- Ovarian follicle matures
- Ovulation
- Corpus luteum formation

Conceptus Period: (Week 3–5)
- Fertilization
- Morula (16 cells)
- Blastocyst
- Trilaminar embryo

Embryonic Period: (Weeks 6–10)
- C-shaped embryo
- Major organs develop
- Yolk sac detaches

Fetal Period: (Weeks 11–12)
- Fetal growth
- Amniotic and chorionic membranes approach each other

Gestational Sac
- Visualized as early as 4.5 wks (TV)
- Intradecidual sign *[Figure 3-6-1]*
- Double decidual sac sign *[Figure 3-6-2]*
  - ➤ Basalis [DB]
  - ➤ Capsularis [DC]
  - ➤ Parietalis [DP]

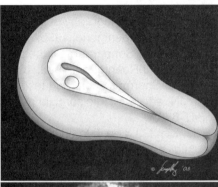

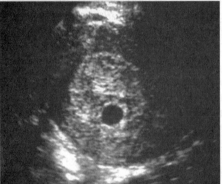

Intradecidual sac sign

Figure 3-6-2

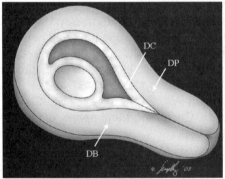

Double decidual sac sign

Gestational Sac = Chorionic Sac

[Figures 3-6-3 and 3-6-4]

- Chorionic laeve = Smooth chorion = Chorionic membrane
- Chorionic frondosum + Decidua basalis = Placenta

Figure 3-6-3

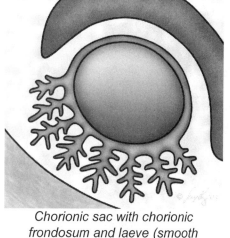

Chorionic sac with chorionic frondosum and laeve (smooth chorion)

Figure 3-6-4

Series of 5 illustrations showing normal 1st trimester development with expansion of the amnion and detachment of the yolk sac

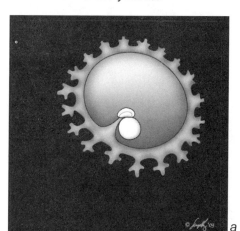

a

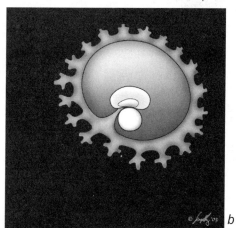

b

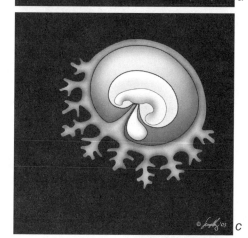

c

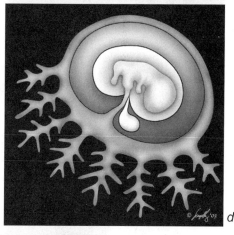

d

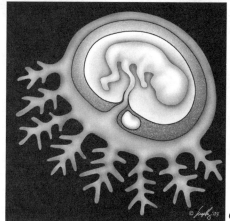

e

Yolk sac [Figures 3-6-5 and 3-6-6]
- Visualized at 5 – 5.5 weeks

Figure 3-6-5

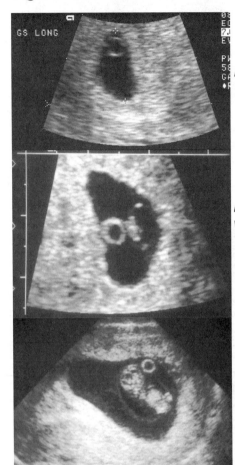

Normal yolk sac at 5.5 wks

Normal 6.5 week embryo with "double bleb" or "diamond ring" sign

7 week embryo surrounded by amnion

Figure 3-6-6

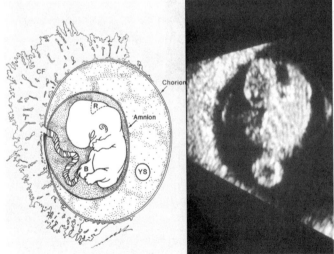

Normal first trimester US including rhombencephalon and bowel herniation

Multiple Gestations
- Types of Twinning
  - Dizygotic (70%)
    2 eggs
  - Monozygotic (70%)
    single egg

Multiple Gestations
- # of chorions equals # of placentas
  - sharing is bad
  - risk for twin/twin transfusion
- # of amnions equals # of separate sacs
  - sharing is really bad
  - risk for cord accidents

Dizygotic Twins *[Figure 3-6-7]*
Dizygotic must be dichorionic (2 placentas) and diamniotic (2 sacs)

Monozygotic Twins
- 1/3 are Dichorionic/Diamniotic
  - cleavage by day 3
- 2/3 are Monochorionic/Diamniotic *[Figure 3-6-8]*
  - cleavage day 4-8
- Rare (approx 1%) Monochorionic/Monoamniotic *[Figure 3-6-9]*]
  - cleavage > 8 days
- Conjoined twins
  - cleavage > 14 days

Figure 3-6-7

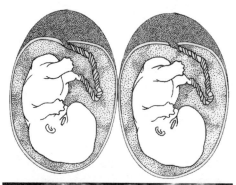
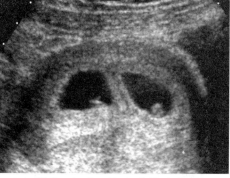

Dichorionic, diamniotic twins

Figure 3-6-8

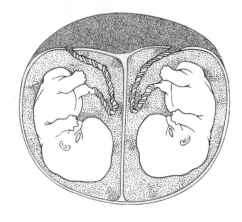
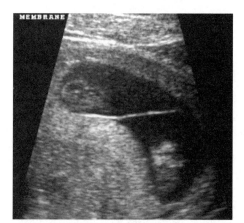

Monochorionic, diamniotic twins

Figure 3-6-9

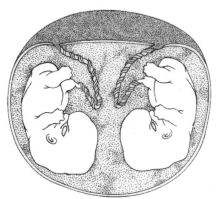

Monochorionic, monoamniotic twins

AIUM Guidelines: First Trimester
- Gestational sac
  - Location
  - Mean Sac Diameter (MSD)
    MSD = (L+W+D)/3
  - Yolk sac
- Embryo
  - Crown rump length
  - Cardiac Activity
- Fetal number
  - Chorionicity/Amnionicity
- Uterus, adnexa, cul-de-sac

- Threshold Level - the size at which a finding may be seen
- Discriminatory Level - the size at which a finding must be seen

	Threshold Level – MSD	Discriminatory Level – MSD
Gestational Sac	2 mm	5 mm
Yolk Sac	TV 4 mm	TV10 mm TA 20 mm
Embryo	TV 8 mm	TV 18 mm TA 25 mm
Heartbeat	2 mm (CRL)	5 mm (CRL)

Major: Discriminators
- MSD > 10 mm **must** have a yolk sac
- MSD > 18 mm **must** have an embryo
- CRL > 5mm **must** have a heartbeat

Cardiac Activity
- Must be present if embryo is >= 5 mm
- 5–6 weeks   100–110 bpm
- 8–9 weeks   150–170 bpm

Abnormal Frist Trimester
- 25% threatened abortion
- Embryonic demise
- Bradycardia
- Anembryonic pregnancy *[Figure 3-6-10]*
- Perigestational hemorrhage *[Figure 3-6-11]*
- Abnormal yolk sac
- Poor growth

Anembryonic Pregnancy *[Figure 3-6-10]*
- Major discriminators
  - MSD > 10 mm without a yolk sac
  - MSD > 18 mm without a fetal pole
- Minor discriminators
  - weak decidual reaction
  - abnormal shape or location
  - empty amnion

Figure 3-6-10

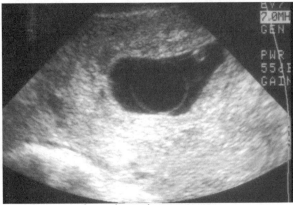

*Anembryonic pregnancy
with empty amnion*

Figure 3-6-11

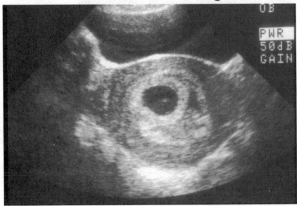

Perigestational hemorrhage

Yolk Sac
- First landmark in gestational sac
- In the chorionic cavity
- Abnormal findings:
  - ➤ >6mm
  - ➤ irregular shape
  - ➤ calcifications
  - ➤ multiple yolk sacs

Growth
- Normal growth rate 1 mm per day

Ectopic pregnancy
- Tubal 95%
- Unusual locations 5%
  - ➤ Interstitial
  - ➤ Cervix
  - ➤ Ovary
  - ➤ Abdominal
- 1:50-1:200 live births
- Risks factors: IUD, prior ectopic, PID, tubal surgery, infertility treatment

Ectopic pregnancy: Uterine Findings *[Figure 3-6-12 and 3-6-13]*
- No gestational sac
- Thickened endometrium
- Pseudogestational sac
- Discriminatory hCG levels
  - ➤ hCG >1,000 IU/L (2nd IS)
  - ➤ hCG >2,000 IU/L (3rd IRP)

Figure 3-6-12

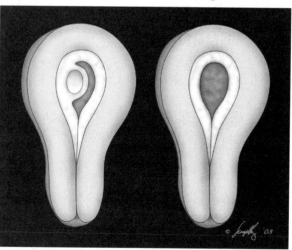

Double decidual sac sign vs. pseudosac

Figure 3-6-13

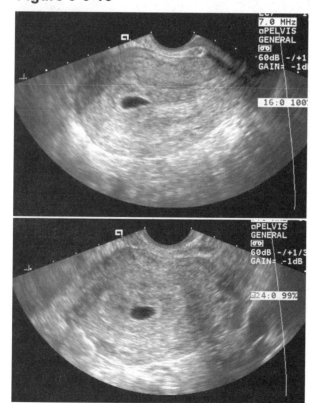

Pseudosac

Ectopic pregnancy: Adnexal Findings [Figure 3-6-14]

- Living extrauterine embryo
- Echogenic ring +/- yolk sac
  - "ring of fire"
- Adnexal mass (clot)
- Cul-de-sac blood
- Normal adnexa

Heterotopic pregnancy

- 1 in 30,000 spontaneous pregnancies
- 1 in 4,000 assisted pregnancies

Interstitial pregnancy [Figure 3-6-15]

- Isthmus
- Rupture later – catastrophic bleeding
- Eccentric
- Lack of encircling myometrium
- Interstitial line sign

Management of Ectopic pregnancy

- Surgical
  - Salpingectomy
  - Salpingostomy
- Medical
  - Systemic methotrexate
  - Intragestational methotrexate
  - Intragestational KCl

Systemic Methotrexate

- Preserves fallopian tube
- Non-invasive
- Outpatient
- Criteria
  - Mass < 4cm
  - No bleeding
  - hCG <3,000 IU/L (2IS)
  - No formed fetal parts

Cutting Edge

- Sonoembryology
- Early diagnosis of major malformations
- Screen for aneuploidy
  - nuchal translucency
  - hypoplastic nasal bone
  - abnormal flow in ductus venosus

Nuchal Translucency
Screen for Trisomy 21 [Figure 3-6-16]

- Accredited lab
- 11-14 weeks
- >3mm abnormal
- Risk assessment based on age, NT, serum screen
- High detection rates (75-90%)
  - nuchal translucency
  - hypoplastic nasal bone
  - abnormal flow in ductus venosus

Figure 3-6-14

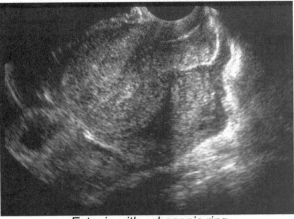

*Ectopic with echogenic ring
and blood in the cul-de-sac*

Figure 3-6-15

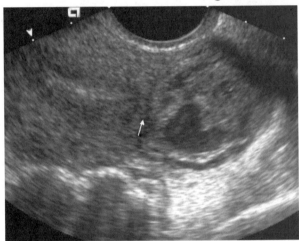

Cornual ectopic with interstitial line sign

Figure 3-6-16

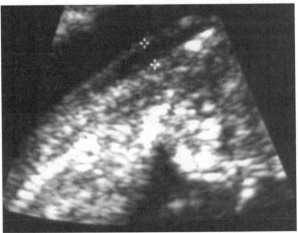

*Increased nuchal translucency in
Down syndrome*

Selected References

1. Ackerman TE, Levi CS, Dashefsky SM, Holt SC, Lindsay DJ. Interstitial line: sonographic finding in interstitial (cornual) ectopic pregnancy. Radiology 1993; 189:83-87.
2. Brown DL, Emerson DS, Felker RE, Cartier MS, Smith WC. Diagnosis of early embryonic demise by endovaginal sonography. J Ultrasound Med 1990; 9:631-636.
3. Brown DL, Doubilet PM. Transvaginal sonography for diagnosing ectopic pregnancy: positivity criteria and performance characteristics. J Ultrasound Med 1994; 13:259-266.
4. Dickey RP, Olar TT, Curole DN, Taylor SN, Matulich EM. Relationship of first-trimester subchorionic bleeding detected by color Doppler ultrasound to subchorionic fluid, clinical bleeding, and pregnancy outcome. Obstet Gynecol 1992; 80:415-420.
5. Frates MC, Brown DL, Doubilet PM, Hornstein MD. Tubal rupture in patients with ectopic pregnancy: diagnosis with transvaginal US. Radiology 1994; 191:769-772.
6. Frates MC, Benson CB, Doubilet PM, et al. Cervical ectopic pregnancy: results of conservative treatment. Radiology 1994; 191:773-775.
7. Frates MC, Laing FC. Sonographic evaluation of ectopic pregnancy: an update. AJR Am J Roentgenol 1995; 165:251-259.
8. Jarjour L, Kletzky OA. Reliability of transvaginal ultrasound in detecting first trimester pregnancy abnormalities. Fertil Steril 1991; 56:202-207.
9. Jurkovic D, Gruboeck K, Campbell S. Ultrasound features of normal early pregnancy development. Curr Opin Obstet Gynecol 1995; 7:493-504.
10. Nyberg DA, Mack LA, Laing FC, Patten RM. Distinguishing normal from abnormal gestational sac growth in early pregnancy. J Ultrasound Med 1987; 6:23-27.
11. Nyberg DA, Filly RA, Laing FC, Mack LA, Zarutskie PW. Ectopic pregnancy. Diagnosis by sonography correlated with quantitative HCG levels. J Ultrasound Med 1987; 6:145-150.
12. Oh JS, Wright G, Coulam CB. Gestational sac diameter in very early pregnancy as a predictor of fetal outcome. Ultrasound Obstet Gynecol 2002; 20:267-269.
13. Rempen A. Diagnosis of viability in early pregnancy with vaginal sonography. J Ultrasound Med 1990; 9:711-716.
14. Sohaey R, Woodward P, Zwiebel WJ. First-trimester ultrasound: the essentials. Semin Ultrasound CT MR 1996; 17:2-14.
15. van Leeuwen I, Branch DW, Scott JR. First-trimester ultrasonography findings in women with a history of recurrent pregnancy loss. Am J Obstet Gynecol 1993; 168:111-114.

Fetal CNS Malformations

Paula J. Woodward, MD
Chief, Genitourinary Radiology
Department of Radiologic Pathology
Armed Forces Institute of Pathology

Figure 3-7-1

Fetal Brain [Figure 3-7-1]

- Ventricular Plane
  - ➤ atrium and choroid
- BPD Plane
  - ➤ thalami
  - ➤ third ventricle
  - ➤ cavum septi pellucidi
- Posterior Fossa
  - ➤ cerebellum
  - ➤ cisterna magna
  - ➤ nuchal skin thickeness

Fetal MRI

- Fast T2WI (SSFSE, HASTE)
- Safety issues
  - ➤ No known deleterious effects
  - ➤ Do not perform in the first trimester
  - ➤ Do not give gadolinium
  - ➤ Obtain informed consent

Congenital CNS Malformations

- Dorsal Induction
  - ➤ anencephaly
  - ➤ encephalocele
  - ➤ spina bifida
- Ventral Induction
  - ➤ holoprosencephaly
  - ➤ Dandy-Walker malformation
- Neuronal Proliferation
  - ➤ microcephaly
  - ➤ macrocephaly
  - ➤ tumors
- Migration
  - ➤ agenesis of corpus callosum

There is too much fluid in there

- Hydrocephalus
- Holoprosencephaly
- Hydranencephaly

Hydranencephaly

- Absent cerebral hemispheres
- Occlusion of ICA -? etiology
  - ➤ infection
  - ➤ vasculitis
  - ➤ emboli
- Falx
- Normal facial development

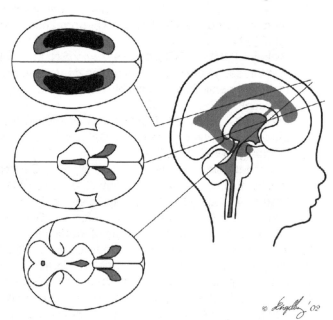

3 required images of the fetal brain

Holoprosencephaly [Figures 3-7-2 to 3-7-4]

- Spectrum of arrested development
  - alobar
  - semilobar
  - lobar
- Absent cavum, absent falx, fused thalami, dorsal sac
- Midline facial defects
  - proboscis
  - cyclopia
  - midline cleft
- Trisomy 13

Figure 3-7-2

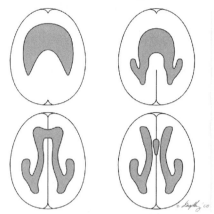

Alobar, semilobar lobar holoprosencephaly compared to normal.

Figure 3-7-3

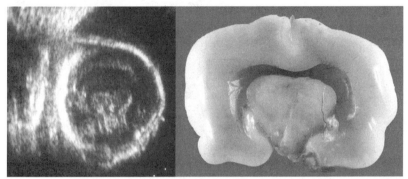

Alobar holoprosencephaly with single ventricle

Hydrocephalus

- Dilated ventricles and enlarged head

Ventriculomegaly

- Dilated ventricles

Signs

- Lateral ventricle > 10mm
- Medial ventricular wall to choroid > 3mm
- Dangling choroid

Hydrocephalus: Differential

- Aqueductal Stenosis
- Dandy-Walker Malformation
- Chiari II
- Communicating Hydrocephalus

Aqueductal Stenosis [Figures 3-7-5]

- Block at aqueduct of Sylvius
- Most common cause of hydrocephalus
- Male predominance (X-linked form)

Figure 3-7-4

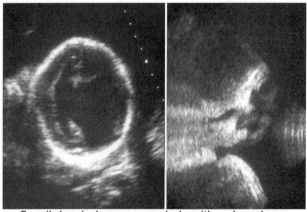

Semilobar holoprosencephaly with a dorsal sac. Face shows a midline cleft.

Figure 3-7-5

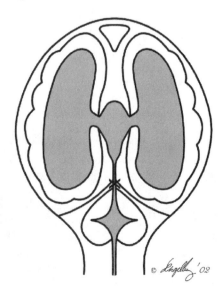

Aqueductal stenosis with dilatation of the lateral and third ventricles.

Dandy-Walker Malformation *[Figures 3-7-6 and 3-7-7]*

- Communicating PF cyst
- Hydrocephalus +/-
- 50 have accociated abnormality

Figure 3-7-6

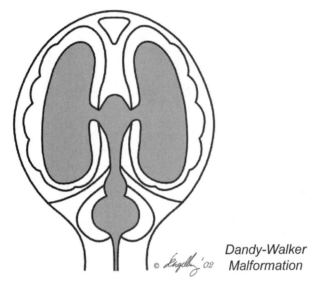

Dandy-Walker Malformation

Figure 3-7-7

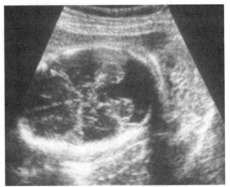

Dandy-Walker Malformation with enlargement of the 4th ventricle and posterior fossa cyst.

Chiari II *[Figures 3-7-8 to 3-7-10]*

- Downward herniation of the 4th ventricle and vermis
- Myelomeningocele
- Hydrocephalus
- "Lemon" and "Banana" sign

Figure

3-7-8

3-7-9

3-7-10

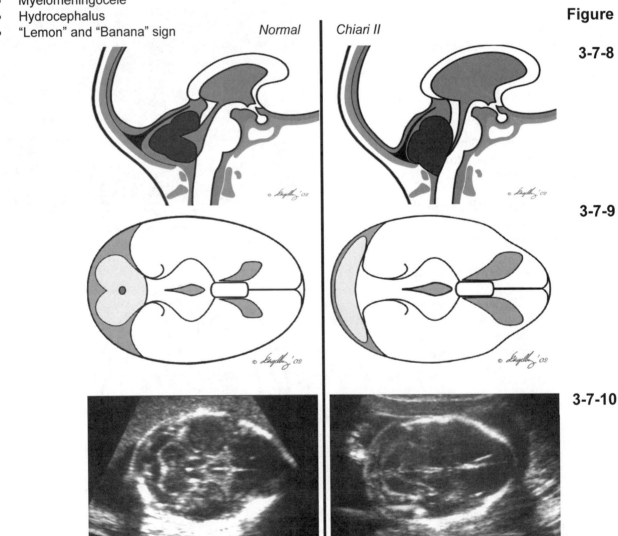

Normal   Chiari II

Communicating Hydrocephalus [Figure 3-7-11]

- Dilatation of all ventricles and subarachnoid space
- Etiology
  - ➢ hemorrhage
  - ➢ ? abnormal arachnoid granulations
  - ➢ ? abnormal superior sagittal sinus

Hydrocephalus: Differential

- Aqueductal Stenosis
- Dandy-Walker Malformation
- Chiari II
- Communicating Hydrocephalus

Agenesis of the Corpus Callosum [Figure 3-7-12]

- Tear-dropped shaped ventricules (Colpocephaly)
- Absent cavum septi pellucidi
- Associated with lipomas and arachnoid cysts
- Often missed or confused with mild ventriculomegaly

Neural Tube Defects

- Anencephaly
- Spina Bifida
- Encephalocele
- Acrania

Anencephaly [Figure 3-7-13]

- Absent cranium and cerebral hemispheres
- Area cerebrovasculosa

Figure 3-7-11

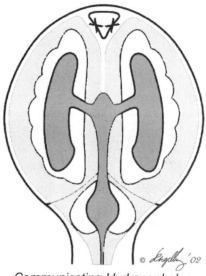

Communicating Hydrocephalus

Figure 3-7-12

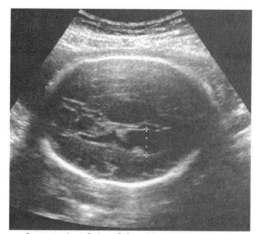

Agenesis of the CC with colpocephaly and arachnoid cyst

Figure 3-7-13

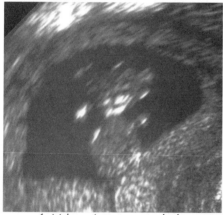

1st trimester anencephaly

Encephalocele [Figure 3-7-14]

- 75% occipital
- Frontal – Southeast Asia
- Evaluate brain tissue
- 80% have associated malformations

Choroid Plexus Cysts

- 30% of trisomy 18
- 1–2% of normals
- 1/500 chance of trisomy 18

Figure 3-7-14

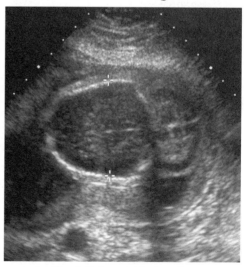

Occipital encephalocele

Trisomy 18 [Figure 3-7-15]

- Overlapping Fingers
- Cardiac Defects
- Omphalocele/Diaphragmatic Hernia
- Choroid plexus cysts

Figure 3-7-15

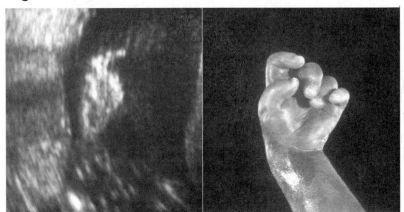

Trisomy 18 with overlapping fingers

Selected references

1. Chang MC, Russell SA, Callen PW, Filly RA, Goldstein RB. Sonographic detection of inferior vermian agenesis in Dandy-Walker malformations: prognostic implications. Radiology 1994; 193:765-770.
2. Chatzipapas IK, Whitlow BJ, Economides DL. The 'Mickey Mouse' sign and the diagnosis of anencephaly in early pregnancy. Ultrasound Obstet Gynecol 1999; 13:196-199.
3. Coleman BG, Adzick NS, Crombleholme TM, et al. Fetal therapy: state of the art. J Ultrasound Med 2002; 21:1257-1288.
4. d'Ercole C, Girard N, Cravello L, et al. Prenatal diagnosis of fetal corpus callosum agenesis by ultrasonography and magnetic resonance imaging. Prenat Diagn 1998; 18:247-253.
5. Ghidini A, Strobelt N, Locatelli A, Mariani E, Piccoli MG, Vergani P. Isolated fetal choroid plexus cysts: role of ultrasonography in establishment of the risk of trisomy 18. Am J Obstet Gynecol 2000; 182:972-977.
6. Goldstein RB, LaPidus AS, Filly RA. Fetal cephaloceles: diagnosis with US. Radiology 1991; 180:803-808.
7. Johnson SP, Sebire NJ, Snijders RJ, Tunkel S, Nicolaides KH. Ultrasound screening for anencephaly at 10-14 weeks of gestation. Ultrasound Obstet Gynecol 1997; 9:14-16.
8. Levitsky DB, Mack LA, Nyberg DA, et al. Fetal aqueductal stenosis diagnosed sonographically: how grave is the prognosis? AJR Am J Roentgenol 1995; 164:725-730.
9. McGahan JP, Nyberg DA, Mack LA. Sonography of facial features of alobar and semilobar holoprosencephaly. AJR Am J Roentgenol 1990; 154:143-148.
10. Pilu G, Romero R, Rizzo N, Jeanty P, Bovicelli L, Hobbins JC. Criteria for the prenatal diagnosis of holoprosencephaly. Am J Perinatol 1987; 4:41-49.
11. Ulm B, Ulm MR, Deutinger J, Bernaschek G. Dandy-Walker malformation diagnosed before 21 weeks of gestation: associated malformations and chromosomal abnormalities. Ultrasound Obstet Gynecol 1997; 10:167-170.
12. Vergani P, Ghidini A, Strobelt N, et al. Prognostic indicators in the prenatal diagnosis of agenesis of corpus callosum. Am J Obstet Gynecol 1994; 170:753-758.

Fetal Anomalies

Paula J. Woodward, MD
Chief, Genitourinary Radiology
Department of Radiologic Pathology
Armed Forces Institute of Pathology

Neck Masses
- Neural Tube Defects
- Cystic Hygroma
- Teratoma (Epignathus)
- Thyroid

Cystic Hygroma *[Figure 3-8-1]*
- Lymphangioma
- Chromosomal Abnormalities
  - ➢ Turners Syndrome XO
  - ➢ Trisomy 21 (2nd trimester nuchal thickening)
- Often associated with hydrops

Iniencephaly *[Figure 3-8-2]*
- Fixed hyperextension of neck ("stargazer" position)
- Rachischisis
- Cephalocele
- Shortened or absent vertebral bodies
- First trimester
  - ➢ head appears large
  - ➢ CRL less than expected

AIUM: Chest *[Figure 3-8-4 and 3-8-5]*
- Four chamber heart
  - ➢ side (stomach and heart both on left)
  - ➢ axis ~35-45°
  - ➢ equal chamber size
  - ➢ excludes 90% of cardiac defect
- LVOT, RVOT if feasible

Figure 3-8-1

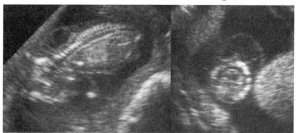

Sagittal and transverse images through the fetal neck show a cystic hygroma

Figure 3-8-2   **Figure 3-8-3**

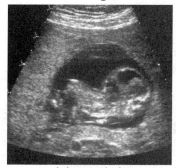   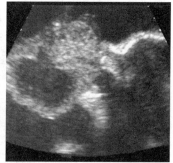

Iniencephaly   *Epignathus (teratoma)*

Figure 3-8-4

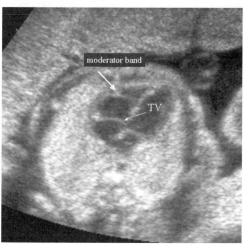

Four-chamber view of normal heart

Figure 3-8-5

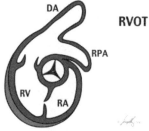

Left ventricular outflow tract and right ventricular outflow tract

Hypoplastic Left Heart [Figure 3-8-6]
- Lethal in neonate if untreated
  - Norwood or transplant
- Small or invisible LV
- Hypoplastic aortic arch
- RA < LA
- Consider Turner syndrome in female fetuses

Chest Masses
- Congenital Diaphragmatic Hernia
- Cystic Adenomatoid Malformation
- Extralobar Sequestration
- Teratoma

Congenital Diaphragmatic Hernia [Figure 3-8-7]
- 90% left-sided through foramen of Bochdalek
- 50% have other anomalies
- Pulmonary hypoplasia
- "Liver-up" poor prognosis

Cystic Adenomatoid Malformation [Figure 3-8-8]
- Lung Hamartoma
- Types I – III
- Arterial supply from pulmonary artery
- May spontaneously regress
- In utero surgery for hydrops

Figure 3-8-8

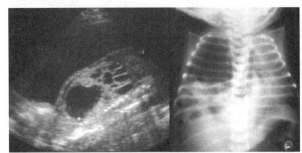

Sagittal scan of the fetal chest and neonatal CXR showing type II CCAM

Extralobar Sequestration [Figure 3-8-9]
- Non-communicating (sequestered) lung segment
- Arterial supply from aorta
- 90% left sided
- 10% below diaphragm

AIUM: Abdomen
- Stomach
- Kidneys
- Bladder
- UC insertion site
- Umbilical cord vessel number

Amniotic Fluid Balance

Production	Removal
Fetal/ Embryo plasma volume	Intramembranous
	Transmembranous
Uterine Perfusion Metanephros (>10 wks)	Swallowing
Lungs	Lungs

Figure 3-8-6

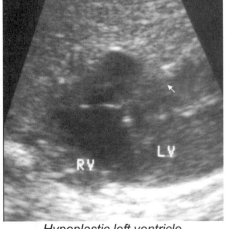

Hypoplastic left ventricle

Figure 3-8-7

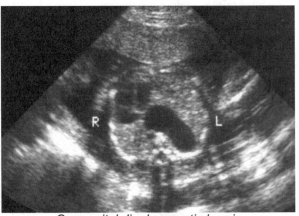

Congenital diaphragmatic hernia with deviation of the heart

Figure 3-8-9

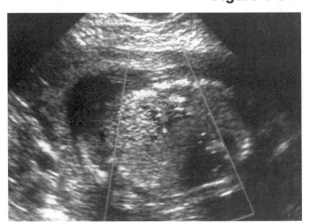

Extralobar sequestration with feeding vessel from the aorta.

Polyhydramnios
- 2/3 idiopathic
- 1/3 definable cause
  - ➤ macroscomia
  - ➤ GI obstruction
  - ➤ CNS malformation
  - ➤ hydrops

Oligohydramnios
- Never normal
- A "DRIP" of fluid
  - ➤ Demise
  - ➤ Renal, also bladder
    often anhydramnios
  - ➤ IUGR
  - ➤ PROM, post dates

Fetal GI Tract
- Atresias
- Abdominal Wall Detect

Atresias
- Esophageal
- Duodenal
- Small Bowel
- Anorectal

Esophageal Atresia
- Stomach may be present but small
- Polyhydramnios after 20 wks
- IUGR common
  - ➤ ingested fluid important for nutrition

Double Bubble [Figure 3-8-10]
- Duodenal Atresia
  - ➤ 30% have trisomy 21
  - ➤ 50% have other structural abnormalities
- Ladd's bands, annular pancreas usually do not present in utero

Jejunal/Ileal Atresia
- 1/3 have cystic fibrosis
- 5-10% may perforate
- Meconium peritonitis
  - ➤ ascites
  - ➤ calcifications
  - ➤ pseudocyst formation

Bowel
- Normal bowel herniation at 8 weeks
- Rotates counterclockwise 270°
- Returns to abdomen in 12 weeks

Abdominal Wall Defects
- Gastroschisis [Figure 3-8-11]
- Omphalocele [Figure 3-8-12 and 3-8-13]
- Limb-body-wall defect

	Gastroschisis	Omphalocele
Location	Right	Central
Membrane	No	Yes
Cord Insertion	NL	On sac
Associated Anomalies	No	50-75%

Figure 3-8-10

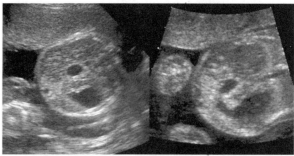

Double bubble, oblique view confirms duodenal atresia

Figure 3-8-11

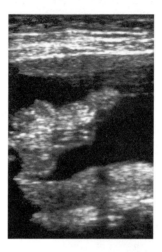

Gastroschisis

Figure 3-8-12

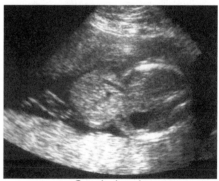

Omphalocele

Figure 3-8-13

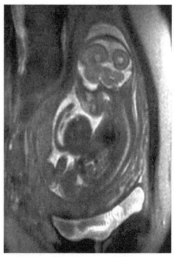

Omphalocele

Limb-Body-Wall Defect (Body Stalk Anomaly)
- Fetus attached to placenta
- Absent or short umbilical cord
- Severe (lethal) malformation
- Scoliosis common

Renal Anomalies [Figure 3-8-14]
- Agenesis
- Renal Cystic Disease
- Hydronephrosis
- Masses

Renal Cystic Disease
- Autosomal recessive polycystic kidney disease [Figure 3-8-15]
- Multicystic dysplastic kidneys [Figures 3-8-16 and 3-8-17]
- Cystic dysplasia due to obstruction
- Autosomal dominant polycystic kidney disease

Associations
- VACTERL Syndrome
  - ➤ Vertebral, anal atresia, cardiac, TE fistula, <u>renal</u>, limb
- Inherited Disorders
  - ➤ Meckel-Gruber (renal cystic dysplasia, encephalocele, polydactyly)
- Chromosomal Abnormalities
  - ➤ Trisomy 13

Hydronephrosis
- UPJ Obstruction
- UVJ Obstruction
- Duplications
- PUV, Urethral Atresia
- Reflux

Hydronephrosis
- Renal Pelvis
  - ➤ $\geq$ 4 mm before 33 weeks
  - ➤ $\geq$ 7 mm after 33 weeks
- AP pelvis diam/AP kidney diam >50%
- Calyceal Dilatation
- Any degree of dilatation accompanied by cystic renal changes

Retroperitoneal Masses
- Renal Cystic Disease
- Renal Tumors
  - ➤ Mesoblastic Nephroma
  - ➤ Wilms Tumor
- Adrenal
  - ➤ Neuroblastoma
  - ➤ Hemorrhage
- Extralobar Sequestration

Cystic Abdominal/Pelvic Collections
- Bladder Obstruction
- Dilated Bowel
- Cysts
  - ➤ Ovarian
  - ➤ Duplication
  - ➤ Mesenteric
  - ➤ Choledochal
  - ➤ Meconium pseudocyst

Figure 3-8-14

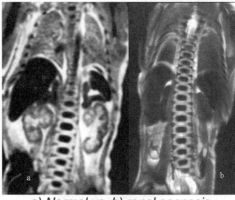

a) Normal vs. b) renal agenesis

Figure 3-8-15

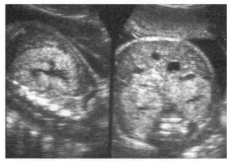

Autosomal recessive polycystic kidney disease

Figure 3-8-16

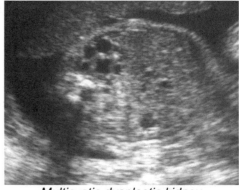

Multicystic dysplastic kidney

Figure 3-8-17

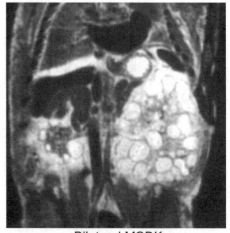

Bilateral MCDK

Posterior Urethral Valves [Figures 3-8-18 and 3-8-19]
- Bladder "funnels" into dilated posterior urethra
- Oligohydramnios common
- Renal dysplasia (echogenic cystic kidneys) bad prognostic sign

Figure 3-8-18

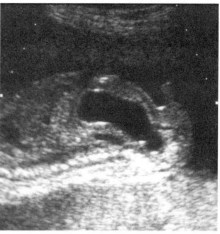

Posterior urethral valves

Figure 3-8-19

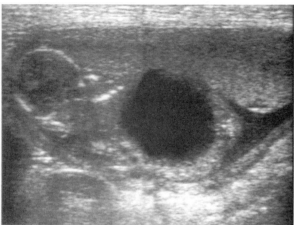

*Severe posterior urethral valves
with oligohydramnios*

Ovarian Cyst [Figure 3-8-20]
- Most common cyst in 3rd trimester
- Anywhere in abdomen
- Complexity suggests torsion or hemorrhage
- Resolve by 6 mos

Figure 3-8-20

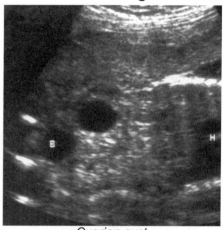

Ovarian cyst

Sacral Mass
- Sacrococcygeal teratoma
- Myelomeningocele

Sacrococcygeal Teratoma [Figures 3-8-21 and 3-8-22]
- Solid, cystic, or mixed
- Location
  - ➣ Type 1: completely external
  - ➣ Type 2: external and internal into pelvis
  - ➣ Type 3: external and internal into abdomen
  - ➣ Type 4: completely internal

Figure 3-8-22

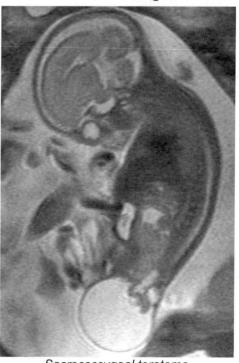

Sacrococcygeal teratoma

Figure 3-8-21

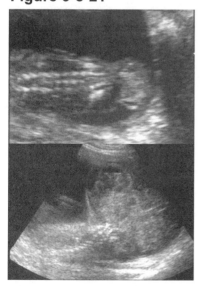

*Solid sacrococcygeal
teratoma with marked
growth*

Selected References

1.   Leung JW, Coakley FV, Hricak H, et al. Prenatal MR imaging of congenital diaphragmatic hernia. AJR Am J Roentgenol 2000; 174:1607-1612.
2.   Coleman BG, Adzick NS, Crombleholme TM, et al. Fetal therapy: state of the art. J Ultrasound Med 2002; 21:1257-1288.
3.   Adzick NS, Harrison MR, Crombleholme TM, Flake AW, Howell LJ. Fetal lung lesions: management and outcome. Am J Obstet Gynecol 1998; 179:884-889.
4.   Lopoo JB, Goldstein RB, Lipshutz GS, Goldberg JD, Harrison MR, Albanese CT. Fetal pulmonary sequestration: a favorable congenital lung lesion. Obstet Gynecol 1999; 94:567-571.
5.   Dalla Vecchia LK, Grosfeld JL, West KW, Rescorla FJ, Scherer LR, Engum SA. Intestinal atresia and stenosis: a 25-year experience with 277 cases. Arch Surg 1998; 133:490-496; discussion 496-497.
6.   Nyberg DA, Resta RG, Luthy DA, Hickok DE, Mahony BS, Hirsch JH. Prenatal sonographic findings of Down syndrome: review of 94 cases. Obstet Gynecol 1990; 76:370-377.
7.   Corteville JE, Gray DL, Langer JC. Bowel abnormalities in the fetus--correlation of prenatal ultrasonographic findings with outcome. Am J Obstet Gynecol 1996; 175:724-729.
8.   Stringer MD, McKenna KM, Goldstein RB, Filly RA, Adzick NS, Harrison MR. Prenatal diagnosis of esophageal atresia. J Pediatr Surg 1995; 30:1258-1263.
9.   Meizner I, Levy A, Katz M, Maresh AJ, Glezerman M. Fetal ovarian cysts: prenatal ultrasonographic detection and postnatal evaluation and treatment. Am J Obstet Gynecol 1991; 164:874-878.
10.   Muller-Leisse C, Bick U, Paulussen K, et al. Ovarian cysts in the fetus and neonate--changes in sonographic pattern in the follow-up and their management. Pediatr Radiol 1992; 22:395-400.
11.   Hutton KA, Thomas DF, Davies BW. Prenatally detected posterior urethral valves: qualitative assessment of second trimester scans and prediction of outcome. J Urol 1997; 158:1022-1025.
12.   James CA, Watson AR, Twining P, Rance CH. Antenatally detected urinary tract abnormalities: changing incidence and management. Eur J Pediatr 1998; 157:508-511.
13.   Abuhamad AZ, Horton CE, Jr., Horton SH, Evans AT. Renal duplication anomalies in the fetus: clues for prenatal diagnosis. Ultrasound Obstet Gynecol 1996; 7:174-177.
14.   Pryde PG, Bardicef M, Treadwell MC, Klein M, Isada NB, Evans MI. Gastroschisis: can antenatal ultrasound predict infant outcomes? Obstet Gynecol 1994; 84:505-510.
15.   Luton D, De Lagausie P, Guibourdenche J, et al. Prognostic factors of prenatally diagnosed gastroschisis. Fetal Diagn Ther 1997; 12:7-14.
16.   Getachew MM, Goldstein RB, Edge V, Goldberg JD, Filly RA. Correlation between omphalocele contents and karyotypic abnormalities: sonographic study in 37 cases. AJR Am J Roentgenol 1992; 158:133-136.
17.   Salihu HM, Boos R, Schmidt W. Omphalocele and gastrochisis. J Obstet Gynaecol 2002; 22:489-492.

Cystic Diseases of the Kidney

Peter L.Choyke, MD
National Institutes of Health

Cystic Disease of the Kidney
- Autosomal Dominant Polycystic Kidney Disease (ADPKD)
- Tuberous Sclerosis Complex (TS or TSC)
- Von Hippel-Lindau Disease (VHL)
- Acquired Cystic Kidney Disease (ACKD)

Inherited Cystic Diseases
- Germline mutation is inherited
- Other allele is damaged during life

ADPKD
- Occurs in 1:1000 Individuals
- Accounts for 5–15% of dialysis patients
- Severity of Disease is variable
  - ESRD in < 50%
  - Risk of Cancer = Not increased

Types of ADPKD
- PKD 1
  - 16p13.3
  - 85–95% of ADPKD
  - Polycystin I
  - Mean age of ESRD=55y
- PKD 2
  - 4q21–23
  - ~5% of ADPKD
  - Polycystin II
  - Mean age of ESRD= 71.5y
- PKD3? PKD4?

ADPKD Pathophysiology

Pathogenesis of PKD
- Only 2–5% of Nephrons are affected:
  - Abnormal Na-K ATP-ase pump may result in secretion into tubule
  - Abnormal cilia (Polycystins I, II)
  - Tubules elongate, tortuous, cyst formation
  - Cysts compromise adjacent parenchyma

Clinical Manifestations
- Pain
- Hypertension
- Infection (Women > Men)
- Stones
- Loss of Renal Function
- Renal Failure

Imaging [Figures 3-9-1 to 3-9-6]

Figure 3-9-1

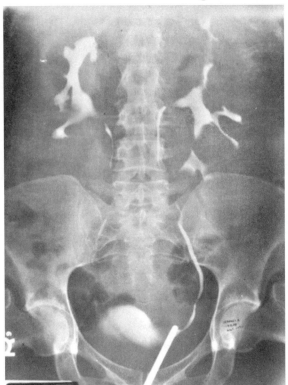

Retrograde pyelogram show distortion of calyces caused by ADPKD

Figure 3-9-4

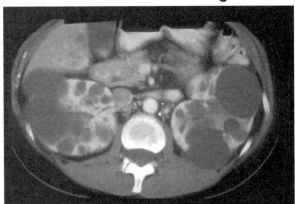

Moderate ADPKD on CT

Figure 3-9-5

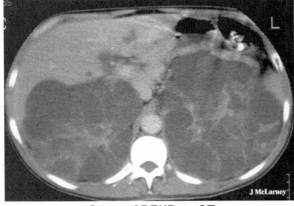

Severe ADPKD on CT

Figure 3-9-2

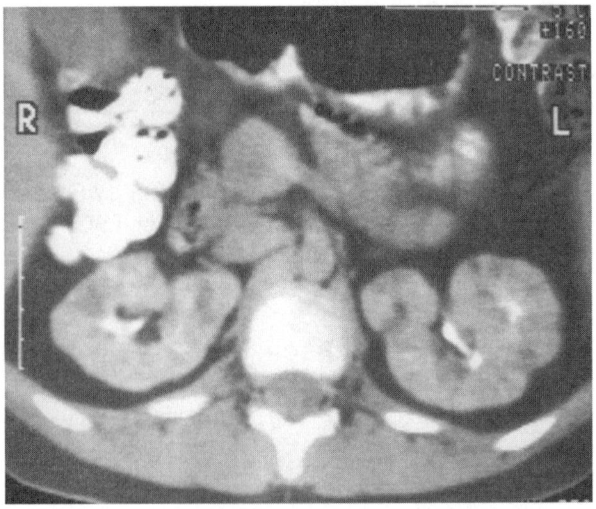

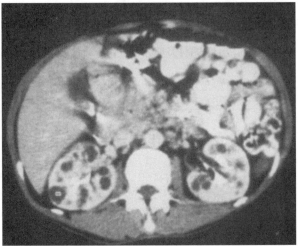

Minimal ADPKD on CT

Figure 3-9-3

Early ADPKD on CT

Figure 3-9-6

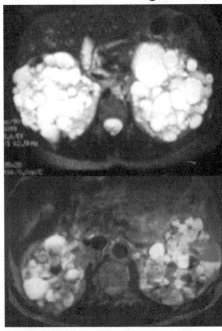

Top: Severe ADPKD on T2 weighted MRI
Bottom: Multiple hemorrhagic cyst within ADPKD kidney on T2 weighted MRI

Manifestations of ADPKD

- Intracranial Aneurysms
- Cysts: Hepatic, Pancreatic, Spleen
- Diverticula: Colon
- Cardiovascular Disease: Mitral, Aortic valve, aortic aneurysm *[Figures 3-9-7]*

Intracranial Aneurysms

- ICA
  - ➢ 18–26% of ADPKD
  - ➢ Rupture ~2–11%
  - ➢ 46–61% Mortality Rate
  - ➢ Mean age 39–47 years of rupture
- Screening (MRA)
  - ➢ Controversy over value in asymptomatic patients with no family history

Liver/Pancreas Cysts

- Occur in 70–75% of ADPKD
- Complications:
  - ➢ Pain
  - ➢ Biliary Obstruction
  - ➢ IVC compression

Screening

- US Screening begins in teenage years
- ~ 2/3 of affected children will show cysts between 11–20
- ~ 95% by age 30

Screening Issues

- Why Screen?
  - ➢ Insurability?
  - ➢ No Rx.
- Genetic Counselling
- Aneurysm, heart disease
- Diet Modification

Localized PKD *[Figures 3-9-8]*

- Unilateral, Segmental
- Non Hereditary
  - ➢ Possible "mosaic" form of ADPKD

Figure 3-9-7

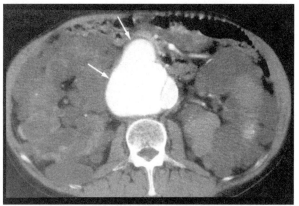

ADPKD with dissecting abdominal aortic aneurysm

Figure 3-9-8

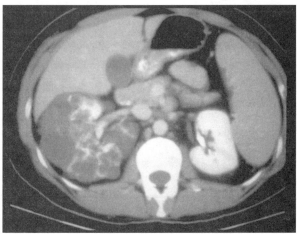

Unilateral polycystic kidney

Autosomal Recessive Polycystic Kidney Disease (ARPKD) [Figures 3-9-9 and 3-9-10]
- Unrelated to ADPKD
- Ductal ectasia, abnormal cilia
  - Few macrocysts
  - Enlarged kidneys
  - Renal Function
    - Infantile form= severe, dialysis from birth
    - Childhood form=milder, non progressive
    - Adult form=hepatic fibrosis predominates

Figure 3-9-9

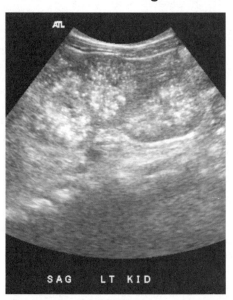

Sonogram of ARPKD kidney showing enlargement and echogenecity

Figure 3-9-10

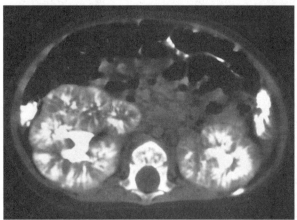

CT of ARPKD kidney showing streaky enhancement pattern

Tuberous Sclerosis
- Prevalence: 1:10,000
- Produces Hamartomas throughout the body:
  - Benign
  - Locally aggressive
- ESRD: 15% (cystic/AML bleeding)
- Risk of Cancer: 1-2% (slight increase)

Genetics
- Autosomal Dominant but..
  - New Mutations account for ~56–80%
  - Inherited form of the disease is less common:
    - Diminished reproductive capacity in affected individuals

Types of TSC
- TSC 1
  - 9q34
  - ~1/3 TSC
  - "Hamartin"
  - Assoc with severe MR
- TSC 2
  - 16p 13.3 !!
  - 2/3 of TSC
  - "Tuberin"
  - Assoc with worse renal disease

Pathogenesis
- Tuberous= nodular, Sclerosis= hard
  - Skin: Adenoma Sebaceum, Angiofibromas
  - CNS: Tubers, Subependymal nodules, Giant Cell Astrocytoma
  - Kidneys: Cysts, Angiomyolipomas
  - Heart: Rhabdomyomas
  - Lungs: Lymphangiomyomatosis (LAM)
  - Bone: Islands

Renal Involvement
[Figures 3-9-11 and 3-9-12]
- Angiomyolipoma predominant
  - Mild to severe
  - Risk of Hemorrhage
  - Treat conservatively
    - Partial nephrectomy
    - RFA
    - Angioembolization

Renal Manifestations
- Carcinoma of the Kidney
  - 1–2% of TS patients
  - Bilateral in 43%
  - Median age 28 years
  - No screening recommendations

Von Hippel Lindau Disease
- Frequency ~ 1:35,000 to 1:45,000
- Target Organs
  - CNS, Retina – Hemangioblastomas
  - Kidney –Cysts and Cancers
  - Pancreas – Cysts and Neuroendocrine tumors
  - Adrenal –Pheochromocytomas
  - Epididymis/ Broad Ligament – Cystadenomas
- ESRD: < 5% Usually due to nephrectomy
- Risk of Cancer: 30-40%

Work-up for VHL
- MRI of the Head and Spine with Gd
- Abdominal CT with Contrast
- Catecholamines (Serum)
- Ophthmalogic Exam
- Audiology
- Mutation Analysis

Genetics
- Sporadic Clear Cell RCC
  - VHL Gene Mutations 3p26

Renal Manifestations [Figures 3-9-13]
- Multiple Cysts
  - Virtually all will have neoplastic clear cell lining
- Cysts containing tumors
- Solid (Clear Cell) tumors

Figure 3-9-11

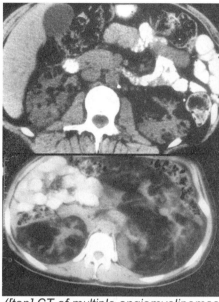

([top] CT of multiple angiomyolipomas in Tuberous Sclerosis

[bottom] CT of large bilateral hemorrhagic angiomyolipomas in TSC

Figure 3-9-12

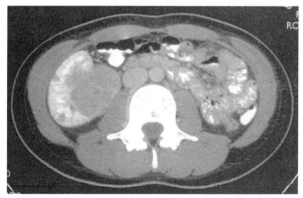

Non fat containing angiomyolipomas in TSC

Figure 3-9-13

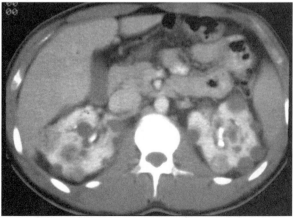

Von Hippel Lindau disease in the kidneys (cystic and solid lesions)

Management
Risk of Metastases - 3 cm rule - Risk of Renal Failure

Acquired Cystic Kidney Disease
- First Described by Dunhill 1977
- Develops in
  - All forms of dialysis
  - Males earlier than Females
- ESRD: 100%
- Risk of Cancer: Increases with duration

Pathogenesis *[Figure 3-9-14]*
- Theory 1: Dialysis Toxin
- Theory 2: Uremic Milieu
  - Mutations which lead to cysts, adenomas, tumors and metastatic cancers

Renal Cancer in ACKD *[Figure 3-9-15]*
- 10–50 Fold Risk of RCC
  - Mean dialysis duration 8 yrs
  - Multifocal & Bilateral
  - 17% Risk of Metastases

Screening
- "Screening is not routinely justified"
  - Relatively low risk of cancer
  - High risk of dying from other causes
  - Reserve screening for pts with good long term prognosis

Levine E, Abdom Imaging 1995 20:569-71

Screening
- "Routine Screening is prudent"
  - Rate of Mets warrant screening
    - Baseline scan
    - Every 1–2 yrs after 3 years of dialysis
    - Men > Women
    - Remove lesions > 2cm

Ishikawa I, Nephron 1991, 58:257-67

ACKD-RCC After Transplant
- Transplantation
  - Cysts Regress
  - New Tumor Formation Decreases
  - Increased Risk of Metastases from Existing RCC
    – Immunosuppression

Take Home Points
- When confronted with a "polycystic kidney"
  - Pure cysts ? Aneurysms ? ADPKD
  - Cysts and AMLs? Brain, skin? TSC
  - Cysts and RCCs? VHL
  - Renal failure on dialysis? ACKD
- Genetic Testing and Screening:
  - PKD1, PKD2
  - TSC1, TSC2
  - VHL
- Risk of Renal Cancer:
  - ADPKD None known
  - TSC ~ 1-2%
  - VHL ~ 35%
  - ACKD ~ 50% (after 8 years of dialysis)

Figure 3-9-14

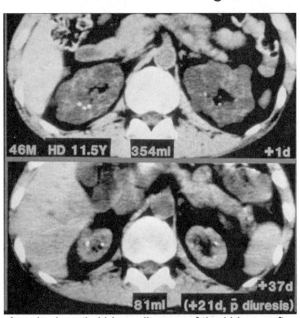

Acquired cystic kidney disease of the kidneys after several years of dialysis

Figure 3-19-15

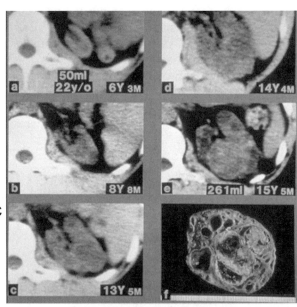

Sequence of images showing development of cystic and neoplastic disease over time in dialysis patients

References:

1. Hughes PD, Becker GJ. Screening for intracranial aneurysms in autosomal dominant polycystic kidney disease. Nephrology (Carlton). 2003 Aug;8(4):163-170.
2. Chapman AB, Guay-Woodford LM, Grantham JJ, Torres VE, Bae KT, Baumgarten DA, Kenney PJ, King BF Jr, Glockner JF, Wetzel LH, Brummer ME, O'Neill WC, Robbin ML, Bennett WM, Klahr S, Hirschman GH, Kimmel PL, Thompson PA, Miller JP; Consortium for Radiologic Imaging Studies of Polycystic Kidney Disease cohort.
3. Renal structure in early autosomal-dominant polycystic kidney disease (ADPKD): The Consortium for Radiologic Imaging Studies of Polycystic Kidney Disease (CRISP) cohort. Kidney Int. 2003 Sep;64(3):1035-45.
4. Mosetti MA, Leonardou P, Motohara T, Kanematsu M, Armao D, Semelka RC. Autosomal dominant polycystic kidney disease: MR imaging evaluation using current techniques. J Magn Reson Imaging. 2003 Aug;18(2):210-5.
5. Narayanan V. Tuberous sclerosis complex: genetics to pathogenesis. Pediatr Neurol. 2003 Nov;29(5):404-9.

Imaging of Prostate Cancer

Peter L. Choyke, MD
National Institutes of Health

Prostate Cancer
- Epidemiology
- Diagnosis
- Staging
- Image guided Therapy

Epidemiology
- ~220,000 new diagnoses per year
  - ~29,000 cancer deaths (USA)
  - 2nd most common cause of cancer deaths in males
  - Slight decrease in cancer deaths

Epidemiology
- Risk Factors for Prostate Cancer
  - Country of Origin
  - Diet
  - Sunlight
  - Hormones

Only a small fraction of prostate cancers cause death

Grading Prostate Cancer
- Gleason Grading System
  - Two predominant cell types
  - Add together for score from 2-10

Screening
- Recommendations:
  - For men > 50 years or > 40 in African Americans or with Family history :
    - ❖ Annual Digital Rectal*
    - ❖ Annual PSA

Prostate Specific Antigen
- Ranges of PSA
  - 0–4ng/ml Normal (PPV=5%)
  - 4–10ng/ml Indeterminate (PPV=22%)
  - > 10 ng/ml Abnormal (PPV=67%)

Adjusted PSA Values
- Age Adjusted PSA
- PSA Density
  - Adjust for volume (PSA/Vol= 0.15)
- PSA Velocity
  - Adjust for increases (0.75ng/ml/yr)
- Free PSA/Total PSA ratio
  - Adjust for ratio of free/bound (~20–25%)
  - Cancer makes a "sticky PSA"

Detecting Prostate Cancer
- Elevated PSA or Abnormal Rectal Exam
- Occasional voiding symptoms
- Transrectal Ultrasound Guided Biopsies
- Biopsy Mapping and Grading

Prostate Ultrasound
- Transrectal Ultrasound-History
  - ➢ The Chair (Watanabe 1968)
  - ➢ Zonal Anatomy (Stamey 1980)
  - ➢ Screening (Lee 1983)
  - ➢ TRUS Guided Biopsy (1985-)
  - ➢ Color Doppler (1995-)
  - ➢ Contrast Enhanced US (2000-)

Anatomy [Figure 3-10-1 and 3-10-2]
- Zonal Anatomy of Prostate
  - ➢ Peripheral Zone
    - ❖ Glandular
    - ❖ 70% of Cancers
  - ➢ Transitional Zone
    - ❖ Stromal/Glandular
    - ❖ 25% of Cancers, 90% of Hyperplastic nodules
  - ➢ Central Zone

The TRUS Examination [Figures 3-10-3 to 3-10-5]
- Examine the PZ for nodules
- Examine the TZ for asymmetry
- Examine Seminal Vesicles
- Determine the Volume

TRUS Guided Biopsy
- Prep:
  - ➢ Antibiotics before and after (Cipro)
  - ➢ Enema (Fleets)
- Core Biopsies with Automatic Cutting Needle
  - ➢ Directed Biopsies at sites of abnormality
  - ➢ Label all specimens; send separately

Tumor Mapping with Biopsy

Figure 3-10-1

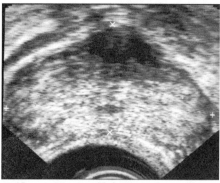

Normal transaxial view of prostate on sonography

Figure 3-10-2

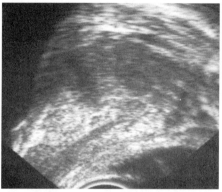

Sagittal view demonstrating ejaculatory ducts and seminal vesicle

Figure 3-10-3

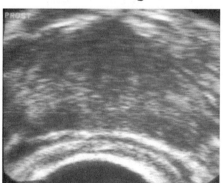

Prostate cancer in right mid prostate gland

Figure 3-10-4

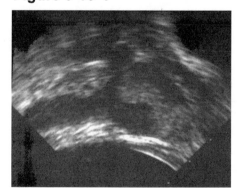

Prostate cancer near base of seminal vesicle

Figure 3-10-5

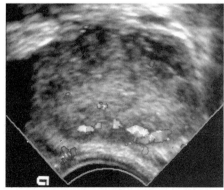

Power Doppler of prostate cancer

Staging (Whitmore-Jewitt)

Staging (TNM)
- Non palpable   A1, 2   T1a, b
- Detected by Bx   **   T1c
- Palpable   B1, 2   T2a, b
- Extracapsular   C1   T3a, b, c(sv)
- Fixed, invasive   C2   T4
- Regional Nodes   D1   Tx, N+
- Distant Mets   D2   Tx, Nx, M+

Treatment
- A1, 2   T1 a-c   Surg/XRT/WW
- B1, 2   T2 a,b   Surg/XRT/WW
- C1, 2   T3 a-c   XRT/WW/Hormonal
- D1   T4   XRT/WW/Hormonal
- D2   Tx, N+, M+   Hormonal/Chemotherapy

Staging with Imaging
- Local Staging (Extracapsular)
  - Ultrasound
  - MRI
- Key Structures:
  - Neurovascular Bundles
  - Seminal Vesicles
  - Apex
  - Periprostatic Venous Plexus

TRUS Staging
- Sensitivity
  - ~40–50%
- Exceptions:
  - Seminal Vesicles
  - Neurovascular Bundle
  - Staging biopsies

Endorectal Coil MRI [Figure 3-10-6]
- Sensitivity:
  - Early Studies ~85–90%
  - Multi institutional Trial ~60–70%
    - ❖ Motion
    - ❖ Microscopic Disease
    - ❖ Operator dependent
    - ❖ Observer dependent

Endorectal Coil MRI [Figure 3-10-7 and 3-10-8]
- Improvements
  - Dynamic contrast enhancement
  - MR Spectroscopy
  - 3-D imaging

Dynamic Enhanced MRI of the Protaste
MRI and 1H-MRSI- Prostate: Metabolic Interrogation

Nodal Staging [Figure 3-10-9]
- CT/MRI only ~ 36% sensitive
  - Size threshold ~8mm + biopsy of nodes
  - Yield improves for high risk pts
  - (PSA >20 ng/ml)
- Prostascint SPECT [Figure 3-202]
- USPIO (Combidex) MR Lymphography

Figure 3-10-6
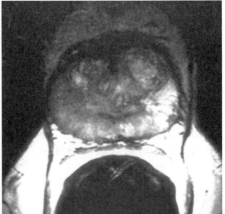
Endorectal coil MRI demonstrating sawtooth pattern

Figure 3-10-7
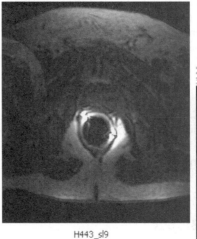
H443_sl9

Dynamic enhanced MRI of prostate cancer

Figure 3-10-8
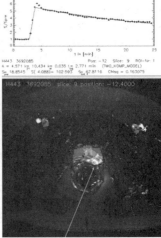
Dynamic enhanced MRI of prostate cancer with color encoding

Figure 3-10-9
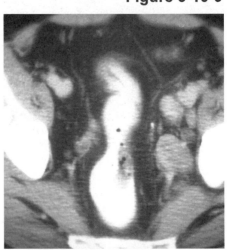
Lymph node metastases from prostate cancer

Staging for Distant Metastases [Figures 3-10-10 to 3-10-12]

- Bone Metastases
  - ➢ Bone Scan
    - ❖ Yield increases after PSA >10
    - ❖ Superscan
    - ❖ Quantitation/Confirmation

Figure 3-10-10

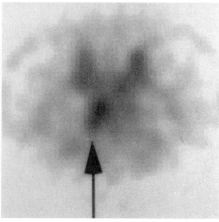

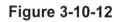

Prostascint SPECT image of pelvis

Figure 3-10-11

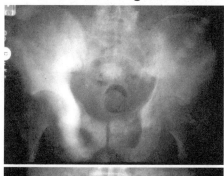

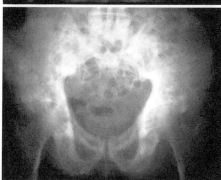

Top: Prostate cancer metastases to pelvis

Bottom: Pagets disease in pelvis

Figure 3-10-12

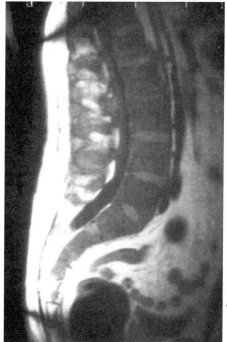

Diffuse bony metastases in lumbar spine on MRI

Radioactive Ablation

- Strontium-89 (Metastron)
  - ➢ ~80% response rate
  - ➢ Up to 6 months relief of bone pain
  - ➢ Samarium and Rhenium

Image Guided Treatment

- Brachytherapy
- Cryotherapy
- Radiofrequency Ablation

Brachytherapy [Figures 3-10-13 and 3-12-14]

- Interstitial Radioactive Seeds (Afterloaded)
  - ➢ Iodine, Iridium, Palladium, Gold
- Introducers are placed within prostate at regular spacing via:
  - ➢ CT
  - ➢ US
  - ➢ MRI

Figure 3-10-13

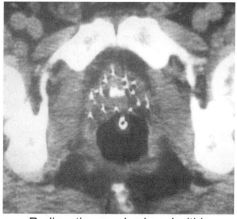

Radioactive seeds placed within prostate for brachytherapy

Figure 3-10-14

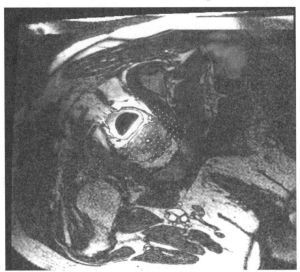

MRI guided brachytherapy

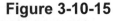

Figure 3-10-15

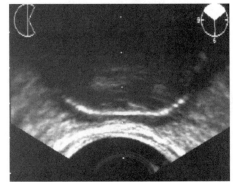

Cryotherapy of prostate

Cryotherapy *[Figure 3-10-15]*
- Liquid Nitrogen instilled via cannulas placed within Prostate under TRUS
- Not enough Data
  - ➢ High rate of impotence
  - ➢ Steep learning curve

Take Home Points
- Imaging currently plays minor role in prostate cancer detection:
  - ➢ MR spectroscopy, Dynamic MRI may change this
- Staging depends on PSA/Grade
  - ➢ MRI for local staging
  - ➢ CT/MRI for nodal staging
  - ➢ Bone Scan/CT/MR for distant staging
- Image Guided therapy is an important trend in treatment

References:

1. Denmeade SR, Isaacs JT. Development of prostate cancer treatment: the good news. Prostate. 2004 Feb 15;58(3):211-24. Review.
2. Fleshner N, Bagnell PS, Klotz L, Venkateswaran V. Dietary fat and prostate cancer. J Urol. 2004 Feb;171(2 Pt 2):S19-24.
3. Engelbrecht MR, Jager GJ, Laheij RJ, Verbeek AL, van Lier HJ, Barentsz JO. Local staging of prostate cancer using magnetic resonance imaging: a meta-analysis. Eur Radiol. 2002 Sep;12(9):2294-302.
4. Harisinghani MG, Barentsz J, Hahn PF, Deserno WM, Tabatabaei S, van de Kaa CH, de la Rosette J, Weissleder R. Noninvasive detection of clinically occult lymph-node metastases in prostate cancer. N Engl J Med. 2003 Jun 19;348(25):2491-9.
5. Onik G, Narayan P, Vaughan D, Dineen M, Brunelle R. Focal "nerve-sparing" cryosurgery for treatment of primary prostate cancer: a new approach to preserving potency. Urology. 2002 Jul;60(1):109-14.
6. Dhingsa R, Qayyum A, Coakley FV, Lu Y, Jones KD, Swanson MG, Carroll PR, Hricak H, Kurhanewicz J. Prostate cancer localization with endorectal MR imaging and MR spectroscopic imaging: effect of clinical data on reader accuracy. Radiology. 2004 Jan;230(1):215-20.

Imaging of Ovarian Masses

Brent J. Wagner, MD
Uniformed Services Univ. of the Health Sciences
The Reading Hospital and Medical Center

Ovarian Masses

- Non-neoplastic
  - ➢ physiologic cyst, endometriosis, etc.
- Neoplastic
  - ➢ epithelial tumors 65%
  - ➢ germ cell tumors 25%
  - ➢ sex-cord stromal tumors 5%
  - ➢ secondary malignancies 5%
  - ➢ gonadoblastoma <1%

Relative Incidence of Ovarian Neoplasms [Figure 3-11-1]

Common Ovarian Epithelial Tumors: Classification

- Serous
- Mucinous
- Endometrioid
- Clear Cell
- Brenner
- Undifferentiated

Ovarian Epithelial Tumors

- 65% of ovarian neoplasms
- 85% of ovarian malignancies
- 60% of epithelial tumors are benign
- 35% of epithelial tumors are malignant
- 5% of epithelial tumors are borderline, low malignant potential

Ovarian Epithelial Tumors

- major risk factor: "incessant ovulation" (Lancet, 1973)
  - ➢ infertility
  - ➢ celibacy
  - ➢ nulliparity
  - ➢ family history
  - ➢ high socioeconomic status
  - ➢ breast cancer
  - ➢ endometrial cancer
  - ➢ lack of oral contraceptive use

Figure 3-11-1

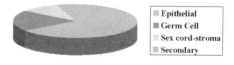

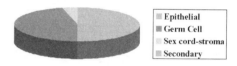

Relative incidence of ovarian neoplasms

CA-125

- abnormally elevated in 85% of ovarian cancer patients
- false negative in 50% of Stage I disease
- false negative in 30% of mucinous tumors
- false positives occur (especially in pre-menopausal patients) with benign neoplasms, endometriosis, etc.
- most commonly used to follow known disease for remission and recurrence
- rarely of use in deciding on surgical vs. non-surgical management at the time of initial presentation of a pelvis mass

Ovarian Epithelial Tumors

- benign
- low malignant potential (LMP)
  - ➢ "borderline" tumors
  - ➢ based on histologic appearance of primary
  - ➢ may be a heterogeneous group (but histologic features overlap)
  - ➢ 95% five year survival overall
- malignant

Epithelial Tumors: Terminology
- adenoma or adenocarcinoma
- add prefix "cyst-" if cystic
- add suffix "-fibroma" if more than 50% fibrous
  - ("cystadenofibroma" or "fibrous cystadenocarcinoma")
  - do not confuse with a true fibroma (one of the sex-cord stromal tumors)

Epithelial Ovarian Neoplasms: Serous
[Figures 3-11-2 to 3-11-6]
- also known as "papillary" tumors
- 25% of benign neoplasms
- 50% of malignant neoplasms
- 63% benign, 30% malignant, 7% LMP
- strongest association with CA-125
- thin-walled cyst, usually unilocular
- papillary soft tissue projections often seen
- psammomatous calcification is more common than with other ovarian neoplasms
- solid or bilateral tumors suggest malignancy

Figure 3-11-2

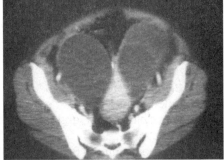

Serous cystadenoma (bilateral)

Figure 3-11-3

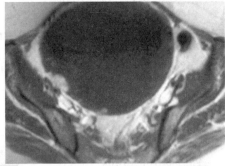

Serous cystadenoma (LMP)

Figure 3-11-4

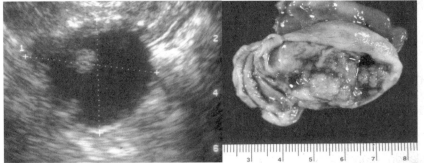

Serous cystadenoma (LMP)

Figure 3-11-5

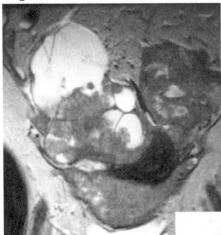

Serous cystadenocarcinoma

Figure 3-11-6

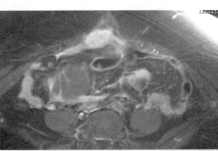

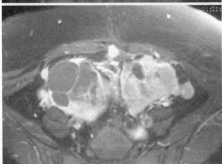

Serous cystadenocarcinoma

Epithelial Ovarian Neoplasms: Mucinous

- mucin-containing cells (cyst content varies)
- up to 20% of benign ovarian neoplasms
- 10% of carcinomas
- 73% benign, 16% malignant, 11% LMP
- serum marker (CA-125) is less reliable (falsely negative) with mucinous tumors

Epithelial Ovarian Neoplasms: Mucinous [Figure 3-11-7]

- thin-walled cyst, usually multilocular
- often large, may be enormous
- occasionally, linear calcifications (but calcifications are LESS frequent than with mucinous tumors of colonic origin)
- solid elements suggest malignancy
- LMP tumors are associated with pseudomyxoma peritonei
  - ➤ cause / effect relationship is often unclear

Pseudomyxoma peritonei [Figure 3-11-8]

- usually arises from appendix
- often difficult to determine whether the process originated from the appendix, ovary, or both (synchronous)
- prolonged, uncomfortable survival (limited treatment options)
- low density, "scalloping" seen on CT
- "Pseudomyxoma peritonei is a poorly understood condition and it is unclear whether its continous production of gelatinous mucin is due to peritoneal implantation of neoplastic mucinous cells or to metaplasia of peritoneal cells into mucinous epithelium, induced by mucin." [1]

[1] Tropé CG et al. Surgery for borderline tumor of the ovary. Seminars in Surgical Oncology 2000; 19:69–75.

Epithelial Ovarian Neoplasms: Endometrioid

- mimics endometrial ca, but is primary to ovary
- may have malignant stroma ("carcinosarcoma" or "malignant mixed mesodermal tumor")
- almost all are malignant
- 10–15% of ovarian cancers
- 25% of patients have an associated uterine abnormality
  - ➤ endometrial carcinoma (separate primary malignancy)
  - ➤ endometrial hyperplasia
- rarely, endometrioid ovarian ca can arise from endometriosis (controversial)

Epithelial Ovarian Tumors: Clear Cell [Figure 3-11-9]

- mimics clear cell cancer of the vagina, but no association with *in utero* DES exposure
- 5% of ovarian cancers (all clear cell tumors are malignant)
- gross appearance is variable:
  - ➤ unilocular cyst with a mural nodule
  - ➤ multilocular
  - ➤ solid, etc.

Ovarian Carcinoma Staging: Local disease (30%)

- Stage I
  - ➤ limited to ovary [subtypes]
- Stage II
  - ➤ extra-ovarian pelvic extension [subtypes]

Figure 3-11-7

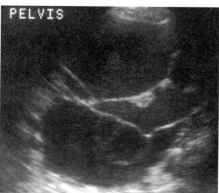

Mucinous cystadenoma (LMP?)

Figure 3-11-8

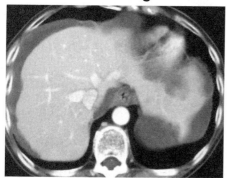

Pseudomyxoma peritonei

Figure 3-11-9

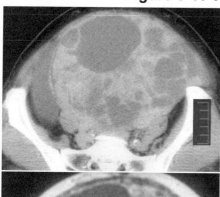

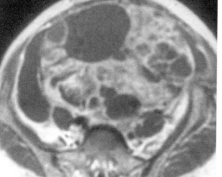

Clear cell carcinoma

Ovarian Carcinoma Staging: Advanced Disease (70%)
- Stage III
  - tumor within the peritoneum (outside the pelvis) [or] retroperitoneal lymph nodes [or] surface of the liver [or] small bowel/omentum (within the pelvis)
- Stage IV
  - distant spread
    - hepatic parenchyma
    - lung
    - etc.

Typical Ovarian Cancer Therapy
- Surgical: hysterectomy, oophorectomy, appendectomy, omentectomy, removal of peritoneal masses
- Medical: 6–8 (monthly) cycles of chemotherapy (a platinum-based agent, plus taxol)
- Second look surgery? (only as part of a structured research protocol)

Ovarian Masses
- Non-neoplastic
  - Physiologic cyst, endometriosis, etc.
- Neoplastic
  - Epithelial tumors   65%
  - Germ cell tumors   25%
  - Sex-cord stromal tumors   5%
  - Secondary malignancies   5%
  - Gonadoblastoma   <1%

Ovarian Germ Cell Neoplasms
- most are mature teratomas:
  - the most common mature teratomas are mature *cystic* teratomas (commonly referred to as "dermoid cysts")
  - less common mature teratomas include carcinoid tumors, struma ovarii, etc.

in the ovary . . .
- all dermoid cysts are mature teratomas (and most, but not all, mature teratomas are dermoid cysts)

Mature Cystic Teratoma *[Figures 3-11-10 and 3-11-11]*
- unilocular cyst
  - cyst fluid is nearly sonolucent
  - posterior acoustic enhancement (fluid at body temperature)
  - images as "fat" (lipid) by CT, MRI – but it is NOT adipose tissue
- Rokitansky nodule
  - contains various tissues (cartilage, gastrointestinal epithelium, etc)
  - echogenic
- child-bearing years
- may undergo:
  - torsion
  - rupture
  - malignant transformation (very rare)
- often discovered as an incidental finding
- 12% bilateral

Figure 3-11-10

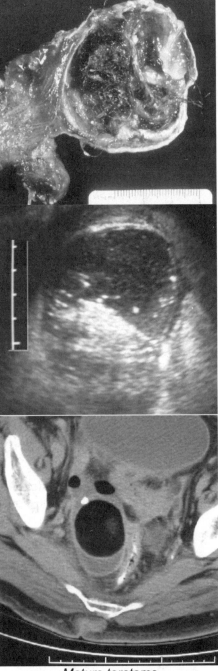

Mature teratoma

Figure 3-11-11

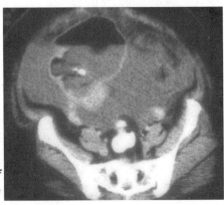

Malignant transformation of mature teratoma

Ovarian Malignant Germ Cell Tumors

- dysgerminoma (similar to seminoma)
- embryonal carcinoma
- endodermal sinus tumor
- immature teratoma
- choriocarcinoma
- mixed germ cell tumor (less common than *testicular* mixed GCT)

Malignant Germ Cell Tumors *[Figure 3-11-12]*

- in general:
  - ➤ younger age group (15–30 years) than epithelial tumors
  - ➤ solid / heterogeneous
  - ➤ highly aggressive
  - ➤ differentiation among the various types is difficult (but immature teratomas are the most likely to have fat, calcification)
  - ➤ may have elevated markers (AFP, HCG)

Sex-cord stromal tumors

- many are very low grade malignancies
- generally diagnosed at Stage I (and therefore surgery is often curative)
- 5–8% of ovarian neoplasms
- hormonal manifestations include:
  - ➤ estrogenic effects: pseudoprecocious puberty, endometrial stimulation
  - ➤ virilization (less common)

Sex-cord stromal tumors

- fibrothecoma
  - ➤ 50% of all sex-cord stromal tumors
  - ➤ more common than either pure thecoma or pure fibroma
- granulosa cell tumors
  - ➤ including juvenile variety
- Sertoli-Leydig
  - ➤ more common than either pure Sertoli or Leydig cell tumors
  - ➤ rare, but the most common virilizing tumor of the ovary

Fibrothecoma *[Figures 3-11-13 and 3-11-14]*

- thecoma component produces estrogen
- fibroma component accounts for low signal on T2-weighted MRI
- sonographically, they tend to be homogeneously hypoechoic but sound-attenuating

Granulosa cell tumors *[Figure 3-11-15]*

- "sponge-like" appearance on imaging
- multicystic lesion with hemorrhage in a patient under 30 suggests juvenile granulosa cell tumor (but these account for only 5% of granulosa cell tumors overall)

Sex-cord stromal tumors

- low signal on T2 suggests fibroma
- hypoechoic sound-attenuating lesion suggests fibroma
- diagnosis of this and other sex-cord stromal tumors may be possible if clinical factors are taken into consideration (morphology is generally solid and non-specific)
- ". . . difficult to suggest a simple algorithm for evaluation of women with ovarian masses" [1]

Figure 3-11-12

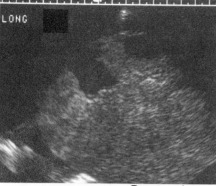

Dysgerminoma

Figure 3-11-13

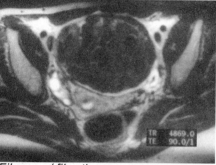

Fibroma / fibrothecoma

Figure 3-11-14

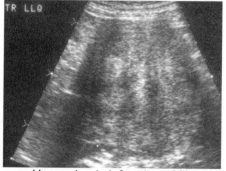

Hemorrhagic infarction of fibroma

Figure 3-11-15

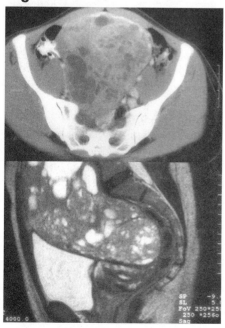

Granulosa cell tumor

- "[Doppler U/S, CT, and MRI] yielded similar [results] for discrimination between benign disease and cancer . . . Although differentiation of benign from malignant disease is obviously clinically important and these detection rates are higher than those previously reported, they are likely still not high enough for surgery to be avoided in most cases." [1]
- "Whatever the modality used, it is hoped that correct staging of advanced disease will lead to appropriate referral to a specialist in gynecologic oncology." [1]

[1] Kurtz A et al Radiology 1999 Jul;212(1):19–27

Scoring systems for ovarian tumors
- wall thickness
- nodularity
- septations
- echogenicity
- ascites?
- size?

Ovarian Masses: Sonographic scoring
- wall irregularities
  - ➢ smooth --> papillary projections
- wall thickness
  - ➢ thin --> thick (< or > 3 mm)
- septa
  - ➢ none --> thin--> thick
- echogenicity
  - ➢ low --> high
- ascites? size?

Doppler sonography*
- ideally, should allow more specificity and sensitivity for malignancy
- based on low resistance flow (high diastolic flow) in malignant neovascularity
- significant overlap with benign processes, especially in pre-menopausal women

* = controversial

Doppler sonography of ovarian masses*
- it *should* work:
  - ➢ in a large series of patients, the presence of high diastolic flow is predictive of malignancy
- however, it is of limited usefulness:
  - ➢ specificity is limited, especially in pre-menopausal patients
  - ➢ there is considerable overlap of benign vs. malignant

* = controversial

Doppler sonography of ovarian masses* [Figure 3-11-16]
- proposed threshold values:
  - ➢ Resistive index (RI) = .45 (or .50)
  - ➢ Pulsatility index (PI) = 1.0
- below these values: suggests malignancy
- corpus luteum may give false positive
- incomplete sampling may give false negative

* = controversial

Figure 3-11-16

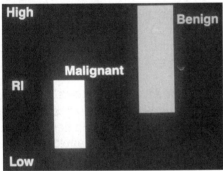

Use of resistive index in assessment of ovarian masses

Doppler sonography of ovarian masses*
- do not use the RI or PI values at the exclusion of the sonographic *morphology*
- color / amplitude Doppler may be of use in characterizing areas that may be confusing or indeterminate morphologically (for example, clot vs. tissue)

* = controversial

Is pre-operative staging of ovarian cancer important? Maybe not, because . . .
- "all" patients go to surgery (cytoreduction)
- in most centers, staging laparotomies are performed by a gynecologic oncologist

Is prediction of malignancy in a neoplastic mass important?
- May determine the surgical approach
- May determine who the surgeon is:
  - ➢ If "probably benign", general gynecologist
  - ➢ If "probably malignant", gynecologic oncologist

Is the differentiation of a neoplasm from a non-neoplastic ovarian mass important?
- Yes (and it's usually accomplished sonography)

Pre-menopausal (ovulating) patient
- Acute symptoms?
  - ➢ check pregnancy test
  - ➢ check for fever, elevated white blood cell count
  - ➢ if severe acute pain, consider torsion

Pre-menopausal (ovulating) patient
- If sub-acute or mild symptoms:
  - ➢ simple cyst < 30 mm, no follow-up
  - ➢ "hemorrhagic cyst" < 25 mm, no follow-up
  - ➢ simple cyst 30–60 mm, follow-up in 6–10 weeks
  - ➢ "hemorrhagic cyst" 25–60 mm, follow-up in 6–10 weeks
  - ➢ any appearance > 60 mm, consider surgery
  - ➢ any soft tissue component (septation, etc), consider surgery

Post-menopausal patient
- simple cyst <16 mm: ignore
- simple cyst 16–50 mm: follow-up 4 months
  - ➢ presumed serous inclusion cyst vs. benign neoplasm
- simple cyst > 50 mm OR any complex lesion: consider surgery

References

DePriest PD, Shenson D, Fried A, Hunter JE, et al. A morphology index based on sonographic findings in ovarian cancer. Gynec Oncol 1993; 51:7-11.

Siegelman ES, Outwater, EK. Tissue Characterization in the Female Pelvis by Means of MR Imaging. Radiology 1999; 212:5.

Outwater EK, Wagner BJ, Mannion C, McLarney JK, Kim B. Sex-cord stromal and steroid cell tumors of the ovary. RadioGraphics 1998; 18:1523.

Kurtz AB, et al. Diagnosis and Staging of Ovarian Cancer: Comparative Values of Doppler and Conventional US, CT, and MR Imaging Correlated with Surgery and Histopathologic Analysis-Report of the Radiology Diagnostic Oncology Group. Radiology 1999; 212:19.

Hricak H, Chen M, Coakley FV. Complex adnexal masses: detection and characterization with MR imaging -- multivariate analysis. Radiology 2000; 214:39.

Kawamoto S, Urban BA, Fishman EK. CT of epithelial ovarian tumors. Radiographics 1999; 19:S85.

Patel MD, Feldstein VA, Lipson SD, Chen DC, and Filly RA. Cystic teratomas of the ovary: diagnostic value of sonography. AJR 1998; 171:1061-1065.

Koonings PP, Campbell K, Mishell DJ, Grimes DA. Relative frequency of primary ovarian neoplasms: a 10-year review. Obstet Gynecol 1989; 74:921-926.

Gajewski W, Legare RD. Ovarian cancer. Surg Onc Clin N Am 1998; 7:317.

Wagner BJ, Buck JL, Seidman JD, McCabe KM. Epithelial Neoplasms of the Ovary: Radiologic-Pathologic Correlation. RadioGraphics 1994; 14:1351.

Adrenal Imaging in Adults:
Radiologic-Pathologic Correlation
Brent J. Wagner, MD
Uniformed Services Univ. of the Health Sciences
The Reading Hospital and Medical Center

Korobkin M. CT characterization of adrenal masses: the time has come. Radiology 2000; 217:629

Caoili EM, Korobkin M, Francis IR, et al. Adrenal masses: characterization with combined unenhanced and delayed enhanced CT. Radiology 2002; 222:629-33

Neoplastic
- Adenoma
- Metastasis
- Lymphoma
- Pheochromocytoma
- Adrenocortical Carcinoma
- Myelolipoma
- Hemangioma (rare)

Non-neoplastic
- Hemorrhage
- Inflammation
- Hyperplasia
- Cyst
- Pseudocyst*

may be secondary to neoplasm (adenoma)

Clinical manifestations of adrenal tumors
- Aldosteronism (hypertension, hypokalemia)
  - 80% due to adenoma (Conn's syndrome)
  - 20% due to hyperplasia
  - < 1% due to adrenal cortical carcinoma
- Virilization
  - most due to hyperplasia
  - 15% due to adenoma
  - 5% due to carcinoma
- Cushing's syndrome (hypertension, obesity, diabetes, etc) may be due to:
  - exogenous steroids (most common)
  - pituitary adenoma → ACTH production → bilateral adrenal hyperplasia
  - non-pituitary tumor → ACTH production → bilateral adrenal hyperplasia
  - 20% due to adrenal adenoma
  - 10% due to carcinoma
- Catecholamine excess (hypertension, tachycardia, flushing, etc.)
  - pheochromocytoma

Adenoma [Figure 3-12-1]
- (3% of the general population)
  - Non-hyperfunctional (vast majority)
  - Hyperfunctional (imaging features are the same as non-hyperfunctional)

Adenoma microscopic pathology
- clear cells (high lipid content)
- cords of fibrovascular tissue

Figure 3-12-1

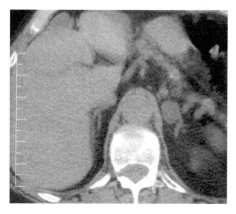

Adrenal adenoma

Adenoma (typical) macroscopic pathology
- well-circumscribed
- homogeneous
- small (usually less than 3 cm)

Adenoma with degeneration (atypical) [Figure 3-12-2]
- heterogeneous
- hemorrhagic
- cystic / necrotic
- calcifications
- (gross and radiologic appearance mimics carcinoma)

Adenoma radiology
- CT findings (NCCT):
  - small, homogeneous
  - hypodense due to lipid content (< 18HU?, <15HU?, <10HU?)
- CT findings (CECT):
  - decreased enhancement compared to metastasis, etc.
  - rapid wash-out of contrast?
- Some adenomas are "lipid poor"
- A mass that does not satisfy the density requirements for an adenoma may still be an adenoma (biopsy or washout study required?)
- A mass that does not decrease in signal on an opposed phase image may still be an adenoma
- MR (opposed phase imaging) [Figure 3-12-3]
  - TE varies with field strength:
    - at 1.5T, TE = 2.1 msec out-of-phase, 4.2msec in phase
  - relies on relatively high lipid content of adenoma
  - voxels which contain both lipid and water will show decreased signal
  - spleen used as internal reference
    - visual assessment is generally adequate, although SI ratios of lesion:spleen may be used
- Opposed phase MRI operates on the same principle (lipid content) as non-contrast CT, therefore will generally add little to the patient work-up (i.e. an indeterminate lesion by CT will likely be indeterminate on opposed phase MRI).

Adrenal Carcinoma [Figure 3-12-4]
- rare
- heterogeneous
- large (mean >10 cm)
- necrotic
- percutaneous biopsy unreliable
- more than 1/3 are calcified
- half are hyperfunctional (these are generally smaller)

Figure 3-12-2

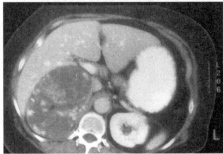

Degenerating adenoma

Figure 3-12-3

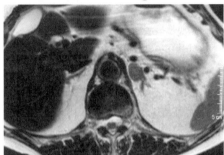
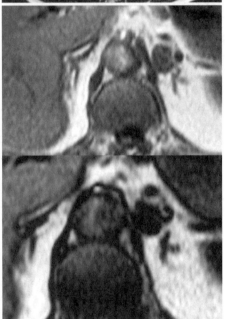

Adrenal adenoma, including opposed phase imaging

Figure 3-12-4   *Adrenocortical carcinoma with extension to inferior vena cava*

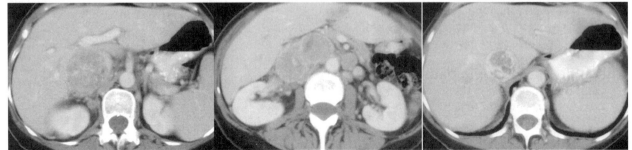

Pheochromocytoma [Figures 3-12-5 and 3-12-6]

- almost all are abdominal
  depends on definition – perhaps all are "adrenal"
- 90% are adrenal (the remainder are "paragangliomas")
- 90% are unilateral
- 90% are "benign" — benignity established by clinical follow-up
- elevated catecholamines
- imaging generally performed for localization, not diagnosis
- CT:
  - ➤ 4 - 6 cm mass
  - ➤ heterogeneous when large (often cystic)
  - ➤ calcification < 5%
- MRI:
  - ➤ historically, characterized as very high signal on T2
  - ➤ not totally specific, but normally needed only for localization
- MIBG:
  - ➤ high sensitivity and specificity
  - ➤ (but generally not needed and availability is limited)

Myelolipoma [Figures 3-12-7 and 3-12-8]

- marrow elements: blood precursors and fat
- benign — no malignant potential
- small lesions very unlikely to bleed
- usually incidental findings, but may present with hemorrhage
- may be diagnosed by needle biopsy (often not needed)
- rarely extra-adrenal (differential diagnosis — liposarcoma)
- most are predominantly fat attenuation (CT) or SI (MR)
- one third have calcification
- occasionally, associated with hormonal activity

Adrenal Mass Evaluation: Helpful features

- Mass is very large: favor adrenocortical carcinoma
- Mass is between 2- 6cm in patient with hypertension: hyperfunctioning adenoma vs. pheochromocytoma
- Mass contains a cystic portion and is less than 6 cm: pheochromocytoma
- Mass is primarily very high signal on T2: suggests pheochromocytoma
- Calcification: inflammatory, old hemorrhage, adrenocortical ca [unlikely: mets, pheo]
- Small, homogeneous, hypodense = adenoma

Figure 3-12-5

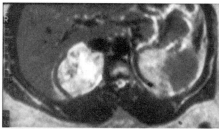
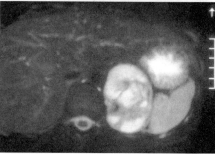

Pheochromocytoma

Figure 3-12-6

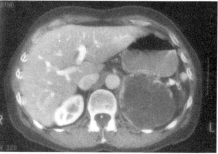

Pheochromocytoma

Figure 3-12-7

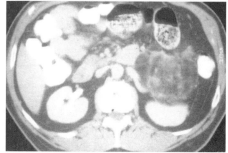

Myelolipoma

Figure 3-12-8

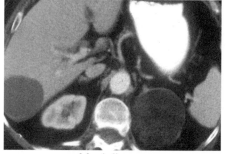

Myelolipoma

Washout calculation [Figure 3-12-9]

$[1 - (HU_{delayed} / HU_{dynamic})] \times 100$

example: if 45 HU at 15 minutes, & 82HU at 70 seconds (dynamic),
$[1 - (45 / 82)] \times 100 = 45\% \neq$ adenoma

Figure 3-12-9

Washout CT of metastasis

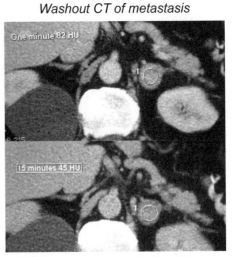

Algorithm

- NCCT:
  - ➢ If less than 10 HU, it's an adenoma [STOP]
  - ➢ If more than 10 HU, proceed to:
    - ❖ CECT: (dynamic and 15* minute delay)
      - ❖ If less than 30* HU on delayed scan = adenoma ?
      - ❖ If more than 30 HU on delayed scan, is relative washout more   than 50% ? If so, it's an adenoma

* = controversial

Mayo-Smith WW. Letter to the Editor: CT Characterization of Adrenal Masses. Radiology 2003;226:289-290

- Opposed phase MRI (OPMRI)
  - ➢ decrease in signal relative to spleen = adenoma → no further evaluation needed
  - ➢ no decrease → biopsy
  - ➢ indeterminate → consider CT evaluation [will probably need "washout"/delay scans because the lipid content is probably too small to make the lesion sufficiently hypodense]

References

Szolar DH, Kammerhuber FH. Adrenal adenomas and nonadenomas: assessment of washout at delayed contrast-enhanced CT. Radiology 1998; 207:369–375

Korobkin M, Brodeur FJ, Francis IR, Quint LE, Dunnick NR, Londy F. CT time-attenuation curves of adrenal adenomas and nonadenomas. AJR 1998; 170:747–752.

Korobkin M. CT characterization of adrenal masses: the time has come. Radiology 2000; 217:629.

Pena CS, et al. Characterization of indeterminate (lipid-poor) adrenal masses: use of washout characteristics at contrast-enhanced CT. Radiology 2000; 217:798.

Kenney PJ, Wagner BJ, Rao P, Heffess CS. Myelolipoma: CT and pathologic features. Radiology 1998; 208: 87-95.

Imaging of the Urinary Bladder and Urethra

Brent J. Wagner, MD
Uniformed Services Univ. of the Health Sciences
The Reading Hospital and Medical Center

Outline
- Bladder
  - ➢ filling defects
  - ➢ wall thickening (+/– calcification)
  - ➢ abnormal contour
- Urethra
  - ➢ anatomy
  - ➢ filling defects
  - ➢ obstructive processes (strictures, valves)

Bladder: Filling defects
- neoplasm
- calculus
- clot
- fungus ball
- ureterocele
- endometriosis
- schistosomiasis
- (prostate)

Bladder: Types of Neoplasms
- transitional cell ca (TCC) (urothelial)
- squamous cell ca
- adenocarcinoma
- leiomyoma/sarcoma
- hemangioma
- metastasis
  - ➢ invasion
  - ➢ other
- embryonal rhabdomyosarcoma (child)

Bladder Neoplasms: (TCC), urothelial carcinoma
[Figure 3-13-1]
- males > females
- 80% over age 50
- typically, projects into lumen
- papilloma = low grade TCC
- irregular surface, "papillary"
- occasionally (30%) multifocal
- CT to assess extraluminal extent
- enhances on early CT scan; filling defect on delayed scan

Bladder neoplasms: Differential features
[Figures 3-13-2 and 3-13-3
- TCC = common
- squamous cell carcinoma = look for associated stones, history of infection (Schistosomiasis?), or chronic indwelling catheter
- adenocarcinoma = often of urachal origin; look for calcified anterior midline mass with prominent extracystic growth

Figure 3-13-1

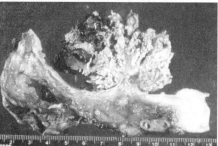
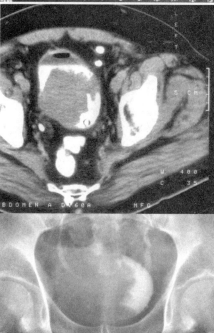

Urothelial carcinoma

Figure 3-13-2

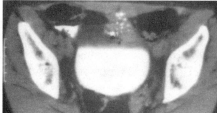
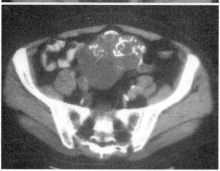

Urachal carcinoma

Filling Defects: (may be mobile)

- clot
  - ➤ often smooth
- stones
  - ➤ shadowing on U/S, midline on supine radiograph
  - ➤ occasionally radiolucent (or obscured) post-contrast
  - ➤ history of infection (and/or)
  - ➤ evidence for bladder outlet obstruction
    - ❖ trabeculation
    - ❖ hydroureter
    - ❖ prostate impression
- fungus ball
  - ➤ laminated, gas-containing

Filling Defects: Miscellaneous: [Figures 3-13-4 and 3-13-5]

- ureterocele
  - ➤ smooth
- prostate
  - ➤ midline, generally smooth
- endometriosis
  - ➤ can look like anything
- gastrointestinal inflammation
  - ➤ Crohn's
  - ➤ diverticulitis

Wall thickening [Figure 3-13-6]

- I. cystitis and variants
  - ➤ infection
    - ❖ TB*
    - ❖ Schistosomiasis*
    - ❖ malakoplakia
    - ❖ cystitis cystica (lobulated, diffuse)
  - ➤ radiation*
  - ➤ post-cytoxan*
- II. Neoplasm (TCC)
- III. Bladder outlet obstruction
- IV. Inflammation/invasion

*may calcify

Malakoplakia

- most common in females with recurrent infection
- mimics infiltrating carcinoma
  - ➤ cysto/bx to diagnose
- Michaelis-Gutman bodies

Cystitis glandularis – is it pre-malignant?

- "Cystitis glandularis is so common that it may be considered a normal feature of the vesical mucosa."
- There are 2 types of cystitis glandularis
  - ➤ "typical"
  - ➤ "intestinal" (less common)
- "Diffuse cystitis glandularis of the intestinal type is termed intestinal metaplasia and usually occurs in chronically irritated bladders such as those of paraplegics or in patients with stones or long term catheterization . . . it is associated with an increased risk of bladder carcinoma."
- "It is only the intestinal type of cystitis glandularis that is associated with adenocarcinoma."

Young RH, Eble JN. Non-neoplastic disorders of the urinary bladder. In: Urologic Surgical Pathology. Mosby 1997. pp 174–5.

Figure 3-13-3

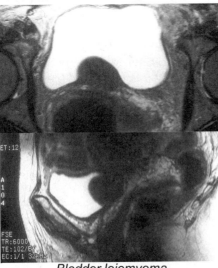

Bladder leiomyoma

Figure 3-13-4

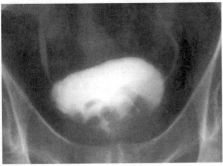

Prostate carcinoma

Figure 3-13-5

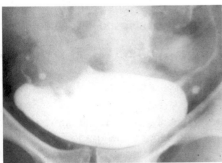

Endometriosis

Figure 3-13-6

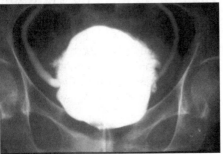

Tuberculosis

Schistosomiasis
- calcification in 50%
- calcification is rare in transitional / urothelial carcinoma
- Schistosomiasis is a risk factor for squamous cell ca of the bladder

Regional enteritis (Crohn's) or other gastrointestinal disease
- combination of regional wall thickening and invasion
- diverticulitis more common than regional enteritis
- associated findings with regional enteritis
  - calculi
  - anterior/right (posterior/left for diverticulitis)
- progression:
  - impression/thickening
  - invasion
  - fistula

Emphysematous cystitis
- urinary tract combined with uncontrolled diabetes mellitus
- air may be intraluminal as well as intramural
  - linear, lucent streaks
- non-surgical condition
- treatment: antibiotics and insulin

Abnormal contour
- smooth narrowing:
  - pelvic lipomatosis
  - pelvic hematoma
  - (irregular narrowing = lymphoma, other mass?)
- focal outpouching (diverticula):
  - bladder outlet obstruction
  - stones/tumors/bleeding
  - reflux/ureteral obstruction
    - ❖ (especially in children)

Urethra: Anatomy
- posterior:
  - prostatic
  - membranous
- anterior:
  - bulbous
  - penile

Urethrography: Technique
- Clamp vs. catheter
- Fluoroscopic guidance
- Hand injection
- Usually, dilute (30%) contrast

Urethra: Masses/filling defects
- urethral carcinoma
  - most are squamous (if proximal, consider transitional/urothelial carcinoma)
  - 70% of cases in males are associated with postinflammatory stricture
  - filling defect or irregular stricturing
- condyloma acuminata [Figure 3-13-7]
  - urethral disease in only 5% of pts with external lesions
  - viral

Figure 3-13-7

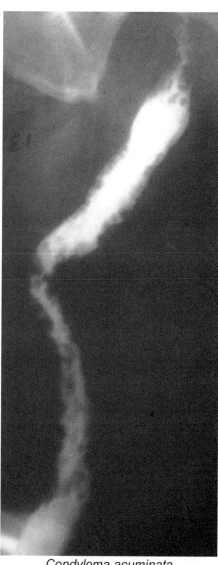

Condyloma acuminata

Urethra: Strictures [Figure 3-13-8]

- post-inflammatory
  - ➤ especially gonococcal (40% of strictures in the U.S.)
- post-traumatic
  - ➤ includes iatrogenic
- may be associated with perineal fistula

Urethra: Obstructive processes [Figure 3-13-9]

- posterior urethral valve
- anterior urethral valve
  - ➤ (vs. diverticulum)
  - ➤ acquired or congenital
  - ➤ may obstruct, or develop calculi

Urethra: Diverticulum of the female urethra [Figure 3-13-10]

- outpouching of contrast
  - ➤ may require double-balloon technique
- fluid-filled mass on CT, MR, or sonography
- associated with carcinoma (usually squamous)

References

Beer A, Saar B, Rummeny EJ. Tumors of the urinary bladder: technique, current use, and perspectives of MR and CT cystography. Abdom Imaging 2003; 28:868.

Pavlica P, Menchi I, Barozzi L. New imaging of the anterior male urethra. Abdom Imaging 2003; 28:180.

Figure 3-13-8

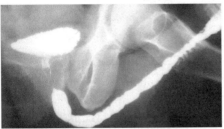

Acute and subacute gonococcal urethritis

Figure 3-13-9

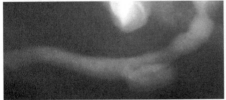

Urethral diverticulum (male)

Figure 3-13-10

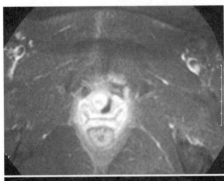

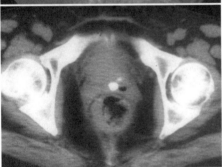

Urethral diverticulum (female)

Non-Neoplastic Disorders Of The Ovary And Adnexae

Jade Wong You Cheong, MD
Associate Professor
University of Maryland School of Medicine

Outline
- Clinical and sonographic characteristics of non neoplastic ovarian and adnexal pathology
- Role of CT / MR
- Gestational trophoblastic disease

Essential Clinical Information
- Age of patient
- Symptoms e.g fever, discharge
- Menstrual status and time in cycle
- Pregnancy status
- Previous surgery and medical history
- Drugs, e.g HRT, ovulation stimulation

Functional ovarian cysts
- Very common incidental findings
- Disordered physiological events
- Most regress spontaneously
- Can present with acute pain and require surgical intervention

Functional ovarian cysts
- Follicular
- Corpus luteal
- Theca lutein

Follicular cyst
- Failure of mature follicle to rupture or regress
- Usually 3–8 cm
- Unilocular simple cyst
- Well defined thin smooth wall
- Regress spontaneously (if <5 cm) or may respond to hormonal suppression
- Clinical or sonographic follow-up in 6–8 weeks

Normal ovaries-MR

Follicular cyst

Corpus luteum cyst
- Persistence of corpus luteum or bleeding into it
- >3 cm
- Acute pain
- Rupture
- Unilocular thick walled cyst
- Vascular wall
- CL cyst of pregancy regresses by 16 wk

Corpus luteum cyst

Corpora lutea

Hemorrhagic functional cysts

- Hemorrage occurs into cyst, presents with acute pain
- More common in luteal cysts
- Imaging spectrum depends on age
- Rapid change
- Thin linear fibrin strands "reticular or fish net"
- Retracting hyperechoic clot
- Fluis – debris level
- Mildly thickened wall
- Diffuse low level echoes with acoustic engancement "ground glass", rarely

Hemorrhagic functional cyst [Figure 3-14-1]

Hemorrhagic Corpus Luteum

Ruptured Cyst [Figure 3-14-2]

Ruptured Cyst with Hemorrhage

Theca lutein cysts

- Gestational trophoblastic disease
  - ➢ Associated with high levels of HCG
- Ovarian hyperstimulation
  - ➢ Secondary to infertility drugs
  - ➢ Abdominal pain, distension, nausea, vomiting

Hyperstimulation Cysts

- Bilateral enlarged ovaries
- Multiple cysts
- May bleed, rupture or torse
- Ascites, pleural effusion, hemorrhage, DIC

OHSS

Theca lutein cysts

Endometriosis

- Functioning ectopic endometrium
- Pelvic peritoneum, ovary, tube

Endometriosis

- Symptoms
  - ➢ Dysmenorrhea
  - ➢ Dyspareunia
  - ➢ Pelvic pain
- Cyclic pain with menses
- Associated with infertility
  - ➢ prevalence 25%

Endometrioma [Figure 3-14-3 next page]

- Thick walled cystic lesion
- "Ground glass" homogeneous low level echoes (highly suggestive)
- Unilocular or multilocular with septations
- Mural reflectors
- Rarely fluid-fluid level

Atypical Endometrioma

Figure 3-14-1

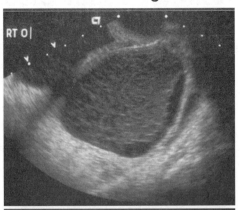

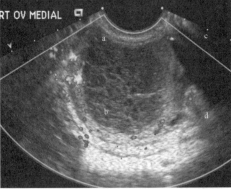

Ultrasound spectrum of hemorrhagic cysts:
top: retracting clot,
bottom: "fish net"

Figure 3-14-2

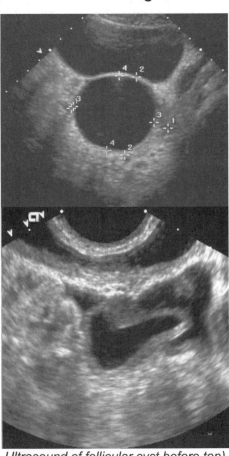

Ultrasound of follicular cyst before top)
and after rupture (bottom)

Diffuse Endometriosis
- More common
- Associated with fibrosis and adhesions
- Laparoscopy is gold standard
- Allows staging and treatment

Endometriosis- MR Technique
- Axial T1-w SE
- Axial/sagittal/coronal T2-w FSE
- Axial fat-suppressed T1-w SE to distinguish fat from blood
- Dynamic enhanced T1-w (optional)

Endometrioma-MR
- Highly accurate, sensitive and specific (90-96%)
- Thick walled cystic lesion
- Hyperintense on T1-w
- Hypointense on T2-w "shading"
- Multiple homogeneous hyperintense lesions T1-w

Endometrioma-MR
- Less specific signs
  - Homogeneously hyperintense lesions T1-w and T2-w
  - Low signal hemosiderin ring
  - Enhancement of cyst wall/peritoneum

Rectus endometriosis

Diffuse Endometriosis-MR
- Poor sensitivity
- Areas of low signal T2-w (fibrosis)
- Areas of high signal T2-w (endometrium)
- Focal peritoneal enhancement
- Adhesions
- MR useful for inaccessible sites or for evaluation of response to medical treatment

Endometrioma or hemorrhagic cyst?
- Clinical history
- Sequential imaging with US
- MR
  - Less bright on T1-w
  - No shading on T2-w
  - Single

"Rule out ovarian torsion"

Ovarian torsion
- 3% of gynecologic emergencies
- Usually premenopausal
- 20% pregnant
- 80% associated mass
- Acute pain, nausea, vomiting
- Previous self limiting episodes

Ovarian torsion
- Gray scale (non specific)
  - Dependent on underlying cause
  - Enlarged hypoechoic ovary with peripheral follicles
  - mass e.g. teratoma, functional cyst
  - Hemorrhagic infarction

Figure 3-14-3

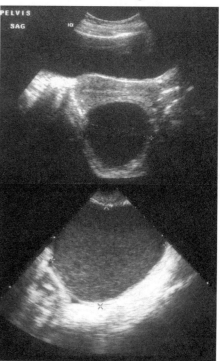

Transabdominal (top) and transvaginal ultrasound (bottom) of endometrioma with ground glass appearance

Ovarian Torsion-enlarged ovary

Adnexal Torsion

Ovarian Torsion - Diagnosis [Figure 3-14-4]
- Doppler is key
  - Absence of arterial and venous flow
  - High resistance arterial flow
  - Loss of venous flow
  - Twisted vascular pedicle
  - Corkscrew vessels

Torsed Teratoma

Adnexal Torsion: CT/MR
- Deviation of uterus to affected side
- Obliteration of fat planes
- Enlarged displaced ovary
- Beak sign with congested vessels
- Lack of enhancement

Torsion of cystadenoma

Ovarian Torsion twisted pedicle [Figure 3-14-5]

Ovarian torsion
- Diagnostic difficulties
  - Dual ovarian arterial supply
  - Incomplete and intermittent torsion
  - False positives
    - Technical
    - Pathologic
- High index of suspicion if symptomatic ovary enlarged
- Rescan early

Hydrosalpinx
- Tubular fluid filled structure
- Folding mimics multilocular lesion
- Sequela of PID, endometriosis, surgery

Pelvic Inflammatory Disease
- Imaging for:
  - Complications
  - Failure to respond to first line treatment
  - Alternative diagnosis
- US first
- CT or MR for difficult / severe cases
- Thick walled tube
- Cog wheel
- Internal echoes
- Tuboovarian complex or abscess
  - Complex adnexal mass with hydro/pyosalpinx

Acute Salpingitis

Pyosalpinx [Figure 3-14-6]

TOA OVT

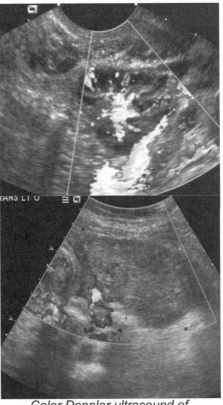

Figure 3-14-4

Color Doppler ultrasound of asymmetric size and blood flow in ovarian torsion
[top]: normal, [bottom]: enlarged ovary with decreased vascularity

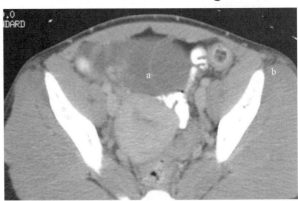

Figure 3-14-5

CT of ovarian torsion with twisted pedicle sign

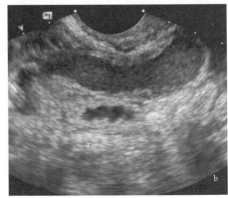

Figure 3-14-6

Ultrasound of pyosalpinx

Ovarian Vein Thrombophlebitis

- Septic thrombosis in ovarian veins
- Post partum or post surgery/pelvic inflammatory disease
- Pain, fever and leucocytosis
- Occult
- Treated with antibiotics and anticoagulants

- Distended ovarian vein
- Thrombus
- Perivenous inflammatory changes
- Edematous adnexa

Ovarian Vein Thrombophlebitis [Figure 3-14-7]

Bilateral Tuboovarian Abscesses

Peritoneal Inclusion Cysts [Figure 3-14-8]
"Benign cystic mesothelioma, multilocular peritoneal cyst"
- Loculated peritoneal fluid within adhesions
- Previous pelvic surgery/endometrosis/PID
- Pre or post menopausal
- Treatment
  - ➢ Surgical (30–50% recurrence)
  - ➢ OCP +/– TV US guided aspiration

- May mimic a cystic ovarian neoplasm
- Septated cystic peritoneal lesion surrounding normal ovary
- Ovary suspended by adhesions
- Flow may be present in septations

Polycystic Ovary Syndrome
- Infertility and hormonal disturbance
- 3–7% of women
- "Stein Leventhal Syndrome"
  - ➢ Amenorrhea, Infertility, Hirsutism
- Absence of mid cycle LH surge
- Increased LH: FSH
- Suspended follicular development
- Androgen production

Polycystic Ovary Syndrome
- Enlarged ovaries (>10–12 cm³)
- Multiple (>10) small (<8–10 mm) peripheral follicles
- Echogenic stroma
- Normal ovaries (30%)

Pache, T., J. Wladimiroff, et al. (1992). "How to discriminate between normal and polycystic ovaries: transvaginal US study." Radiology 183(2): 421-423.

Polycystic ovaries

Paraovarian/paratubal Cysts
- 10–20% of adnexal masses
- Arise in broad ligament from mesothelial and paramesonephric remnants
- Any age (3rd–4th decades most common)
- Complicated by
  - ➢ Hemorrhage
  - ➢ Torsion
  - ➢ Rupture
  - ➢ Neoplasm

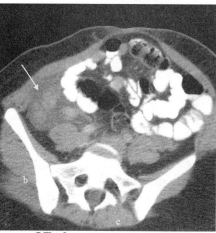

Figure 3-14-7

CT of post partum ovarian thrombophlebitis c: arrow on dilated thrombosed ovarian vein with perivenous edema

Figure 3-14-8

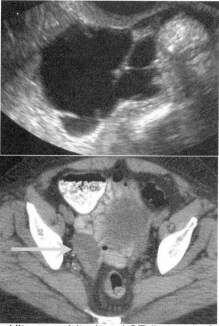

Ultrasound (top) and CT (bottom) of peritoneal inclusion cyst

Paraovarian Cysts

- Simple unilocular adnexal cyst
- Separate from (but adjacent to) ovary
- Lack of change with time
- Rarely bilateral or multiple
- Rarely complex

Serous Inclusion Cysts

- 17% of asymptomatic post menopausal women
- <3 cm, thin walled unilocular cysts
- Cyclic variation
- Secondary to repeated ovulation with trapping of surface epithelium in ovarian cortex
- Majority resolve, follow-up sonography

Levine D. Simple adnexal cysts: the natural history in postmenopausal women. Radiology, 1992; 184, 653-659

Gestational Trophoblastic Disease

- Heterogenous group of disorders
- Abnormal proliferation of chorionic tissues
- Varying propensity to invade and metastasize
- Elevated beta HCG
  - ➤ Hyperemesis, toxemia, bleeding

Gestational Trophoblastic Disease

- Benign
  - ➤ Hydatidiform mole
- Malignant
  - ➤ Invasive mole
  - ➤ Choriocarcinoma
  - ➤ Placental site trophoblastic disease

Gestational Trophoblastic Disease

- Chorionic villi of blighted ovum persist
- Hydropic change

Benign Hydatidiform Mole

- Most common (80%)
- 1 in 1200–2000 pregnancies (US)
- Extremes of reproductive life
- Previous mole (risk of recurrence 1% after 1 mole, 23% after 2 molar pregnancies)

Molar Pregnancy

Classic "complete" mole	Partial mole
➤ 80%	Triploid
➤ 46 XX	69 XXY 80%
➤ Complete molar change	69 XXX
➤ No fetal tissue	Hydropic placenta
➤ Nuclear DNA paternal	
➤ Cytoplasmic DNA maternal	

Figure 3-14-9

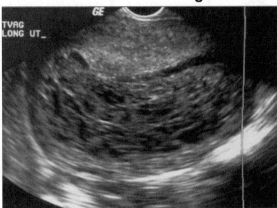

Transvaginal ultrasound of a complete mole

Complete mole: sonography [Figure 3-14-9]

- Enlarged uterus
- Echogenic mass in endometrial cavity
- Small cystic spaces
- Low impedance flow
- Theca lutein cysts (20–50%)
- May mimic incomplete abortion, hydropic placenta

Complete Hydatidiform Mole

Partial mole
- Triploid fetus
  - IUGR, anomalies
- Hydropic placenta
- Spontaneous abortion

GTD
- Management
  - D & C
  - Monitoring of beta HCG levels
    - ❖ Exponential drop (near zero by 10–12 weeks)
  - US to exclude pregnancy
  - Invasive mole 10%
  - Choriocarcinoma 5% → Chemotherapy

Recurrent Complete Mole

Malignant GTD
- Invasive mole
  - Locally invasive, non metastatic, <10%
  - Vesicular chorionic villi with myometrial invasion
- Choriocarcinoma
  - 5%, hematogenous metastases to lungs, brain, liver, etc.
  - May not necessary follow a gestation
  - No villous structure

Choriocarcinoma [Figure 3-14-10]

Summary
- Characteristic sonographic features allow diagnosis of most benign adnexal masses
- MR useful for indeterminate adnexal mass

Figure 3-14-10

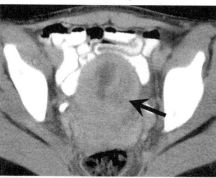
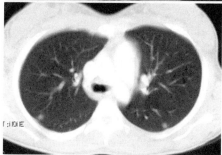

CT of choriocarcinoma: (top) myometrial invasion, (bottom) lung metastases

References

Patel, M. D., V. A. Feldstein, et al. (1999). "Endometriomas: Diagnostic Performance of US." Radiology 210(3): 739-74

Togashi K. Endometrial cysts: diagnosis with MR imaging. Radiology 1991,180: 73-78

Sugimura K. Pelvic endometriosis: detection and diagnosis with chemical shift MR imaging. Radiology 1993; 188: 435-438.

Woodward, P. J., R. Sohaey, et al. (2001). "Endometriosis: Radiologic-Pathologic Correlation." RadioGraphics 21(1): 193-216.

Siegelman, E. S. and E. K. Outwater (1999). "Tissue Characterization in the Female Pelvis by Means of MR Imaging." Radiology 212(1): 5-18.

Albayram F, Hamper UM. Ovarian and adnexal torsion. Spectrum of sonographic findings with pathologic correlation. J Ultrasound Med 2001; 20:1083-1089

Descargues G, et al. Adnexal torsion: a report on forty five cases. Eur J Obstet Gynecol Reprod Biol 2001; 98:91-96

Lee EJ, et al. Diagnosis of ovarian torsion with color Doppler sonography: depiction of twisted vascular pedicle. J Ultrasound Med 1998; 17:83-89

Rha SE et al. CT and MR features of adnexal torsion. RadioGraphics 2002; 22:283-294 Hertzberg BS. Ovarian cyst rupture causing hemoperitoneum: imaging features and the potential for misdiagnosis. Abdominal imaging 1999; 24:304-308

Bennett, G. L. et al. (2002). "Gynecologic Causes of Acute Pelvic Pain: Spectrum of CT Findings." RadioGraphics 22(4): 785-801.

Jain, K. A. (2000). "Imaging of Peritoneal Inclusion Cysts." Am. J. Roentgenol. 174(6): 1559-1563

Sohaey, R., T. L. Gardner, et al. (1995). "Sonographic diagnosis of peritoneal inclusion cysts." J Ultrasound Med 14(12): 913-7.

Wagner BJ, Woodward PJ, Dickey GE. From the archives of the AFIP. Gestational trophoblastic disease: radiologic-pathologic correlation.Radiographics. 1996 Jan;16(1):131-48.

Green, C., T. Angtuaco, et al. (1996). "Gestational trophoblastic disease: a spectrum of radiologic diagnosis." RadioGraphics 16(6): 1371-1384.

Imaging of Solid Organ Transplants

Jade Wong-You-Cheong, MD
Associate Professor
University of Maryland School of Medicine

Transplantation
- Higher success rates with better anti rejection therapy, patient selection and surgical techniques
- Rejection remains major cause of graft loss
- Immunosuppression predisposes to infection and neoplasm
- Symptoms and signs of infection subtle
- High index of suspicion

Types of Transplants
- Renal
- Pancreas
- Liver

Post-transplantation Imaging
- Ultrasound is the primary modality
  - Echotexture
  - Fluid collections
  - Blood flow
  - Guidance for interventional procedures

Post-transplantation Imaging
- CT
  - Collections
  - Infection
  - Surgical Complications
  - Neoplasm
  - Guidance for procedures

Post-transplantation Imaging
- MRI and MRA
  - Parenchyma
  - Vascular complications
  - Perfusion
  - Masses
  - Rejection

Post-transplantation Imaging
- Other
  - Scintigraphy
  - Cystography
  - Cholangiography
  - Arteriography and intervention

Renal Transplants
- CRT: Cadaveric renal transplant
- LRT: Living related renal transplant
- LNRT: Living non-related renal transplant
- Dual: "En bloc" pediatric or two adult
- SPK: Simultaneous pancreas-kidney

Renal Transplantation: Surgical Technique
- Iliac fossa extraperitoneal placement
- Arterial anastomosis
  - ➤ End to side to external iliac artery
- Venous anastomosis
  - ➤ End to side to external iliac vein
- Ureteral anastomosis very variable

Renal Transplants: Sonography
- Gray scale: hydronephrosis, echotexture, collections
- Color Doppler: identify vessels
- Duplex Doppler of
  - ➤ MRA, MRV
  - ➤ Segmental, interlobar and arcuate arteries
  - ➤ Measure RI – x3
- Real time guidance for biopsy

Normal Renal Transplant

Resistive Index $RI = (PSV-EDV) / PSV$

Renal Transplant Complications
- Perinephric fluid collections (50%)
- Rejection – acute and chronic
- Obstruction (1–10%)
- Vascular Complications (10%)
- Acute tubular necrosis (DGF)
- Cyclosporine toxicity
- PTLD (1%)
- Torsion

Perinephric Fluid Collections
- Early
  - ➤ Hematomas 9%
  - ➤ Seromas
  - ➤ Urinary leak 18% (1–2 weeks)
- Later
  - ➤ Abscess 30%
  - ➤ Lymphoceles 43% (4–8 weeks)
- Aspirate for diagnosis

Hematoma [Figure 3-15-1]

Hemorrhage

Urinoma

Lymphocele

Abscess [Figure 3-15-2]

Hydronephrosis
- 1–10%
- Early: edema of UVJ
- Late:
  Compression by fluid collections
  - ➤ Denervation (non obstructive
  - ➤ Full bladder (repeat with empty bladder)
  - ➤ Ureteric ischemia, surgical technique (kinks)
  - ➤ Rejection
  - ➤ Intraluminal clot or calculi

Figure 3-15-1

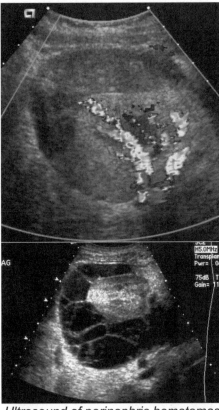

Ultrasound of perinephric hematomas of various ages

Figure 3-15-2

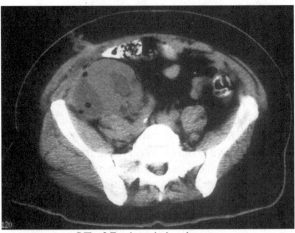

CT of Perinephric abscess

Hydronephrosis

Ureteral stricture [Figure 3-15-3]

Hydronephrosis
- Dilatation does not equal obstruction
- RI not reliable in differentiating dilatation from obstruction

Echoes Within Collecting System
- Hemonephrosis
  - ➢ Low level echoes
  - ➢ Move with patient
  - ➢ Hematuria
  - ➢ Post biopsy
  - ➢ Urinary infection

Hemonephrosis

Candidiasis
- Fungus balls
  - ➢ Highly echogenic, weakly shadowing
  - ➢ Candida in urine

Echoes Within Collecting System
- Calculi or nepohrocalcinosis
  - ➢ Echogenic structures with acoustic shadowing

Nephrocalcinosis

Calculi

Gas
- Emphysematous pyelonephritis
- Reflux from catheterization

Rejection
- Non specific elevation of creatinine
- Fever, white count, pain over transplant
- Decreased urine outpout
- Acute (> day 5) reversible with treament
- Chronic (months to years) irreversible

Acute Rejection Gray Scale
- Non specific
  - ➢ Enlargement
  - ➢ Increased cortical echogenicity
  - ➢ Decreased echogenicity of central sinus
  - ➢ Loss of corticomedullary differentiation
  - ➢ Prominent pyramids
  - ➢ Thickening of collecting system

Thick urothelium

Acute Rejection
- Vascular rejection results in increased resistance with increase in resistive index
- Correlation highly variable
- Threshold? 0.7 or 0.9
- BIOPSY: only reliable method to determine cause of renal dysfunction

Figure 3-15-3

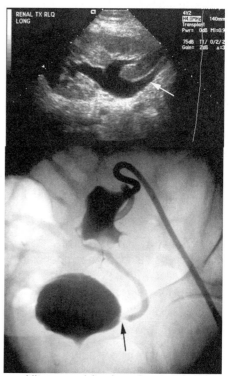

Ultrasound (top) and antegrade ureterogram (bottom) of transplant ureteral stricture

Chronic Rejection
- Small allograft
- Echogenic from fibrosis
- Fatty replacement
- Calcification
- Decreased blood flow

Vascular Complications
- Early (Surgical emergencies)
  - Renal vein thrombosis
  - Renal artery occlusion
- Later
  - Renal artery stenosis (10%)
  - Post biopsy complications (AVF, PSA)
  - Renal vein stenosis

Renal Vein Thrombosis
- Gray-scale: swollen hypoechoic
- Doppler:
  - Absent venous flow
  - Reversed plateauing of diastole
  - High resistance

Renal Vein thrombosis [Figure 3-15-4]

Renal Artery Occlusion
- Gray-scale: swollen kidney
- Doppler
  - Absent intrarenal arterial
  - High resistance, high PSV, no diastolic flow
  - Spiked preocclusive wave form
- NB: Severe acute rejection can cause diminished flow

Figure 3-15-4

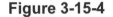
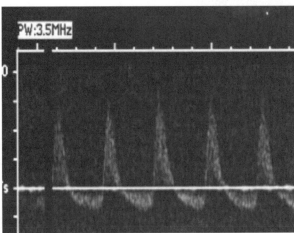

Doppler ultrasound of renal vein thrombosis

Renal Artery Stenosis
- Hypertension, graft dysfunction and bruit
- Conventional angiography
  - Reference standard (invasive contrast)
  - Allows angioplasty
- Sonography
- MR Angiography

MRA normal

Sonographic criteria
- PSV >2 m/s
- Velocity gradient >2:1
- Post stenotic spectral broadening
- Pulsus tardus-parvus(prolonged early acceleration, diminished amplitude SAT >0.07s, AI <3 M/s^2 ,RI <0.56

Renal artery stenosis

Tardus parvus

Intrarenal Arteriovenous Fistulae/Pseudoaneurysms
- Secondary to percutaneous biopsy
- Most clinically insignificant and resolve
- May be treated conservatively if small and asymptomatic
- Embolized if large or causing ischemia and severe hematuria

Intrarenal Arteriovenous Fistulae
- Gray scale
  - Usually invisible
- Color Doppler
  - Flurry/perivascular bleeding
  - Feeding artery – draining vein if large
  - Aliasing
- Duplex
  - High velocity/low resistance
  - Arterialized venous flow

Arteriovenous fistula

Pseudoaneurysms *[Figure 3-15-5]*
- Gray scale
  - Simple or complex cyst
- Doppler
  - Yin yang swirling flow
  - To and fro (neck)
  - Disorganized flow within
- May rupture

Renal Vein Stenosis
- Perivascular fibrosis
- Compression by fluid collections
- Doppler
  - Aliasing
  - Velocity increase (x3–4)

Pancreas Transplants
- SPK: Simultaneous pancreas-kidney
- PAK: Pancreas after kidney
- PTA: Pancreas transplant alone
- OLT: Orthotopic liver transplant

Pancreatic Transplantation: Surgical Technique
- Endocrine Drainage (Venous)
  - Systemic (iliac vein)
  - Portal vein
- Exocrine Drainage
  - Bladder
  - Enteric
- Arterial supply from common iliac artery

Simultaneous Pancreas and Kidney Transplantation

Pancreatic Transplant Complications
- Rejection
  - Acute
  - Chronic
- Surgical complications
  - Infection
  - Anastomotic Leak
- Vascular thrombosis
  - Arterial
  - Venous
- Pancreatitis

Figure 3-15-5

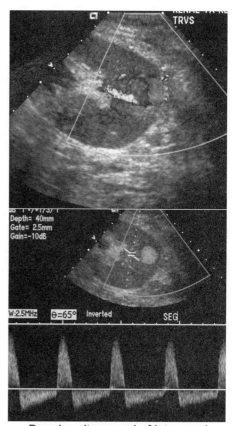

Doppler ultrasound of intrarenal pseudoaneurysm

Normal Pancreas Transplant

Pancreas Transplant CT

Pancreatic Transplant MR [Figure 3-15-6]

Pancreas Transplant MRA

Figure 3-15-6

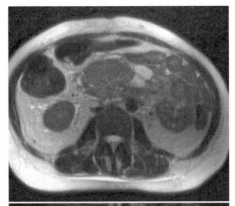

Peripancreatic Collections
- 2-10%
- Hematoma, seroma, anastomotic leak, abscess
- Nonspecific appearance
- Aspiration needed for diagnosis

Anastomotic leak with abscess [Figure 3-15-7]

Pancreatic Transplant Rejection
- 40% of graft loss
- Enlargement and heterogeneity of gland
- US Doppler RI – no correlation
- Diagnosed by percutaneous US guided biopsy

Pancreatic Transplant Vascular Thrombosis
- 6–10% of graft loss
- Venous more common than arterial
- US and MRA most useful
- Swollen heterogenous gland
- No flow or enhancement
- Thrombosed vessels

Pancreatic Thrombosis

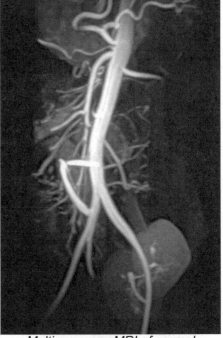

Multisequence MRI of normal pancreas transplant: (top) T2 axial, (bottom) MRA

Liver Transplantation
- Established or fulminant liver failure (hepatitis C, PBC, PSC, alcolhol, cryptogenic cirrhosis, etc.)
- Cadaveric
- Living or cadaveric split liver (right lobe)

Liver Transplantation
- Gray scale evaluation includes
  - Fluid collections
  - Free fluid (ascites or bile)
  - Biliary dilatation – choledochojejunostomy or choledocholedochostomy
  - Parenchyma

Post Operative Imaging
- Sonography
- CT
- MRI MRA
- Angiography
- Scintigraphy – bile leaks
- Cholangiography

Liver Transplantation
- Doppler evaluation includes
- MPV, LPV, RPV
- CHA, LHA, RHA
- HV x 3
- IVC above and below anastomosis

Figure 3-15-7

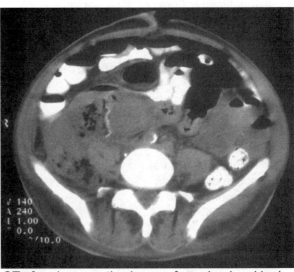

CT of peripancreatic abscess from duodenal leak

Biliary Tree

Complications
- Rejection
- Vascular thrombosis or stenosis
- Biliary obstruction or leak
- Recurrent hepatitis
- Fatty infiltration
- Neoplasm

Hepatic Artery Thrombosis

Portal Vein Thrombosis

Cavernous Transformation

Fatty Infiltration

Biliary

Parenchyma
- Hematoma
- Abscess

Bilomas after arterial thrombosis

Post Transplant Lymphoproliferative Disorder
- Related to Epstein Barr virus
- Any time (mean = 15 months)
- Spectrum
  - ➤ Polyclonla diffuse B cell proliferation
  - ➤ Malignant monoclonal lymphoma
- Treatment
  - ➤ Decreased immunosuppression
  - ➤ Antiviral agents
  - ➤ Chemotherapy

Post Transplant Lymphoproliferative Disorder *[Figure 3-15-8]*
- Radiology
  - ➤ Lymphadenopathy
  - ➤ Solid/hollow visceral involvement
    - ❖ Liver
    - ❖ Lungs
    - ❖ Spleen
    - ❖ Bowel

PTLD SBO

Post Transplant Malignancy
- Kaposi's sarcoma   x 400–500
- Lymphoma   x 20–350
- Vulva/perineum   x 100
- Lip   x 29
- Skin (squamous)   x 7–40
- Cervix   x 4–14

Figure 3-15-8

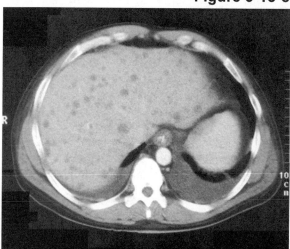

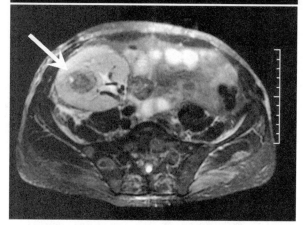

Post transplant lymphoproliferative disorder in liver (top) and renal transplant (bottom)

Lymphadenopathy

Summary

- Ultrasound with color and duplex Doppler is an ideal first line modality for renal , pancreas and liver transplants
- Sensitive for vascular complications, fluid collections and hydronephrosis
- Biopsy needed for diagnosis of rejection
- CT for infection, fluid collections, procedures, malignancy
- MR for evaluation of vascular and parenchymal abnormalities

References

Baxter GM. Ultrasound of renal transplantation. Clin Radiol 2001; 56:802-818
Hohenwalter MD et al. Renal transplant evaluation with MR angiography and MR imaging. RadioGraphics. 2001; 21:1505-1517

Middleton WDE, et al Post-biopsy renal transplant arteriovenous fistulas: color Doppler ultrasound characteristics. Radiology, 1989; 171:253-257

Tobben PJ, et al. Pseudoaneurysms complicating organ transplantation: roles of CT, duplex sonography and angiography. Radiology 1988; 169:65-70

Linkowski GD, et al: Sonography in the diagnosis of acute renal allograft rejection and cyclosporin toxicity Am J Roentgenol 1987; 148:291-295

Vrachliotis TG, et al. CT findings in posttransplantation lymphoproliferative disorder of renal transplants. AJR 2000; 175:183-188

Sebastia C, et al. Helical CT in renal transplantation: normal findings and early and late complications. RadioGraphics 2001; 21:1103-1117

Kaushik S, et al. Posttransplantation lymphoproliferative disorder: osseous and hepatic involvement. AJR 2001; 177:1057-1059

Dachman AH, et al. Imaging of pancreatic transplantation using portal venous and enteric exocrine drainage. AJR 1998 Jul;171(1):157-63

Boeve WJ, et al. Comparison of contrast enhanced MR-angiography-MRI and digital subtraction angiography in the evaluation of pancreas and/or kidney transplantation patients: initial experience. Magn Reson Imaging. 2001 Jun;19(5):595-607

Crossin JD, Muradali D, Wilson SR. US of liver transplants: normal and abnormal. Radiographics. 2003 Sep-Oct;23(5):1093-114

The Neglected Nephrogram

David S. Hartman, MD
Penn State
College Of Medicine

Nephrogram
- Excretory Urography
- CT
- MR
- Nuclear Medicine
- Angiography
- ? Ultrasound

Normal Nephrographic Pysiology
- The main driving force for urine production is filtartion pressure (blood pressure)
- Contrast is filtered, it is not excreted or reabsorbed by the tubules
- Contrast which gets into the nephron will eventually get to the collecting system

Nephrographic Density
- Iodine concentration
- GFR
- Transit time

Normal Nephrogram requires
- Kidney
- Blood in
- Blood out
- Urine out
- Nephrons

Normal Pyelogram
- Symmetric
- 3 minute film
- Delayed side is the diseased side

CT
- Vascular (cortical)
- Nephrographic
- Pyelographic

Nephrographic Patterns (6)
- Absent
- Delayed pyelogram (unilateral)
- Unilateral hyperdense
- Persistent (bilateral)
- Rim
- Striated

Absent Nephrogram *[Figures 3-16-1]*
- No kidney
- No blood in
- No blood out
- No urine out
- No nephrons

Figure 3-16-1

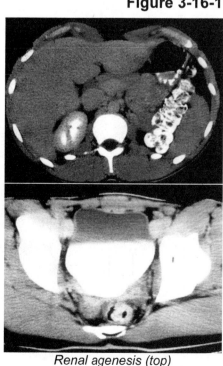

Renal agenesis (top)
Seminal Vesicle Cyst (bottom)

Unilateral Delayed Pyelogram [Figures 3-16-2 and 3-16-3]

- Slow blood in
- Slow blood out
- Slow urine out
- Poor nephron function

Unilateral Hyperdense Nephrogram

- Slow urine out
- Slow blood in
- Slow blood out

Pyelonephritis

- Rarely produces a unilateral hyperdense nephrogram

ATN

- Tubular damage and obstruction
- Decrease blood flow
- "Acute vasomotor nephropathy"

Persistent Bilateral Nephrogram

- Hypotension
- Obstruction
  - ➢ ATN
  - ➢ Urate
  - ➢ Protein
  - ➢ Myoglobin
- Less likely
  - ➢ Bilateral Ureteral Obstruction
  - ➢ Bilateral Renal Artery Stenosis
  - ➢ Bilateral Renal Vein Thrombosis

Rim Nephrogram [Figure 3-16-4]

- Vascular occlusion
- Days to a week to develop

Figure 3-16-2

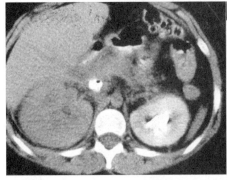
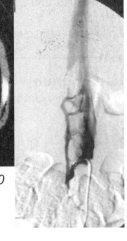

Acute renal vein thrombosis in a 20 YO woman with Antiphospholipid Syndrome (SLE)

Figure 3-16-3

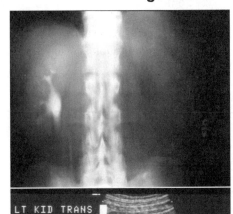
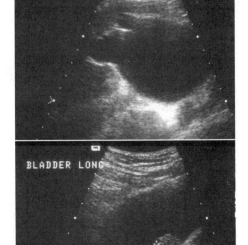

TCC of left UVJ (slow urine out in a 71YO Man with hematuria

Figure 3-16-4

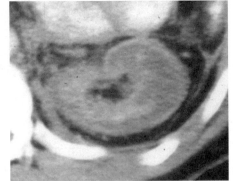

Rim nephrogram in a 21 YO Man with trauma 10 days ago

Striated Nephrogram *[Figure 3-16-5]*

- ARPCK
- Acute pyelonephritis
- Obstruction
- RVT
- Contusion
- Hypotension
- Tubular Obstruction

Striated Nephrogram

- May be normal
- Is non specific
- Many entities with tubular stasis or edema

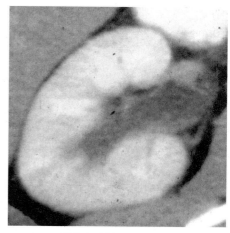

Figure 3-16-5

Striated Nephrogram

References

Davidson, AJ, Hartman, DS, Choyke PL, Wagner BJ. Davidson's Radiology of the Kidney and Genitourinary Tract. Philadelphia, W.B. Saunders 1999; Chapter 27 Nephrographic Analysis.

Amis ES, Epitaph for the urogram. Radiology 1999; 213:639–640.

Yuh BI, Cohan RH. Different phases of renal enhancement: role in detecting and characterizing renal masses during helical CT. AJR 1999; 173:747–755.

Birnbaum BA, Jacobs JE, Langlotz CP, Ramchandani P. Assessment of a bolus-tracking technique in helical renal CT to optimize nephrographic phase imaging. Radiology 1999; 211:87–94.

Saunders HS, Dyer RB, Shifrin RY, Scharling ES, Bechtold RE, Zagoria RJ. The CT nephrogram: implications for evaluation of urinary tract disease. RadioGraphics 1995; 15:1069–1085.

Kim SH, Han MC, Han JS, Kim S, Lee JS. Exercise-induced acute renal failure and patchy renal vasoconstriction: CT and MR findings. J Comput Assist Tomogr 1991; 15:985–988.

Problem Renal Masses

David S. Hartman, MD
Penn State
College Of Medicine

Problem Renal Masses
- Basic Principles of Renal Neoplasia
- Small Renal Mass
- Cystic Renal Mass

Centennial Sounding Board
Personal Refelection on Growth of Diagnostic Imaging
- "As we accurately image and inspect the human body with thinner and more detailed sections, we approach the 1–2 mm serial sections of the pathologist, who can find evidence of "disease" in almost every organ and everyone."
- "The radiologist of the future will need to understand the implications of their findings and know the natural history of each disease detected."

Robert J. Stanley, AJR 2000;174:609

4 Arbitrary Steps
- Carcinoma In Situ (CIS)
- Angiogenesis
- Vascular invasion
- Metastasis

Cell Cycle
- Proliferation
- Programmed death (Apoptosis)

Normally Cell Proliferation and Apoptosis are Activated in Parallel
- Controlled by genes
  - ➢ Oncogene = Accelerator
  - ➢ Suppressor gene = Brake

Neoplasia
- Results from disequilibrium of proliferation and cell death
- Controlled by Genes

Chromosomal Instability Pathway
- Multi-step process
- 4–10 genetic events
- Can stop at any point

Carcinoma In Situ
- Confined by basement membrane
- Stops expanding after reaching diffusion limit of the nearest vessel
- "No" metastatic potential
- Very, very common

Carcinoma In Situ
- Most human tumors exist as in situ lesions
  - ➢ 0.2– 2 mm
- Renal CIS is found in 22% of autopsies

Angiogenic Phenotype
- Ability to recruit host blood supply
- Penetrate basement membrane
- May enlarge to become macroscopic

Virtually All Solid Tumors Which are Visible Are Angiogenesis Dependent

VEGF Vascular, Endothelial, Growth, Factor

17,000 Age matched American Down's Patients
- No prostate cancer
- No breast cancer
- No pancreatic cancer
- mild leukemia
- same incidence of testicular cancer

- have an extra copy of Collagen 18 on Chromosome 21
- Endostatin is an integral component of Collagen 18
- AMT of circulating Endostatin is 10 X Normal Population

Vascular Invasion
- Tumor shedding and vascular invasion may occur relatively early
- In animal models, tumors shed 3-6 million cells per Gram per 24 hours
- Most cells which are shed do not progress to viable metastases

Critical Feature of RCC: Metastasis
- Very imprecise at knowing which, where and when RCC will metastasize
- Mets are controlled by genes
- Each metastasis must become angiogenic to grow

Genes Crucial For Growth Of Metastases
- Angiogenic gene
- "New roots" gene
- BRMS gene

Nonangiogenic Metastases May Remain Microscopic and Dormant for many Years

Renal Tumors < 3cm uncommonly have detectable Metastases
- The renal tumor doesn't "know" how large it is
- The larger the renal tumor, the more undifferentiated it "may" be
- The more undifferentiated, the greater the likelihood that a metastatis can become angiogenic

The small (< 3 cm) Renal Mass [Figure 3-17-1]
- 1.5 - 3.0 cm
    - A . cyst
    - B . cystic
    - C . solid
- < 1.5 cm (often TSTC)

The small solid Renal Mass 1.5-3cm
- Fat = AML
- No Fat
    - A . Renal Epithelial Tumor with low metastatic potential
    - B. Cannot diagnose Adenoma (Oncocytoma)

Figure 3-17-1

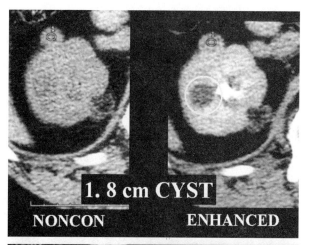

1. 8 cm CYST

NONCON   ENHANCED

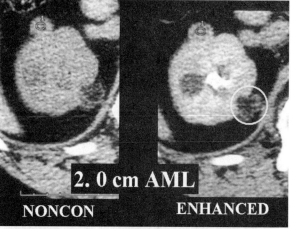

2. 0 cm AML

NONCON   ENHANCED

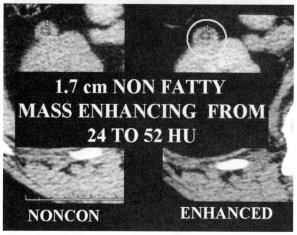

1.7 cm NON FATTY MASS ENHANCING FROM 24 TO 52 HU

NONCON   ENHANCED

Best Diagnosis
Renal Epothelial Tumor with low (< 5%) p[robability of Metastasis

Management Options
- Excise
- Ablation
- Follow
- Biopsy
- Nephrectomy
- Ignore

Figure 3-17-2

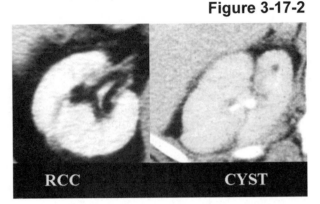

Too small to characterize *[Figure 3-17-2]*
No Single Algorithm for Every Case
Risks and Benefits of Any Strategy

Always Consider
- Pretest probability
- Patient's ability to tolerate uncertainty
- Your ability to tolerate uncertainty

How Should The TSTC Mass Be Evaluated?
- There is no large, prospective, pathologically proven series which indicates correct management

Figure 3-17-3

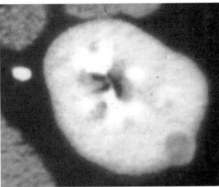

Too Small to Characterize (< 1.5 cm)
1. Ignore
2. Follow *[Figure 3-17-3]*
3. Get another study

How Often Should Small Lesions Be Followed?
- The smaller the lesion, the longer the followup interval
- If following a lesion, compare oldest comparable study available

Small Lesion Considered Aggressive
- Size > 3cm
- Doubling time faster than 6 months

How Is Doubling Time Calculated?
http://www.chestx-ray.com/index.html

Get the Referring Doctor Involved

Get the Patient Involved

Cystic Renal Mass
- 5-10% of cases of Renal Carcinoma present as a Fluid-Filled mass
- The Simple Cyst can be confidently diagnosed (US, CT, MR)
- Rarely Simple Cysts become complicated (Hemorrhage, infection, ischemia)
- Complicated Simple Cyst is grossly indistinguishable from Cystic RCC
- RCC is a Histologic Diagnosis

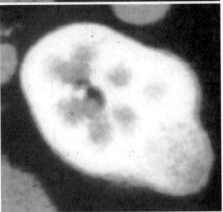

51 YO Man followed for AAA
Top: 1cm
Bottom: 4 years later, 3cm RCC

Most effective treatment for Renal Cell Carcinoma: Surgery or Ablation

Papillary Renal Cell Carcinoma
- may present as a homogeneous hyperdense mass
- may enhance uniformly
- enhances less than non papillary RCC
- may be "avascular" at angiography

Cyst Not Simple If It Has. . . . .should be termed CYSTIC LESION
- Calcification
- Septation
- Hyperdensity
- Multiple Locules
- Thick Wall
- Nodularity
- Enhancement

Calcified Cystic Mass
- Benign *[Figure 3-17-4]*
  - ➤ Peripheral or septal
  - ➤ Thin
  - ➤ Smooth
  - ➤ Milk of calcium
- Surgical *[Figure 3-17-5]*
  - ➤ Central
  - ➤ Thick
  - ➤ Irregular

Benign Calcification Can Be Recognized
Surgical Calcification May Be Benign Or Malignant

Hyperdense Mass
- Most Are Cystic
  - ➤ Blood
  - ➤ Protein
  - ➤ Colloid
- May Be Solid
  - ➤ Lymphoma
  - ➤ RCC
  - ➤ Hamartoma

Benign Hyperdense
- Homogeneous
- No "Significant" Enhancement
- US: cyst

What constitutes "Significant" Enhancement ?
- < 10 HU   Beam Hardening
- 10-15 HU   ????
- > 15 HU   Vascular

Surgical Hyperdense
- Heterogeneous
- Enhancement
- US: not a cyst

Hyperdense Masses Are Surgical
- Enhancement
- Heterogeneous
- Solid on US

Figure 3-17-4

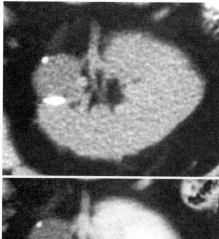
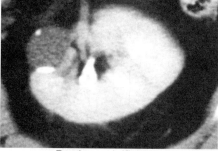

Benign calcification

Figure 3-17-5

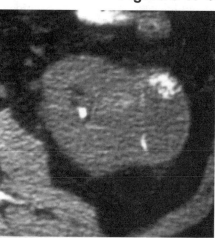
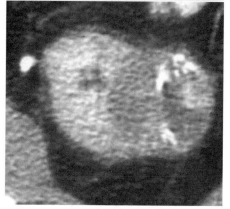

Surgical calcifications

Septations

Benign Septations
- Thin ,<2mm
- No nodularity
- May calcify

Surgical Septations
- Thick,>2mm
- Nodular
- Irregular

Benign Septations Can Be Recognized [Figure 3-17-5]

Surgical Septations May Be Benign or Malignant [Figure 3-17-6]

Multiloculated Renal Mass
- More than 3 or 4 septa
- Two most common multiloculated masses in adults
  - Multilocular cystic nephroma (MLCN)
  - Renal cell Ca (ML RCC)

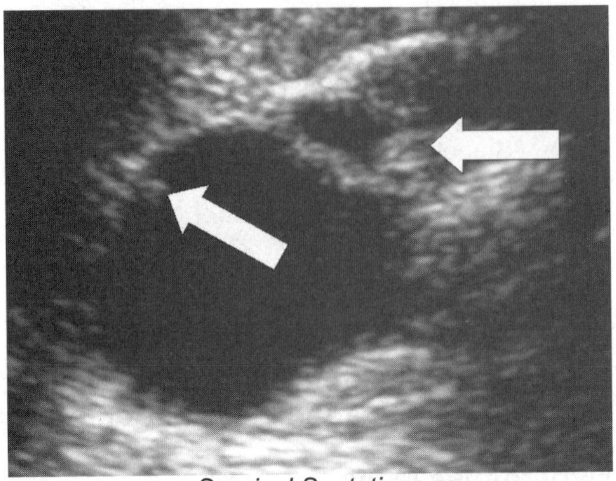

MLCN	ML-RCC
Female	Male
No Blood	Blood
Pelvic Herniation	Venous Invasion
Usually Benign	Malignant

Multiloculated Masses should be excised

Deenhancement
- enhanced scan, wait 20 minutes, rescan, evaluate decreased CT numbers
- same significance as enhancement

Most Cystic Masses With Nodularity, Wall Thickening or Enhancement Are Malignant

Cannot Distinguish Benign From Malignant Radiologically

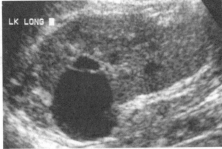

Figure 3-17-5

LK LONG

Benign Septations

Figure 3-17-6

Surgical Septations

Cystic Renal Masses

	Benign	Surgical
Calcification	Thin Peripheral Milk of calcium	? Thick ? Central Enhancement
Hyperdense	Homogeneous No enhancement Cyst or cystic	Heterogeneous Enhancement Solid
Septations	<2mm No nodularity Bosniak II F	>2mm Nodularity Bosniak III

Cystic Renal Masses

	Benign	Surgical
Multi-loculated		All
Enhancement		All
Nodularity		All
Thick wall		All
		Bosniak III or IV

Category II F (Follow) [1]

Septa	Minimal INCR number
	Minimal enhancement
Calcifications	Thick and nodular
Hyperdense	Totally intrarenal
	> 3 cm
Wall	"Minimal" thickening

[1] Gary M. Israel and Morton A. Bosniak . Follow-Up of Moderately Complex Cystic Lesions of the Kidney (Bosniak Category IIF). AJR 2003

References

Zagoria RJ. Imaging of small renal masses: A medical success story. AJR 2000; 175:9456-955
Hartman DS, Choyke PL, Hartman MS. A practical approach to the cystic renal mass. RadioGraphics Oct 2004
Israel GM, Bosniak MA. Follow up CT of moderately complex cystic lesions of the kidney Bosniak category IIF. AJR 2003; 181:627-633
Ho VB, Allen SF, Hood MN, Choyke PL. Renal masses: quantitative assessment of enhancement with dynamic MR imaging. Radiology 2002;224:695-700

Seminar: MSAFP

All of the following scans were ordered following a routine blood test.
- What was the test?
- Was it high or low?

Elevated Maternal Serum Alpha-Fetoprotein (MSAFP)

Fetal Alpha-fetoprotein
- Glycoprotein produced by fetal liver, GI tract, and yolk sac
- Excreted through the urinary tract into the amniotic fluid
- Peaks at 14–16 wks
- Small amounts leak into maternal circulation

Maternal Serum Alpha-fetoprotein (MSAFP)
- Screening in second trimester (16–18 weeks)
- Elevated if 2.5 MOM (multiples-of-the-median)
- 10–15% risk of open neural tube defect

Case 1

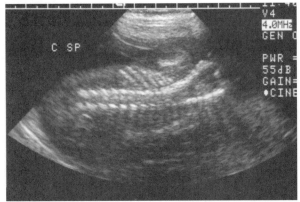

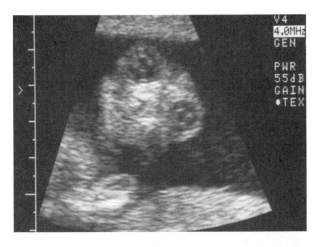

Case 2

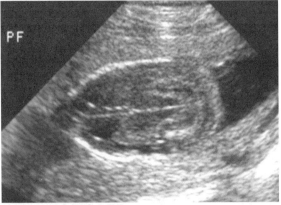

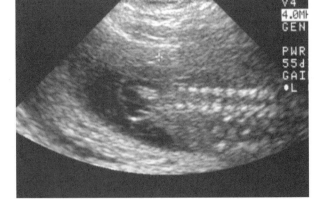

Elevated MSAFP
- Incorrect dates
- Twins
- Fetal death
- Open neural tube defect
- Abdominal wall defect
- Subchorionic hemorrhage

Case 3

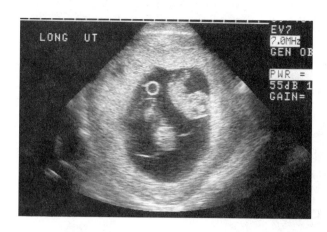

Case 4

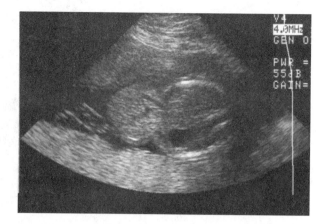

Case 5

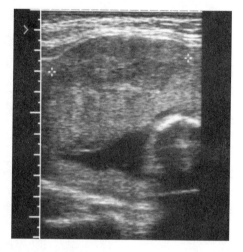

Elevated MSAFP
- Can perform amniocetesis and measure direct AFP and ACE
- Acetylcholinesterase (ACE) – neural tissue specific

Elevated MSAFP
- Inc AFP, inc ACE – ONTD
- Inc AFP, nl ACE – abdominal wall defect
- Nl AFP, nl ACE – prior bleed

Decreased MSAFP
- Trisomy 21,18
- Combine with human chorionic gonadotropin (hCG) and estriol (uE3) for increased specificity – triple screen

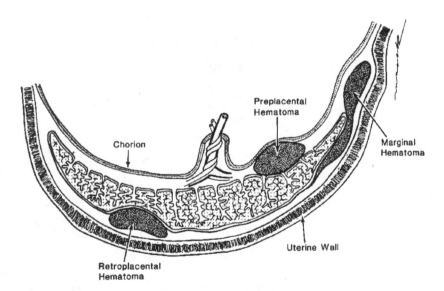

Placental hemorrhages

Seminar: Renal Calcifications

Renal Calcifications
- Dystrophic calcification
- Nephrocalcinosis
  - ➢ cortical
  - ➢ medullary
- Nephrolithiasis

Dystrophic Calcification
- Calcification of abnormal tissue
- DDx
  - ➢ tumor
  - ➢ inflammatory mass (TB)
  - ➢ hematoma
  - ➢ cysts

66 yo man with hematuria

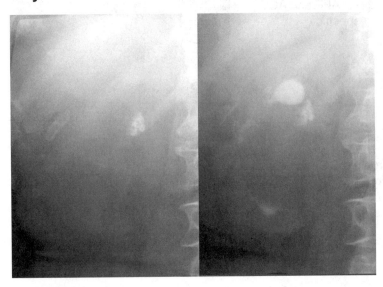

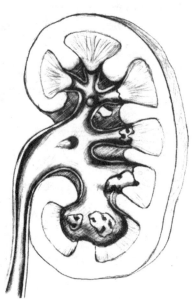

Papillary necrosis

Renal Tuberculosis
- Hematogenous spread
- Bacilli lodge in corticomedullary jct.
- Progress along nephron into pelvo-calyceal system

Renal Tuberculosis
- History of TB elsewhere
- Active disease coexistent
  in only 10% of cases

Symptoms
- Asymptomatic
- Frequency
- Hematuria
- "Sterile" pyuria

Radiologic Findings
- 10% normal
- Papillary irregularity
- Papillary necrosis

Radiologic Findings
- Infundibular stenosis
- Amputated calyx
- Parenchymal scarring

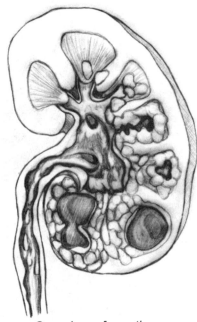

Granuloma formation

Calcifications

- Present in 30–50%
- Variable appearance
  - ➢ punctate – healed granulomas
  - ➢ amorphous – granulomatous masses
  - ➢ extensive reniform – autonephrectomy
- 20% have calculi
- Ureter and bladder may also be involved

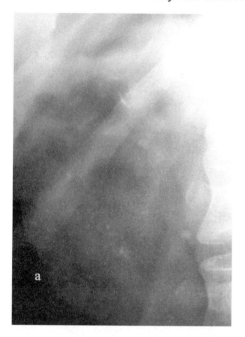

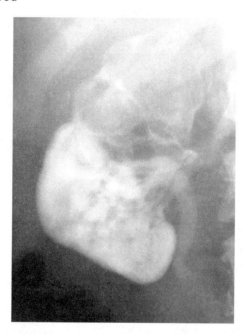

45 yo woman from Mexico with pyuria

Cortical Nephrocalcinosis

- Egg-shell calcification
- Generally small kidneys
- Renal function usually impaired

Cortical Nephrocalcinosis

- Chronic glomerulonephritis
- Acute cortical necrosis
  - ➢ pregnancy, sepsis, trauma, nephrotoxins (ethylene glycol)
- Chronic transplant rejection
- Alport's syndrome
  - ➢ nephritis, nerve deafness, hematuria, ocular abnormalities

33 yo in aircraft accident with severe chest and skeletal trauma

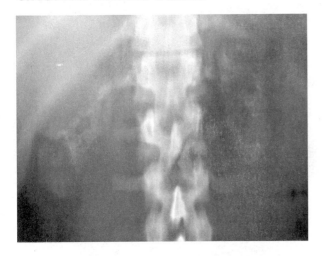

47 yo male admitted with an abdominal abscess. What is the renal disease?

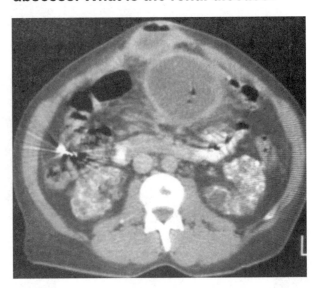

Medullary Nephrocalcinosis
- Metastatic calcification – calcification in normal tissue
- Triangular deposition conforming to pyramids
- Renal function usually not impaired
- Often associated with nephrolithiasis

Medullary Nephrocalcinosis
- Hypercalcemic states
  - ➢ hyperparathyroidism, paraneoplastic, sarcoidosis, milk-alkali syndrome, hyper-vitaminosis D
- Medullary sponge kidney (renal tubular ectasia)
  - ➢ may be unilateral or focal

27 yo man with a history of stone disease

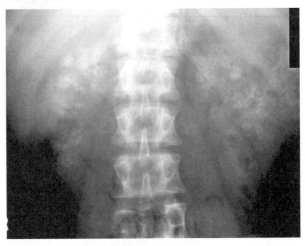

Medullary Nephrocalcinosis
- Renal tubular acidosis – Type I (distal)
  - ➢ distal tubule can not secrete hydrogen ion, urine becomes alkaline
  - ➢ symmetric
- Oxalosis
  - ➢ primary (children) -severe may also see cortical calcification
  - ➢ seconday – distal small bowel resection

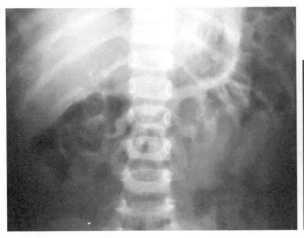

5 yo boy with an inherited disorder

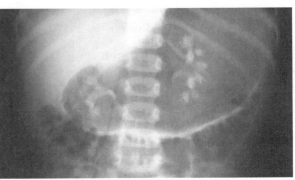